Pharmacology and Therapeutics

Pharmacology and Therapeutics

THIRD EDITION

RUTH D. MUSSER, A.B., M.S.
*Assistant Professor in Pharmacology,
School of Medicine, and Chairman of
Pharmacology, School of Nursing,
University of Maryland, Baltimore*

AND

BETTY LOU SHUBKAGEL, B.S., M.N., R.N.
*Assistant Professor of Medical-Surgical Nursing,
School of Nursing, University of Maryland, Baltimore*

THE MACMILLAN COMPANY, NEW YORK
COLLIER—MACMILLAN LIMITED, LONDON

FOREWORD

The Third Edition of *Pharmacology and Therapeutics* will be a welcome and timely contribution to the instructional program of student nurses in the ever-expanding field of pharmacology. The book has enjoyed a deserved widespread acceptance since the appearance of the First Edition in 1958. The Third Edition has been completely revised by Professors Musser and Shubkagel in consultation with specialists in the various fields of medical science and practice. The authors have made an effective effort to present the subject matter from the nurse's point of view with special emphasis on the nurse's responsibilities in the medication of the patient. This was achieved through the splendid cooperation of Professor Shubkagel of the faculty of the School of Nursing of the University of Maryland.

The authors have admirably adhered to the policy of presentation which was the hallmark of success of the former editions. This is expressed in the *principles of drug therapy*, i.e., *what to do and why*; associated with the *practice of drug therapy*, i.e., *how to do it and when*. Each of these facets is delineated with succinctness and accuracy.

The excellent training and experience of the authors again are manifested in the Third Edition of the text. Professor Musser has taught pharmacology to student nurses and medical students for more than two decades in the Department of Pharmacology of the School of Medicine of the University of Maryland. Her record in teaching student nurses has been a paragon of excellence and was recognized as such by the Middle (Atlantic) States Association.

Professor Shubkagel, who has served effectively for ten years as a member of the Department of Medical and Surgical Nursing of the School of Nursing of the University of Maryland, is recognized as an expert clinical nurse practitioner and competent teacher. Each of these skills finds its expression in the new revision of the text on which she worked with indefatigable energy.

In addition, as previously mentioned, the authors have obtained expert advice in various medical specialties which they have skillfully embodied in the text. This has endowed the Third Edition with breadth of vision and authenticity. It is my firm opinion that this edition of *Pharmacology and Therapeutics* will make a significant contribution to nursing education and receive the widespread acceptance and acclaim it so eminently deserves.

JOHN C. KRANTZ, JR.
Professor and Head of
Pharmacology
University of Maryland School of Medicine

PREFACE

The advances in pharmacologic and therapeutic knowledge have necessitated a thorough revision of this book, formerly titled *Modern Pharmacology and Therapeutics*, bringing something new to nearly every page. The advances in the basic nursing sciences and a broader interpretation of the functions of nurses have brought changes in the curriculum that are reflected throughout this text.

The accepted features of this book and the order of presentation have been retained. As in other editions, there have been revisions or additions of materials and features suggested by teachers and students. Their suggestions have been evaluated and utilized to enhance the original objectives—a practical, comprehensive, and current textbook especially adaptable to clinical nursing courses.

Some of the new features of this edition include material on the revised system of naming drugs; the Federal Food and Drug Act; Kefauver-Harris Amendments; additional sites for hypodermic injections; vital role of DNA and RNA; additional penicillins; gonorrhea and chemotherapy; additional material on neoplasms and drug therapy; radioactive isotopes; table of specific agents used in cancer chemotherapy; additional material on the action of morphine on all body systems; nursing implications in the administration of analgesics; preoperative and postoperative sedation; expanded discussion of epilepsy and its control; premature infants and the toxic effects of oxygen; nerve impulse mechanisms in respect to new drugs developed to increase or decrease transmission; shock conditions and chemotherapy; additional material on the astringents; oral contraceptives; nursing responsibilities related to the administration of whole blood; teaching suggestions for patient's guidance; and a new chapter, "Drugs Acting Locally on the Eye, Ear, and Nose."

Along with the introduction of new drugs, new treatments, and additional information developed in the practice of medicine and nursing, other changes have been made in many of the chapters. Greater emphasis has been given to anatomy, physiology, pathology, and biochemistry. The beginning student, the advanced student, and the graduate nurse can use the basic information and concepts as a frame of reference which will better enable them to comprehend relationships between pharmacology and the other health sciences. Particular attention has been given to the human reactions to the drugs administered, the reactions normally to be expected, those that may produce adverse effects, and the nurse's responsibilities in the administration of all medications, thus providing greater understanding of the nurse's functions in the therapeutic milieu.

Drugs are grouped according to their action. It is believed this is the logical method of presentation and lends value to the book not only as a text for the course in pharmacology, but also as a reference in any situation in which medications are used. Since numerous drugs have the same action, the prototype of each group is presented in detail, and the unique qualities of related drugs are noted. If the drug has several actions or is used in various situations, it is mentioned briefly in subsidiary discussions, and the reader is referred to the main presentation in which the information regarding the action of the drug, its side and toxic effects, precautions and contraindications, usual dosage, and various preparations is complete.

Those concepts that have long since been supplanted by newer ideas and methods are included only if they offer important contributions to the advance of pharmacology, thus eliminating traditional descriptions that have outlived their usefulness.

The material that is needed and used by nurses as they work with and teach patients who are receiving drugs is included in this text. However, the manner of teaching a patient is not included since it is the opinion of the authors that each nurse-patient relationship is unique and that there is no one way of teaching or assisting the patient.

Some of the diagrams have been simplified, and others added to supplement the text. The questions at the end of the chapters are designed primarily to stimulate and encourage further thought rather than to test the student's factual knowledge. References at the end of the chapters and at the end of the book will be useful to those searching for additional information.

Many of the chapters were submitted to instructors for their opinions and suggestions. Their appraisals have contributed greatly to the orientation and completeness of this textbook. The authors wish to express their appreciation to those medical and nursing specialists, and will welcome additional suggestions from teachers, students, and reviewers for use in future editions.

The many new drugs that have been incorporated in this edition have been selected because they offer a new dimension in drug therapy, because of the need they fulfill, and because of the interest they have aroused. Approved names, the dose and dosage forms of the drugs in the U.S.P. XVII, N.F. XII, and B.P. IX are given. Trade names used both in the United States and Great Britain follow the approved names. The doses are given in the metric system.

The index includes page references to disease conditions and their chemo-therapy, providing a quick reference for students in clinical nursing: medical; surgical; obstetrical; gynecological; pediatric; geriatric; psychiatric; eye, ear, nose, and throat; emergency; recovery room; and other nursing services.

ACKNOWLEDGMENTS

We express our deepest appreciation to Dr. Joseph G. Bird who withdrew from this and future editions because of his increasing responsibilities as Director, Division of Clinical Research, Sterling-Winthrop Research Institute, Rensselaer, New York, and who generously gave permission to use whatever we wished of his contributions.

We wish to thank members of the faculty of the School of Medicine and the School of Nursing, University of Maryland, who have read and contributed their knowledge to portions of the manuscript:

SCHOOL OF MEDICINE

Department of Pharmacology:

Frederick K. Bell, Ph.D., Research Associate
Raymond M. Burgision, Ph.D., Professor of Pharmacology
John J. O'Neill, Ph.D., Associate Professor
Robert Rozman, Ph.D., Assistant Professor

Department of Medicine

Theodore E. Woodward, M.D., Professor of Medicine, and Head of the Department
Joseph B. Workman, Associate Professor of Medicine, and Head of the Radioactive Isotope Laboratory

Department of Anatomy

Frank H. J. Figge, Ph.D., Professor of Anatomy and Histology

SCHOOL OF NURSING

Shirley L. Hale, Assistant Professor of Psychiatric Nursing
Janet E. Burchett, Instructor of Maternal and Child Nursing

Karin E. Larsen, Assistant Instructor of Maternal and Child Nursing
F. Patricia Koontz, Assistant Professor of Tuberculosis Nursing
M. Rita Dy, Instructor of Medical and Surgical Nursing
Katherine Wohlson, Associate Professor of Public Health Nursing
E. Ann Seymour, Instructor of Medical and Surgical Nursing
Hector J. Cardellino, Instructor of Urological Nursing

We also express our appreciation to James Certa, M.D., Department of Gastroenterology, School of Medicine, University of Pennsylvania, Philadelphia; to Gilbert Duritz, Ph.D., the University of Maryland, School of Medicine; and to Patricia K. Leather, Assistant Instructor of Cardiovascular Nursing, who prepared the sketches for some of the drawings.

We especially express our gratitude to Dr. John C. Krantz, Jr., Professor of Pharmacology, School of Medicine, and to Dr. Florence M. Gipe, Professor of Nursing and Dean of the School of Nursing, University of Maryland, for their inspiration and cooperation in the production of this book and to Dr. Krantz for writing the Foreword.

It is not feasible to list the names of all persons who gave so generously of their time and talents in the preparation of this book. However, the authors wish especially to thank the following for their advice, help, and encouragement: Dr. William S. Stone, Dean, School of Medicine, University of Maryland; Miss Virginia Conley, Chairman, Baccalaureate Program, School of Nursing, University of Maryland; and Dr. Mary K. Carl, Chairman, Graduate Program, School of Nursing, University of Maryland.

Finally, the authors wish to express their warm appreciation to the staff of The Macmillan Company, particularly to Mr. Henry Van Swearingen, Editor, for their fine cooperation and the use of their wide experience in producing this book.

RUTH D. MUSSER
BETTY LOU SHUBKAGEL

CONTENTS

I INTRODUCTION

EARLY BEGINNINGS OF PHARMACOLOGY

Briefly stated, pharmacology is the study of drugs and their effects on the body and its diseases. A description of this basic science will be given in Chapter 1 with definitions of its subdivisions and closely related fields. Pharmacology has, as has medicine itself, existed from days before history was recorded, when man first administered substances to an ailing person or animal. The earliest recordings of civilization in the Near East and Egypt reveal a progressive interest in using materials at hand in attempts to restore health. More often than not, the measures were useless or harmful, and failures were ascribed to supernatural influences.

The practice of the healing arts became increasingly more sophisticated but only slowly more helpful. The physician-priests of ancient Egypt used mainly plant materials or botanicals, with a few minerals and animal preparations to complete their armamentarium.

MILESTONES IN THE DISCOVERY OF ACTIVE DRUGS

Early Egyptian papyri, manuscripts, and prescriptions included materials still in use today, such as magnesia, lime, soda, iron salts, and sulfur. Simple compounds of arsenic and poisons found in plants, such as hemlock and strychnine, were used by the ancient Greeks and Romans. Quinine, an antimalarial drug, was discovered as the result of the use of the bark of the cinchona tree in Peru. In 1630 the fever and chills of a Spanish official quickly subsided upon its use, it is said, whereupon it was brought to Europe and used as a drug for fevers of various causes. However, the fever of malaria alone responds to quinine.

The very important heart drug, digitalis, was brought into rational medical use in 1783 by a physician who had become curious about the remarkable effects seen in the medical use of a number of herbs mixed together by an Englishwoman. In 1803 morphine was extracted in pure form from the dried juice, called opium, of the oriental poppy which had been used in medicine by the Egyptians and subsequent civilizations. There then followed a series of

1

important chemical extractions of the active ingredients of many of the botanical drugs: caffeine in 1821, from the tea leaf, long and widely used as a beverage; atropine, in 1831, from belladonna leaves; and codeine, also from opium, in 1832. Until recent times most of our medicinal agents were portions of plants, such as roots, bark, leaves, and sap, but now many of the active principles have been isolated and made available in very pure form. Hundreds of plant materials have been used in medicine, the more useful of which will be described in the text. The remainder have been practically abandoned, being of little or no value, or replaced by more recent discoveries.

In medical schools the subject of pharmacology was titled Materia Medica *until 1890, when the new term began to come into use. Study material then began to change from elaborate descriptions of plants, their medicinal products, and alleged uses to a modern science. Modern pharmacology necessarily awaited the development of modern chemistry and physiology, both of which grew rapidly in the nineteenth century. The selection over the centuries of medicinal agents by trial and error, which may be called the* empirical *method, began near the close of the past century to be replaced by the development of drugs by experimentation.*

One of the pioneers in the development of pharmacology was Dr. John J. Abel, who became professor of pharmacology at the Johns Hopkins School of Medicine in 1892. To him and his associates is due the credit for isolating and studying epinephrine (Adrenalin) and acetylcholine from the adrenal glands of animals. The discovery of these hormones was of considerable importance, as we shall see. Dr. Abel's illustrious career was climaxed by the isolation of pure insulin, the antidiabetic hormone of the pancreas, in 1926. His studies of the actions of these hormones and many other biological and synthetic agents are classics in American biochemistry and pharmacology. The discovery of the anesthetic activity of ether, the discovery of arsphenamine, penicillin, and the host of synthetic medicinals now in use, and the development of increasingly accurate methods for finding better drugs, are additional examples of the innumerable milestones in medicinal science, the more important of which will be presented in the text.

THE NURSE'S RELATIONSHIP TO PHARMACOLOGY

The nurse's responsibility in administering drugs must include not only correct preparation and method of administration of drugs, but also observation of the patients for evidence of effectiveness, manifestations of side or toxic effects, and allergic reactions to drugs. If untoward effects occur, the nurse must initiate action to correct them. This action may take a variety of forms from reporting facts to the physician to engaging in emergency resuscitation procedures. In order to be able to make pertinent observations and take appropriate action, the nurse's knowledge of drugs must portray depth and breadth, for if she is unaware of the side effects of a drug, it is unlikely she will recognize their signs and symptoms as such and intelligent action then cannot be undertaken.

1

The Scope of Pharmacology.
Nature and Sources of Drugs

DEFINITIONS

Pharmacology may be defined most simply as the study of drugs. In the broadest sense it includes all the scientific knowledge of drugs, such as the name, source, physical and chemical properties, and the mixing or preparing of drugs in the form of medicine. It is concerned also with physiological actions of drugs—their absorption, action, and fate in the body—and with their therapeutic uses, as well as the poisonous effects that result from overdosage.

A drug is a chemical substance that affects living protoplasm and does not act as a food. It is used in the cure, treatment, or prevention of disease in man or animals. In addition, drugs alleviate suffering and pain.

The subject of pharmacology may be divided into a number of distinct sciences such as pharmacognosy, pharmacy, posology, pharmacodynamics, pharmacotherapeutics, and toxicology.

Pharmacognosy is a descriptive science and is concerned with the recognition, quality, purity by macroscopic and microscopic means, and identification of plants and animal drugs.

Pharmacy deals with the preparation, stability, preservation, and storage of drugs. From these drugs the pharmacist prepares, compounds, and dispenses medicines. Most drugs are prepared by pharmaceutical manufacturers and are distributed to the pharmacy or hospital in such suitable dosage forms as tablets, capsules, liquid preparations, or sterile solutions for injection. The pharmacist now has no less a responsible role in properly dispensing the preparations in finished forms than when he powdered, dissolved, mixed, and otherwise compounded prescriptions. He still performs these functions for many of these orders.

Posology is concerned with the dosage or amount of a drug given in the treatment of disease. There is a minimum, maximum, usual or therapeutic, and toxic dose for each drug. The most important is the usual dose, which is the oral dose for an adult weighing 70 kg. There are a number of conditions that modify the dose of a drug. See pages 85–87.

4

Pharmacodynamics is concerned with the response of living tissues to chemical stimuli, that is, the action of drugs on the living organism in the absence of disease. It is one of the newest biological sciences and is closely associated with physiology, biochemistry, pathology, and microbiology. It is unique in that its interest is focused on drugs. It is a study of the absorption, fate, excretion, and action of a foreign substance in the body.

Pharmacotherapeutics deals with the action of drugs in the presence of disease. It involves the treatment of the sick. Drugs are used to bring comfort, relieve pain, induce sleep, and restore the patient to health.

Toxicology deals with the toxic or poisonous effects produced by overdosage. This science is concerned with the identification of the poison, the symptoms of poisoning, and their treatment with suitable antidotes.

PURPOSE OF PHARMACOLOGY

The purpose of pharmacology as a pure science is to determine the response of living organisms to chemical stimuli in the presence or absence of disease, for example, in inducing sleep in insomnia or obtunding pain in surgical procedures. It attempts to correlate chemical structure with biological activity and to classify chemically related drugs into groups such as the barbiturates and the sulfonamides.

As an applied or practical science, it has the following functions: (1) to test drugs quantitatively and standardize them so that they are available to the doctor and patient in a uniform and dependable form; (2) to determine how drugs produce their effects on the animal body; (3) to develop new drugs; and (4) to establish the rational and safe dosage.

NATURE AND SOURCES OF DRUGS

There are four sources for obtaining drugs. They are: (1) plant parts or plant products, (2) mineral products, (3) animal products, and (4) pure chemicals or synthetic drugs that are prepared in the laboratory of the organic chemist.

PLANTS

Various parts of plants are used, such as the leaves, roots, fruit, and the bark of trees. These are variously processed, and the resulting products are known as *crude drugs*. Pure chemical substances may be extracted from the crude drugs. These are called *active principles,* or active constituents, and they are responsible for the main activity of the crude drug. These active principles may be classified according to their physicochemical properties into the following groups:

1. Alkaloids
2. Glycosides
3. Oils
   a. Fixed oils
   b. Volatile oils

4. Resins
5. Gums
6. Gum resins
7. Balsams
8. Tannins

Alkaloids. Alkaloids are basic organic substances containing carbon, hydrogen, nitrogen, and oxygen. They occur in almost all parts of plants but are most often found in the seeds, roots, and leaves. They are very active substances and many are violent poisons. There is a wide variation in the structure and in the response of these compounds. Most of the alkaloids are white crystalline compounds, such as atropine and morphine, and combine with acids to form salts. The salts are usually much more soluble in water than the alkaloid base itself. To a large extent the soluble salts of the alkaloids have replaced the crude drugs because of their rapidity of action, dependability, and purity, thus permitting their use by injection. Examples: atropine, from the leaves and roots of the belladonna plant; quinine, from the bark of the cinchona tree; and morphine, from the juice of the Oriental poppy. Many alkaloids have been prepared synthetically. Examples: caffeine, atropine, and cocaine.

Glycosides. Glycosides are ether-like combinations of sugar with some other organic substances. Glycosides are referred to as glucosides if the sugar in combination is glucose. Glycosides do not react with acids to form salts. When they are warmed with mineral acids, the sugar or sugars are split off. The remaining substance is called the aglycone, or *genin*. The most important glycosides are those found in the leaves of digitalis. Of these, digitoxin is the most widely used.

Oils. The two types of oils used medicinally are the fixed and the volatile oils.

Fixed Oils. Fixed oils are greasy substances that leave a stain. Generally they are more dietetic than medicinal. Like olive oil and cottonseed oil they are digested and serve as food. Some fixed oils, however, are medicinal agents, like castor oil, which is used as a cathartic. Others are used as vehicles for drugs that are injected intramuscularly.

Volatile Oils. Volatile oils evaporate readily without leaving a stain. They have a pleasant aromatic odor and taste and are often used as flavoring agents. They are found mainly in the fruit, flowering parts, or leaves of plants and are responsible for plant aroma. Examples: oil of peppermint, from the leaves; and oil of rose, from the rose petals.

Some of the volatile oils are used as carminatives (oil of peppermint), some have a mild bacteriostatic action and are used in mouthwashes (oil of thyme), and others exert an anodyne effect (such as oil of cloves for the relief of toothache, and oil of wintergreen for pain in arthralgias).

Resins. Resins are rosin-like substances and are usually formed by the oxidation of volatile oils. Saps from many trees and roots of some plants contain resins. Certain of these are regarded as crude drugs; in other cases the crude drug must be extracted, as in the preparation of podophyllin from podophyllum. Most of the resins are used as cathartics.

Gums. Gums are secretory products from plants. They are carbohydrates that absorb water and swell to form thick, mucilaginous colloid solutions. Gums are either digested and used as carbohydrates in the body or they remain unchanged and are not absorbed from the gastrointestinal tract. They are hydrophilic colloids, and those that are not digested remain in the gastrointestinal tract where they absorb water and increase the bulk, which produces evacuation of the bowel. Typical laxative gums are obtained from agar and psyllium seeds.

Gums are used in aqueous solutions as emulsifying agents for oils and to suspend insoluble substances in water. Examples: gum acacia and gum tragacanth.

Gum Resins. Gum resins are mixtures of gums and resins in varying proportions. Example: myrrh.

Balsams. Balsams are resinous, aromatic liquids, or semisolid substances containing benzoic acid or cinnamic acid, or both. Example: benzoin.

Tannins. Tannins are complex plant principles found widely distributed in plants. They have an astringent action and are used in the treatment of diarrhea and hemorrhoids.

Antibiotics. Antibiotics, which have a lethal or inhibitory action on microorganisms, are substances produced by or derived from living cells. These substances are produced by living bacteria, yeasts, molds, and other plants. Examples: penicillin, streptomycin, chlortetracycline, oxytetracycline, and tetracycline.

MINERAL DRUGS

Mineral drugs have an important place in therapeutics. Elementary substances (oxygen, iodine, iron), free acids (boric acid and hydrochloric acid), metallic hydroxides (aluminum hydroxide), and salts (Epsom salt as a cathartic and magnesium trisilicate as an antacid) are frequently used.

ANIMAL DRUGS

For centuries the organs of animals have been used in the treatment of disease. At first their use was empirical. The lungs of the fox were dried and given as a potion to persons who had difficulty in breathing. Today glands such as the liver and thyroid are dried and powdered and are administered orally as replacement therapy. Frequently it is necessary to purify and process the animal source of the drug through many intricate chemical and physical procedures to obtain the active constituent in a suitable dosage form.

Some of our greatest successes in modern medicine have resulted from the use of animal products: (1) liver in the treatment of pernicious anemia, (2) thyroid in the treatment of hypothyroidism, (3) insulin in the treatment of diabetes, and (4) cortisone and ACTH in the treatment of arthritis and other diseases. Immune serums and serum fractions, which are used in the prevention and treatment of infectious diseases, are obtained from human beings and animals (horses and rabbits) following natural or artificial infection with bacteria, viruses, or rickettsiae. The use of these substances in producing immunity comes within the purview of immunology rather than pharmacology. However, because serums and vaccines are administered by the nurse, they are discussed in Chapter 49, "Vaccines and Serums."

Synthetic Drugs

Synthetic drugs are pure chemical substances produced in the laboratory by the organic chemist. They may be made by emulating or imitating substances found in nature. The alkaloids cocaine and atropine and the hormone epinephrine have been made synthetically. Synthetic alkaloids also are prepared by modifying and improving upon substances found in nature. Examples are dihydromorphinone and homatropine. There are many other new chemical substances that are prepared synthetically, such as the barbiturates, the sulfonamides, and the general anesthetics. The laboratory of the organic chemist is a most important source of new drugs.

REVIEW QUESTIONS

1. *What is a drug?*
2. *Define pharmacology and discuss its purpose as a pure and as an applied science.*
3. *Name four sources for obtaining drugs and give two examples of each.*
4. *What are active principles? Name and define four different types obtained from plant drugs. Give two examples of each.*
5. *Name five drugs obtained from animal products. Discuss their importance in therapeutics.*
6. *What are synthetic drugs? Discuss their importance in pharmacology. Give four examples of synthetic drugs.*

2

Dosage Forms and Naming of Drugs

DOSAGE FORMS

Pharmaceutical preparations are the forms in which drugs are prepared by the pharmacist or pharmaceutical chemist for administration in the treatment of the sick. A knowledge of some of the most important dosage forms is essential to those administering drugs.

FLAVORED VEHICLES AND COLORING SUBSTANCES

Vehicles or solvents are used to dissolve or suspend drugs and make them more palatable. Waters, syrups, and elixirs are important groups under this heading. Spirits and tinctures may also be used as flavored vehicles.

Waters. Aromatic or flavored waters are saturated solutions of volatile substances, usually volatile oils, dissolved in water. They are used as solvents and mask the disagreeable taste of drugs, especially salts. They have no marked therapeutic activity, as the solutions are very dilute. Examples: Peppermint Water, U.S.P.; Cinnamon Water, N.F.

Syrups. Simple syrup is an almost saturated solution of sugar in water. It is thick and viscid and is used as a diluent for making other syrups which are soothing or demulcent to the mucous membrane of the throat.

There are two classes of syrups:

1. *Flavored syrups* are employed to mask the taste of unpleasant-tasting drugs and to add stability to preparations. Examples: Acacia Syrup, N.F.; Cocoa Syrup, U.S.P.; Cherry Syrup, U.S.P.; Orange Syrup, U.S.P.; Raspberry Syrup, U.S.P.

2. *Medicated syrups* such as Ipecac Syrup, U.S.P. (emetic, expectorant), and Chloral Hydrate Syrup, U.S.P. (hypnotic), contain some added medicinal substance.

Elixirs. Elixirs are sweetened, pleasantly flavored hydroalcoholic solutions. Because of the alcoholic content, they are miscible with tinctures.

1. *Aromatic Elixir, U.S.P. (Simple Elixir)*, and *Iso-alcoholic Elixir, N.F. (Iso-Elixir)*, are used mainly for diluting other liquid preparations.

9

2. *Medicated elixirs* include Phenobarbital Elixir, U.S.P.; Diphenhydramine Hydrochloride Elixir, U.S.P.; and Terpin Hydrate and Codeine Elixir, N.F.

Coloring Substances

Many of the flavored vehicles possess their own distinctive color. When coloring agents are added to colorless solutions to make them more pleasing or acceptable to the patients, they must be either an official preparation or a coal tar color certified as harmless and suitable for the purpose of coloring drugs by the Federal Food, Drug, and Cosmetic Act. Amaranth Solution, U.S.P., and Compound Amaranth Solution, N.F., are used to color solutions red. They have replaced cudbear tincture and compound cudbear tincture. Carmine solution, a red solution prepared from cochineal, is still used in some preparations. Other colors frequently used are brown and green.

Today, capsules, powders, and tablets are also tinted with a variety of colors.

Solid Sweetening Substances

Sucrose, U.S.P., B.P. (Saccharum, Sugar). Sucrose is the sugar widely used in sweetening and preparing food. It is used pharmaceutically in the preparation of syrups, elixirs, and some hypodermic tablets. Other names are cane sugar and beet sugar.

Saccharin, U.S.P., B.P. (Benzosulfimide, Gluside). Saccharin is an artificial sweetener which is much sweeter than sugar. The sixteenth revision of the *United States Pharmacopeia* (U.S.P. XVI) states that saccharin in dilute solution is about 500 times sweeter than sucrose (sugar); hence 15 mg. are equivalent in sweetening power to approximately 7.5 Gm. of sucrose. To some persons, it also has a bitter taste, especially in high concentrations.

Calcium Saccharin, N.F., Sodium Saccharin, N.F., B.P. (Soluble Saccharin, Soluble Gluside), has the advantage of greater water solubility than saccharin, which is only slightly soluble in water. Medicinally these substances are used as sweeteners in diabetes and obesity and where sugar is contraindicated.

Preparation

Sodium Saccharin Tablets, N.F.   15, 30, and 60 mg.

Calcium Cyclamate, N.F. (Sucaryl Calcium), and Sodium Cyclamate, N.F. (Sucaryl Sodium). These official salts are synthetic noncaloric sweeteners for use in the diet of the diabetic and other patients who must restrict their carbohydrate intake. The calcium salt is available for persons on a restricted sodium diet. The sodium salt is used to sweeten oral dosage forms of drugs. It is about 30 times as sweet as sugar.

Preparations

Calcium Cyclamate and Calcium Saccharin Solution, N.F.	5.4 to 6.6 Gm. calcium cyclamate and 540 to 660 mg. saccharin calcium in 100 ml.
Calcium Cyclamate and Calcium Saccharin Tablets, N.F.	50 mg. calcium cyclamate and 5 mg. saccharin calcium
Sodium Cyclamate and Sodium Saccharin Solution, N.F.	5.4 to 6.6 Gm. sodium cyclamate and 540 to 660 mg. saccharin sodium in 100 ml.
Sodium Cyclamate and Sodium Sacchrarin Tables, N.F.	50 mg. sodium cyclamate and 5 mg. saccharin sodium

Trade name: Sucaryl

AQUEOUS SOLUTIONS

Aqueous solutions contain one or more chemical substances dissolved in water. They are prepared (1) by dissolving mineral or organic substances in water (e.g., Strong Iodine Solution, U.S.P.; Benzalkonium Chloride Solution, U.S.P.) or (2) by extracting the medicinal material from mammalian organs and glands (e.g., Oxytocin Injection, U.S.P.; Epinephrine Solution, U.S.P.). They are administered topically, orally, or parenterally (see discussion of injections, pp. 12, 76–82).

AQUEOUS SUSPENSIONS

Aqueous solutions contain one or more chemical substances dissolved in in water by means of harmless suspending or dispersing agents. Suspensions, emulsions, gels, mixtures, and magmas are discussed with this group of substances.

Suspensions. Suspensions are preparations of finely divided, undissolved drugs dispersed in liquids. Powders for suspensions are preparations of finely divided drugs intended for suspension in liquid vehicles. They are available for (1) oral administration, (2) parenteral administration (see discussion of injections, pp. 76–82), and (3) ophthalmic use. Suspensions for oral administration are: Tetracycline Oral Suspension, U.S.P.; Trisulfapyrimidines Oral Suspension, U.S.P. Those intended for ophthalmic use are: Ophthalmic Oxytetracycline Hydrochloride, N.F.; Cortisone Acetate Ophthalmic Suspension, N.F. For sterile suspensions intended for injection, see below.

Emulsions. Emulsions are suspensions of fats or oils in water. The oil is dispersed through an aqueous solution of an emulsifying agent. The oil particles are coated with gum so that they will not coalesce and so are in permanent suspension. Gelatin may also be used in preparing emulsions. Example: Liquid Petrolatum Emulsion, N.F.

Gels. Gels are colloidal aqueous suspensions of hydrated inorganic substances. Example: Aluminum Hydroxide Gel, U.S.P.

Mixtures. A mixture is a suspension of a solid material in a liquid. Example: Chalk Mixture.

Magmas.   Magmas are bulky suspensions of poorly soluble substances in water which resemble milk or cream. They tend to separate on standing and require a "SHAKE WELL" label. Example: Milk of Magnesia, U.S.P., Magnesium Hydroxide Mixture, B.P.

INJECTIONS

The sterile preparations intended for parenteral administration have been divided by U.S.P. XVII into five groups:

1. **Injections,** which are sterile solutions of drugs suitable for injection. Examples: Digitoxin Injection, N.F.; Epinephrine Injection, U.S.P.
2. **Dry solids** from which are obtained, upon the addition of a suitable solvent, sterile solutions suitable for injection. Examples: Sterile Potassium Penicillin G, U.S.P.; Hyaluronidase for Injection, N.F.
3. **Sterile suspensions** are solids suspended in suitable solvents which are never injected intravenously or intrathecally. They are available only for intramuscular or subcutaneous injection. Example: Sterile Benzathine Penicillin G Suspension, U.S.P.
4. **Dry solids,** which are mixed with certain suitable harmless buffer and suspending agents to produce preparations comparable to sterile suspensions when suitable vehicles are added. Example: Sterile Chloramphenicol for Suspension, N.F.
5. **Emulsions** of fluids in a fluid medium suitable for parenteral administration, which are not to be injected into the spinal canal. Example: Sterile Phytonadione Emulsion, U.S.P.

The aqueous vehicles used for preparing injections are: Water for Injection, U.S.P.; Sodium Chloride Injection, U.S.P.; and Ringer's Injection, U.S.P. Other vehicles used are fixed oils of vegetable origin, certain mono- or diglycerides, and oleic acid.

Injections are available in sealed glass ampuls or multiple-dose vials complete with rubber stopper through which the hypodermic needle may be inserted to remove the contents of the vials. Examples of preparations available in sealed glass ampuls are: Nikethamide (Coramine) Injection, N.F.; Nalorphine (Nalline) Hydrochloride Injection, U.S.P. Examples of preparations in multiple-dose vials are: Insulin Injection, U.S.P.; Isophane Insulin Suspension, U.S.P.

ALCOHOLIC SOLUTIONS

Spirits or Essences.   Spirits are alcoholic solutions of volatile substances, usually volatile oils. Many are flavoring agents (e.g., Peppermint Spirit, N.F., B.P.; Compound Orange Spirit, U.S.P.). Aromatic Ammonia

Spirit, N.F., which is a medicated spirit, is used as a reflex stimulant. Peppermint spirit is also used as a carminative.

EXTRACTIVE PREPARATIONS

Extractive preparations are made from vegetable drugs and contain the active principles from crude drugs in a hydroalcoholic solvent called the *menstruum*. These preparations are made by two processes, maceration and percolation. In the first method the coarsely divided drug is mixed and agitated frequently with the solvent. After three or four days, the solution is filtered and made up to a suitable volume. Example: Compound Benzoin Tincture, U.S.P. In the percolation method, the solvent trickles through a column of coarsely divided drug and extracts the medicinal substances from the crude drug. The drug residue is called the *marc*.

Tinctures, fluidextracts, and extracts are examples of extractive preparations.

Tinctures. Tinctures are hydroalcoholic solutions of medicinal substances usually obtained by extraction of vegetable drugs. Pharmacologically potent drugs are prepared in 10 per cent strength in tinctures. Examples: Belladonna Tincture, U.S.P.; Digitalis Tincture, N.F. Drugs having very little pharmacological action may be prepared in 50 per cent strength. These tinctures are used as flavoring agents. Examples: Lemon Tincture, U.S.P.; Sweet Orange Peel Tincture, U.S.P.; Vanilla Tincture, N.F. Hydroalcoholic solutions of inorganic or organic substances are used as antiseptics. Examples: Iodine Tincture, U.S.P.; Nitromersol Tincture, N.F.

Fluidextracts. Fluidextracts are hydroalcoholic extracts of vegetable drugs made by percolation so that 1 ml. of the fluidextract represents the active principles in 1 Gm. of the crude drug. This highly concentrated form of vegetable drugs is ten times stronger than the tinctures described above. One fluidextract widely used medicinally is Aromatic Cascara Sagrada Fluidextract, U.S.P.

Extracts. Extracts are concentrated, solid or semisolid preparations made by percolation and evaporation of the percolate. They are adjusted to a specific strength and are generally two to six times stronger than the crude drugs from which they are prepared. There are two kinds of extracts: the semisolid, or pilular; and the dry, powdered extract. The pilular extracts are used in making ointments and pills. The powdered extract is prescribed in capsules or tablets along with other drugs. Example: Belladonna Extract, N.F.

SOLID DOSAGE FORMS

Many drugs are more stable and more conveniently marketed in powder or crystalline form. These may be dispensed as powders, capsules, spansules, tablets, pellets, or pills.

Effervescent Powders. Powders may be mixed in the dry state with sodium bicarbonate, tartaric acid, and citric acid. When water is added, the drugs dissolve, carbon dioxide is liberated, the mixture effervesces, and the drug becomes more palatable. Example: Fizrin (nonofficial drug).

Capsules. Capsules are small soluble containers made of tasteless gelatin. They are hard or soft, flexible shells that are used to enclose doses of drugs for oral administration. The hard capsules are used for dispensing powdered drugs, and the soft ones are used for oils and solutions of active drugs. They are readily swallowed, are effective in disguising drug tastes, and dissolve rapidly in the stomach. However, they may be coated with substances that prevent their disintegration in the stomach. These enteric capsules then dissolve in the alkaline juices of the intestines. Capsules are available in many sizes and are one of the most popular forms of medication. Examples: Sodium Amobarbital Capsules, U.S.P.; Halibut Liver Oil Capsules.

Spansules. A spansule is prepared by variably coating particles of the active ingredient with a substance that permits gradual release of the drug in the gastrointestinal tract. A number of these tiny particles, or *beads,* are placed in one capsule. After ingestion, some of the particles disintegrate immediately, others after two to four hours, and still others in six to eight hours. Thus uniform medication is assured over a period of 10 to 12 hours. Example: Spansule Sustained Release Capsules Dexedrine Sulfate (nonofficial drug).

Tablets. Tablets are solid dosage forms containing granulated or powdered drugs that are compressed or molded into round or discoid shapes. They vary greatly in size and shape, and many are scored so that they may be easily divided to afford smaller doses.

Compressed Tablets. Solid drugs, usually after being converted to granules, may be subjected to mechanical pressure and compressed into tablets. Many compressed tablets contain a filler such as dried starch, which acts as a disintegrating agent. The starch swells when it comes in contact with water and causes disintegration of the tablet. Tablets may be coated with chocolate, gelatin, or other suitable substances to improve their taste. Clear plastic coatings may be colored for the purpose of identification or patient acceptance. If the coating is made of keratin, shellac, phenyl salicylate, or cellulose acetate phthalate, which does not dissolve in the acid juices of the stomach, it is called an *enteric-coated* tablet. Such coatings protect acid-sensitive drugs from the action of the gastric juices and also prevent certain drugs from irritating the stomach, with ensuing discomfort. The coatings then dissolve in the alkaline juices of the intestinal tract, and the drug is liberated and produces the desired effect. Compressed tablets are administered orally. Examples: Aspirin Tablets, U.S.P.; Erythromycin Tablets, U.S.P.

Tablet Triturates or Molded Tablets. These are small, usually cylindrical, molded or compressed disks of various sizes. Powders may be mixed with dextrose or a mixture of lactose and sucrose and diluted alcohol. The resulting mass is shaped by means of a tablet mold. The alcohol evaporates, whereupon the tablet is ejected and dried. Most tablet triturates weigh about 60 mg. They may be used for oral, sublingual, or buccal administration (sublingual or buccal tablets). Examples: Ergotamine Tartrate Tablets, U.S.P.; Nitroglycerin Tablets, U.S.P.

Hypodermic Tablets. Hypodermic tablets are tablet triturates that are completely and readily soluble in water. These tablets, dissolved in Water for Injection, U.S.P., are available for parenteral administration.[1] Examples: Atropine Sulfate Tablets; Morphine Sulfate Tablets.

Pellets. Pellets are small sterile spheres formed by the compression of certain steroid hormones. They are implanted subcutaneously in the body tissue and form a depot from which the hormone is slowly released. Pellets are marketed in individual sterile vials. Examples: Desoxycorticosterone Acetate Pellets, N.F.; Testosterone Pellets, N.F.

Pills. When powdered drugs are mixed with adhesive substances like glucose or honey, they may be molded in spherical or ovoid forms called *pills.* In recent years pills have been replaced to a large extent by tablets and capsules.

Dosage Forms for External Administration

The dosage forms for application to the skin and mucous membranes are ophthalmic solutions (collyria), sprays, inhalants, inhalations (aerosols), liniments, lotions, ointments, pastes, plasters, and suppositories.

Ophthalmic Solutions (Collyria). These are sterile, usually isotonic, buffered solutions prepared for instillation in the eye. For rapid therapeutic effects, small amounts of a hypertonic solution that may be quickly diluted by tears may be used. To prevent irritation, solutions used to wash the eyes should be approximately isotonic because of the large volume used. Examples: Isoflurophate Ophthalmic Solution, N.F.; Silver Nitrate Ophthalmic Solution, U.S.P.

Sprays. Sprays are solutions of one or more drugs in oil or water, usually administered by atomizers. Air forced through the atomizer by squeezing the bulb carries with it a coarse liquid spray, containing the drug, into the nose and throat. Example: Tyrothricin Spray, N.F.

Inhalants. Inhalants are drugs or combinations of drugs that, because of their high vapor pressure, may be carried into the nasal passages with

---

[1] The difficulties of preparing sterile, suitably clear solutions from such tablets offset to a great extent the convenience claimed for their use. No hypodermic tablets are official in the United States Pharmacopeia.

the inhaled air. They are available in portable inhalers. Example: Propylhexedrine Inhalant, N.F.

Inhalations (Aerosols). Aerosols (Gr. *aero-*, referring to air) are rather stable suspensions of extremely small liquid or solid particles (0.5 to 5 μ in diameter) in a gas such as air or oxygen. They are produced and administered by nebulizers. This nebulized mist may reach the bronchi and even the alveoli.

Types of Aerosols. There are two types of aerosols prepared by nebulization: liquid aerosols and solid aerosols.

LIQUID AEROSOLS. Water is used to dissolve the drug, and a fine stable mist is formed. There is an increase in relative humidity, which aids in liquefying secretions and correcting local dehydration. Examples: Epinephrine Inhalation, U.S.P.; Isoproterenol Hydrochloride Inhalation, U.S.P.

SOLID AEROSOLS. These are composed of micropulverized penicillin, streptomycin, and the sulfonamides. They are administered with nebulizers or Aerohalors and are used for lung infections.

Liniments. Liniments are liquid preparations applied to the skin with rubbing. They consist of one or more active ingredients and a liniment base or vehicle. The base is generally a fixed oil, soap, or alcohol. The oil and soap of liniments adhere to the skin and serve as lubricants in rubbing, whereas the alcohol is miscible with the sebaceous layer of the skin and permits absorption of the active ingredient. Most liniments are anodyne (to relieve pain) and rubefacient (to make red). Examples: Camphor Liniment, N.F.; Camphor aud Soap Liniment, N.F.

Lotions. Lotions are aqueous suspensions of insoluble substances. Glycerin is frequently used in lotions. After lotion is applied to the skin, the fluid evaporates, leaving a film of the suspended ingredients. Lotions are used for soothing, astringent, and antipruritic effects. Example: Phenolated Calamine Lotion, U.S.P.

Ointments. Ointments are semisolid greasy substances through which one or more substances are distributed. They are applied locally to the skin and mucous membranes. The usual ointment has a petrolatum base, which consists of petrolatum (petroleum jelly or mineral oil), emulsifying or dispersing agents, and thickening substances. Some ointment bases are miscible with water. One of these is Hydrophilic Ointment, U.S.P. Ointments serve as soothing agents, astringents, and antiseptics. Examples: Zinc Oxide Ointment, U.S.P.; Bacitracin Ointment, U.S.P. The ointment bases are discussed on page 724.

Ophthalmic Ointments. These are sterile ointments to be used in the eye. Examples: Ammoniated Mercury Ophthalmic Ointment, U.S.P.; Epinephrine Bitartrate Ophthalmic Ointment, N.F.

Plasters. Plasters are solid adhesive preparations that are applied to the skin to protect, soothe, and lessen pain. Substances having adhesive properties are spread evenly on certain fabrics that may or may not be coated with a water-repellent film. Examples: Adhesive Tape, U.S.P.; Mustard Plaster.

Pastes. Pastes are ointment-like preparations of one or more medicaments and some adhesive material that are applied to oozing surfaces. They afford greater protection and are more absorptive than ointments. Examples: Aluminum Paste, U.S.P.; Zinc Oxide Paste, U.S.P.

Suppositories. Suppositories are mixtures of substances with a firm base suitable for insertion into the body cavities. The base may be glycerinated gelatin, hard soap, or cocoa butter. They melt at body temperature and allow the active ingredient to come in contact with the mucous membrane to produce local or systemic effects. There are rectal, vaginal, and urethral suppositories.

Rectal Suppositories. These are conical or bullet-shaped and usually weigh about 2 Gm. They are used to produce local and systemic effects and to produce catharsis. When used for systemic effects, the rectal dose is usually much larger than the oral dose.

Vaginal Suppositories. These are conical or spherical in shape and weigh from 4 to 10 Gm. They are used to confer antisepsis, to combat various infections, and as spermatocides.

Urethral Suppositories. These are pencil-shaped and weigh from 2 to 4 Gm. They are used mainly for local treatment of the female urethra.

NAMING OF DRUGS

The use of several names for a given drug makes the subject of pharmacology and the practice of medicine and nursing more complicated than they would be if a single name were used for each agent. Some medications, for example, morphine sulfate, codeine phosphate, and sulfadiazine, have but one name. These names are for older, well-known drugs and may be used by any manufacturer, since they are not trade-mark names.

When a new drug is manufactured and patented, three names are involved: the chemical, the approved, and the trade-mark names. The nurse is rarely concerned with the chemical name, which is usually much longer than the other names for the same compound. In addition to the names, each compound is characterized by a definite structural formula that depicts the relative positions of all atoms in the molecule when this is known.

There are two classes of nonproprietary names: the generic name, which is official and appears in the *United States Pharmacopeia* and the *National Formulary,* and the United States Adopted Name (U.S.A.N.). The American Medical Association–U.S. Pharmacopeia (AMA–USP) Nomenclature Committee was established in 1961 to select names for new compounds. These names are publicized in the *Journal of the American Medical Association* and in various medical and pharmaceutical journals. After the U.S.A.N. is published, the Committee urges the FDA and the producers of the drug to adopt that name as quickly as possible by using it on labels and in all literature discussing the drug. The U.S.A.N. names should be regarded in the same manner as the U.S.P. and N.F. designations.

As an example involving the three names for a patented drug, we may consider chlorpromazine (generic name). The *chemical name* for the drug is 3-chloro-10-(3-dimethyl-aminopropyl) phenothiazine. This describes exactly to the trained chemists of many nations the positions of the 40 atoms of carbon, hydrogen, nitrogen, sulfur, and chlorine in the molecule. It is so precise as not to be applicable to any other chemical compound. It is because of its length and complexity that its manufacturer gives it a coined name which can be learned and remembered more easily. In this case "chlorpromazine" was selected as the *generic name*. When the compound is patented, this name and a third, the *trade-mark* ("brand" or "registered") *name*, are listed with the patent office. The trade-mark name for our example is Thorazine®. It is spelled with a capital first letter, and is followed by the letter R (meaning "registered," thus legally protected), encircled and usually somewhat elevated.

The life of a patent is 17 years, after which other manufacturers may produce the product. However, they may not use the trade-mark name Thorazine®, for this remains the property of the legal owner. They must use the generic name chlorpromazine or secure some trade-mark name of their own. Sometimes two or more companies market the same patented drug, in which case each will attach a different trade-mark or "brand" name. In other cases, where no patent exists, the drug may be offered by a large number of firms under as many names. Regardless of the number of trade names, there is only one generic name in each country. It is selected for reasons of simplicity as a substitute for the chemical name and in order that a reasonably short name can become public property upon termination of the patent rights of the inventor.

In other countries firms may select trade names that are more appropriate by reason of language or other differences. Thus chlorpromazine is known as Largactyl in France and Great Britain. In this text, generic names are used predominantly, with outstanding trade names included in parentheses for aiding the student in associating the two. The nurse is often given orders for drugs with the trade or brand name, rather than the generic. These trade names are capitalized in the text, but the encircled R is omitted for convenience. Both the generic and trade names are used for labeling the various products.

There are far more combinations of drugs sold in both the solid and liquid forms than there are single agents. These are usually given a trade name. Combinations are useful but are not usually discussed in textbooks of pharmacology except in certain cases of augmentation or synergism.

The Index of this book gives several names for the same drug wherever available, with cross-listing to the generic name used in the United States, or to another generally acceptable term. The various synonyms in this and other countries and various trade names are given at the end of the individual drug sections where appropriate.

The magnitude of the problem of providing the nurse with an easy reference to the identification of any medicinal product with which she may come in contact is evidenced by the fact that there are more than 7000 registered medications on the market in the United States alone. Most of these are multiple formulations, i.e., combinations of several ingredients. It is obviously impossible even to list this number of products.

REVIEW QUESTIONS

1. *What are pharmaceutical preparations or dosage forms? Name four dosage forms and give an example of each.*
2. *What are flavored vehicles? Why are they used in preparing dosage forms? Why are coloring agents used in preparing dosage forms?*
3. *In what available forms are drugs to be used as suspensions? Give three therapeutic uses.*
4. *What are injections? Name four groups and give an example of each.*
5. *Define tablets and describe three kinds. How are they used?*
6. *What are inhalations (aerosols)? How are they administered and for what purposes are they used?*
7. *What is a generic name for a drug? What is the U.S.A.N. name? What are trade-mark (brand) names? Give examples of both types.*

3

Drug Standards and Drug Legislation

Drugs occurring in nature, such as opium, digitalis, and epinephrine, show wide variations in strength and activity. These variations occur among different specimens of the same drug and even among different leaves grown on the same plant. Reliable results in the treatment of disease demand that these drugs should be of uniform strength. Therefore, drug standardization methods have been developed, not only to ensure uniformity among the natural drugs but also to establish standards for their identification and purity in order to prevent purposeful adulteration.

Chemistry has played an important role in the standardization of drugs. The potency of some natural or crude drugs may be determined by extracting the pure chemical substances, or *active principles,* contained therein and purifying and weighing them, or by extracting them and titrating them. However, these *chemical methods* are inadequate to standardize some drugs. The activity of this type can be determined quantitatively by *bio-assay,* or the effect of the drug on animals or man. Dr. E. B. Houghton, one of the first to employ a living animal to test the potency of a drug, used the frog's heart to assay digitalis, a heart-tonic drug. The application of pharmacological methods to determine the potency of drugs has also been made in the case of insulin, ergot, epinephrine, the sex hormones, and many other drugs.

DRUG STANDARDS

UNITED STATES

The legal standards for drugs used in the United States are established by the *United States Pharmacopeia* (U.S.P.), the *National Formulary* (N.F.), and the *Homeopathic Pharmacopeia of the United States.* The preparations contained in these books are known as "official" preparations.

United States Pharmacopeia (U.S.P.). The first *United States Pharmacopeia* was published in 1820 under the leadership of Dr. Lyman Spalding. It contained a relatively small list of therapeutic agents, which were mostly vegetable drugs collected by the apothecary and made into suitable preparations such as tinctures, syrups, and elixirs. Provision was made for its revision every ten years. In 1940 the period of revision was reduced to five

20

years, with provisions for supplements or interim revisions. In 1820 the U.S.P. was a private medical effort. In 1850, however, the pharmacists took part and have had an important role ever since. In 1880, by which time the chemical and pharmaceutical houses had become well established, tests and assays and official standards of strength and purity of drugs were added. Today, these tests and assays are a major part of the U.S.P.

In 1910 the enterprise was incorporated under the laws of the District of Columbia as the United States Pharmacopeial Convention.

The first Food and Drugs Act, passed by the United States Congress in 1906, gave official status to the *United States Pharmacopeia* and the *National Formulary*. The same status was continued under the Food, Drug, and Cosmetic Act of 1938. Thus these books contain standards for drugs, and these standards are enforced by the federal government.

The revision of the U.S.P. is supervised by a full-time Director of Pharmacopeial Revision, who is appointed by the Board of Trustees. Delegates from all parts of the country meet in Washington, D.C., every five years. These delegates are physicians, medical scientists, and pharmacists, who are sent from the colleges of medicine and pharmacy, incorporated medical and pharmaceutical societies, and certain governmental agencies. The General Committee of Revision is made up of voluntary workers, who are elected by the national convention; it includes many physicians and scientists (including bacteriologists, organic and physical chemists, physicists, and pharmacists). The Subcommittee on Scope, which includes physicians, pharmacologists, and medical specialists, is responsible for the selection of newer remedies to be included and decides which drugs should be deleted. The current edition of the U.S.P., the seventeenth, was published in 1965.

The purpose and scope of the U.S.P. are to provide standards for drugs of therapeutic usefulness and pharmaceutical necessity. The drugs of pharmaceutical necessity are preparations such as alcohol, glycerin, and orange tincture, which are used in making dosage forms. The U.S.P. also provides tests to ensure the identity, strength, quality, and purity of medicinal substances. Some patented drugs are now included, provided their composition and mode of manufacture are not secret, as exemplified by reserpine and certain of the antihistaminics.

The drugs in the U.S.P. are arranged alphabetically according to their official names. The following information is given for each drug:

1. Official name.
2. Purity rubric (purity recognized by the U.S.P.).
3. Description of the product and the structural formula, when known.
4. Assays, both chemical and biological.
5. Methods of preservation and storage.

6. Dose—the *usual dose* and the *usual dose range* (in the metric system) as well as the method and frequency of administration. The usual dose is the amount of drug that is required to produce the desired therapeutic effect for which the drug is most usually employed. Unless otherwise specified, it is the adult oral dose. It is intended to guide the physician, who may vary it according to the needs of his patient. The *usual dose range* is given to guide the pharmacist in seeking confirmation of prescriptions containing unusually large doses. It may also guide the nurse in checking the dose given on orders for administering the drugs.

7. Dosage forms for the U.S.P. drugs, such as tablets, capsules, injections, etc.

8. Category—classification of drugs according to their therapeutic uses as antibiotics, tranquilizers, anticoagulants, sedatives, analgesics, narcotic analgesics, etc.

National Formulary (N.F.). The *National Formulary*, first published by the American Phamaceutical Association in 1888, attained official status under the Federal Food and Drugs Act of 1906. It is revised and published simultaneously with the U.S.P.; the current edition is the twelfth, which became official in 1965. Drugs and dosage forms admitted to the N.F. are selected on the basis of therapeutic efficacy. Standards are included for older drugs that still are widely used. Also included are many vehicles that are used as diluents. All doses are expressed in the metric system. A statement of category is provided with each monograph for useful information.

New and Nonofficial Drugs (N.N.D.). This book is issued annually under the supervision of the Council on Drugs of the American Medical Association, a body that analyzes carefully all pertinent data found in the medical literature, reports from laboratories, and its own investigations concerning newly introduced drugs.

Most physicians are unable to make an exhaustive appraisal of the reports describing all new agents, even in a particular field of specialization. Reports in medical journals are at times confusing, if not conflicting, with regard to the evidence of usefulness of a new substance. There are many examples of the enthusiastic use in some quarters of questionably effective new drugs. Critical evaluation by some physicians eventually reduces such a product to its appropriately limited place or to deserved oblivion. This elimination often requires much time, and in the meanwhile considerable use of the drug may have been made on erroneous faith generated by early favorable reports. The Council is the one national body that at the earliest appropriate time presents impartially the available facts concerning the pharmacology, toxicity, and results of clinical usage of new drugs, thus enabling physicians to prescribe as wisely as possible at that time. Monographs are written on clearly useful products as well as on agents of unestablished value. Thus, inclusion in *New and Nonofficial Drugs* does not necessarily sanction the use of a compound in the diagnosis, prevention, or treatment of disease.

The critiques which are first published in the Council's section of the weekly *Journal of the American Medical Association* (J.A.M.A.) appear in the next edition of the book *New and Nonofficial Drugs*. Their publication follows, after varying periods of time, the actual use of the agents being described, but precedes, often by years, their appearance in the official compendia, the U.S.P. or the N.F. Through the medium of the J.A.M.A. and of N.N.D., the Council is able to protect, to a great extent, the public and the medical, dental, and pharmacy professions against the effects of premature or unjustifiable conclusions in medical literature, misleading advertising, and occasional fraud in product promotion. It is no longer appropriate to use the letters N.N.D. following the drug names in the manner that the letters U.S.P. and N.F. are used because neither official status nor approval is signified by inclusion in N.N.D.

Dispensatory of the United States of America. This large book, encyclopedic in character, contains practical and modern information about drugs. The twenty-sixth edition, published in 1960, includes drugs that were official in U.S.P. XV, N.F. X, the *British Pharmacopoeia* (B.P. VIII), and the *Pharmacopoea Internationalis* (I.P.), as well as many new and nonofficial drugs. In addition, it contains many general-survey articles on such subjects as adrenergic blocking agents, antibiotics, radioisotopes, etc.

Hospital Formularies and Handbooks. These are often published by large hospitals and contain the drugs and dosage forms often prescribed in a particular institution.

BRITISH COMMONWEALTH OF NATIONS

British Pharmacopoeia (B.P.). This book, which is similar in scope to the U.S.P., contains standards for drugs that are official in the United Kingdom, the British dominions, and the Crown colonies. It is published by the British Pharmacopoeia Commission, under the general direction of the General Medical Council, pursuant to the Medical Act of 1956. All doses are given in the metric system. The drugs included in the *British Pharmacopoeia* are labeled B.P.

New monographs include a wide range of synthetic drugs, antibiotics, hormones, and biological products together with preparations such as injections and tablets. This book has included for the first time monographs on radioactive chemicals such as sodium radio-phosphate and sodium radio-iodide. The tenth *British Pharmacopoeia*, published in 1963, became official in January, 1964. It contains nearly 1000 monographs including 211 which did not appear in the ninth edition.

British Pharmaceutical Codex (B.P.C.). The *British Pharmaceutical Codex*, published by the Pharmaceutical Society of Great Britain, is similar in scope to the N.F.

Canadian Formulary (C.F.). This book contains formulas for preparations widely used in Canada as well as standards for new medicines that are prescribed there but are not included in the B.P. The seventh revision was published in 1949 by the Canadian Pharmaceutical Association and was given official status by the Canadian Food and Drug Act.[1]

Physicians' Formulary. The *Physicians' Formulary*, published by the Canadian Medical Association, contains many formulas for drugs used in medical practice in Canada.

Other International Standards

The drug standards of other nations include the *German Pharmacopeia*, revised in 1926; the *French Codex*, revised in 1938; and the pharmacopeias of Czechoslovakia, Estonia, Yugoslavia, Turkey, and Poland. The Spanish translation of the *United States Pharmacopeia* is widely used in South America.

Pharmacopoea Internationalis (I.P.). Because the various national pharmacopeias have varying standards, strengths, and nomenclature for widely used drugs, these differences have accounted for much confusion and have been sources of inconvenience and even danger to travelers. Therefore, to satisfy a desire for unification of terms, strengths, and composition of drugs used throughout the world, the World Health Organization, in 1951, published the first volume of an international pharmacopeia. The *Pharmacopoea Internationalis*, published in English, French, and Spanish, is not intended to have official status in any country unless adopted by the pharmacopeial authority of that country. The nomenclature is in Latin; the doses are in the metric system; and included are long-established drugs, drugs official in other national pharmacopeias, and drugs recently introduced that are likely to be accepted later by national pharmacopeias. Dosage tables for adults contain the method of administration and the usual and maximum single and daily doses for drugs. Tables of usual daily doses for children up to 30 months and from 30 months to five years are also included.

DRUG LEGISLATION

Drug standards have been available for many years. Cities such as London (1618), Paris (1639), and Edinburgh (1699) had their own pharmacopeias. The Continental Army of the United States had a pharmacopeia in 1777, and

---

[1] The U.S.P. and N.N.D. are rather widely used in Canada because many of the drugs employed in that country are obtained from the United States.

the first pharmacopeia of the United States, national in scope, was published in 1820. However, there were no provisions to enforce these standards. Unscrupulous persons could adulterate drugs to defraud the public for profit, or market unsuitable or unreliable drugs.

In 1887, Dr. E. R. Squibb, who had been purchasing agent of drugs for the United States Navy, turned to private life and founded a drug company for the purpose of providing physicians with reliable and dependable drugs. Physicians could not obtain good results with drugs that were too weak to produce the therapeutic effects desired or so strong that they produced poisoning and even death. Dr. Squibb voiced the need for controls for food and drugs in New York State and wrote a food and drugs act that was adopted by the New York State Legislature in 1881. Other states soon adopted food and drug acts similar to that of New York. Thus *within the states* the standards for drugs could be enforced by the state officials. The enforcement necessitated the establishment of laboratories for testing drugs manufactured and sold in the state.

FEDERAL FOOD AND DRUGS ACT OF 1906

Since drugs that were shipped from one state to another were not covered by state laws, the Food and Drugs Act of 1906 was enacted by Congress to enforce standards for drugs in *interstate commerce*. This act named the *United States Pharmacopeia* and the *National Formulary* as the official standards, and the federal government was given the power to enforce these standards. It could confiscate an objectionable or adulterated drug.

The 1906 Act was essentially a "label" law and required the contents of the bottle or container to conform with the label statement. It defined a drug as a substance used in the prevention, cure, or mitigation of disease in man or animals. As time passed, this law proved inadequate for the ever-increasing number of drugs and cosmetics; therefore, a new law was enacted in 1938, which was much broader in scope.

FEDERAL FOOD, DRUG, AND COSMETIC ACT OF 1938

The Federal Food, Drug, and Cosmetic Act of 1938, amended in 1952 by the Durham-Humphrey Law, and in 1962 by the Kefauver-Harris amendments, sets forth standards for drugs, therapeutic devices, and cosmetics, and is enforced by the Food and Drug Administration of the Department of Health, Education, and Welfare. This law also makes the *United States Pharmacopeia*, the *National Formulary*, and the *Homeopathic Pharmacopeia of the United States* the official standards.

A drug or therapeutic material must meet the following provisions of the Act:

1. The article must conform with the strength and purity it is represented to possess.

2. Labeling (including all printed and graphic matter accompanying the article) must be truthful.

3. The label must contain the name and address of the manufacturer, packer, or distributor, as well as a statement of the contents.

4. The label must bear the statement, "CAUTION, FEDERAL LAW PROHIBITS DISPENSING WITHOUT PRESCRIPTION," if the drug falls in any of the following three categories:

a. Narcotic, hypnotic, or habit-forming drug or one of its derivatives specified in the Act.

b. Any drug which because of its toxicity or potentiality for harmful effect, or method of its use, is not safe except under supervision of a practitioner licensed by law to administer the drug. Under the definition, all drugs for injection except insulin preparations are regarded as prescription drugs.

c. Any drug limited to preliminary investigational use under professional supervision by an effective new-drug application.

5. If the drug is not required to be labeled as a prescription drug, it must bear adequate directions for lay use.

6. Labeling must bear adequate warnings against unsafe use in pathological conditions.

7. The article must not be dangerous to health when used in dosage or with frequency or duration prescribed.

8. It must bear labels warning against habit formation if it contains narcotic or hypnotic habit-forming substances or any derivative which possesses the same properties.

9. It must conform to the specifications in the *United States Pharmacopeia*, *National Formulary*, or *Homeopathic Pharmacopeia*, including packaging and labeling requirements. However, deviations in strength, quality, and purity are permitted, provided the labels bear statements of the extent of such deviation.

10. A new drug may not be distributed until applications establishing its safety, after adequate tests, have been submitted and become effective. During the period that the new drug is under investigation by experts, the label of the drug must bear the statement, "CAUTION: NEW DRUG, LIMITED BY FEDERAL LAW TO INVESTIGATIONAL USE."

11. A drug consisting wholly or in part of insulin or any kind of penicillin, streptomycin, chlortetracycline, bacitracin, or other antibiotic must be made from a batch certified by the Food and Drug Administration.

12. The following provisions of the Act relate to prescriptions:

a. A prescription is an order to the pharmacist, for single filling unless otherwise designated by the physician.

b. Prescription for most drugs may be telephoned to the pharmacist.

c. Authority for refilling a prescription may be telephoned.

d. The pharmacist must keep a record of telephoned prescriptions and refills.

e. Labeling of a prescription drug must include a package insert to accompany the drug to the retail pharmacy, which will include full information as to directions for use, dosage levels, warnings, hazards, contraindications, and other information necessary for safe and effective use of the drug. Such full-disclosure information is also required in the labeling of sample packages, etc., sent to the doctors in separate brochures.

Exceptions may be made only for prescription drugs for which all such information is commonly known to all practitioners.

f. The label of every drug must carry the "established name" of the drug and each active ingredient in the product, and, whether active or not, the quantity, kind, and proportion of certain specified ingredients such as alcohol, bromides, and other drugs whose presence must be known for safe administration.

g. The labels of prescription drugs must bear, in addition to the above, the quantity of each active ingredient. On prescription drug labels, the "established name" must appear in direct association with the corresponding proprietary name and in type at least half as large as that used for the proprietary name.

There are several regulations in the amended act that are of special importance to physicians. They are set forth as follows:

1. New drugs must be effective as well as safe before marketing.
2. Experimental drugs.

a. Animal tests reasonably establishing safety must be submitted to the FDA before human clinical trial. Animal test data, plus other information regarding safety or efficacy of drug, must be made available to clinical investigators.

b. Clinical trials must be conducted only by persons qualified by training and experience. Patients must be informed that an experimental drug is being used, and consent obtained unless this is not feasible or, in the professional judgment of the investigator, would not be in the patient's best interest.

c. The investigator must maintain complete records of the use or other disposition of the drug, and the case histories of his patients.

3. Cancellation of new drug approvals.

a. New drug approvals may be canceled immediately if the Secretary finds there is imminent danger to health.

b. A previous approval can also be revoked, after opportunity for a hearing, if it appears that safety is not established, or manufacturing methods, facilities, or controls are inadequate.

4. Drug names.

a. FDA may establish "official" names for drugs and ingredients when desirable in the interest of usefulness and simplicity.

b. The established name—whether the name in the official compendium, or the officially designated name, or the common or usual name—must be used on labels and in labeling.

c. In addition, all labels, labeling, and advertising of prescription drugs must carry the established name of the drug and its active ingredients whereever a brand name of drug or ingredient appears. The established name must be printed in type at least half as large as the brand name.

d. Labeling and advertising of prescription drugs must also give the amount of each effective ingredient, and information about side effects, contraindications, and effectiveness of the drug, for the guidance of the physician. This information must be summarized briefly in advertisements.

In addition to specific requirements for drugs, the following provisions are made:

1. Dyes used in coloring foods, drugs, or cosmetics must be made from batches certified by the Food and Drug Administration.

2. Food must not be injurious to health. Addition of poisonous or deleterious substances to food is prohibited unless such substances are necessary or cannot be avoided in good manufacturing practice, in which case a safe tolerance is established.

3. Definite labeling requirements and special dietary regulations must be met before marketing foods for special dietary uses.

4. A cosmetic must not contain any substance harmful to users, when employed under directions for use on the label.

5. Residues of pesticides used on growing crops and of food additives used in processing, packaging, storage, or transportation of foods must be proved safe by the manufacturer, and must be used in accordance with safe tolerances and regulations established by the Food and Drug Administration.

HARRISON NARCOTIC ACT OF 1914

The Harrison Narcotic Act of 1914, amended in 1919, 1946, and 1956, regulates the importation, manufacture, sale, dispensing or prescribing, and use of opium and cocaine and all their derivatives. It now includes synthetic remedies known to produce addiction. Drug manufacturers are licensed to manufacture; retail and wholesale druggists are licensed to sell; physicians, dentists, and veterinarians are licensed to prescribe; and hospitals and institutions of learning are licensed to use narcotics. They must register and pay a fee annually to the Internal Revenue Service. Special blanks are required to purchase these drugs; accurate records must be kept of the drugs used, and inventories are subject to inspection. Violations are subject to fine and imprisonment.

NARCOTIC CONTROL ACT OF 1956

The Narcotic Control Act of 1956 provides more effective control of narcotic drugs and marihuana. All heroin in the hands of physicians, hospitals, institutions, etc., must be surrendered to the federal government. The Act provides stern penalties for persons over 18 years who give, sell, or dispense narcotics to juveniles (persons under 18 years). These offenders may be fined $10,000 to $20,000, imprisoned for ten years to life, or, at the discretion of the jury, given the death penalty.

MARIHUANA TAX ACT OF 1937

The Marihuana Tax Act of 1937 regulates the growing of hemp and the manufacture of hemp products. Further provisions for the control of marihuana are included in the Narcotic Control Act of 1956.

REVIEW QUESTIONS

1. *Why is it necessary to have standards for drugs?*
2. *What is the scope of the* United States Pharmacopeia?
3. *Discuss the value of* New *and* Nonofficial Drugs *to the nurse and practicing physician.*
4. *What is the* Pharmacopoea Internationalis? *Discuss its importance in drug administration.*
5. *Discuss some of the provisions of the Federal Food, Drug, and Cosmetic Act as amended in 1952; in 1962.*
6. *What is the purpose of the Harrison Narcotic Act?*

REFERENCES

OFFICIAL DRUG COMPENDIA

The Pharmacopeia of the United States of America, 17th rev. Mack Publishing Company, Easton Pa., 1965.
The National Formulary, 12th ed. Mack Publishing Company, Easton, Pa., 1965.
The Dispensatory of the United States of America, 25th ed. J. B. Lippincott Company, Philadelphia, 1960.
The British Pharmacopoeia, 10th ed. The Pharmaceutical Press, London, 1963.
The Canadian Formulary, 7th ed. Canadian Pharmaceutical Association, Toronto, 1949.
Pharmacopoea Internationalis, 1st ed. World Health Organization, Geneva, Switzerland, Vol. 1, 1951; Vol. 2, 1955.

NONOFFICIAL DRUG COMPENDIA

New and Nonofficial Drugs (formerly entitled *New and Nonofficial Remedies*). Published annually by J. B. Lippincott Company, Philadelphia, 1964.

Reports of the Council on Drugs of the American Medical Association with the comments that have appeared in the *Journal of the American Medical Association*. Published annually by J. B. Lippincott Company, Philadelphia.

Goodhart, R. S. (ed.): *Modern Drug Encyclopedia and Therapeutic Index*, 9th ed. Drug Publications, Inc., New York, 1961. Supplements every month.

The Merck Index of Chemicals and Drugs: an Encyclopedia for the Chemist, Pharmacist, Physician, and Allied Professions, 7th ed. Merck & Company, Inc., Rahway, N.J., 1960.

Physicians' Desk Reference to Pharmaceutical Specialties & Biologicals, 14th ed. Medical Economics, Inc., Oradell, N.J., 1965.

Smith, R.G.: "The Development and Control of New Drugs," *Amer. J. Nurs.*, **62**:56, 1962.

4

Arithmetic Review. Weights and Measures. Preparation of Solutions. Calculations of Dosages. Prescriptions and Orders

ARITHMETIC REVIEW

The ability of the nurse and others handling drugs to make accurate calculations is essential for the administration of correct doses of drugs to patients. This requires a working knowledge of the fundamental principles of arithmetic such as addition, subtraction, multiplication, and division as applied to fractions, decimals, percentage, ratio, and proportion. A familiarity with the systems of weights and measures and their approximate equivalents, as used by physicians in writing their prescriptions and orders, is also indispensable. The objective of this arithmetic review is to recall the simplest mathematical principles because these are necessary for the preparation of medications, the calculation of dosages, and the conversion of doses from one system to the other. Speed and accuracy with mathematical procedures are gained through frequent practice in solving problems.

ARABIC AND ROMAN NUMERALS

The Arabic system of numerals uses the symbols 0, 1, 2, 3, 4, 5, 6, 7, 8, and 9. All possible numerical values may be expressed by combinations of these symbols, which are called integers, or whole numbers. These same symbols may express values of less than one by the use of fractions and decimals. This system of numbers is used in expressing doses in both the metric and the apothcaries' systems. In the metric system the whole number precedes the symbol (e.g., 1 Gm., 2 mg.), and fractions are expressed decimally (e.g., 1.5 Gm.).

The Roman system of numerals uses the following letters as symbols and combines them in a definite way to make all values of whole numbers.

I—1	C—100
V—5	D—500
X—10	M—1000
L—50	

31

Doctors, nurses, and pharmacists use the small letters i, v, x, and l with the apothecaries' system for the values 1, 5, 10, and 50, respectively, in connection with the writing, filling, and labeling of prescriptions and orders for medications. They are used for expressing whole units and follow the abbreviation or symbol (e.g., gr. v). A dot is placed over the Roman numeral *i* to prevent mistaking it for the Roman numeral *l* (small-case L for 50) (e.g., gr. iv, gr. ix). A fraction of a grain is expressed by using a common fraction (e.g., gr. ¼, gr. ⅓); the symbol "ss" (meaning *semis*) is often used to designate ½. The capital letters are commonly used in outlines, for chapter designations in books, on the dials of timepieces, for dates on public buildings, etc.

The following rules are used for expressing numbers by the Roman system:

1. Two or three numerals of equal value written in a series are added: II or ii means 2; XXX or xxx means 30. V, L, and D are not repeated because their values when doubled are represented by X, C, and M, respectively.

2. A number of lesser value that follows one of greater value is added to the latter: xiii means 10 plus 1 plus 1 plus 1, or 13.

3. When a number is immediately followed by one of greater value, the first number is subtracted from the second: iv means that 1 is subtracted from 5 and so its value is 4; xl means that 10 is subtracted from 50 and so its value is 40.

4. A number of lesser value placed between numbers of higher value is read in connection with the number following it: xxix means 29, that is, "20" plus "1 subtracted from 10."

Problems

Write as small Roman numerals:

1. 8 __viii__

2. 4 __iv__

3. 16 __xvi__

4. 60 __lx__

5. 35 __xxxv__

6. 49 __il__

7. 75 __l__

8. 52 _____

9. 90 _____

10. 87 _____

Write as Arabic numbers:

1. iii _____

2. xx _____

3. xix _____

4. lx _____

5. iv _____

6. xvi _____

7. lxv _____

8. xiv _____

9. xxx _____

10. lxxxi _____

COMMON FRACTIONS

A common fraction is one or more aliquot parts of a unit or whole number. It is expressed by two numbers, the numerator above and the denominator below the line:

$$\frac{numerator}{denominator}$$

The denominator is the term of the fraction that shows the number of equal parts into which the unit is divided. The numerator is that term of the fraction which shows how many parts are taken.

Kinds of Fractions.   A *proper fraction* is one having a numerator less than the denominator, such as $\frac{1}{4}$, $\frac{2}{3}$.

An *improper fraction* is one having a numerator greater than the denominator, such as $\frac{6}{5}$, $\frac{3}{2}$.

A *complex fraction* is one whose numerator or denominator, or both, are fractions, such as:

$$\frac{\frac{1}{2}}{\frac{2}{3}} \quad or \quad \frac{\frac{2}{3}}{5}$$

A mixed number is composed of a whole number, or integer, and a fraction, such as $5\frac{1}{2}$, $4\frac{2}{3}$.

Changing an Improper Fraction to a Mixed Number.   To change an improper fraction to a mixed number, divide the numerator by the denominator and place the remainder over the denominator.

$$\frac{13}{5} = 5\overline{)\,\begin{matrix}2\\13\\-10\\\hline 3\end{matrix}} = 2\tfrac{3}{5}$$

Problems

Change improper fractions to mixed numbers:

1. $\frac{18}{5}$ _____
2. $\frac{89}{7}$ _____
3. $\frac{13}{6}$ _____
4. $\frac{21}{4}$ _____
5. $\frac{39}{4}$ _____

6. $\frac{7}{3}$ _____
7. $\frac{43}{5}$ _____
8. $\frac{60}{8}$ _____
9. $\frac{77}{5}$ _____
10. $\frac{11}{3}$ _____

Changing a Mixed Number to an Improper Fraction.   To change a mixed number to an improper fraction, multiply the denominator by the whole number and add to the numerator and place the sum over the denominator. $3\frac{1}{2} = \frac{7}{2}$.

$$3 \times 2 = 6$$
$$6 + 1 = 7$$

$$3\frac{1}{2} = \frac{7}{2}$$

Problems

Change mixed numbers to improper fractions:

1. $6\frac{1}{6}$ _____

2. $7\frac{9}{10}$ _____

3. $8\frac{1}{2}$ _____

4. $9\frac{1}{8}$ _____

5. $40\frac{2}{3}$ _____

6. $5\frac{3}{4}$ _____

7. $66\frac{2}{3}$ _____

8. $7\frac{3}{8}$ _____

9. $33\frac{1}{3}$ _____

10. $2\frac{5}{6}$ _____

Reduction of Fractions. Fractions are reduced to their lowest or simplest terms by dividing both the numerator and denominator by the greatest number that is contained in them evenly (greatest common divisor). When both the numerator and the denominator are divided by the same number, the value of the fraction does not change. Fractions are usually written in their lowest terms.

$$\frac{6}{12} = \frac{1}{2}$$

Problems

Reduce the following fractions to their lowest terms:

1. $\frac{12}{60}$ _____

2. $\frac{6}{15}$ _____

3. $\frac{27}{36}$ _____

4. $\frac{5}{25}$ _____

5. $\frac{4}{36}$ _____

6. $\frac{500}{2500}$ _____

7. $\frac{6}{16}$ _____

8. $\frac{12}{15}$ _____

9. $\frac{8}{32}$ _____

10. $\frac{5}{20}$ _____

Change the following fractions to higher terms:

1. $\frac{5}{8} =$ /48

2. $\frac{3}{4} =$ /24

3. $\frac{1}{3} =$ /9

4. $\frac{4}{5} =$ /15

5. $\frac{2}{3} =$ /12

6. $\frac{5}{7} =$ /35

7. $\frac{1}{2} =$ /20

8. $\frac{1}{5} =$ /30

9. $\frac{3}{4} =$ /8

10. $\frac{5}{6} =$ /36

Simplifying a Complex Fraction. To simplify a complex fraction, divide the numerator by the denominator.

$$\frac{\frac{3}{4}}{\frac{7}{8}} = \frac{3}{4} \div \frac{7}{8} = \frac{3}{4} \times \frac{8}{7} = \frac{24}{28} = \frac{6}{7}$$

$$\frac{\frac{1}{3}}{7} = \frac{1}{3} \div 7 = \frac{1 \times 1}{3 \times 7} = \frac{1}{21}$$

Problems

Simplify the following complex fractions:

1. $\dfrac{\frac{7}{9}}{\frac{3}{5}}$ _____

2. $\dfrac{\frac{3}{8}}{\frac{4}{7}}$ _____

3. $\dfrac{\frac{6}{7}}{\frac{2}{3}}$ _____

4. $\dfrac{\frac{5}{3}}{\frac{1}{9}}$ _____

5. $\dfrac{\frac{3}{4}}{\frac{1}{2}}$ _____

6. $\dfrac{\frac{5}{11}}{\frac{1}{10}}$ _____

7. $\dfrac{\frac{3}{16}}{\frac{5}{4}}$ _____

8. $\dfrac{\frac{1}{3}}{\frac{4}{25}}$ _____

9. $\dfrac{\frac{1}{8}}{\frac{1}{2}}$ _____

10. $\dfrac{\frac{9}{10}}{\frac{1}{4}}$ _____

Changing a Series of Fractions to Ones That Have the Same Denominator. Fractions may be multiplied or divided when their denominators are not alike; but before addition or subtraction, fractions must have the same denominator. Fractions having a common denominator may be combined in one fraction by adding the numerators.

Problems

Change the following fractions to ones which have the same denominator:

1. ½, ¼ _____

2. ¾, ⅛ _____

3. ⅔, 1/15 _____

4. ⅜, 5/16 _____

5. 2/7, 3/14 _____

6. ⅗, 4/10 _____

7. ⅘, 2/20 _____

8. ⅚, 4/12 _____

9. ½, ⅓ _____

10. ⅔, ⅗ _____

Least Common Denominator (LCD). The least common denominator (least common multiple of the denominators given) may usually be determined by inspection. If not, all the denominators are written in a row and divided by a number that will go evenly into two or more of them. The numbers that are not evenly divisible by that number are brought down to the second line with the quotients resulting from the possible even divisions, and the procedure is repeated with another divisor until there are no pairs of numbers evenly divisible by the same number.

To find the LCD of the following fractions:

$$\frac{5}{6},\ \frac{3}{4},\ \frac{1}{5},\ \frac{2}{3}$$

```
3)6  4  5  3
2)2  4  5  1
  1  2  5  1
```

multiply the divisors and divisible remainders, 3 × 2 × 2 × 5, to obtain the LCD, which is 60. To change each fraction to an equal fraction having the common denominator, divide the denominator into the LCD and multiply the original numerator and denominator by this quotient.

$$60 \div 6 = 10,\quad \frac{5}{6} \times \frac{10}{10} = \frac{50}{60};\quad 60 \div 4 = 15,\quad \frac{3}{4} \times \frac{15}{15} = \frac{45}{60}$$

$$60 \div 5 = 12,\quad \frac{1}{5} \times \frac{12}{12} = \frac{12}{60};\quad 60 \div 3 = 20,\quad \frac{2}{3} \times \frac{20}{20} = \frac{40}{60}$$

Therefore, the original fractions now have a common denominator and have become

$$\frac{50}{60},\ \frac{45}{60},\ \frac{12}{60},\ \frac{40}{60}$$

Problems

Convert these fractions to ones with LCD:

1. 1/3, 3/7, 4/5 ________
2. 5/9, 3/5, 2/3 ________
3. 1/8, 3/4, 3/7 ________
4. 1/6, 4/9, 3/8 ________
5. 2/5, 3/10, 2/3 ________
6. 2/6, 3/4, 4/5 ________
7. 1/2, 4/5, 2/3 ________
8. 4/8, 3/4, 5/6 ________
9. 4/7, 5/9, 2/5 ________
10. 3/4, 2/3, 3/9 ________

Addition of Fractions. Fractions must be converted to fractions with a common denominator before they can be added or subtracted. The sum of fractions having a common denominator is equal to the sum of the numerators over the common denominator.

$$\frac{50}{60} + \frac{45}{60} + \frac{12}{60} + \frac{40}{60} = \frac{147}{60} = 2^{27}\!/_{60} = 2^{9}\!/_{20}$$

Problems

Add the following fractions and reduce the resulting fractions to the lowest terms:

1. $\frac{1}{4} + \frac{5}{8} + \frac{3}{4} + \frac{4}{9}$ = _____ = _____

2. $\frac{4}{6} + \frac{1}{3} + \frac{3}{4} + \frac{7}{12}$ = _____ = _____

3. $\frac{3}{8} + \frac{4}{32} + \frac{2}{3} + \frac{1}{4}$ = _____ = _____

4. $\frac{3}{5} + \frac{4}{10} + \frac{3}{4} + \frac{1}{2}$ = _____ = _____

5. $\frac{2}{3} + \frac{5}{12} + \frac{7}{16} + \frac{3}{4}$ = _____ = _____

6. $\frac{5}{6} + \frac{3}{5} + \frac{3}{4} + \frac{6}{15}$ = _____ = _____

Subtraction of Fractions.   The difference between two fractions having a common denominator is equal to the difference between the numerators over the common denominator.

$$\frac{2}{3} - \frac{1}{6} = \frac{4}{6} - \frac{1}{6} = \frac{3}{6} = \frac{1}{2}$$

Problems

Subtract the following fractions and reduce the resulting fractions to the lowest terms:

1. $\frac{7}{8} - \frac{2}{3}$ = _____   4. $\frac{5}{8} - \frac{1}{12}$ = _____

2. $\frac{4}{25} - \frac{2}{50}$ = _____   5. $\frac{5}{7} - \frac{1}{5}$ = _____

3. $\frac{3}{4} - \frac{1}{3}$ = _____   6. $\frac{13}{16} - \frac{4}{32}$ = _____

Multiplication of Fractions.   To multiply a fraction by a whole number, multiply the numerator by the whole number and place the product over the denominator. Convert the fraction obtained to a whole or mixed number.

$$4 \times \frac{3}{8} = \frac{4 \times 3}{8} = \frac{12}{8} = 1\frac{1}{8} = 1\frac{1}{2}$$

To multiply a fraction by another fraction, multiply the numerators and place their product over the product obtained by multiplying the denominators. Reduce the fraction to its lowest terms.

$$\frac{5}{6} \times \frac{3}{4} = \frac{15}{24} = \frac{5}{8}$$

Problems

Multiply the following fractions and reduce the resulting fractions to the lowest terms:

1. $\frac{2}{3} \times \frac{7}{8} =$ __________ 4. $6 \times \frac{7}{8} =$ __________

2. $\frac{3}{7} \times 4 =$ __________ 5. $\frac{8}{9} \times \frac{4}{6} =$ __________

3. $\frac{3}{4} \times \frac{2}{3} =$ __________ 6. $\frac{1}{5} \times \frac{5}{6} =$ __________

Division of Fractions. To divide a whole number by a fraction or a fraction by another fraction or a fraction by a whole number, invert the terms of the divisor and then multiply.

$$4 \div \frac{5}{6} = 4 \times \frac{6}{5} = \frac{24}{5} = 4\tfrac{4}{5}$$

$$\frac{2}{3} \div \frac{1}{2} = \frac{2}{3} \times \frac{2}{1} = \frac{4}{3} = 1\tfrac{1}{3}$$

$$\frac{5}{6} \div 4 = \frac{5}{6} \times \frac{1}{4} = \frac{5}{24}$$

Problems

Divide the following fractions and reduce the resulting fractions to the lowest terms:

1. $\frac{2}{3} \div 6 =$ __________ 4. $\frac{3}{8} \div \frac{1}{64} =$ __________

2. $\frac{3}{4} \div \frac{2}{9} =$ __________ 5. $\frac{1}{2} \div \frac{1}{3} =$ __________

3. $\frac{1}{3} \div \frac{2}{5} =$ __________ 6. $\frac{3}{4} \div 7 =$ __________

Decimal Fractions

A decimal fraction is a simple fraction whose denominator is some power of ten. The denominator is not written, but a dot (the decimal point) is placed before the numerator, and the denominator is indicated by the number of digits after the decimal point. One digit after the decimal means a denominator of 10. Thus, $\frac{4}{10}$ is written .4, or 0.4. Two digits indicate a denominator of 100, as $\frac{9}{100}$, or 0.09. Three digits shows thousandths, as $\frac{126}{1000}$, or 0.126, etc.

Decimal Fractions	*Common Fractions*
0.1	$\frac{1}{10}$
0.01	$\frac{1}{100}$

$$0.001 \qquad\qquad \frac{1}{1000}$$

$$0.0001 \qquad\qquad \frac{1}{10,000}$$

Reading and Writing Decimals.   Mixed decimals contain whole numbers and decimal fractions, such as 436.78 and 35.7. Reading from the left from a decimal point, the first digit is a simple integer, the value of the second is multipled by ten, the third by one hundred, etc. One hundred twenty-six is written 126. Reading to the right decreases the values in the same progression, as shown in the above table. One hundred twenty-six and $\frac{3}{10}$ is 126.3; one hundred twenty-six and $\frac{34}{100}$ is 126.34.

Problems

Write in words the following decimal fractions:

1. 0.06 ——————   4. 12.598 ——————

2. 0.004 ——————   5. 318.07 ——————

3. 0.064 ——————   6. 0.0162 ——————

Addition of Decimal Fractions.   The numbers are written so that the decimal points are directly under each other. They are then added as whole numbers and the decimal point in the sum is placed under the other decimal points.

$$
\begin{array}{r}
5.69 \\
10.004 \\
+1106.542 \\
\hline
1122.236
\end{array}
$$

Problems

Add the following decimal fractions:

1. 327.94, 8262.34, 287.05, 417.43
2. 7.20, 9.736, 12.895, 0.25
3. 0.064, 0.001, 0.0002
4. 17.756, 9.0623, 0.987, 0.0062
5. 204.125, 14.321, 98.346, 452.06

Multiplication of Decimals.   Decimal fractions are multiplied in the same manner as two whole numbers, but the product must have the same number of decimal places as the decimal fraction multiplied. Decimal places are counted from right to left.

$$\begin{array}{r} 275 \\ \times\,0.03 \\ \hline 8.25 \end{array}$$

A decimal fraction can be multipled by 10, 100, 1000, etc., by moving the decimal point as many places to the right as there are zeros in the multiplier.

Decimals are multipled by each other in the same manner as whole numbers, but the product must contain as many decimal places as the sum of the decimal places in the two numbers multipled.

$$\begin{array}{rl} 9.756 & \text{3 decimal places} \\ \times\quad 0.8 & \text{1 decimal place} \\ \hline 7.8048 & \text{4 decimal places} \end{array}$$

Problems

Multiply the following decimal fractions:

1. 234.43 × 0.256 = _____   4. 0.7 × 0.008   = _____

2. 12.42 × 213.89 = _____   5. 0.5 × 0.4   = _____

3. 0.5 × 0.016   = _____   6. 1.75 × 0.005 = _____

Division of Decimal Fractions.   Decimal fractions are divided by one another in the same manner as whole numbers, but the number of decimal places in the dividend must equal or exceed the number in the divisor. If the dividend does not have enough decimal places, zeros can be added as final figures beyond the decimal point without changing the value of the dividend. After the division, the number of decimal places in the divisor is subtracted from the number in the dividend, and the difference is the number of decimal points to be pointed off in the quotient. Thus, to divide 595.4 by 0.26 we have:

$$\begin{array}{r} 2290 \\ \hline 0.26\,)\,595.40 \end{array}$$ with no decimal in the quotient

Another example is:

$$\begin{array}{r} 36.4 \\ \hline 0.2\,)\,7.28 \end{array}$$

A number may be divided by 10, 100, 1000, etc., by moving the decimal point as many places to the left as there are zeros in the divisor.

$$1 \div 10 = 0.1; \quad 1 \div 100 = 0.01; \quad 1 \div 1000 = 0.001$$

Problems

Divide the following decimal fractions:

1. 21 by 0.025
2. 639.028 by 98.312
3. 25.95 by 3.46
4. 16.15 by 4.25
5. 67 by 32.524
6. 3002 by 75.05

Divide the following numbers by each of the following—0.1, 0.01, 10, 100:

7. 16.14
8. 50.65
9. 963.456
10. 0.568

Converting Common Fractions to Decimal Fractions. To convert a common fraction into a decimal fraction, divide the numerator of the fraction by the denominator:

$$\frac{1}{4} \text{ means } 1 \div 4 \text{ or } 4\overline{)1.00}^{\,0.25}; \text{ may be written } 0.25$$

To convert a decimal fraction into a common fraction, drop the decimal point and write the denominator in the proper multiple of 10.

$$0.5 = \frac{5}{10} = \frac{1}{2}, \quad 0.05 = \frac{5}{100} = \frac{1}{20}$$

Problems

Convert the following common fractions to decimal fractions:

1. ¾
2. ⅟₂₅
3. ⅚

4. ⅜
5. ⁹⁄₁₇
6. ⁵⁄₂₂

Convert the following decimal fractions to common fractions:

1. 0.50
2. 0.45
3. 0.2045

4. 0.75
5. 0.04
6. 0.00654

PERCENTAGE AND RATIO

Percentage and ratio are other terms for expressing parts of a unit.

Percentage.   Percentage means "parts in 100." The term "per cent" is generally indicated by the symbol %. A 5% solution of a drug means that $\frac{5}{100}$, or 0.05, of the total amount of the solution is drug. Since strengths of solutions used in preparing drugs are expressed sometimes as per cent and sometimes as a ratio, it is essential for the nurse to know how to change per cent to ratio and ratio to per cent, to change per cent to decimal and common fractions, and to determine any required percentage of any number.

Ratio.   Ratio is another method of expressing fractions, decimals, and percentage. It is the quotient of one number divided by the other. The ratio of 1 to 4 may be written 1:4, $\frac{1}{4}$, 0.25, or 25%. They all mean the same; i.e., for every 1 part of drug there are 4 parts of solution. The numbers 1 and 4 are the terms of the ratio. The first term of a true ratio is always 1.

Rules for Making Conversions.   (1) To change ratio to per cent, make the first term of the ratio the numerator of a fraction, make the second term of the ratio the denominator. Divide the numerator by the denominator, and multiply by 100.

$$1:4 = \frac{1}{4} \times 100 = 25\%$$

2. To change per cent to a ratio, change the per cent to a fraction and reduce to its lowest terms. The numerator of the fraction is the first term of the ratio and the denominator is the second term.

$$50\% = \frac{50}{100} = \frac{1}{2} = 1:2$$

3. To change per cent to a decimal fraction, drop the per cent sign and express decimally as hundredths.

$$2\% \text{ becomes } 0.02 \text{ and } 10\% \text{ becomes } 0.10, \text{ or } 0.1$$

4. To change per cent to a common fraction, drop the per cent sign and put the number over 100 to make the fraction.

$$5\% \text{ becomes } \frac{5}{100}$$

5. To change a decimal fraction to per cent, multiply by 100 and write as a whole number with the per cent sign.

$$0.5 \times 100 = 50\%$$

6. To change a decimal fraction to a ratio, write the decimal as a common fraction. Then the numerator of the fraction will be the first term and the denominator of the fraction will be the second term.

$$0.5 \text{ becomes } \frac{5}{10} \text{ and the ratio } 5:10, \text{ or } 1:2$$

7. To change a common fraction to per cent, divide the numerator by the denominator and multiply the resulting decimal by 100.

$$\frac{1}{25} = 0.04, \quad 0.04 \times 100 = 4\%$$

8. To find a certain per cent of any number, multiply the number by the per cent expressed as a common or as a decimal fraction.

$$5\% \text{ of } 200 = 200 \times \frac{5}{100} = 10 \text{ or } 200 \times 0.05 = 10$$

9. To determine what per cent any amount is of a larger amount, divide the smaller number by the larger number and multiply the quotient by 100.

Problems

Change the following ratios to per cent:

1. 1:1000
2. 3:5
3. 1:500

4. 8:250
5. 1:20
6. 1:2

Change the following percentages to ratio, decimal fractions, and common fractions:

	Ratio	Decimal Fractions	Common Fractions
1. 45%	_____	_____	_____
2. ½%	_____	_____	_____
3. 2%	_____	_____	_____
4. 67%	_____	_____	_____
5. 33⅛%	_____	_____	_____
6. 75%	_____	_____	_____
7. ¾%	_____	_____	_____
8. 89%	_____	_____	_____
9. ⅛%	_____	_____	_____
10. 68%	_____	_____	_____

Change the following decimal fractions to per cent and ratio:

1. 0.3 _____ _____
2. 0.75 _____ _____
3. 0.532 _____ _____

4. 0.413 _____ _____
5. 0.8 _____ _____
6. 0.5 _____ _____

Change the following common fractions to per cent:

1. ⅞ _____   4. ⅔ _____

2. ⅖ _____   5. ⁵⁄₁₂ _____

3. ¾ _____   6. ⁷⁄₁₅ _____

Find a given per cent of the following numbers:

1. 5% of 650 _____   4. 0.1% of 2000 _____

2. ¼% of 25 _____   5. 1⅔% of 216 _____

3. 10% of 3500 _____   6. 12½% of 400 _____

What per cent of:

1. 75 is 15 _____   4. 9 is 3 _____
2. 40 is 2 _____   5. 18 is 9 _____
3. 1.5 is 0.5 _____   6. 60 is 12 _____

PROPORTION

A proportion is an expression of the equality between two ratios: 1 is to 4 as 5 is to 20, or 1:4::5:20. It may also be written as an equation between equal fractions: ¼ = ⁵⁄₂₀. The first and last terms are called the extremes; the second and third terms are the means. In any proportion the product of the means equals the product of the extremes.

$$1:4::5:20 \qquad 1 \times 20 = 4 \times 5$$

When one of the extremes in a proportion is not known, it can be found by multiplying the two means and dividing this product by the known extreme. Similarly if a mean is not known, it can be determined by multiplying the extremes and dividing by the known mean. The unknown factor is usually designated as x.

$$1:4::5:x \qquad\qquad 1:4::x:20$$
$$x = 20 \qquad\qquad 4x = 20$$
$$x = 5$$

Most of the problems in solutions and dosage involve finding the third term of a proportion.

Problems

Find the value of x:

Substitute the value of x in the proportion to check your answer:

1. 0.75:100::x:1000

2. $\dfrac{1/4}{1/6} = \dfrac{x}{1}$

3. 8:4::x:9

4. 30:x::10:15

5. 0.1:10::x:3

SHORT CUTS

The use of short cuts in arithmetical procedures increases both speed and accuracy in mental calculations. A short cut to find the third term of a proportion is to express the first and second terms as a common fraction and multiply by the fourth term. From this the following formula may be derived:

$$\underset{\substack{\text{Have per cent or ratio} \\ \text{(2nd term)}}}{\overset{\substack{\text{(1st term)} \\ \text{Desired per cent or ratio}}}{\frac{\rule{0pt}{0pt}}{\rule{0pt}{0pt}}}} \times \underset{\text{(4th term)}}{\text{Quantity of solution}} = \underset{\text{(3rd term, } x)}{\text{Quantity of drug}}$$

$$1:200::x:2000$$

$$200x = 2000$$

$$x = 10$$

or

$$\frac{D}{H} \times Q = q(x)$$

$$\tfrac{1}{200} \times 2000 = 10$$

Proof: $1 \times 2000 = 2000$ $200 \times 10 = 2000$

WEIGHTS AND MEASURES

In the United States there are two systems for weighing and measuring drugs, the metric and the apothecaries' systems. Although the metric system is used almost exclusively in countries abroad, in the United States it has not yet entirely replaced the apothecaries' system. It is, however, the official system of the present *United States Pharmacopeia, British Pharmacopoeia, Pharmacopoea Internationalis,* and *National Formulary,* and it is also used in *New and Nonofficial Drugs.* Since at the present time the two systems are used interchangeably in the United States in many hospitals and by many physicians for writing prescriptions and orders for medicines, it is imperative for the nurse to be able to convert measurements from one sytem to the other rapidly and accurately.

THE METRIC SYSTEM

Our daily living finds us constantly using a decimal system of calculating as we handle our money. This is the basic advantage of the metric system, for it, too, is a decimal system for measuring length, capacity, and weight. The unit of length is the meter. The unit of capacity is the liter. The weight unit is the gram. Prefixes of Greek origin indicate multiples of the basic units as follows: *deca* multiplies the unit by 10, *hecto* by 100, *kilo* by 1000. Fractions of the units are indicated by the following prefixes from the Latin: *deci* divides by 10, *centi* by 100, and *milli* by 1000.

—————————————————— Table 1 ——————————————————

Decimal System	Thou-sands	Hun-dreds	Tens	Units	One Tenth	One Hun-dredth	One Thou-sandth
Metric System	Kilo-1000.0	Hecto-100.0	Deca-10.0	Meter Liter Gram	Deci-0.1	Centi-0.01	Milli-0.001

In the metric system of measurement, the *meter* is the basic unit from which the other measurements were derived. It is longer than a *yard*, measuring about 39.37 in. It is divided into 100 parts and gives us the convenient length the centimeter. This is abbreviated to cm. and is less than ½ in. (1 in. equals 2.5 cm.).

Liquids in this system are measured by the *liter* (abbreviated L.), which is approximately 2 pt. or 1 qt. A very frequently used measure in medicine is the *milliliter* (abbreviated ml.), which is one thousandth of a liter. A milliliter is the approximate equivalent of a *cubic centimeter* (abbreviated cc.); however, it should be noted that it is the general practice of pharmacopeias throughout the world to use the milliliter rather than the cubic centimeter.

Weights in this system are based upon the *gram* (abbreviated Gm.) as the fundamental unit. This is the weight of 1 ml. of water at a temperature of 4° C. For medical purposes, no differentiation between this temperature and room temperature is necessary. A milliliter of other liquids, such as alcohol and ether, will weigh less than 1 Gm. because they are lighter than water. A very frequently used measure in medicine is the *milligram* (abbreviated mg.), one thousandth of a gram. Some drugs are so potent that their doses are of the order of 0.1 mg. to 50 mg. Such quantities are so small that inert filler powders are used in manufacturing tablets or capsules containing doses of this size. Thus, a tablet labeled as containing 0.1 mg. or another containing 25 mg. of a certain drug may contain up to 300 mg. of an inert material to make it the size of an aspirin tablet. It may have considerably less filler and be only one tenth of that size, as in the case of tablets to be dissolved and administered by syringe and needle.

The milligram and the gram are the only weight units in the metric system that are used in drug dispensing. In some rarer cases, a millionth of a gram (one thousandth of a milligram) is used. This fraction is called the microgram (abbreviated mcg.), or gamma. The kilogram (abbreviated kg.), 1000 Gm., is often used in recording the weights of patients.

Problems

Convert liters to milliliters:

3.75 liters ——————

2.46 liters ——————

0.35 liters ——————

Convert grams to milligrams:

0.350 Gm. ——————

0.0015 Gm. ——————

0.060 Gm. ——————

0.001 Gm. ——————

0.0003 Gm. ——————

Convert milliliters to liters:

1753 ml. ——————

8736 ml. ——————

1500 ml. ——————

Convert milligrams to grams:

30   mg. ——————

500   mg. ——————

0.4   mg. ——————

0.05 mg. ——————

2   mg. ——————

THE APOTHECARIES' SYSTEM

The unit of weight in this ancient system is the *grain*. It has no fundamental relationship to any other constant, as does the meter of the metric system, which originated as one ten-millionth of the distance from the equator to the pole. It came into use purely on some arbitrary basis. When compared to the far more satisfactory metric system, one finds that 1 grain weighs about 65 mg. Many drugs are ordered in fractions of a grain (e.g., ⅙ grain of morphine sulfate) or in several grains (e.g., 10 grains of aspirin). While all such doses can be ordered in the metric system, using the same tablets, the older system, so long associated with the older drugs, will continue to be employed for some time to come. Hence it is necessary to learn both systems, and, what is somewhat more difficult, one must know how to convert a number in one system to an equivalent in the other. Conversion is nearly always from the old to the new system. Much reviewing from time to time is necessary in developing this ability. Familiarity with the tables that follow should be acquired.

Two other weight units in this system are the *dram* (ℨ), equal to 60 grains, and the *ounce* (℥), or 480 grains (8 drams, or 28.35 Gm.). All may apply to dry materials.

Liquids are measured in this system in *minims* (roughly "drop-sized"), *drams, ounces,* and *pints*. More specifically, one may state fluid drams and fluid ounces to distinguish liquid from solid measurements. No misunderstanding is to be expected in dropping the designation "fluid" because the name of the material ordered generally denotes whether it is fluid or solid. Many physicians delete the term "fluid." Hence it is incumbent upon the nurse to use the correct measuring device. This will be a graduated vessel, a syringe, or a teaspoon or tablespoon, as the case may be.

CONVERSION OF OTHER DENOMINATIONS IN THE SAME SYSTEM

There are no intermediate units of weight between milligrams and grams in the metric system. The weight of a substance in this system may be expressed in grams, decimal fractions of grams, milligrams, or decimal fractions of milligrams. Remembering always that 1 Gm. contains 1000 mg., it is easy to change grams to milligrams by multiplying the number of grams by 1000. To change milligrams to grams, divide the number of milligrams by 1000. The same applies to units of volume in this system. There are no intermediate units of volume between the liter and the milliliter. To change liters to milliliters, multiply the number of liters by 1000. To change milliliters to liters, divide the number of milliliters by 1000. One liter may be expressed as a unit (1 liter), but it is more frequently expressed in milliliters (1000 ml.). Units larger than 1 liter or fractions of a liter are also expressed in milliliters; for example, 1500 ml., 2500 ml., 800 ml., or 300 ml.

In the apothecaries' system it is often necessary to convert the units on hand to comparable units that may be readily calculated, measured, and dispensed. Therefore, one must know how many smaller units are contained in the larger units, and vice versa, to convert from one unit to another. It is more practical to weigh solids or measure liquids in the highest possible denomination in this system.

Table 2 may be used for converting units in the apothecaries' system.

Table 2

Weights

60 grains = 1 dram
480 grains, or 8 drams = 1 ounce

Volume

60 minims = 1 fluid dram (℥)
480 minims, or 8 fluid drams = 1 fluid ounce (℥)
7680 minims, or 16 fluid ounces = 1 pint (O)
2 pints = 1 quart

In changing a lower denomination to a higher one, the lower denomination is divided by the number of units in the highest denomination. Thus grains or drams may be converted to ounces, while minims, drams, or ounces may be changed to comparable larger units by division. To convert from a higher denomination to a lower, the number is multiplied by the number of smaller units contained in 1 unit of the higher denomination. Thus ounces may be converted into smaller units such as drams or grains, while pints may be converted to smaller units such as ounces, drams, or minims by multiplication. In solving problems or calculating dosages, one cannot compare grains with ounces or minims with pints, because both terms of a ratio must be in the same category.

Before measuring 330 minims, it should be converted to the highest denomination possible. Since 330 minims is less than 1 ounce, a dram is the highest possible denomination. There are 60 minims in 1 dram; therefore,

$$\frac{330}{60} = 5\frac{1}{2} \text{ drams, or 5 drams and 30 minims}$$

The highest denomination contained in 560 grains is 1 ounce, or 480 grains; therefore,

$$\frac{560}{480} = 1 \text{ ounce and 80 grains}$$

There are 60 grains in 1 dram; therefore,

$$\frac{80}{60} = 1 \text{ dram and 20 grains}$$

Therefore, 560 grains = 1 ounce, 1 dram, and 20 grains.

Problems

Convert to higher denominations:

430 minims —————   —————
16 drams   —————   —————
18 ounces   —————   —————

Convert to lower denominations:

6 fluid drams   —————
5½ fluid ounces —————
2 pints   —————
1½ quarts   —————

CONVERTING UNITS FROM ONE SYSTEM TO ANOTHER

Because of their complexity, exact metric equivalents of units in the apothecaries' system are not used by the nurse or even by the physician in writing prescriptions. Indeed, the exact equivalents are used only by the pharmacist in compounding prescriptions or in converting a pharmaceutical formula. The reason is evidenced by a brief comparison of the exact equivalents. One gram in the metric system equals 15.432 grains in the apothecaries' system; or 1 grain is equal to 0.0648 Gm. (64.8 mg.); 15.43 minims equal 1 ml. and 0.0616 ml. equals 1 minim.

Approximate equivalents are provided as a convenience to physicians in prescribing, and these are used by the nurse for conversion from one system

Table 3

Metric Doses with Approximate Apothecary Equivalents*

Metric	Approximate Apothecary Equivalents	Metric	Approximate Apothecary Equivalents
LIQUID MEASURE		**LIQUID MEASURE**	
1000 ml.†	1 quart	3 ml.	45 minims
750 ml.	1½ pints	2 ml.	30 minims
500 ml.	1 pint	1 ml.	15 minims
250 ml.	8 fluid ounces	0.75 ml.	12 minims
200 ml.	7 fluid ounces	0.6 ml.	10 minims
100 ml.	3½ fluid ounces	0.5 ml.	8 minims
50 ml.	1¾ fluid ounces	0.3 ml.	5 minims
30 ml.	1 fluid ounce	0.25 ml.	4 minims
15 ml.	4 fluid drams	0.2 ml.	3 minims
10 ml.	2½ fluid drams	0.1 ml.	1½ minims
8 ml.	2 fluid drams	0.06 ml.	1 minim
5 ml.	1¼ fluid drams	0.05 ml.	¾ minim
4 ml.	1 fluid dram	0.03 ml.	½ minim
WEIGHT		**WEIGHT**	
30 Gm.	1 ounce	30 mg.	½ grain
15 Gm.	4 drams	25 mg.	⅜ grain
10 Gm.	2½ drams	20 mg.	⅓ grain
7.5 Gm.	2 drams	15 mg.	¼ grain
6 Gm.	90 grains	12 mg.	⅕ grain
5 Gm.	75 grains	10 mg.	⅙ grain
4 Gm.	60 grains (1 dram)	8 mg.	⅛ grain
3 Gm.	45 grains	6 mg.	⅒ grain
2 Gm.	30 grains	5 mg.	1/12 grain
1.5 Gm.	22 grains	4 mg.	1/15 grain
1 Gm.	15 grains	3 mg.	1/20 grain
0.75 Gm.	12 grains	2 mg.	1/30 grain
0.6 Gm.	10 grains	1.5 mg.	1/40 grain
0.5 Gm.	7½ grains	1.2 mg.	1/50 grain
0.4 Gm.	6 grains	1 mg.	1/60 grain
0.3 Gm.	5 grains	0.8 mg.	1/80 grain
0.25 Gm.	4 grains	0.6 mg.	1/100 grain
0.2 Gm.	3 grains	0.5 mg.	1/120 grain
0.15 Gm.	2½ grains	0.4 mg.	1/150 grain
0.12 Gm.	2 grains	0.3 mg.	1/200 grain
0.1 Gm.	1½ grains	0.25 mg.	1/250 grain
75 mg.	1¼ grains	0.2 mg.	1/300 grain
60 mg.	1 grain	0.15 mg.	1/400 grain
50 mg.	¾ grain	0.12 mg.	1/500 grain
40 mg.	⅔ grain	0.1 mg.	1/600 grain

* Reprinted from U.S.P. XVI.

† A milliliter (ml.) is the approximate equivalent of a cubic centimeter (cc.).

to the other in preparing solutions and calculating dosage. These simplified equivalents, which are much easier to learn and to manipulate, have been adopted by the *United States Pharmacopeia,* the *National Formulary,* and *New and Non official Drugs* and therefore have the approval of the Federal Food and Drug Administration. These equivalents are given in Table 3.

It is always good practice to refer to tables of equivalents when calculating dosage, but it is also desirable to remember certain equivalents to be able to convert doses from one system to the other without reference to tables.

Table 4

Metric Weights with Approximate Apothecary Equivalents

Weight

1	Gm.	15 grains
0.06	Gm.	1 grain
4	Gm.	1 dram
30	Gm.	1 ounce

Volume

1	ml.	15 minims
0.06	ml.	1 minim
4	ml.	1 fluid dram
30	ml.	1 fluid ounce
500	ml.	1 pint
1000	ml.	1 quart

Rules for Conversion Using the Above Equivalents. (1) To convert grams to grains or milliliters to minims, multiply the number of grams or milliliters by 15 or divide by 0.06.

2. To convert grains to grams or minims to milliliters, multiply the number of grains or minims by 0.06 or divide by 15.

3. To convert grams to ounces or milliliters to fluid ounces, divide the number of grams or ounces by 30.

4. To convert ounces to grams or fluid ounces to milliliters, multiply the number of grams or fluid ounces by 30.

Problems

Convert the following metric quantities to their apothecaries' equivalents:

1. 500 ml. _____

2. 30 ml. _____

3. 4 ml. _____

4. 0.06 ml. _____

5. 0.1 ml. _____

6. 40 mg. _____

7. 2 mg. _____

8. 15 Gm. _____

9. 0.3 Gm. _____

10. 0.4 mg. _____

Convert the following apothecaries' quantities to their metric equivalents:

1. 1 quart _____   6. 75 grains _____

2. 7 fluid ounces _____   7. 10 grains _____

3. 2½ fluid drams _____   8. 2½ grains _____

4. 12 minims _____   9. 1/150 grain _____

5. ½ minim _____   10. 1/400 grain _____

Conversion Problems

1. A bottle contains 5-gr. tablets of aspirin. How many tablets are needed to give 600 mg. of the drug?

2. How many tablets are necessary to dispense 20 mg. of morphine sulfate from a bottle of ⅙-gr. tablets of the drug?

3. Dispense gr. 1/150 from a bottle of glyceryl trinitrate 0.4-mg. tablets.

4. Prepare 1 pt. of a 1:5000 solution. How many grams are necessary?

HOUSEHOLD MEASURES

It is sometimes necessary to use household measures that approximate apothecaries' and metric measures. Teaspoons, tablespoons, and cups vary so in size that their use for measuring medications should be avoided except in cases of necessity. Teaspoons ordinarily available in the home today contain approximately 5 ml.; consequently, for practical purposes the teaspoon may be regarded as representing 5 ml. In this case there would be 3 teaspoonfuls in each tablespoon.

═══════════════════ **Table 5** ═══════════════════

| | **Approximate Household Equivalents** | |
Household Measures	*Apothecaries' Units*	*Metric Units*
1 teaspoonful (tsp.)	1 fluid dram (60 minims)	4 ml. (5 ml.)
1 dessertspoonful	2 fluid drams	8 ml.
1 tablespoonful (tbsp.)	4 fluid drams	16 ml. (15 ml.)
2 tablespoonfuls	1 fluid ounce	30 ml.
1 teacupful	6 fluid ounces	180 ml.
1 glassful	8 fluid ounces	240 ml.

For more accurate measurements, 1-ounce measuring glasses and 1-dram minim glasses are available for hospital use. The ounce glasses are graduated in teaspoonfuls, dessertspoonfuls, tablespoonfuls, and in 5, 10, 15, 20, 25, and 30 ml. The minim glasses are graduated in units of 5 minims.

Problems

Convert the following quantities to household equivalents:

6 fluid ounces _____   5 ml.   _____

30 ml.   _____   240 ml.   _____

2 fluid drams   _____

PREPARATION OF SOLUTIONS

The strength or concentration of a solution is expressed by percentage or by ratio. Solutions are prepared by three methods.

1. Per cent weight in weight (W/W) expresses the grams of drug (solute) in 100 Gm. of solution (solvent).

2. Per cent weight in volume (W/V) expresses the grams of drugs in 100 ml. of solution.

3. Per cent volume in volume (V/V) expresses the milliliters of drug in 100 ml. of solution.

The percentage or ratio expresses the quantity of drug in relation to the total quantity of solution. Therefore, solutions are made by placing a known weight of drug or a measured amount of solution in a graduated container and adding sufficient water or other liquid to bring the total volume to the desired amount.

Solutions are made from (1) full-strength drugs, (2) tablets, or (3) stock solutions.

1. **Full-Strength Drugs** (often referred to as pure drugs.). These may be in solid or liquid form and are 100 per cent in strength unless otherwise stated.

a. *Powders or Crystalline Substances* (such as sodium chloride, boric acid, or sodium bicarbonate). The nurse often measures rather than weighs such solid drugs. Thus sodium chloride (table salt) may be measured in a teaspoon or graduate when preparing a solution to be used as a gargle.

Antibiotics, such as penicillin, streptomycin, erythromycin, etc., are marketed in weighed amounts in vials. The drug may be dissolved by injecting into the vial a sterile isotonic salt solution, 5 per cent dextrose, or water for injection. The desired dose is withdrawn into a syringe and the unused portion of the solution in the vial should be labeled as to dilution and stored in the refrigerator for later use.

b. *Liquids.* Alcohol that contains 5 per cent water is often classified as a full-strength drug.

2. **Tablets.** These contain a definite quantity of drug.

3. **Stock Solutions.** These are relatively strong solutions from which weaker solutions are made. The strength of these solutions may be expressed

as a percentage or as a ratio. Various dilutions may be made rapidly without weighing the full-strength drug. Many of the new drugs are marketed in concentrated solutions in vials or ampuls and must be diluted before administration to the patient. Examples: Levarterenol Bitartrate Injection, U.S.P.; Succinylcholine Chloride Injection, U.S.P.

ARITHMETIC OF DOSAGE AND SOLUTIONS

Most problems in preparing solutions and calculating dosage are solved by proportion, in which three factors are known. The unknown factor is represented by x. The following rules should be observed in setting up a proportion:

1. Both terms in a ratio must be expressed in the units of measurement.

a. The strength of the desired solution and the strength of the drug used must both be expressed as either per cent or ratio (e.g., 2%:4%, or 1:2). It is easy to convert from per cent to ratio or ratio to per cent (see p. 42).

b. Both the amount of drug to be used and the total amount of solution must be expressed in either the metric or the apothecaries' system.

c. Units of measurement must be expressed in equivalent terms, i.e., grams and milliliters, or grains and minims, etc. Liters, quarts, and pints must be changed to smaller units. Liters are always changed to milliliters. Quarts and pints may be converted to ounces, drams, or minims, depending upon the quantity of drug.

2. The terms in each ratio should be in the same order of value, i.e., small:large: :small:large (e.g., 2:4: :6:12, or 4:2: :12:6).

3. Each term should be labeled as per cent, grams and milliters, or grains and minims, as the case may be (e.g., 5%:100%: :x Gm.:500 ml.).

After the calculations are made, the answer should be proved by substituting the answer for x and multiplying the means and the extremes. If the product of the means equals the product of the extremes, the answer is correct.

A short-cut method may be employed by using the formula

$$\frac{D}{H} \times Q = q \quad \text{(see p. 45)}.$$

In solving problems involving dosage and the preparation of solutions, a variation of not more than 10 per cent in dosage is permitted. The answer may contain a fraction or whole number that is not practical to measure. It is then common practice to round off that quantity if it can be done without changing the amount of drug more than 10 per cent. By "rounding off a quantity" we mean *adding to* or *subtracting from* the answer enough to obtain a resultant quantity that can be conveniently measured with the equipment available.

It is therefore necessary to determine whether the amount you wish to add or subtract is, in fact, less than 10 per cent of the number you wish to round off. The simplest way to do this is to calculate 10 per cent of the number and then compare that quantity with the amount you wish to add or subtract. If the number is a fraction or mixed number, it should be converted to a decimal fraction. Then 10 per cent can be found by moving the decimal point one place to the left.

Examples

1. The number in the answer is 22.

    Can you round off to 20 or 25?
    10 per cent of 22 is 2.2.
    To round off to 20 it is necessary to subtract 2.   2 is less than 2.2, so 22 may be rounded off to 20.
    To round off to 25 it is necessary to add 3.   3 is more than 2.2, so 22 may not be rounded off to 25.

2. The number in the answer is 12¾.

    Convert to a decimal fraction 12.75.
    10 per cent of 12.75 is 1.275.
    0.75 is less than 1.275, so the fraction can be dropped.

3. The number in the answer is 4.8.

    10 per cent of 4.8 is 0.48.
    The fraction 0.8 is more than 0.48, so the fraction cannot be dropped; but 0.2, which is less than 0.8, may be added to make 5.

Preparing Solutions from Full-Strength Drugs

Problem.   To find the quantity of drug required to make a desired amount of solution. Convert the terms or measurements as necessary and set up a proportion. Since the quantity of drug is not known, it is represented by x.

1. To prepare 500 ml. of a 5 per cent solution of boric acid.

$$\left(\begin{array}{c} \text{Desired} \\ \text{strength} \end{array} \right) : \text{available strength} :: \text{quantity of drug} : \left(\begin{array}{c} \text{quantity of} \\ \text{solution} \end{array} \right)$$

$$5\% : 100\% \qquad\qquad :: x \text{ Gm.} \qquad\qquad : 500 \text{ ml.}$$

$$100\,x = 2500 \text{ Gm.}$$

$$x = 25 \text{ Gm.}$$

or

$$\frac{\text{Desired strength}}{\text{Available strength}} = \frac{\text{quantity of drug } (x)}{\text{quantity of solution}}$$

$$\frac{5}{100} = \frac{\text{quantity of drug } (x)}{500 \text{ ml.}}$$

$$5 \times \frac{1}{100} \times 500 = 25 \text{ Gm.}$$

or, using the formula,

$$\frac{D}{H} \times Q = q$$

$$\frac{5}{100} \times 500 = 25 \text{ Gm.}$$

a. 25 Gm. plus sufficient water to make 500 ml. are required.
b. Place 25 Gm. of boric acid in a 500-ml. graduate; add water to 500 ml.
c. To prove: multiply the means and extremes of the equation.
d. If the two products are equal, the solution is correct.

$$5 \times 500 \text{ ml.} = 2500 \qquad 25 \text{ Gm.} \times 100 = 2500$$

2. To prepare 8 ounces of a 25 per cent solution of glycerin.
   a. Convert 8 ounces to 250 ml.

$$25\% : 100\% :: x \text{ ml.} : 250 \text{ ml.}$$
$$100 \ x = 6250$$
$$x = 62.50$$

or

$$\frac{25}{100} \times 250 \text{ ml.} = 62.50 \text{ ml.}$$

b. 62.50 may be rounded off to 60 ml. because 2.50 is less than 10 per cent of 62.50.
   c. Pour 60 ml. of glycerin into a graduate and add water up to 250 ml.
3. To prepare a pint of 2 per cent sodium chloride.
   a. Convert 1 pint to minims.

$$1 \text{ pint} = 7680 \text{ minims}$$
$$\frac{2\%}{100\%} \times 7680 \text{ minims} = \frac{1536}{10} = 153.6 \text{ grains}$$
$$\frac{2.5 \text{ drams}}{60) \, 156.3}$$

b. 2.5 drams of sodium chloride are necessary to prepare 1 pint of a 2 per cent solution.

Preparing Solutions from Tablets

Problem. To find the amount of drug to be used. To find the number of tablets equivalent to that amount of drug.

1. To prepare 1 quart of 0.85 per cent sodium chloride from $2\frac{1}{8}$-Gm. tablets.

a. Convert 1 quart to 1000 ml.

$$\frac{0.85\%}{100\%} = \frac{x \text{ Gm.}}{1000 \text{ ml.}}$$
$$100 \ x = 850$$
$$x = 8.5 \text{ Gm.}$$

b. The number of tablets required may be obtained by dividing the weight of the drug to be used by the weight of the tablet.

c. Convert $2\frac{1}{8}$ to a decimal fraction, 2.125.

$$2.125 \overline{)8.500} \quad \text{4 tablets}$$

d. Four tablets ($2\frac{1}{8}$ Gm. each) of sodium chloride are required to prepare 1 quart of 0.85 per cent solution.

Problem. To find the amount of water in which to dissolve a tablet of known strength to make a solution of desired strength.

1. To prepare a 1:4000 solution from tablets containing 0.5 Gm.

$$\frac{\text{Strength of tablet}}{\text{Strength of desired solution}} = \left(\begin{array}{c} \text{amount of water in which} \\ \text{to dissolve the tablet} \end{array} \right)$$
$$\frac{0.5}{\dfrac{1}{4000}} \text{ or } 0.5 \times \frac{4000}{1} = 2000 \text{ ml. of water}$$

a. 2000 ml. of water is required to prepare a 1:4000 solution from a 0.5-Gm. tablet.

Percentage Problems

1. How many grams are necessary to prepare 0.5 liter of a 4 per cent boric acid solution?

2. Prepare 4000 ml. of a 1:1000 mercuric chloride solution from 0.5-Gm. tablets of the drug. How many tablets are necessary?

3. Prepare 1000 ml. of a 0.1 per cent solution of a drug from gr. viiss tablets. How many tablets are needed?

4. How many grains x sodium bicarbonate tablets would be needed to prepare 50 ml. of a 5 per cent solution?

5. How much 5 per cent potassium iodide solution can be prepared from 60 ml. of an 80 per cent solution of the drug?

Preparing Solutions from Stock Solutions

Problem. To find the amount of stock solution of known strength required to make a weaker solution of desired strength. The unknown quantity is the number of milliliters of stock solution to be diluted.

1. To prepare 1000 ml. of 0.1 per cent benzalkonium chloride solution from a 12.8 per cent (concentrated) solution.

$$\frac{0.1\%}{12.8\%} = \frac{x \text{ ml.}}{1000 \text{ ml.}}$$
$$12.8 \, x = 100, \quad x = 7.81 \text{ ml.}$$

a. Since 0.19 is less than 10 per cent of 7.81, it may be added to it to make a total of 8 ml.

b. 8 ml. of the stock solution are poured into a liter graduate and water is added to make the total volume 1000 ml.

2. To prepare solutions for intravenous infusion from concentrated solutions.

a. Levarterenol Bitartrate, U.S.P. (Levophed), is supplied in sterile aqueous solution in 4-ml. ampuls. Each milliliter of this 0.2 per cent solution contains 2 mg. of levarterenol bitartrate equivalent to 1 mg. of the base. This is a *concentrated solution* and *must be diluted* before use. Four milliliters (the contents of one ampul) are added to 1000 ml. of 5 per cent dextrose solution or 5 per cent dextrose in saline solution. The resulting dilution, which contains 4 mcg. of the base in each milliliter, is given by intravenous infusion.

b. Succinylcholine Chloride, U.S.P. (Anectine), is marketed in 10-ml. ampuls as a sterile solution containing 50 mg. in each milliliter. It is a *concentrated solution* and *must be diluted*. Solutions of 0.1 per cent or 0.2 per cent are conveniently prepared by adding 500 mg. (the contents of one 10-ml. vial containing 50 mg. in each milliliter) to 500 or 250 ml. of 5 per cent dextrose solution or sterile isotonic saline solution.

Problems

From full-strength drugs:

1. Prepare 2500 ml. of 1:5000 potassium permanganate solution from the crystals.

2. Prepare 1 quart of normal physiological salt solution (0.85 per cent) for mouthwash or irrigation.

3. Prepare 1500 ml. of 4 per cent boric acid solution.

4. Prepare 2 liters of 70 per cent alcohol.

From tablets:

1. Prepare 2 liters of normal physiological salt solution using 1-Gm. salt tablets.

2. Prepare 200 ml. of a 5 per cent solution of sodium bicarbonate from tablets gr. v.

3. Prepare 1 liter of 1:3000 potassium permanganate solution from tablets gr. v.

From stock solutions:

1. Prepare 1½ quarts of physiological salt solution (0.85 per cent) from a 10 per cent stock solution.

2. Prepare 500 ml. of a 1 per cent phenol solution from a solution labeled 5 per cent.

3. Prepare 1000 ml. of a 50 per cent alcohol solution from a stock solution of 70 per cent.

4. Prepare a liter of 1:5000 benzalkonium chloride solution from a stock solution of 1:1000.

CALCULATIONS OF DOSAGES

MEASURING MEDICATIONS (ORAL)

The drug manufacturers supply solid drugs in the form of capsules and tablets in the doses usually prescribed. Sometimes it is necessary to give several tablets or capsules at the same time, to obtain the desired dose. On the other hand, because smaller doses may be needed, tablets are scored so that they may easily be broken into halves or quarters. These tablets or capsules should be shaken into the cap of the bottle and dropped into the medicine glass in which it is carried to the patient.

Stock solutions are often diluted to prepare doses for oral administration.

Liquid Doses. Small doses of liquid drugs are measured in 60-minim glasses calibrated in 5 minims (i.e., 5, 10, 15, etc.). Ounce glasses calibrated in 5 ml. are used for the administration of doses over 4 ml. (1 dram).

The measurement of minim doses that are multiples of 5 is simple and quite accurate. However, if the number of minims prescribed is less than 5 (e.g., 4) or more than 5 and less than 10, the drug is diluted and the fraction of the dilution that contains the desired dose is administered to the patient.

1. To measure 4 minims.

a. Measure 5 minims of drug and dilute five times, making 25 minims, a 1:5 dilution.

b. To obtain the prescribed dose, multiply the number of minims ordered by 5.

$$4 \times 5 = 20 \text{ minims}$$

c. 20 minims of the dilution contain the prescribed dose. Discard 5 minims and administer 20.

2. To measure 8 minims.

a. Measure 10 minims and dilute five times, making 50 minims, a 1:5 dilution.

b. To obtain the prescribed dose multiply the number of minims ordered by 5.

$$8 \times 5 = 40 \text{ minims}$$

c. 40 minims of the dilution contain the prescribed dose. Discard 10 minims and administer 40.

3. To measure 1 minim.

a. Measure 5 minims and dilute five times, making 25 minims.

b. Each 5 minims contains 1 minim of drug; 5 minims constitute the dose administered.

4. To measure a fraction of a minim such as ½ minim.

a. Measure 5 minims of drug and dilute ten times, making 50 minims.

b. Each 10 minims contains 1 minim of the drug; therefore each 5 minims contains ½ minim. The dose administered is 5 minims of the dilution.

5. To measure ⅓ minim.

a. Measure 5 minims and dilute 15 times, making 75 minims.

b. Each 15 minims contains 1 minim of the drug; 5 minims contain ⅓ minim.

c. The dose administered is 5 minims of the dilution.

PROBLEMS IN DOSAGE

Doses prescribed in physicians' orders for subcutaneous administration may be the same or an exact multiple of the dose available in hypodermic tablets. On the other hand, the desired dose may be larger or smaller and not an exact multiple of the dose on hand. When the prescribed dose differs in strength from that of the tablets available, it is necessary to determine how many tablets or what part of a tablet should be used in preparing the solution. These solutions are usually administered in 0.6 to 1 ml., or 10 to 16 minims, of water. Injections of amounts larger than 1 ml. or 16 minims may be painful, whereas injections of amounts smaller than 0.6 ml. or 10 minims increase the margin of error if a drop or two is expelled from the needle of the syringe accidentally.

PREPARATION OF DOSAGES

When the Strength of the Tablet on Hand is Greater Than That of the Desired Dose

To prepare gr. $\frac{1}{4}$ from gr. $\frac{1}{3}$ tablets.

$$\text{gr. } \tfrac{1}{4} : \text{gr. } \tfrac{1}{3} :: x \text{ tablet} : 1 \text{ tablet}$$
$$\tfrac{1}{3} \, x = \tfrac{1}{4}$$
$$x = \tfrac{1}{4} \div \tfrac{1}{3} = \tfrac{1}{4} \times \tfrac{3}{1} = \tfrac{3}{4} \text{ of a gr. } \tfrac{1}{3} \text{ tablet}$$

or, using the formula,

$$\frac{\tfrac{1}{4} \, (D)}{\tfrac{1}{3} \, (H)} \times 1 \text{ tablet} = \tfrac{3}{4} \text{ of a gr. } \tfrac{1}{3} \text{ tablet.}$$

To prepare the solution, dissolve $\frac{1}{3}$-grain tablet in the number of minims indicated by the denominator and give the number of minims indicated by the numerator. As the solutions injected subcutaneously are generally dissolved in 10 to 16 minims, if the number indicated by the numerator is less than 10, multiply the numerator and denominator by the same number so that the numerator will be 10 or more. To prepare a dose from $\frac{3}{4}$ of the tablet,

$$\tfrac{3}{4} \times \tfrac{4}{4} = \tfrac{12}{16}$$

Dissolve the tablet in 16 minims of water. Discard 4 minims and inject the remaining 12 minims.

When the Strength of the Tablet on Hand Is Less Than the Desired Dose

To prepare gr. $\frac{1}{6}$ morphine from gr. $\frac{1}{8}$ tablets: Since $\frac{1}{6}$ is greater than $\frac{1}{8}$, it will be necessary to use 2 tablets.

$$\text{gr. } \tfrac{1}{6} : \tfrac{2}{8} \text{ tablets} :: x : 1 \text{ tablet}$$
$$\tfrac{2}{8} \, x = \tfrac{1}{6}$$
$$x = \tfrac{1}{6} \div \tfrac{2}{8} \quad \text{or} \quad \tfrac{1}{6} \times \tfrac{8}{2} = \tfrac{8}{12} = \tfrac{2}{3} \text{ of 2 tablets (gr. } \tfrac{1}{8})$$

or

$$\frac{\tfrac{1}{6} \, (D)}{\tfrac{2}{8} \, (H)} = \frac{q}{\text{tablet } (Q)} \qquad \frac{\tfrac{1}{6}}{\tfrac{2}{8}} = \tfrac{1}{6} \times \tfrac{8}{2} = \tfrac{8}{12} = \tfrac{2}{3}$$
$$\tfrac{2}{3} \times \tfrac{5}{5} = \tfrac{10}{15}$$

Dissolve 2 (gr. $\frac{1}{8}$) tablets in 15 minims of water. Discard 5 minims and administer 10 minims.

Calculating a Dose Using a Stock Solution. The label on a rubber-capped vial of penicillin G sodium states that there are 1,000,000 units in 10 ml. The dose ordered is 50,000 units.

$$50,000 \text{ units} : 1,000,000 \text{ units} :: x \text{ ml.} : 10$$
$$1,000,000 \; x = 500,000 \text{ ml.}$$
$$x = 0.5 \text{ ml.}$$

or

$$\frac{50,000 \text{ units}}{1,000,000 \text{ units}} \times 10 \text{ ml.} = 0.5 \text{ ml.}$$

Therefore 0.5 ml. of the solution is the dose to be administered.

Problems

Tell how to measure the following doses:

1. minims ix _____

2. minims iii _____

3. ⅛ minim _____

4. ⅕ minim _____

5. 23 minims _____

To prepare doses from tablets:

1. Prepare atropine sulfate gr. ½₀₀ (*H*) from tablets labeled gr. ¹⁄₁₀₀.
2. Prepare codeine sulfate gr. ⅙ from tablets labeled gr. ⅓.
3. Prepare morphine sulfate 0.01 Gm. from tablets gr. ⅛.

To calculate doses using stock solutions:

1. Give meperidine hydrochloride (Demerol) 25 mg. from an ampul labeled 100 mg. in 2 ml.
2. Give crystalline digitoxin (Crystodigin) 0.15 mg. intramuscularly from an ampul labeled 0.2 mg. in 1 ml.
3. Give atropine sulfate gr. ½₀₀ from a 1:1000 solution.
4. Give morphine sulfate 15 mg. from a 1 per cent solution.

To prepare doses from full-strength drugs:

1. Prepare oxytetracycline 250 mg. for intravenous injection from Oxytetracycline Hydrochloride for Injection, U.S.P., which contains 500 mg. in a vial.
2. Prepare 400,000 units of procaine penicillin G and buffered crystalline penicillin G for intramuscular injection from Sterile Procaine Penicillin G and Buffered Crystalline Penicillin G for Suspension, U.S.P., which contains 2,000,000 units. Label the strength of the solution remaining in the vial after the dose has been administered.

MEASURING DOSAGES OF INSULIN

Various preparations of insulin are available which provide either 40 or 80 U.S.P. units for each milliliter of the injection. The dose that is given in units is easily measured, using insulin syringes graduated in units. There are three types of insulin syringes: (1) those graduated in 40 units; (2) those graduated in 80 units; and (3) those having a double scale, U 40 on one side and U 80 on the other. Great care must be exercised to use the scale calibrated for the strength of insulin being used.

Syringes that are available to measure any strength of insulin are (1) 1-ml. syringes calibrated in tenths of milliliters and (2) the 1-ml. tuberculin syringe calibrated in tenths and hundredths of a milliliter and in minims. When these syringes are used, it is necessary to determine the number of minims or the fraction of a milliliter which contains the dose. This amount may be obtained by using the following formula:

$$\frac{\text{Units in the dose}}{\text{Units on hand}} \times 16 \text{ minims or 1 ml.}$$

$$\frac{\text{U 30—dose}}{\text{U 40—on hand}} \times 16 \text{ minims} = 12 \text{ minims containing the dose prescribed}$$

$$\frac{\text{U 30—dose}}{\text{U 40—on hand}} \times 1 \text{ ml.} = \tfrac{3}{4} \text{ or 0.75 ml. containing the dose prescribed}$$

Problems

The following doses of insulin have been ordered. Calculate the fraction of a milliliter required when using a 1-ml syringe, or the number of minims when using a 16-minim syringe.

Units ordered	Strength of insulin used	ml.	minims
U 15	U 40	_____	_____
U 10	U 40	_____	_____
U 35	U 80	_____	_____
U 45	U 80	_____	_____
U 25	U 40	_____	_____
U 16	U 40	_____	_____

CHILDREN'S DOSAGE

As a general rule, children are more sensitive to drugs than adults; consequently they require smaller doses. There are several rules based on either age or weight which are available for use in calculating the fraction of the adult dose to be given to infants and children. The ones most frequently used are the following.

Young's Rule. This is used for children from 2 to 12 years old.

$$\frac{\text{Age}}{\text{Age} + 12} \times \text{adult dose} = \text{child's dose}$$

The adult dose of a certain drug is gr. xx. What is the dose for a child four years old?

$$\frac{4}{4 + 12} \times \text{adult dose} = \frac{1}{4} \text{ of } 20, \text{ or gr. v}$$

Fried's Rule. This is used for infants.

$$\frac{\text{Age in months}}{150 \text{ (average adult weight)}} \times \text{adult dose} = \text{infant dose}$$

The usual adult dose of a certain drug is 50 mg. What is the dose for an infant 15 months old?

$$\frac{15}{150} \times 50 = 5 \text{ mg.}$$

Clark's Rule. This rule uses the weight of the child to determine the dose.

$$\frac{\text{Weight of child in pounds}}{150} \times \text{adult dose} = \text{child's dose}$$

The usual adult dose of a given drug is 60 mg. What is the dose[1] for a child weighing 50 pounds?

$$\frac{50}{150} \times 60 = \frac{100}{5} = 20 \text{ mg.}$$

Problems

1. The usual adult dose for aspirin is 600 mg. What is the dose for a child weighing 50 pounds?

2. The usual adult dose for phenobarbital is 30 mg. What is the dose for a child three years old?

---

[1] This method of calculating children's dosage according to age and weight is no longer suitable in many cases. Each child and each drug should be considered individually. Children may require the same dose as adults of certain drugs such as the antihistaminics, amphetamine, and isoniazid. On the other hand, it is necessary to reduce the adult dose considerably when such drugs as morphine are administered to children. Gaisford, W.: "Paediatric Prescribing," *Brit. M. J.*, **1**:794, 1960.

3. The usual adult dose for chloral hydrate is 600 mg. What is the dose for a child weighing 25 pounds?

4. The usual adult dose of erythromycin is 300 mg. What is the dose for an infant 15 months old?

5. The usual adult dose for sulfadiazine is 1 Gm. What is the dose for a child four years old?

PRESCRIPTIONS AND ORDERS

The nurse will want to understand prescriptions, for, although she will never write one, she will constantly be executing the physician's written orders. We may apply the name "prescription" to an order, written by a physician to a pharmacist, calling for medication for the patient, with all necessary directions to the pharmacist for the patient. We may apply the term "order" to the direction by the physician to the nurse to dispense certain medication to the patient. This, too, should always be written. Both prescriptions and orders should be written in ink and be legible. If an order or a prescription cannot be understood, it should not be dispensed.

The prescription is actually a legal document. The writer must be licensed by the state; only doctors of medicine, dentistry, and veterinary medicine who successfully pass examinations given by licensing boards of medical examiners are permitted to write for "prescription drugs." This term will be explained after a discussion of prescriptions and orders.

PARTS OF A PRESCRIPTION

A prescription must bear the name of the patient to ensure delivery of the medication to the correct individual. The date and physician's address and telephone number are important as a means of guaranteeing authenticity. A narcotic number is required if the medication is a narcotic or contains any narcotic ingredients. Prescriptions should be written in ink for many reasons. Primarily, ink is more legible than pencil. Secondly, some patients may desire to change the amount of the prescribed drug. This is especially true of some narcotic addicts. Lastly, prescriptions are filed for a number of years as prescribed by law and the permanency of ink is desirable.

The body of a prescription consists of four parts: the superscription, the inscription, the subscription, and the signature.

The Superscription.   This consists of the symbol ℞. It is of historical origin, generally understood as representing the contraction of the Latin "recipe"—"take thou." It is the beginning of a direct order from the physician to the compounder, directing him to use the ingredients listed and the quantities described therein.

The Inscription.   The inscription, body, is the principal part of the prescription. The ingredients are listed below one another, the smaller amounts often appearing above those of larger amounts. Symbols and abbreviations are commonly employed. Quantities may be represented in either the metric or apothecaries' system. Legally, the U.S.P. and N.F. have adopted the metric system, i.e., grams and milliliters. In the prescription listed below, the solid ingredients are weighed (in grams) and liquid substances are measured (in milliliters). To avoid error due to decimal points and imperfections in the paper, the vertical line shown below has been adopted. In the apothecaries' prescription, the units (grains, etc.) are listed before the quantities, and the quantities are often written in small-case Roman numerals.

The Subscription. The first line beneath the list of drugs contains the physician's directions to the pharmacist. Often no directions are given and it is assumed that the pharmacist will prepare the medication according to his art (S.A.—*secundem artem*). The letter "M" is an abbreviation for the Latin *misce* and is interpreted as "mix" (see abbreviations, Table 6). Other abbreviations listed in the subscription would be:

M. et. fiat Cap. No. 10

(Mix and make ten capsules)

Metric Prescription

Tel. 2-6980	Mary Elizabeth Bosley, M.D.*	Reg. No. 490
	1201 Center Avenue	
Appointments	Denver, Colorado	

Name: Mrs. J. L. Smythe*   Age: Date: June 3, 1965

Address: 1709 Ridgeway Road

℞

Phenobarbital Sodium		2	5
Belladonna Tincture		45	
Cardamom Tincture, Compound		45	
Peppermint Water	q.s.	240	

M.
Sig. One teaspoonful in water t.i.d. p.c.

Refill 0 - 1 - 2 - 3   (Signature)   M.D.

*Fictitious names.

Apothecary Prescription

```
┌────────────────────────────────────────────────────────────────────────┐
│  Tel. 2-6980          Mary Elizabeth Bosley, M.D.*         Reg. No. 490  │
│                           1201 Center Avenue                             │
│  Appointments             Denver, Colorado                               │
├────────────────────────────────────────────────────────────────────────┤
│                                                                          │
│  Name: Mrs. J. L. Smythe*            Age:          Date: June 3, 1965    │
│                                                                          │
│  Address: 1709 Ridgeway Road                                             │
│                                                                          │
│        ℞                                                                 │
│                                                                          │
│                 Codeine phosphate      gr. i                             │
│                 Aspirin                gr. v                             │
│                 Phenacetin             gr. iii                           │
│                                                                          │
│                 M. ft. caps. No. 10                                      │
│                 Sig. Take 2 caps. h.s.                                   │
│                                                                          │
│  Refill 0 - 1 - 2 - 3                (Signature)                  M.D.   │
│                                                                          │
└────────────────────────────────────────────────────────────────────────┘
```

* Fictitious names.

Table 6

Abbreviations of Latin Words Commonly Used in Orders and Prescriptions

Abbreviation	Latin Derivation	Meaning
āā	ana	of each
a.c.	ante cibum	before meals
ad	ad	to, up to
ad lib.	ad libitum	as desired
aq.	aqua	water
aq. dest.	aqua destillata	distilled water
amp.		ampul
b.i.d.	bis in die	twice a day
c.	cum	with
caps.	capsula	capsule
comp.	compositus	compound
cong.	Congium	a gallon
dil.	dilutus	dilute
E.C.		enteric coated
elix.	elixir	elixir
et		and
ext.	extractum	extract

Table 6 (Continued)

Abbreviations of Latin Words Commonly Used in Orders and Prescriptions

Abbreviation	Latin Derivation	Meaning
fl. or fld.	fluidus	fluid
Ft.	fiat	make
Gm.	gramme	gram
gr.	granum	grain
gtt.	gutta	a drop
h.	hora	hour
h.s.	hora somni	hour of sleep, or at bedtime
hypo		hypodermically
H.T.		hypodermic tablet
i.m.		intramuscularly
i.v.		intravenously
Lin.	linimentum	liniment
Lot.	lotio	lotion
M.	misce	mix
mist.	mistura	mixture
n.r.	non repetatur	do not repeat
o.d.	omni die	every day
o.d.	oculus dexter	right eye
o.s.	oculus sinister	left eye
p.c.	post cibum	after meals
pil.	pilula	pill
p.r.n.	pro re nata	when required
pulv.	pulvis	powder
q.h.	quaque hora	every hour
q. 2 h., q. 3 h.	quaque 2 or 3 hora	every 2 or 3 hours
q.i.d.	quatuor in die	four times a day
q.s.	quantum sufficit	as much as is required
℞	recipe	take
s	sine	without
s.a.	secundum artem	according to the arts
Sig. or S.	signa	write on label
sol.		solution
s.o.s.	si opus sit	if necessary
sp.	spiritus	spirit
ss.	semis	one half
stat.	statim	at once
s.v.r.	spiritus vini rectificatus	alcohol
syr.	syrupus	syrup
tab.	tabella	tablet
t.i.d.	ter in die	three times a day
tinct.	tinctura	tincture
T.T.		tablet triturate
ung.	unguentum	ointment
ut dict.	ut dictum	as directed

If the powder or mixture of powders is available, already prepared, in tablets or capsules from pharmaceutical manufacturers, the physician merely writes "Tablets No. 50" or "Caps. No. 24" or any number he wishes.

The word "Sig." on prescriptions actually means "write on the label." It is the abbreviation of the Latin *signa*. The various directions used under this heading are of great importance to the nurse. This is the portion of the prescription she must know well in all its variations. It is the portion that the intern and other physicians write in the order book or patient's chart for the nurse to carry out. The various abbreviations will be listed. In our example, the "Sig." contains the letters "t.i.d., p.c.," meaning "three times daily after meals."

Prescriptions formerly were written in Latin by all physicians. Many are still so written. However, English names for drugs are now preferred. Trade names or official names should be used. Latin abbreviations in the signature are still used because of their brevity and popularity. Likewise the metric system of weights and measures is now preferred and is growing in its usage, although the centuries-old apothecaries' system is still used in the case of older drugs.

There are a number of abbreviations of Latin words which are commonly used in doctors' orders and prescriptions. They save time. They are considered standard terms and are well understood by the pharmacist. It is essential for the nurse to know their meaning.

ORDERS

An order is a direction to a nurse for dispensing medication. It differs from a prescription in that there is no specific form. Like a prescription, an order may be a written or an oral instruction, or a telephone message. In each instance, the instructions are recorded by a nurse who, after administration of the medication, records the amount given and other necessary information. Quite often the directions of an order are written in Latin abbreviations, similar to that of the subscription of the prescription. Examples are:

Tablets and Capsules

Codeine	30 mg.	} of each q.4h. p.r.n.
Aspirin	600 mg.	
Madribon	500 mg. b.i.d.	
Phenobarbital	30 mg. t.i.d.	
Digoxin	0.25 mg. q.d. in A.M.	

Liquid

Kondremul	30 ml. stat.
Milk of Magnesia	30 ml. h.s.
Tr. of Belladonna	gtts.x q.i.d. (a.c. and h.s.)

Injections

| Chloromycetin | 1 Gm. i.m. q.6h. |
| Demerol | 75 mg. i.m. q.4h. p.r.n. |

Abbreviations Used in Orders and Prescriptions

Example 1. Sig: cap. ii b.i.d.

Example 2. Sig: dram i q.4h. cum. aq.

Example 3. Sig: gtt.iii stat. gtt.i p.r.n.

Example 4. Sig: 5 ml. q.4h. et h.s.

Example 5. Sig: Apply ung. ut. dict.

PRESCRIPTION DRUGS

Many medicinal products, both old and new, are available from licensed pharmacists without a prescription from the physician. The majority of medicinal products are sold in this way. The Federal Food, Drug, and Cosmetic Act of 1938, amended in 1952 and 1962, sets rules for the protection of the public which must be adhered to by all manufacturers, dealers, and others who handle these products. The Act is enforced by the Food and Drug Administration. This body decides whether to allow over-the-counter sales of a medicinal product or to require that it be dispensed only on the prescription of a physician. The law requires prescriptions for drugs which can be safely or effectively used only under the supervision of physicians, dentists, or veterinarians. The manufacturer must use such a statement on his label under these conditions.

Theoretically no prescription item, under the above definition, should be refillable without another written or verbal approval by the physician. The physician may, however, indicate on the original prescription the number of times he wishes it to be refilled. If the physician does not indicate a certain number of refills, the druggist may not refill the prescription on the request of the patient without calling the physician for the specific authorization.

One group of drugs for which a prescription cannot be refilled under the law without the writing of a new prescription is the narcotic group. Here the physician may not authorize even a refill without rewriting the prescription.

Other provisions of the Federal Food, Drug, and Cosmetic Act have already been discussed.

REFERENCES

Fitch, Grace E.: *Arithmetic Review and Drug Therapy for Practical Nurses.* The Macmillan Company, New York, 1961.

Goostray, S.: *Mathematics and Measurements in Nursing Practice.* The Macmillan Company, New York, 1963.

Sackheim, G. I.: *Applied Mathematics for Nurses.* The Macmillan Company, New York, 1961.

5

Methods of Administration of Drugs. Distribution, Detoxification, and Excretion of Drugs. Dosage and Modification of Drug Action

The method or route of administration of drugs modifies their effects and also their rate of absorption into the blood stream. Drugs are administered for their local or general effects.

All hospitals have certain procedures to be followed in the administration of drugs. These vary greatly from place to place. There is no one most correct way to prepare and administer medications. The procedures which are developed by the personnel of various hospitals are based on many factors including: their unique situation, their past experience with medication errors, the types of medicine most frequently administered, the types of patients hospitalized, and the status of the people who administer medications. The reason a procedure is written is to provide safe effective care in one particular setting.

The process of preparing and administering medications is indeed a simple one—perhaps one of the easiest tasks a nurse performs. The goal of the process is to see that the right person receives the right medication in the right amount at the right time by the right method. Because the nurse is not licensed to prescribe medications, an order for each drug to be given must be obtained from a qualified person (a physician or dentist). The order should include the route and frequency of administration and the amount to be given. The nurse must then prepare the drug either by placing the required number of pills or capsules in a small container or by measuring the ordered amount of a liquid or powder in a calibrated container. If the route of administration is parental, sterile technique must be used during preparation.

This is a simple process, yet one which is not always done correctly. Errors occur in relation to each of the "rights" mentioned above. There are numerous reasons why errors are made. Many occur because the nurse is not following the accepted procedure, others because the task becomes a habit and the nurse's thoughts are elsewhere when she is preparing medications.

71

Poor communication among nurses and between doctors and nurses and the nurse's inadequate knowledge of the drugs she is administering are other possible sources of error.

The use of certain general practices can reduce the number of errors made. Medications should be prepared in a quiet environment with the nurse's entire attention focused upon the task at hand. If interruptions occur or the nurse is expected to accomplish several tasks at one time, then errors are likely to result. Only medicines for which there are doctor's orders should be given. Although the nurse has many medicines available to her, she is not permitted to prescribe.

Despite a variation in medication procedures among different hospitals, there is usually a specific sheet on which the physicians' orders are written. If this sheet is on the patient's chart or in a special book, the orders are transcribed onto individual medicine cards in order to facilitate ease in handling. On the medicine card must be:

1. The name of the patient
2. The location of the patient
3. The name of the drug
4. The dosage of the drug
5. The time and frequency of administration
6. The route of administration
7. The date ordered
8. The name of the person transcribing the order
9. The termination date if included in the order

Room 112

Jones, Jane

Phenobarbital

mg. 30

P.O.

q.i.d.

8-12-4-8

DC 9/8/64 @ 8 p.m.

S. Smith, R.N.

9/6/64

FRONT   BACK

Although the nurse's task may be simplified through the use of the medicine card, the addition of steps to any procedure increases the possibility of error.

When a dose requires calculation, it is advisable to check the answers and to have another person compute the problem if any doubt exists. Fluids or powders are measured by holding a graduated container at eye level and by estimating the amount of liquid present as indicated by the lower level of the miniscus. Any medicine which is in a suspension must be shaken before using it. Otherwise the drug will not be distributed equally throughout the solution and an incorrect dose will be given. Awareness that the correct drug has been selected from the medicine cabinet is possible only if the container is properly labeled. On the label should be not only the name of the drug but the amount found in the typical quantities to be administered. For example:

Aspirin   Demerol
1 tablet contains 300 mg.   or   1 ml. equals 50 mg.

Because many drugs are identical in appearance or have similar names, the identity of the medicine to be used should be verified several times during the prepartion by checking the label of the container with the appropriate medicine card.

A medicine card or similar identification must be kept with the drug until it is administered. If the period of time between preparation and administration is prolonged, the possibility of error is increased because the nurse's attention may have been focused elsewhere during that time. Another factor of merit when considering the safety of the patient is the assurance that comes from giving only medicine which you have prepared.

Before administering any medication, the nurse must be fully aware of the identity of the patient. Methods other than calling a patient by name should be utilized as there are instances when patients may respond to names other than their own. This may occur, for example, if the patient is irrational or has difficulty in hearing. Depending on their physical or emotional condition, patients may need various degrees of assistance when taking their medicines. Most hospitals require that the nurse remain with the patient until the drug is taken. This is obviously necessary if the nurse is to record the medicine as having been administered. It also prevents the possibility of medicines being misplaced or accumulated by the patient. If the objectives of the hospital are to prepare the patient to care for himself at home, then other policies may apply. For example, the drugs may be kept at the patient's bedside so that he may become accustomed to administering his own medications.

Many medication errors and untoward drug reactions are prevented by nurses who investigate seemingly unimportant comments patients make when receiving drugs. The patient may report symptoms of side or toxic effects which will require the drug to be discontinued or the dosage altered. On exploring a patient's simple comment such as "What, more medication?" one may find that the doctor has just discontinued the drug or that another nurse has given it. By investigating the situation, the nurse demonstrates to the patient her concern for him and her acceptance of him as a responsible person.

ADMINISTRATION FOR GENERAL OR SYSTEMIC EFFECTS

General or systemic effects are produced after a drug is absorbed by the blood and is carried by the circulation to the tissue or organ on which it has a selective action. To produce these effects, drugs are administered (1) orally, (2) parenterally, (3) by inhalation, (4) sublingually, (5) rectally, or (6), in some cases, by topical administration to the skin or mucous membranes. The most popular method of administering medications for systemic effects is by mouth, since it is the easiest and simplest way. Parenteral administration requires special equipment and techniques, but it is often preferred because of the rapid and reliable effects obtained. It is also available for administering drugs that are not effective when given orally, such as insulin.

ORAL ADMINISTRATION

Many drugs are readily absorbed from the gastrointestinal tract and are very effective when given by mouth. These may be administered as tablets, capsules, pills, or as a liquid. Drugs in solution are more quickly absorbed than solids; therefore, if a rapid effect is desirable, the substance should be diluted or given with water immediately before meals.

Taste is an important factor from the viewpoint of the patient. Many drugs have a disagreeable, salty, or bitter taste, which may be disguised by giving them in a large amount of fluid, such as fruit juices or effervescent drinks; in syrups or emulsions; or as tablets or capsules, etc. Fluids that have an unpleasant taste should be given cold, often with ice, followed by a large drink of water. If a medication is given for its local effect on the mucous membrane of the mouth or upper respiratory tract, it should not be diluted or followed with water. Drugs which may corrode or discolor the teeth should be given through a straw which is placed in the mouth behind the teeth. The use of sterile technique is not necessary when drugs are given orally since the gastrointestinal tract is not sterile. However, cleanliness is essential.

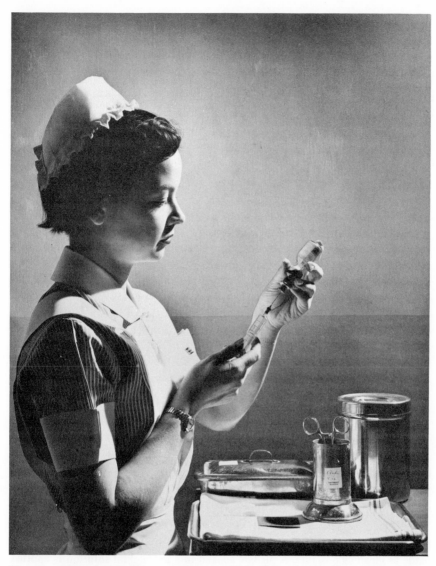

Fig. 1. Method of holding a syringe to fill it with solution from a vial. Before the needle enters the vial, the rubber stopper is cleaned with a germicidal sponge. Then the plunger is withdrawn from the syringe to the point indicating the amount of medication to be administered; thus, it is possible to inject into the vial an amount of air equivalent to the amount of drug to be withdrawn. The tray holds a covered syringe pan containing sterile syringes, a container for alcohol sponges, and sterile pickups, the container for which is marked with a date indicating the expiration of sterility. *(Courtesy of University Hospital and School of Nursing, University of Maryland.)*

PARENTERAL ADMINISTRATION

Administration of medications by injection is termed parenteral. The three most frequently used routes are intramuscular, subcutaneous, and intravenous. These may be selected when the drug is poorly absorbed from the gastrointestinal tract or made inactive by the intestinal and gastric enzymes, if the patient is unable to tolerate oral medications, or if a rapid effect is desired. Sterile technique must be applied whenever a medicine is given

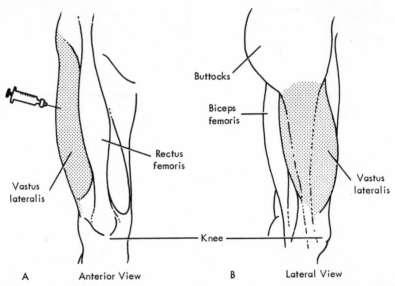

Fig. 2. *A.* Laterofemoral injections. Anterior view. The injection site is on the outer lateral surface of the thigh, between the knee and the head of the femur. The drug is deposited into the vastus lateralis.

B. Laterofemoral injection. Lateral view.

parenterally (see Fig. 1). Although the skin cannot be made sterile, it must be made as clean as possible. A pledget soaked in a germicidal solution is applied in a firm circular motion, moving from the center outward. All equipment used in the preparation of the injection must be sterile and handled in such a manner as to maintain this sterility. Poor technique may result in an infection at the site of injection or, in case of intravenous administration, systemically. Knowledge of the anatomy of the area in which the injection is to be made is essential. Bleeding can occur if large vessels are punctured unintentionally, and injury to a nerve may result in paralysis. To penetrate the skin with a minimal amount of pain, the injection should be made with a rapid smooth motion. Pain on injection occurs when the nerve fibers in the skin are touched. In case of subcutaneous and intramuscular administration, pain may also be felt if the fluid is injected rapidly causing a sudden increased pressure on the nerve fiber. Thus the drug should be injected slowly and the area should be massaged after the needle is withdrawn. This promotes the spread of the fluid in the tissue. An exception to this general rule is when the drug which is irritating to the subcutaneous tissue is given intramuscularly. Massage in this situation could allow the medicine to spread to the subcutaneous tissue via the tract made by the needle, causing pain

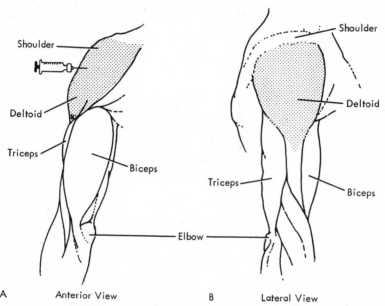

Fig. 3. *A*. Deltoid injection. Anterior view. The injection site is on the lateral aspect of the arm into the body of the deltoid muscle, the shape of which can be seen through the skin. Large amounts of fluid should not be injected into this muscle.

B. Deltoid injection. Lateral view.

and possible abscess formation or fibrous infiltration. When the needle is thought to be in the correct location, and before any drug is injected, a negative pressure should be created in the syringe (aspiration) to more accurately ascertain its location. If the drug is to be injected intramuscularly or subcutaneously, and blood is aspirated, indicating puncture of a vessel, then the needle should be withdrawn. When a series of injections is given, the insertion sites must be rotated to prevent severe tissue trauma.

Subcutaneous (Hypodermic) Injections. In general, only solutions are given into the subcutaneous tissue. Modified insulins (N.P.H. and P.Z.I.)

are exceptions. Medications administered by this route are absorbed more rapidly than those given orally. The injection is usually made into the outer surface of the upper arm. However, areas such as the anterior surface of the thigh, the abdomen, or the buttock may also be used. Since the solutions are usually thin and the subcutaneous tissue is that layer just under the skin, a small short needle is used (25 to 28 gage). After the skin is cleansed, an area approximately 2 in. in width is pinched between the finger and thumb. While a 45- to 60-degree angle to the skin, depending on the amount of tissue present, is maintained, the needle is inserted. Small amounts of solution (0.5 to 2 ml.) may be injected by this method.

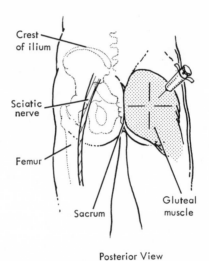

Posterior View

Fig. 4. Dorsogluteal intramusclar injection. The dorsogluteal injection is given in the upper outer quadrant of the buttock. In this area, which is about 1½ to 2 in. below the iliac crest, the nurse is least likely to hit bones, large nerves, and blood vessels. The site of injection is varied by using not only alternate buttocks but also a number of points within the safety zone.

Intramuscular Injections. Suspensions of drugs as well as true solutions can be injected into the skeletal muscle. Owing to the greater blood supply, medicines are absorbed more rapidly from muscles than subcutaneous tissue. When drugs in suspension are injected, a depot is established causing the onset of action to be slow and the duration of response prolonged. The choice of the injection site depends on the amount and type of drug being given and the size of the patient's muscle. Frequent sites employed include the buttock (gluteus maximus), laterofemoral muscle (vastus lateralis), upper arm (deltoid), and anterior gluteal muscle (gluteus medius and gluteus minimus). After the skin is cleansed, the layer of subcutaneous tissue which lies between the skin and the muscle is compressed by stretching the skin between the thumb and forefinger or by displacing the skin firmly to one side. The needle is then inserted perpendicular to the skin. The size of the needle used depends on the thickness of the fluid to be injected and the depth of the injection, the usual length being 1 to 3 in.

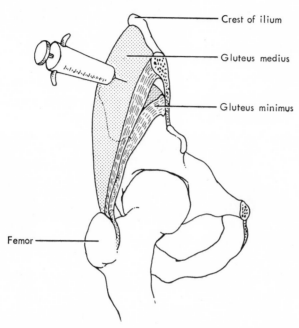

Crest of ilium

Gluteus medius

Gluteus minimus

Femor

Fig. 5. Anterior gluteal injection. The site of this injection is found by placing one finger on the iliac spine and the thumb or another finger just below the iliac crest with the palm of the hand on the patient's hip. There is a large amount of muscle in this area and no large blood vessels or nerves.

Intravenous Injections and Infusions. Most superficial veins in the body are suitable for intravenous injection. However, those in the ante-cubital fossa are most frequently used because they are large and easily accessible. If an infusion is being given, other sites which allow the patient more normal movement may be preferred.

In order to insert a needle into a vein, the vessel must be distended with blood. This is usually accomplished by applying a tourniquet above the injection site. The pressure applied by the tourniquet should be such that the venous return, but not the arterial supply, is obstructed. Other techniques that are useful in obtaining proper venous distention include: lightly slapping the veins, opening and closing the hand by patient, holding the extremity

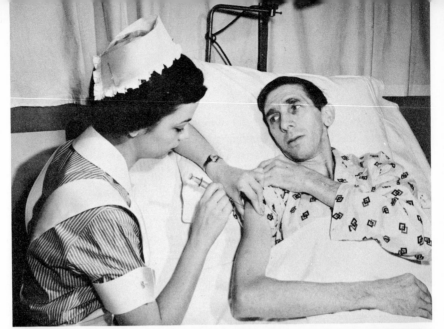

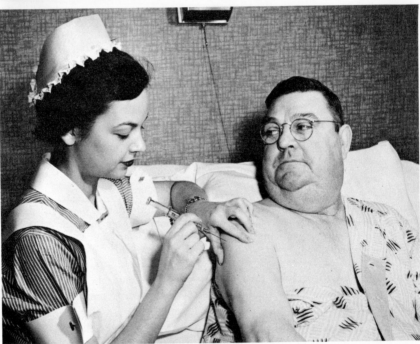

Fig. 6. Methods of administering intramusclar injections into the arm. When the patient has an emaciated muscle structure *(above)*, the tissue should be lifted up and the needle inserted perpendicularly through the subcutaneous tissue into the muscle. In the obese patient *(below)*, the tissue should be distended before the insertion of the needle; in this type of patient there is much more tissue into which the needle may be inserted. The second method of administration seems to be less painful than the first. *(Courtesy of University Hospital and School of Nursing, University of Maryland.)*

in a dependent position, and applying heat. After the vein is distended, the skin over the site is cleansed and stretched tight over the vein. Then the needle is inserted through the skin in the same direction as the course of the vein. As the needle enters the vein, its angle to the skin should be very slight so that it may be advanced into the vein rather than through it. As the needle enters the vein, a backflow of blood will be seen in the syringe or plastic tubing. Releasing the tourniquet allows the blood to flow freely in the vein. The infusion flow rate should then be regulated or the drug in the syringe should be slowly inserted. If swelling or other signs of extravasation are observed, the needle is removed and another site is chosen. The patient must be

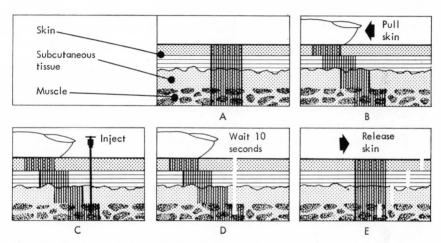

Fig. 7. Z-tract technique. This injection technique is recommended to avoid leakage of a drug into the subcutaneous tissue. By displacement of the skin laterally prior to injection, the site is sealed off.

carefully observed for any untoward reaction to the drug given. The rapid rate of infusion obtained on intravenous administration allows more such reactions. Whenever antidotes are available, the nurse must be aware of what and where they are.

Intradermal Injections.   Very small amounts of a solution are injected into the upper layers of the skin in intradermal injections. This method is primarily used to determine the patient's sensitivity to a substance such as tetanus antitoxin or penicillin. This procedure is usually the responsibility of a physician.

Intrathecal or Intraspinal Injections.   These injections are made by inserting the needle through the interspinous spaces into the spinal fluid. They are useful in the treatment of infectious diseases such as meningitis and in producing spinal anesthesia.

Intrasternal Injections. These injections are made by inserting the needle into the marrow of the sternum and are used when veins are not available. They are comparable to intravenous injections. The response is immediate.

Syringes and Needles. Drugs in solution are injected into the body by means of a syringe and needle. The Luer type, which is most commonly used, is made of Pyrex glass and consists of a plunger and barrel. The barrel has a narrow neck to which the needle is attached. These syringes, which vary in size from 1 to 50 cc. (ml.), are calibrated on the barrel so that the solution to be injected may be accurately measured. The tuberculin syringe, which is used for the measurement of very small quantities of drug, is calibrated in 0.01 cc. (ml.) and in minims. The plunger is colored blue. Insulin syringes are calibrated in units for ease in measuring the dosage of insulin, which is expressed in units. The calibrations are red on the syringes used for measuring 40 units; they are green on those measuring 80 units. This differentiation by color is particularly useful for the diabetic patient who makes his own injections.

The needles most commonly used are made of stainless steel and vary in length from ½ to 3 in. and in the diameter of the bore from 27 to 13 gage. The higher-gage numbers indicate smaller bores. The needles must be sharp and smooth for satisfactory injections.

Drugs for injection are available in ampuls, rubber-stoppered vials, and hypodermic tablets, which are all prepared under aseptic conditions. Reusable syringes and needles should be sterilized by steam under pressure. Many types of disposable presterilized needles and syringes are also available.

INHALATION

Volatile substances are administered by inhalation. Gaseous anesthetics, the vapors of liquid anesthetics, such gases as oxygen, carbon dioxide, and helium, and such drugs as aromatic ammonia spirit and amyl nitrite produce very rapid responses upon their administration by this method. Nonvolatile substances must be nebulized before being inhaled.

Method of Administration. The exact dose of the drug to be administered is placed in the nebulizer, the mask nose- or mouthpiece is fitted to the patient's face, and oxygen or compressed air is allowed to flow through the nebulizer at the rate of 5 or 6 L. per minute. The drug is carried by the gas to the bronchial tree. Compressed air is used for long-term therapy. Oxygen is indicated in hypoxia and under certain special conditions.

The Aerohalor is a device for the administration of solid aerosols to the upper respiratory tract and lungs. It consists of a discharge chamber with interchangeable mouth- and nosepieces. The drug is dispensed in Aerohalor Cartridges which fit into the Aerohalor. As the patient inhales, a stream of air enters the device. A small amount of drug enters the air stream and is carried to the respiratory tract.

The Dispolator is a plastic inhaler containing a micropulverized powder which the patient inhales through the nose or mouth. It is discarded after use.

The Medihaler is a nebulizer used for the administration of liquid medi-

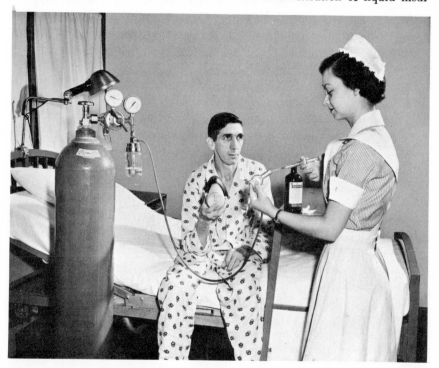

Fig. 8. Administration of aerosol using oxygen. The liquid aerosol is withdrawn by syringe from a stock bottle and is injected into the nebulizer. The nebulizer is then attached to a facial mask that covers the oronasal passages, whereupon the oxygen supply is turned on. In the beginning, the oxygen flow is 5 liters per minute, but this is increased as the drug nebulizes. The oxygen, which is humidified by passing through the water in the jar, enters the nebulizer and carries the drug, in the form of a dry mist, to the bronchopulmonary tree. *(Courtesy of University Hospital and School of Nursing, University of Maryland.)*

cations. The drug, in an inert aerosol vehicle, is available in a "leakproof, spillproof" plastic-coated bottle or vial. The bottle fits into an unbreakable plastic oral adapter. Each inhalation delivers a uniform measured dose of the drug. The medication and the adapter are combined in a small plastic case. Examples: Medihaler-Epi and Medihaler-Iso for use in asthma. The Mistometer is a similar device containing isoproterenol (Isuprel).

SUBLINGUAL ADMINISTRATION

Some hypodermic tablets are placed under the tongue, where they dissolve rapidly and are absorbed quickly in the general circulation. Drugs administered by this method do not reach the liver, and a small dose is effective. The patient must be instructed not to swallow the tablet nor should water be taken immediately following the tablet. Glyceryl trinitrate tablets are administered in this way.

RECTAL ADMINISTRATION

Rectal absorption is, in some cases, prompt and useful. Drugs are administered by enema or suppositories. Larger doses are necessary when drugs are administered in this manner.

ADMINISTRATION FOR LOCAL EFFECTS

For their local effects, drugs are administered topically to the skin and mucous membranes. They may also be injected under the skin, into the spinal canal, or around the nerve trunk to produce local anesthesia. Drugs which upon oral administration are poorly absorbed from the gastrointestinal tract may be given in this manner for their local effect.

Drugs are applied topically to the skin to produce a variety of local effects (antiseptic, soothing, antipruritic, analgesic, and irritant effects) in the form of ointments, lotions, solutions, sprays, liniments, plasters, and pastes (see Chaps. 44 and 46).

Drugs are applied to the mucous membranes of the nose, throat, eye, urinary bladder, etc., by irrigation, instillation, and painting or swabbing of the surface. For their effects in the respiratory tract, drugs may also be administered by inhalation or spraying. Steam medicated with benzoin or volatile oils, discrete droplets, mists, and nebulae are inhaled. Medicated steam is administered by means of an inhalator; coarse sprays, which are used for their local action in the upper passages of the respiratory tract, are applied by means of an atomizer; fine sprays, mists, nebulae, and aerosols, which are used for their effect in the bronchi, are inhaled by using nebulizers or Aerohalors. Aerosols of penicillin or epinephrine are examples.

DRUG RESPONSE MODIFIED BY METHOD OF ADMINISTRATION

One drug may produce several different effects in accord with the different methods of administration. When the insoluble bismuth salts, such as bismuth subcarbonate, are administered orally, they serve as protectives to the gastrointestinal tract. They have been administered intramuscularly in the treatment of syphilis, but they are too toxic for intravenous use. When Epsom salt (magnesium sulfate) is taken orally, it acts as a cathartic. When it is administered locally in heated solution, it relieves pain and reduces swelling by withdrawing fluid from the affected part of the body. Magnesium sulfate injected intravenously produces depression of the central nervous system and is used in some cases of convulsions in toxemias of pregnancy (eclampsia). Thus, some drugs are used in one way for one type of action and in another way for an entirely different purpose.

DISTRIBUTION, DETOXIFICATION, AND EXCRETION OF DRUGS

Distribution.   Drugs, as a rule, are distributed throughout the body by the circulation of the blood and other fluids. Some accumulate in certain tissues and body fluids in greater concentrations than in others. Drugs may be stored in certain tissues or organs and may be slowly released to other tissues.

Detoxification.   Many drugs are inactivated or detoxified in the body by various enzymatic activities. They may be oxidized, reduced, or hydrolyzed. Other drugs may be conjugated with other chemical substances in the body and are thus rendered inactive. Some drugs are not metabolized, destroyed, or inactivated and are excreted unchanged.

Excretion.   Drugs may be excreted unchanged, or in conjugated form, or in the form of their metabolites (end products) by one or more channels. The most important organs of excretion are the kidneys, colon, and lungs. Drugs may reach sufficient concentrations in the organs in which they are excreted to be useful, (1) as in the case of x-ray contrast materials, or (2) as anti-infective drugs; or they may be detrimental, as in the case of crystal formation in the kidney tubules when the older sulfonamide drugs were used.

DOSAGE AND MODIFICATION OF DRUG ACTION

The dose is the amount of a drug needed to produce a desired therapeutic effect. This amount varies with the disease as well as with the weight, age, and other characteristics of the patient. The usual U.S.P. doses are those that may be expected ordinarily to produce the therapeutic effect for which the preparation is most commonly used. They are the oral adult doses unless otherwise specified.

CONDITIONS THAT MODIFY DOSAGE

Weight.   Persons of smaller size requires less drug.

Age.   Children and older people require smaller doses. There is a relationship between age and weight. Weight is a better criterion than age. There are a number of rules for the calculation of dosage for the child (see p. 64).

It is well to remember that the child is not always a "small adult" with respect to drugs.

Sex Factors. During pregnancy the diabetic mother may not require insulin because insulin is in the fetal circulation. Since the placenta is not a barrier to drugs, those substances that may affect the fetus should be avoided. Violent cathartics are contraindicated, as they may produce abortion.

During menstruation full doses of cathartics should be avoided, since they increase the flow and pain in the pelvic area.

During lactation, bitter drugs, opiates, and hypnotics should not be given to nursing mothers because they could appear in the milk.

Temporary Factors or the Condition of the Patient. The presence of food in the stomach delays absorption. A drug is absorbed more rapidly from an empty stomach. In pylorospasm the drug remains in the stomach and does not reach the intestine, where most of the absorption takes place.

Time, Place, and Temperature Factors. The time of day has a tremendous influence on the amount of sedatives and stimulants administered. Smaller doses of sedatives are required at night and larger doses are given in the morning to produce the same degree of quieting. Larger doses of stimulants are required at night, if necessary at that time, and smaller doses are equally effective in the morning. If sodium bicarbonate is given after meals, it neutralizes gastric acidity; if given before breakfast or one-half hour before meals, it is absorbed and augments the alkaline reserve. If irritant drugs are given before meals, they irritate the mucosa of the stomach and may cause nausea. If they are given after meals, irritation is prevented but absorption is slower.

At high altitudes the dose of potent drugs should be decreased because the capacity of the cells of the body to oxidize them is diminished.

In hot weather, drugs produce greater and more prolonged effects because the patient's metabolism is depressed and his resistance is lowered. Here, again, smaller doses are indicated.

Idiosyncrasy or Drug Allergy. Idiosyncrasy is an unusual and often unpredictable response to a drug by an individual. Small doses of relatively harmless drugs may produce toxic effects in some people. An example is the rash and other untoward (undesirable) effects produced in a minority of patients by the administration of penicillin.

Tolerance. Tolerance is the resistance of a patient to drugs in ordinary doses. After taking a drug over a period of time, larger doses are required to produce the desired therapeutic effect. Increasingly large doses of morphine are necessary to relieve pain if it is necessary to give it regularly over prolonged periods of time.

Cumulative Effect. A cumulative effect is the response produced by *continued* dosage with certain drugs. The first dose produces little or no effect. When the second dose is given, there is the combined effect of two doses. A definite concentration of the drug in the body is required to produce a response. The concentration depends on the amount of drug absorbed, destroyed, and excreted. Several doses of digitalis may be given before the desired therapeutic effect is obtained. Then one sixth to one tenth of the dose will maintain the effect.

Synergism. Drugs may potentiate or increase the action of each other. They produce a degree of action greater than the sum of the effects of the separate drugs.

Antagonism. Drugs that produce opposite effects or counteract the action of each other are antagonists. The effect produced by an overdose of a drugs or poison may thus be antagonized by an antidote. Nalorphine is given to increase the respiration that has been depressed by overdosage with morphine.

PLACEBO THERAPY

A placebo is a tablet, capsule, injection, or any dosage form that does not contain a medically active ingredient. It often contains merely milk sugar (lactose) or starch. Placebos came into use long ago when physicians found it highly desirable under certain circumstances to pretend to be giving effective treatment when there were no drugs available for the condition.

With the increasing advances in the fields of pharmacology and psychiatry, the use of placebos seems to be diminishing. Emphasis is directed toward spending more time with the patient, listening to what the patient may be communicating through his description of his symptoms, and helping to meet his psychological needs through this interaction. At the present time placebos are used primarily in double-blind studies. These studies are used to test the effectiveness of a new drug. In this method of research the doctor is aware that some of the medicines being used are placebos. However, he does not know which patient is receiving them.

The placebo effect is defined as the changes produced by a placebo. This can be a positive or negative effect; i.e., the symptoms may be relieved or made worse. Since there is no ingredient in the placebo to account for these changes, it is felt that they have a psychological basis. Various factors that influence this effect have been identified including: the meaning of the medicine to the patient and the doctor-patient and the nurse-patient relationship. This effect can occur not only with placebos but with all medications and other types of treatment. The nurse must use this knowledge when caring for patients if she is to be helpful to them.

REVIEW QUESTIONS

1. *Give several methods for administering drugs locally. What are some of the desired therapeutic effects which may be obtained by these methods?*
2. *In what ways are drugs administered by injection? What are the advantages for parenteral administration? In what forms are drugs available for parenteral administration?*
3. *Name several types of drugs that are given by inhalation to produce systemic effects.*
4. *How are drugs inactivated or detoxified in the body? In what ways may they be excreted?*
5. *Name several conditions that may modify dosage.*
6. *Explain the following terms: idiosyncrasy, tolerance, antagonism.*

REFERENCES

Adriani, John: "Venipuncture," *Am. J. Nursing*, **62**:66, 1962.

Baker-Bates, E. T., and Cadman, E. F. B.: "Aerosol Therapy in Pulmonary Disease," *Practitioner*, **175**:736, 1955.

Barker, Kenneth, and McConnell, Warren: "How to Detect Medication Errors," *Modern Hospital*, **99**:1, 1962.

Chow, Rita: "Innovations in IV Equipment," *Am. J. Nursing*, **62**:80, 1962.

Drew, J. A., and Blumberg, M. S.: "What Happens to Medication Orders?" *Am. J. Nursing*, **62**:59, 1962.

Fuerst, E. V., and Wolff, L. V.: *Fundamentals of Nursing.* J. B. Lippincott Co., Philadelphia, 1956, p. 371.

Harmer, B., and Henderson, V.: *Textbook of the Principles and Practice of Nursing*, 5th ed. The Macmillan Company, New York, 1955.

Hershey, N.: "Question That Drug Order," *Am. J. Nursing*, **63**:96, 1963.

"Intravenous Technique," *Spectrum*, 1961.

Kron, Thora: "Stepping Beyond the 5 Rights of Administering Drugs," *Am. J. Nursing*, **62**:62, 1962.

Lief, H. I., *et al.*: *The Psychological Basis of Medical Practice*, Harper & Row, New York, 1963, pp. 163-177.

Parenteral Administration. Abbott Laboratories, North Chicago, Ill., 1959.

Pitel, M., and Wemett, M.: "The Intramuscular Injection," *Am. J. Nursing*, **64**:104, 1964.

6

The Response of Cells to Drugs

Drugs used clinically are arranged in two main categories: those substances normally present and those foreign to the body. They are simple or complex chemical substances which may be either natural in origin or man-made. When naturally occurring substances such as hormones, vitamins, and minerals are deficient or entirely absent, they may be augmented or replaced by drugs of either category. Drugs may modify what the cells of the body do quantitatively, but they cannot change cell functions. They may exert *specific effects,* such as stimulation or depression, or *nonspecific effects,* such as irritation.

Stimulation. An increase in the activity of the specialized cells of the body is called *stimulation.* A tissue may be stimulated to the point of in-activity or paralysis, which is similar to physiological fatigue. When the drug is metabolized or excreted, the activity of the tissue usually returns to normal. There is a temporary loss of function, but the tissue is not destroyed. For ex-ample, dextro amphetamine increases the activity of the cells of the cerebral cortex and produces "brighter spirits" and increased mental alacrity.

Depression. A decrease in the activity of specialized cells is called *de-pression.* Frequently this effect may be produced by large doses of a stimulant. In some cases, stimulation may be a matter of dosage. Drugs have a *selective* action and, in therapeutic doses, usually exert their primary effect on a definite structure or tissue. In larger doses the action of the drug extends to other areas. The depressant action of drugs on the central nervous system is of clinical value because the degree of activity can be regulated by dosage so that any desired intensity of depression, from mild sedation or hypnosis to gen-eral anethesia, may be produced. Examples of depressants of the central nervous system are phenobarbital, which is often used to produce sedation; pentobarbital, which is used as a hypnotic; and thiopental, which is used as a general anesthetic.

Irritation. Irritation is usually an adverse and nonspecific effect that may influence growth, nutrition, and anatomical structure of cells, such as the epithelial and connective tissue cells. Mild degrees of irritation are bene-ficial in stimulating indolent groups of cells to normal activity, but if irritants are applied too long or in too high concentrations, they may cause destruction of tissues.

Irritation occurs in three stages: (1) reddening of the skin, owing to vasodilatation of the blood vessels (rubefacient action); (2) blistering (vesicant action); and (3) destruction of tissues (caustic or corrosive action).

Irritation of the skin may produce a reflex action and effects on tissues remote from the site of application. Drugs that produce this type of action are used to relieve referred pain.

Mercury salts are irritant to the tubules of the kidneys and may cause death of cells (necrosis) and loss of kidney function. In small doses, this irritant action of mercury compounds is used to increase the flow of urine (diuresis).

Replacement Therapy. The active hormone or the dried, powdered gland from some other species may be used to replace a secretion or substance that is absent or deficient and has upset the hormonal balance in an otherwise healthy person. Insulin, the active extract of the pancreas, is used in the treatment of diabetes mellitus, and the dried, powdered thyroid gland is used in the treatment of hypothyroidism.

Anti-infective Drugs. In addition to the direct effects of drugs on man's body cells, drugs are used to kill or attenuate parasitic invaders that produce disease in man. Here, drugs are administered for their toxic or detrimental effects on individual microorganisms. They are more toxic for the invading organisms than for man, the host, and so can be used to bring about cures in infectious diseases. Quinine and chloroquine are used in the treatment of malaria; penicillin is used in the treatment of syphilis, certain types of pneumonia, and many other infectious diseases. Drugs are also used to suppress neoplastic (malignant) growths. The effects here are transient rather than permanent.

Chemotherapy, in its original sense, was the treatment of infectious diseases with chemical agents designed or found to kill or inhibit the invading organisms. In its more modern, broader usage, it is, as the word denotes, treatment in general by means of chemical compounds (drugs). Enzyme systems within the cell play an important part in the response of cells to drugs. Physical and physicochemical properties and chemical constitution of drugs are also vital factors in drug action.

PHYSIOLOGY OF THE CELL

The human body contains hundreds of billions of cells, which are structural as well as functional units composed of the material which these cells have made. Cells depend upon the blood and tissue fluids for nourishment and oxygen and for carrying away the waste products of their metabolism. They are all alike in certain fundamental structures and properties (i.e., they are all composed of protoplasm, the substance common to all life), but they vary greatly in size, shape, and specialization of function. They are mostly micro-scopic in size; however, some muscle and nerve cells are visible to the naked eye. Cells of one kind can be distinguished by a similar size and shape.

Organization of Cells. Groups of cells and often the structural products formed by them may be grouped together to accomplish a certain purpose. Such larger organizations are known as *tissues*. Various tissues become further specialized and are organized into *organs*, such as the heart, which acts mainly as a pump to propel blood into the blood vessels. The *systems*, which are the main functioning divisions of the body, are made up of one or more organs and specialized tissues; for example, the entire nervous system is made up of the brain, ganglia, spinal cord, and nerves. All systems are interrelated and interdependent; the circulatory and nervous systems integrate the work of other systems, and the hormones regulate the activity of various tissues and organs.

If there is a disturbance in the normal balance of various systems and tissues of the body, drugs that antagonize the effects of this abnormal condition may be used to return the patient to normal balance. Thus, if the brain is over-active and the patient is excited and disturbed, drugs may be used to quiet him. If blood clots in the blood vessels, as in thrombophlebitis, anticoagulants may be used to prevent further clotting. A majority of drugs are used to alleviate symptoms or conditions caused by disease. Many drugs discussed in the following chapters are classified according to the systems of the body on which they exert their effects.

Properties of Cell Membranes. The cell membrane is a mosaic com-posed of proteins and emulsions of fat with small openings between. Water and dissolved particles move across cells and cell membranes if there is no obstruction to them. The tendency for substances to move from a region of higher concentration to one of lower concentration is known as *diffusion*. The membranes of the body are permiselective; i.e., they permit some substances to pass into the cell, whereas they keep out other substances. Small molecules (some proteins, amino acids, and glucose), water, and oxygen, which readily diffuse into cells, likely enter through small openings in the cell membrane. Chemicals, foods, and drugs that are soluble in fats may be dissolved in the fat in the membrane and thus enter the cells.

Osmosis is the selective flow of water through a permiselective membrane. If solutions on either side of a membrane permeable only to water are unequal in concentration, there is a tendency to equalize the concentration. Water will tend to flow from the weaker solution to the more concentrated one. The pres-sure exerted by the water is called *osmotic pressure*. Solutions that have equal concentrations of the solute on either side of a permiselective membrane have established an equilibrium and are called *isotonic solutions*. If red blood cells are placed in solutions containing a higher concentration of sodium chloride (hypertonic solutions), water is drawn from the cells, causing them to shrink. They typically assume rough, tented shapes. This effect is called *crenation.* If the cells are placed in solutions containing lower concentrations of salt (hypotonic solutions), water is drawn into the cells, and they burst from increased pressure, i.e., hemolyze. Isotonic salt solutions are used for the instillation of drugs into the body cavities because they are nonirritating to the mucous membrane linings. In addition, solutions isotonic with blood are used for preparing drugs for intravenous injection because they do not alter the character of the red blood cells. A solution containing 0.85 or 0.9 per cent sodium chloride is often used for this purpose.

The cells of the body are bathed in the interstitial fluid which serves as the internal environment for the cell. The intracellular and extracellular[1] fluids are composed largely of water in which certain salts are dissolved in concentrations that remain relatively constant. Salts in solution separate into particles called ions which migrate toward positive (anode) and negative (cathode) electrodes in an electrical field. The positively charged ions go to the cathode and are called cations; the negatively charged ions attracted to the anode are called anions. The most prevalent cations in body fluids are Na^+ and K^+; the most prevalent anions are Cl^- and the bicarbonate and phosphate ions. Potassium (K^+) is largely confined to the intracellular space (inside the cell); Cl^- is found almost exclusively outside the cell except for the red blood cells. Sodium (Na^+) like Cl^- is concentrated in the extracellular fluid. The presence of these ions in body fluids is associated with conduction of electricity and assists in promoting differences in electrical potential in the cell membrane and between the interior and exterior of the cell.

The cell membrane separates solutions of quite different composition. Protein molecules, because of their size, are normally retained within the cell, since they cannot pass through openings in the membranes. Their presence tends to draw water into the cell, and a colloidal osmotic pressure is exerted. However, differences in the ionic concentrations of the cellular and external solutions compensate for differences in colloidal osmotic pressure, and so internal and external osmotic pressures are similar. As a result, the cell maintains its normal volume.

The ability of the cell to regulate its own composition and maintain the constancy of the extracellular fluid is assured by the transport of certain ions from a lower to a higher concentration across its membrane. This requires work and the utilization of energy. Energy derived from cellular metabolism is stored in the form of adenosine triphosphate (ATP) until needed. The "active transport" of Na^+ out of the cell and K^+ into the cell consumes ATP. Thus Na^+ is maintained at low level in the cell and K^+ is kept high. The mechanism by

---

[1] The extracellular fluid refers to all fluids not inside the cells. It includes the interstitial fluid as well as the cerebrospinal fluid, blood plasma, lymph, etc.

which these concentration gradients are regulated requires a functioning membrane and is referred to as the "sodium pump." An enzyme called *ATPase* has been demonstrated which acts on ATP and increases in activity in the presence of Na^+ and K^+. Drugs known to alter Na^+-K^+ movement and to regulate cell excitability, e.g., ouabain, prevent this enzyme from acting on ATP.

During the active transport of Na^+ across certain cell membranes, a spontaneous electrical potential is developed. This difference in electrical potential is due to the preponderance of negatively charged substances inside the cell and positively charged ions outside the cell. In addition, the charge on the membrane itself contributes to the capacity of ions to cross the membrane.

To summarize: There are four factors that control the flow of ions across membranes:

1. The structure of the cell membrane.
2. Active Na^+–K^+ transport.
3. Transmembrane concentration differences.
4. Transmembrane potential differences.

Metabolism of Cells.   The living cell is a very minute amount of protoplasm and is composed of a nucleus and cytoplasm, surrounded by a cell membrane (animal) or cell wall (plants, bacteria). It is a very complex dispersion of proteins, fats, and carbohydrates in water, containing essential minerals and vitamins. It is a biochemical laboratory in which many physicochemical reactions are continually taking place, largely owing to the presence of enzymes essential to the life of the cell.

Outstanding research in recent years has resulted in the elucidation of the vital role played by deoxyribonucleic acid (DNA) in the chemical control system which governs heredity and, therefore, life itself. This substance, which is a complex polynucleotide of high molecular weight, is found in the nucleus of every cell of living matter. DNA duplicates itself exactly and stores genetic information in the form of a code controlling the development of the organism which it transmits to daughter cells and to the next generation. Under the direction of DNA, ribonucleic acid (RNA), which is a similar compound, regulates the structure of various proteins made by the cells and thus controls their growth, multiplication, and functions. DNA and RNA are composed of code units of certain purines and pyrimidines in combination with a sugar and phosphate. DNA contains the purines adenine and guanine and the pyrimidines cytosine and thymine, in combination with a sugar, deoxyribose; RNA contains adenine, guanine, cytosine, and the pyrimidine uracil with ribose.

Illnesses resulting from inborn errors in metabolism have been traced to defects in DNA, and it appears probable that diabetes, muscular dystrophy, and cancer will be found to result from the transmission of faulty DNA information. An abnormality in the DNA of the reproductive cells of the parents may result in the birth of an infant lacking the ability to produce a crucial enzyme. For example, hereditary defects in the metabolism of phenylalanine due to the absence or deficiency of the enzyme phenylalanine oxidase are phenylketonuria or phenylpyruvic oligophrenia. This condition is characterized by an impaired mental ability and the excretion in the urine of phenylpyruvic acid, excessive amounts of phenylalanine, and small amounts of phenyllactic acid.

Nourishing material and oxygen diffuse from the capillaries through the intervening tissue fluids and into the cells. From these materials the cell builds up characteristic protoplasm. Proteins are used mainly for growth and repair. Carbohydrates and fats are oxidized, thus releasing energy that is vital for carrying out various activities of the cells and for the body as a whole. Waste products formed during metabolism (carbon dioxide, water, and nitrogenous products) are excreted from the cells into the tissue fluids.

The proteins, present in the cell in colloidal suspension, are distributed homogeneously throughout the cytoplasm. The number of particles is very large, so that the total amount of surface provided is tremendous. The change that this suspension undergoes from a fluid (sol) to a semisolid (gel) state is one of rearrangement of the solid particles and is readily reversible. Muscular contraction is an example of this phenomenon. The electric charges on the surfaces of proteins in the cells are probably responsible for the dispersion of particles in the cells. Since like charges repel each other, the particles are held apart.

Energy Liberated by Cells. Energy is supplied to cells by oxidation of foodstuffs. There are two types of oxidation: (1) fermentation or glycolysis and (2) cell respiration. Each type involves electron transfer and the release of energy. Glycolysis is the conversion of simple sugars (glucose, fructose) and complex ones (starch, glycogen) to lactic acid with the release of a portion of the available chemical energy. In respiration, the cell utilizes available oxygen to oxidize foodstuffs and complete the process of energy release. Unlike simple combustion in which energy is released as heat energy, biochemically, energy is transferred to "high-energy" phosphorus compounds, e.g., adenosine triphosphate (ATP). The over-all oxidation-reduction process is catalyzed by enzymes and coenzymes present in tissues and is referred to as *oxidative phosphorylation*, i.e., the formation of high-energy phosphorus compounds coupled with oxidation of foodstuffs. Glycolysis provides only one twentieth of the energy derived from a sugar molecule, the major portion coming from oxidative phosphorylation. The functioning brain and nervous system cannot long survive in the absence of either oxygen (anoxia) or sugar (hypoglycemia), and unconsciousness or tissue death follows quickly.

Summary. A knowledge of the essential functions of the cell membrane in controlling continuous interchange of ions and other substances between the cell and surrounding fluid is of fundamental importance to the study of pharmacology, i.e., the action of drugs on cells. The physiological concepts discussed in this chapter are necessary for the understanding and explanation of the many basic phenomena such as (1) electrical excitability of nerve and muscle cells, the conduction and transmission across synapses, (2) secretion and absorption in the gastrointestinal tract, (3) formation of urine by the kidney, and (4) distribution of ions and water in the various body fluids.

HOW AND WHERE DRUGS ACT

A drug is a substance usually foreign to the cell. The drug may (1) be adsorbed on the surface of the cell, (2) penetrate the cell membrane, or (3) combine chemically with some components of the cell.

Drugs may act locally at the site of application, as on the skin or a mucous membrane, to produce a protective, soothing, antiseptic, irritant, or neutralizing action. These effects may also be produced within the gastrointestinal tract. Drugs may produce a reflex action remote from the site of application, as exemplified by counterirritants. The majority of our therapeutic agents exert their action after they reach certain specialized sites in the body, such as the cells of the brain, liver, heart, blood vessels, nerve ganglia or endings, and kidney tubules. The anti-infective drugs exert their principal, if not exclusive, effects upon the invading organisms.

Drugs and Cellular Oxidation. The interference with cellular oxidation may be illustrated best by the following examples: Some chemical agents produce their action on cells by decreasing the oxygen available to them. Carbon monoxide combines with the hemoglobin of the red blood cells to form carbonylhemoglobin, which does not readily take up oxygen and consequently blocks the carrying of oxygen to the tissues. The activity of the cells is depressed and they may die from want of oxygen.

If the cyanide ion is absorbed, it inactivates the enzyme cytochrome oxidase, and so breaks the chain in a series of oxidations essential to the cell. Oxygen is not taken up from oxyhemoglobin and is therefore not available for use by the cells, which are also depressed and die from lack of oxygen.

Physical Properties of Drugs. Volatile anesthetics enter the body, produce their effects, and are excreted unchanged (see p. 293). They dissolve in the lipids of the cell, and their presence diminishes the oxygen uptake of the cell and decreases its activity. In addition, the electrical properties of membranes, i.e., electrical resistance or impedance, may temporarily change and as a consequence cells may become less responsive to stimuli until the anesthetic is removed. These drugs may also affect enzyme systems of the cell, but it is doubtful whether this explains their mechanism of action.

Chemical Structure and Biological Activity.   Drugs may either stimulate or depress cell activity. This property depends on the nature and complexity of the chemical structure of the drug molecule. Some drug action is rather nonspecific, and a broad spectrum of molecules can elicit a response. For example, general anesthesia may be observed with simple molecules such as xenon and nitrous oxide and by highly complex structures such as steroid anesthetics. High specificity of action is seen on the other hand, e.g., stimulation of the adrenal cortex by adrenocorticotrophic hormone (ACTH), a complex polypeptide. Although structure-activity relationships (S-A-R) can be predicted with some certainty, the biological activity of the parent compound is usually discovered by accident or only after exhaustive study.

Competitive Inhibition.   Drugs that act directly to prevent the action of other substances but do not have a definite action of their own are known as *blocking agents*. They compete with these substances for certain receptor sites. Diphenhydramine (Benadryl) will prevent the action of histamine on the bronchi of the guinea pig and will cause the bronchi constricted by histamine to relax, but it will not dilate or relax the bronchi in the direct way in which epinephrine does (see p. 450).

Enzyme Inhibition.   Some drugs act directly to inhibit the function of some enzyme system. Physostigmine inhibits the action of the enzyme cholinesterase, which normally destroys acetylcholine and terminates its action. When this enzyme is inactivated, acetylcholine can accumulate in the tissues and produce a more prolonged effect.

Metabolite Antagonism.   Para-aminobenzoic acid (PABA), an essential metabolite in some bacteria, inhibits the bacteriostatic action of the sulfonamides. Drs. D. D. Woods and P. A. Fildes (see p. 164) have suggested that the sulfonamides, because of their similarity in structure to PABA, might block folic acid formation in the bacteria and thereby prevent their multiplication.

Drugs of Similar Structure.   Drugs of similar structure often produce the same types of response, with variations as to intensity of action, rapidity, and duration of response. Thus the barbiturates, which have similar structures with slight modifications, are used as sedatives, hypnotics, or general anesthetics. Their action is one of depression of the central nervous system (see p. 316). The fact that many drugs of the same or like structure produce similar responses has resulted in the introduction of many new drugs into clinical medicine.

However, at times even slight variation in structure alters tissue response to drugs.

1. *Side-Chain Modification.*   In the morphine molecule, replacement of the N-methyl side chain by the unsaturated allyl group results in a very useful morphine antagonist (N-allyl morphine, Nalline).

Isoproterenol (Isuprel), a very useful drug for treating asthmatic attacks, differs from epinephrine only by replacement of N-methyl by an isopropyl group.

2. *Ring Substitution.* Many useful diuretics resulted from the chance observation that an inactive sulfonamide-like compound increased renal output. Most of these are substituted thiazides of the chloro-compound, chlorothiazide (Diuril), i.e., hydrochlorothiazide (Esidrix).

Phenothiazines, derivatives of which are too numerous to mention, were designed as a modification of methylene blue, a dyestuff of high biological activity. Replacement of hydrogen by chlorine (chlorpromazine) resulted in a most potent and perhaps one of the most useful drugs in the management of psychiatric patients; replacement of ring sulfur in the same molecule by carbon yielded compounds having very mild tranquilizing or calmative action, e.g., Elavil.

Osmosis.   Magnesium sulfate is poorly absorbed and so retains water in the gastrointestinal tract or causes diffusion by osmotic properties from the blood and tissues into the intestinal tract. The increase in water content in the bowel causes peristalsis and purgative action.

REVIEW QUESTIONS

1. *Explain stimulation and give an example of a stimulant drug.*
2. *Explain depression and discuss the clinical value of this action.*
3. *Explain irritation and list three stages. Discuss how irritant drugs are used in clinical medicine.*
4. *What is replacement therapy?*
5. *Define chemotherapy.*
6. *Explain briefly the action of drugs on the cells of the body.*

REFERENCES

Clark, A. J.: *The Mode of Action of Drugs on Cells.* A. E. Arnold & Company, London, 1933.

Danielli, J. F.: *Cell Physiology and Pharmacology.* Elsevier Press, Inc., New York, 1950.

Davson, H., and Danielli, J. F.: *The Permeability of Natural Membranes.* Cambridge University Press, Cambridge, 1943.

Hsia, D. Y.: *Inborn Errors in Metabolism.* Year Book Publishers, Inc., Chicago, 1959.

Marsh, D. F.: *Outline of Fundamental Pharmacology: the Mechanics of the Interaction of Chemicals and Living Things.* Charles C. Thomas, Publisher, Springfield, Ill., 1951.

Ruch, T. C., and Fulton, J. F.: *Medical Physiology and Biophysics.* W. B. Saunders Company, Philadelphia and London, 1960.

II THE ANTI-INFECTIVE DRUGS

The discovery of pathogenic organisms and the recognition of their part in disease have resulted in the science of chemotherapy. *The term "chemotherapy," in its original sense, denotes the treatment of infectious diseases with chemicals that will destroy or inhibit the growth of the causative microorganisms, with little or no injury to the host. This modern science was founded in 1906 by Dr. Paul Ehrlich and co-workers, who, after years of systematic research, synthesized and introduced into medicine the drug Salvarsan, or 606, later known as arsphenamine. This organic arsenical, which was effective in bringing about cures in syphilis, was the first synthetic drug with a definite specificity for an invading pathogenic organism.*

The advent of the antibiotics *is one of the most outstanding medical achievements since the discovery and identification of bacteria, which began in the past century. After the discoveries of the causes of man's infections, medical science learned to combat the invaders one by one. In some cases, the method was the administration of serum taken from animals that had been caused to develop high resistance to a particular bacterium. In other cases, the method was preventive; persons were caused to develop their own immunity in advance. This is still an important measure for preventing many diseases. Immunization is discussed in Chapter 49.*

For still other diseases, drugs were developed to combat infections. For localized infections, as in lacerations, incised abscesses, empyema, etc., a very large number of bactericidal materials have been used. These local anti-infectives, which are used to destroy microorganisms outside the body, are discussed in Chapter 46. For systemic infections such as pneumonia and meningitis, little progress was made before the advent of the sulfonamides. Although syphilis has been treated for more than half a century by the use of arsenic, bismuth, and mercury compounds, this is a crude method compared to the efficiency of penicillin in this disease.

By the use of sulfonamides, available after 1935, many infectious diseases were brought under control and untold lives saved. Penicillin, introduced in 1943, gave us control over many additional diseases and surpassed the sulfonamides in many of their own spheres of usefulness. Except for persons with a hypersensitivity to the drug, penicillin has the advantage of having no serious toxicity, whereas the sulfonamides have grave potentialities if not used carefully. Many diseases still had to be conquered. Some of these, such as the rickettsial and certain viral diseases, became amenable to treatment with the introduction of streptomycin, tetracycline and its analogs, chloramphenicol, and many others.

Legs and arms were often amputated because of infections that can now be cured with drugs. Other surgical procedures in all parts of the body have been drastically reduced because of the antibiotics. Many infectious agents have yet to be brought under adequate chemotherapeutic control, notably certain viruses, protozoa, and metazoa, and some bacteria and fungi. Considerable progress has been made recently in the treatment of intestinal worm and protozoal infections. Within the last few years substances or extracts obtained from microorganisms have been reported to have antitumor or antineoplastic activity in experimental animals.

The future offers great challenge in this field, as there are still many goals to be attained. We need chemotherapeutic agents with lower toxicity which do not produce allergies and have less tendency to produce resistant strains of bacteria. We also need (1) drugs of greater potency that will be bactericidal rather than bacteriostatic; (2) drugs with greater specificity for infectious agents such as the tubercle bacillus and many other organisms for which we do not now have sufficiently effective therapeutic measures; and (3) drugs that would be useful in the treatment or prevention of cancer and diseases caused by the small viruses (e.g., the common cold) which still evade chemotherapeutic control.

The hope for the future looks bright. New antibiotics are often reported every week, and thousands of new chemical compounds are prepared every year. In addition, many physicians and scientists are working ceaselessly to discover drugs that will produce cures in the still unconquered infections.

7

Introduction to the Antibiotics.
Penicillin. Syphilotherapy

THE ANTIBIOTICS

The medical profession formerly had many disinfectants. One of these was carbolic acid, introduced by Lord Lister in 1865. Also known as *phenol,* this substance became the standard of reference with which a large number of subsequent disinfectants could be compared. The early materials were more toxic to human cells than to bacteria, but were still required in helping over come localized infections. Research led to more satisfactory agents. However, all such compounds were more toxic to the white blood cells, the leukocytes, than to the bacteria. The leukocytes which gather at the site of infections congregate in huge numbers to combat the infections. It was not until the antibiotics became available that we possessed material that was toxic to the bacteria and often completely nontoxic to the leukocytes and other cells and tissues.

The number and varieties of bacteria which inhabit the earth are tremendous. Many of them excrete from their cells a chemical substance which diffuses through the medium in which they are growing. The material may be toxic to bacteria of other varieties, or it may not affect them. In some cases it seems to benefit other bacterial types. Thus we may have two different species of bacteria commonly existing as a team. In many cases they grow more easily together than alone. Some of our diseases are caused by a pair of organisms seemingly cooperating. This phenomenon is known as *symbiosis,* and the arrangement may be termed a *symbiotic* one.

The opposite situation also exists, with one species of microorganisms— whether it is bacteria, fungi, or another type—antagonizing growth of others. The excretion of one causes inhibition or death of the others which are susceptible. This is termed *antibiosis.* Man is quite often very susceptible to poisonous products or toxins elaborated by bacteria. This is exemplified in diseases such as tetanus ("lockjaw") and diphtheria. In general, we are made ill by the circulating toxins of the microorganisms that successfully invade our tissues. These toxins, as the name implies, are poisonous to various tissues of our bodies.

101

However, it has been found that toxins produced by certain fungi have a remarkable power in stopping the growth of bacteria and have limited or no adverse effect upon the patient. These toxins are called antibiotics.

In some cases the antibiotics are *bacteriostatic;* i.e., they stop the multiplication of existing bacteria. The leukocytes and other defense measures in time eradicate the infection. In other cases the antibiotics are *bactericidal,* causing death of the bacteria. The latter, of course, is more satisfactory, but the former action gives us a good method of control over the disease involved.

Use and Abuse of Antibiotics.   The widespread use of antibiotics has resulted in microorganisms that are resistant to many of them. Resistance occurs when the drug loses its effectiveness on the organism. It often results from the rapid multiplication of resistant mutants already present in the flora which survive after the sensitive organisms have been destroyed. It may also occur when the infecting organism develops a mechanism to oppose the antibiotic activity of the drug by (1) preventing the attachment or entry of the drug, (2) developing an alternate pathway to that blocked by the drug, or (3) secreting an antagonist which inactivates the drug.

Sensitivity studies throughout the world show that penicillin-resistant staphylococci are continuing to increase and that many of these organisms also become resistant to the broad-spectrum antibiotics. Resistant strains occur frequently among the tubercle bacilli as well as among other classes of microorganisms associated with acute and chronic diseases.

A second disadvantage in the extensive and indiscriminate use of antibiotic therapy is the danger of severe allergic reactions, superinfections, both bacterial and fungal, and direct toxic effects. Superinfections may occur in patients when the normal bacteria are altered by prolonged antibiotic therapy which disturbs the bacterial balance in the body. As a result there is overgrowth of resistant organisms which cause more serious infections than those which were suppressed. The infections generally occur when the patient's resistance is lowered by debility, old age, malnutrition, certain disease conditions or with the administration of drugs such as cortisone or related compounds or antineoplastic agents. The organisms most often responsible for these infections are staphylococci, *Aerobacter, Klebsiella, Proteus, Pseudomonas,* fungi, *M. tuberculosis,* and enterococci. For best clinical results treatment should be carefully selected on the basis of the specific organism and its vulnerability to one or more antibiotics. Many outstanding scientists in this field believe that fixed antibiotic combinations may be undesirable and that their ability to prevent the emergence of resistant strains may only be delayed.

THE PROBLEM OF ANTIBIOTIC-RESISTANT BACTERIA

Physicians, nurses, public health officials, and hospital administrators are greatly concerned about the increasing number of serious, and often fatal, bacterial infections in hospitalized patients. Although mutant strains of staphylococci are the chief offenders, certain gram-negative bacteria—particularly species of *Proteus, Pseudomonas,* and the coliform bacteria—must share the blame. Their mutant strains are no longer sensitive to the common antibiotics and, consequently, are free to cause wound infections, bronchopneumonia, urinary tract infections, osteomyelitis, enteritis, septicemias, and many other disease conditions; they invade hospital nurseries and produce serious outbreaks of gastroenteritis and acute mastitis.

The infections occur much more frequently in hospitals than in the general population. Following the introduction and widespread use of an antibiotic in the hospital, the organisms that are endemic, particularly the staphylococci, develop a resistance to the drug. When the hospital use of a particular antibiotic is restricted for a period of time, a strain that had been resistant to the drug may again become sensitive to it.

Most hospital infections are either (1) cross-infections or (2) superinfections. Antibiotic therapy in hospitals promotes the colonization of resistant strains in the nasopharynx and on the skin of patients, doctors, nurses, and other personnel. These organisms are spread from patient to personnel and from personnel to patient. The persons who harbor the organisms (carriers) and the hospital areas that shelter them (bedding, curtains, floors) are the chief factors in the spread of bacterial infections.

According to many workers in the field, these hospital infections are generally preventable, and the following methods have been suggested to control their spread:

1. Improved housecleaning, sanitation, and laundry processing and improved aseptic conditions. Furniture should be cleaned with liquid or treated cloths, while floors should be flooded with a disinfectant solution, which is removed by a wet vacuuming process. Benzalkonium chloride (see pp. 742–43), an effective quaternary ammonium antiseptic, is available as Roccal for hospital use; laundry can be rinsed in this agent for a disinfectant effect that will last during use. Hexachlorophene Soap, U.S.P., has the disadvantage of not affecting gram-negative organisms.

2. Segregation of certain patients.

3. Protection of patients, as far as possible, from direct contact with carriers.

4. Reduction of the prophylactic use of antibiotics.

5. Detection of carriers and eradication of their organisms.

PENICILLIN

The first antibiotic discovered and introduced into medicine was penicillin. Sir Alexander Fleming observed in London, in 1928, the absence of bacterial growth near a contaminating mold (fungus) colony on one of his culture plates. As the mold was *Penicillium notatum*, he named the substance it secreted penicillin. The mold was grown in broth which then was found to possess antibacterial action against many common pathological organisms both in vitro (in the test tube) and in vivo (in the animal body). Much was learned about penicillin during the next few years, but its rise to prominence began only after energetic research was revived in 1940 by Drs. Chain and Florey at Oxford.

Penicillin is an antibacterial agent secreted by species of molds belonging to the genus *Penicillium*. These are common molds found on bread, cheese, fruits, and vegetables. *Penicillium notatum* and *P. chrysogenum* produce the highest yields of the antibiotic.

Production of Penicillin. Penicillin is prepared by the extraction of cultures of the mold grown in special liquid media. At first all the penicillin available was obtained from subcultures of Dr. Fleming's strain, which was grown in broth by the surface-culture method. Commercial preparations today are obtained generally by growing in corn-steep liquor a strain of *P. chrysogenum* developed from a mold found on a cantaloupe in Peoria, Illinois. By this method much larger yields of penicillin are obtained more rapidly and much less expensively.

The various forms of penicillin so far isolated are designated as F, G, K, O, V, and X. All are derivatives of 6-aminopenicillanic acid. They are closely related chemically but differ in their antibacterial effects in the body. The penicillins are white crystalline acids which lose their activity slowly in solution or in the presence of moisture. Penicillin G, U.S.P. (benzyl penicillin), which is easily manufactured and is most generally effective, is available as either the potassium or sodium salt. The dry crystalline salts are stable without refrigeration for long periods of time. Once in solution, the drug is not stable and must be refrigerated. Buffered solutions of penicillin G are more stable than the unbuffered ones and may be kept for three days.

By the addition of intermediates to the media or by subjection of the cultures to x-rays, mutants have been obtained which have increased the yield of penicillin 60 to 100 per cent. Penicillin O is obtained by growing the mold in a medium containing allylmercaptoacetic acid. This antibiotic is useful in cases where patients are sensitive to penicillin G. The 2-chloroprocaine salt of penicillin O is the insoluble form. Phenoxymethyl penicillin (penicillin V) is produced biosynthetically by *P. chrysogenum* in a special culture medium.

In 1957, Dr. John C. Sheehan prepared phenoxymethyl penicillin by total chemical synthesis. The following year he converted penicillin G to 6-aminopenicillanic acid, the basic compound of the mold-grown penicillin G now in use. In 1959 a group of British scientists, headed by Drs. F. R.

Batchelor and G. N. Rolison, isolated this compound, 6-aminopenicillanic acid, from the fermentation broth of penicillin G and thus made it available for commercial use. Since that time many hundreds of penicillins have been prepared by the addition of different side chains to this compound. Six of these semisynthetic penicillins which are available for clinical use today are phenethicillin (Broxil, Chemipen, Maxipen, Ro-cillin, Syncillin), methicillin (Celbenin, Staphcillin), and oxacillin (Prostaphlin), nafcillin (Unipen), and cloxacillin (Orbenin) for resistant strains of staphylococci and ampicillin (Penbritin) for the treatment of gram-negative infections.

Biological Features of Penicillin

Potency and Assay of Penicillin. In order to determine the potency of various penicillin preparations, growth inhibition of standard test organisms such as *Bacillus subtilis* or certain staphylococci produced by a suitable dilution of standard penicillin is compared with inhibition produced by solutions of unknown penicillins to be tested. The amount of growth inhibition is determined by the measurement of clear zones surrounding the cups containing the penicillin solutions or disks impregnated with penicillin on an agar plate inoculated with the test organism.

The potency of penicillin is expressed in *units*. One U.S.P. Unit is the antibiotic activity of 0.6 mcg. of U.S.P. Sodium Penicillin G Reference Standard, 1 mg. of which represents 1667 units. This is used as a standard of comparison of the potency of other preparations of penicillin. The dosage of penicillin is expressed in milligrams and units. The use of weights rather than units in the calculation of dosage is increasing. In such calculations, 600 mg. may be regarded as the equivalent of 1,000,000 units. Chemical assays for penicillin are described in U.S.P.

Mechanism of Action. Penicillin, in adequate concentrations, not only inhibits the growth of penicillin-sensitive bacteria but also kills the organisms. Penicillin acts by blocking the synthesis of the bacterial cell wall. Bizarre giant forms are produced which undergo lysis. Rapidly multiplying bacteria are the most susceptible to the killing effect of penicillin.

Antibacterial Spectrum. This is the range of activity against different bacteria. Penicillin is chiefly effective against such gram-positive organisms as the streptococcus, pneumococcus, staphylococcus, and species of the genus *Clostridium*, and such gram-negative cocci as the gonococcus and meningococcus. It is also effective in bacterial endocarditis due to susceptible organisms, anthrax, actinomycosis, and Vincent's angina, and is the drug of choice in the treatment of syphilis and gonorrhea. It is not useful in tuberculosis, bacillary diseases, viral infections, rickettsial diseases, and most fungus infections. (See Table 7, pp. 108, 109.)

Bacterial Resistance. The strains of staphylococci resistant to penicillin are continuing to increase. This may be due to two causes: (1) organisms sensitive to penicillin were killed off and the highly resistant organisms present at that time in small numbers have multiplied; and (2) when bacteria were exposed to inadequate amounts of the drug, there occurred in later generations of the organisms adaptive biochemical changes which were not present in the parents. It has also been shown that some organisms which are penicillin-resistant produce an enzyme, penicillinase, which destroys penicillin. It is fortunate that other antibiotics have been developed which are effective in combating infections caused by these resistant organisms.

Absorption and Excretion.   Penicillin G is rapidly absorbed upon intramuscular injection in aqueous solution, and therapeutic blood levels are obtained in 15 to 30 minutes. It is also rapidly and partially absorbed from the gastrointestinal tract upon oral administration, and maximum concentrations are obtained in 30 to 60 minutes. However, the oral dose must be four to five times the parenteral dose as about two thirds of that ingested is destroyed by the gastric juice and by penicillinase, an enzyme produced by bacteria in the intestinal tract. A small amount is excreted in the feces.

Penicillin is rapidly excreted by the kidneys under normal conditions. About one third of the parenterally administered drug is metabolized and the rest is excreted unchanged in the urine. About 60 to 90 per cent of the unchanged drug may be excreted in the first hour and only traces are found in the urine after two hours. The concentration of active drug in the urine is much higher than in the blood. Thus penicillin G may be used for the treatment of urinary tract infections caused by *E. coli* and *Proteus mirabilis*. The drug is generally administered every three or four hours and sometimes every two hours to maintain adequate concentrations in the blood and tissues. In order to prolong therapeutic concentrations in the blood and to lessen the number of necessary injections, probenecid (Benemid), which inhibits tubule excretion of penicillin, has been given orally at six- to eight-hour intervals simultaneously with penicillin therapy. This method is rarely used today. Larger doses of penicillin are preferred.

Distribution of Penicillin.   After administration penicillin is widely distributed throughout the fluids and tissues of the body, and its ready permeability to most tissues is important. Large amounts appear in the kidneys, lungs, bronchi, skeletal and intestinal musculature, and mucosa. Very small amounts, sometimes none at all, appear in the bone marrow, brain, cornea, lens, and cerebrospinal fluid. However, when the meninges are inflamed, penicillin may penetrate the cerebrospinal fluid in therapeutic concentrations.

Toxicity and Hypersensitivity.   Penicillin is a nontoxic drug, in the usual sense, in the vast majority of persons. However, in some patients allergic responses occur which vary from mild urticaria, dermatitis, ulcerated mucous membranes, or drug fever to fatal anaphylactic shock. Some physicians routinely test the patients for allergic reactions to the drug before giving it. This can be done by placing one drop of the solution into the conjunctival sac or by a scratch test on the forearm. If the reaction is positive, then the drug should not be given. Knowledge of the allergy history of the patient is also helpful. Most hospitals have allergy sheets for the doctors' and nurses' information. Repeated exposure to the drug by any method of administration is usually responsible for sensitization of these patients. The incidence of the reactions is greatest upon topical administration and least when the drug is taken orally. However, the severity of the reactions is greater with systemic use. Many severe anaphylactoid reactions and deaths have resulted from penicillin sensitivity. Death may occur instantly or after several hours and generally follows parenteral administration of the antibiotic. These reactions are occurring more frequently with the more widespread use of the antibiotic.

Treatment. The mild reactions may be combated with the administration of one of the antihistaminic drugs. Treatment for the more severe reactions includes the intravenous or intramuscular injection of epinephrine, the establishment of a free airway, and the administration of oxygen when available. Pressor substances such as levarterenol (Levophed) may be injected intravenously for the treatment of shock, and isoproterenol (Isuprel) or aminophylline may be given for the relief of bronchospasm. Parenteral cortisone-like steroids and antihistaminics are also indicated.

Penicillinase (Neutrapen) is an enzyme prepared from *Bacillus cereus*. It is used to destroy penicillin in the patient undergoing severe delayed penicillin reactions. Destruction of penicillin in the body fluids begins within one hour and the effects persist for three to four days. A second injection may be given at the end of that time, if necessary. Penicillinase may cause febrile reactions and local pain and tenderness. It should not be used in the treatment of anaphylactic shock as it may itself be antigenic and cause such reaction. It is available in vials as a lypholized, purified powder. The contents of the vial (800,000 units) are dissolved in 2 ml. of sterile water and administered intramuscularly and at times intravenously. The powder is stable at room temperature, but solutions must be refrigerated and should be discarded after one week.

Preparation

Penicillinase Injection	Neutrapen
Vials containing 800,000 units	1 unit neutralizes 1 unit of penicillin

Therapeutic Uses. Penicillin is the drug of choice in the following conditions, provided the organism is and remains sensitive to it:

1. Streptococcal and staphylococcal infections.
2. Many cases of pneumonia, with the exception of the virus types.
3. Tetanus, gas gangrene, and diphtheria, with full doses of antitoxin.

---- **Table 7** ----

Summary of Clinical Use of Antibiotics and the Sulfonamides

Micro-organism	Disease	Drugs of Choice
Streptococcus		
β-hemolytic	Various infections	Penicillin, erythromycin
α-hemolytic	Subacute bacterial endocarditis	Penicillin with streptomycin
anaerobic	Various infections	Penicillin with streptomycin
Staphylococcus	Pyogenic infections	Penicillin, erythromycin
Staph. aureus	Various infections	Penicillin, erythromycin, tetracycline, chloramphenicol
	Penicillinase producing	Methicillin, oxacillin, nafcillin, cloxacillin, cephalothin, vancomycin, and others based on sensitivity such as erythromycin, novobiocin, chloramphenicol, tetracycline and bacitracin
Pneumococcus	Lobar pneumonia; meningitis	Penicillin, erythromycin, tetracycline Penicillin, sulfonamides, erythromycin
Gonococcus	Gonorrhea	Penicillin, erythromycin, tetracycline
Meningococcus	Epidemic meningitis	Penicillin, sulfonamides, tetracycline
C. diphtheriae	Diphtheria, with antitoxin	Penicillin, erythromycin, tetracycline
B. anthracis	Anthrax	Penicillin, tetracycline, sulfonamides
Clostridium	Tetanus, with antitoxin	Penicillin, erythromycin
	Gas gangrene, with antitoxin	Penicillin, erythromycin
E. coli	Various infections	Tetracyclines, sulfonamides, chloramphenicol, polymixin B, cephalothin
Proteus	Urinary tract infections	Kanamycin, neomycin, chloramphenicol (penicillin for *P. mirabilis*), cephalothin
Ps. aeruginosa	Urinary tract infections	Polymixin B or colisthimethate
A. aerogenes	Urinary tract infections	Tetracycline with streptomycin, chloramphenicol, polymixin B or cephalothin
K. pneumoniae	Friedländer's pneumonia	Tetracycline with streptomycin, chloramphenicol, polymixin B, cephalothin, or colisthimate
H. influenza	Meningitis	Tetracycline, chloramphenicol, ampicillin, cephalothin
H. pertussis	Whooping cough	Tetracycline, chloramphenicol, streptomycin with sulfonamides
S. typhi	Typhoid fever	Chloramphenicol
S. paratyphi	Paratyphoid fever	Chloramphenicol
Shigella	Bacillary dysentery	Sulfonamides, tetracycline, chloramphenicol, oral neomycin
V. cholerae	Cholera	Sulfonamides, penicillin
Brucella	Brucellosis	Tetracycline with streptomycin, chloramphenicol
P. pestis	Plague	Streptomycin, sulfonamides
P. tularensis	Tularemia	Tetracyclines, streptomycin
H. ducreyi	Chancroid	Tetracycline, sulfonamides, streptomycin
T. pallidum	Syphilis	Penicillin, erythromycin, tetracycline

108

─────────── **Table 7** (*continued*) ───────────

Summary of Clinical Use of Antibiotics and the Sulfonamides

Micro-organism	Disease	Drugs of Choice
T. pertenue	Yaws	Penicillin, tetracycline
Leptospira	Weil's disease	Penicillin, tetracycline
Borrelia	Vincent's angina	Penicillin, tetracycline
M. tuberculosis	Tuberculosis	Streptomycin
M. leprae	Leprosy	Streptomycin
Actinomyces	Actinomycosis	Penicillin with tetracycline, sulfonamides
Rickettsiae	Typhus and related fevers	Tetracycline, chloramphenicol
Viruses	Psittacosis and ornithosis	Tetracycline, chloramphenicol
	Lymphogranuloma inguinale	Tetracycline, chloramphenicol, penicillin
	Primary atypical pneumonia	Tetracycline
	Herpes zoster	Tetracycline
	Trachoma	Tetracycline
E. histolytica	Amebiasis	Tetracycline
D. granulomatosis	Granuloma inguinale	Streptomycin, tetracycline, sulfonamides
Candida	Moniliasis	Amphotericin B, nystatin
Blastomyces		Amphotericin B
Cryptococcus	Cryptococcosis	Amphotericin B
Coccidioides	Coccidioidomycosis	Amphotericin B
H. capsulatum	Histoplasmosis	Amphotericin B
Microsporum	Ringworm	Griseofulvin
Trichophyton	Trichophytosis	Griseofulvin

4. Anthrax infections, even after bacteremia.

5. Syphilis.

6. Gonorrhea.

7. Subacute bacterial endocarditis (penicillin-susceptible organisms). Controlling the infection prevents destructive myocardial changes, which are responsible for the high mortality.

8. Prophylactically in persons who have rheumatic fever to prevent upper respiratory infections.

9. Yaws.

10. Urinary tract infections produced by *E. coli* or *Proteus mirabilis*.

11. Gram-negative infections caused by organisms sensitive to ampicillin.

Dosage and Methods of Administration.   Adequate blood concentrations of penicillin are necessary for the satisfactory control of systemic infections and to prevent the emergence of resistant strains of organisms. The microbiological laboratory can determine, with cultures from the patient, what blood levels should be maintained for treatment. Clinical judgment and responsiveness of the patient are also of vital importance in determining dosage. Doses for the various preparations are given on pages 111–16.

Penicillin is administered intramuscularly, intravenously, intrathecally, orally, sublingually, locally, or by inhalation.

Intramuscular Injections.   Aqueous solutions of sodium or potassium penicillin G (sterile crystalline buffered salts) are administered intramuscularly to produce rapid effects. For prolonged action, procaine penicillin G, benzathine penicillin G, or combinations of these preparations, with or without sodium or potassium penicillin G, are injected.

Intravenous Administration.   For rapid action, either sodium or potassium penicillin G is dissolved in water for injection, isotonic salt solution, or 5 per cent dextrose solution, and is injected intravenously.

Continuous intravenous infusion has been employed in severe infections, and penicillin is administered in these cases as a solution containing 25 to 50 units per milliliter at the rate of 5000 to 10,000 units every hour. The total daily dose may be 1 million to 50 million units. Table 8 shows the blood levels obtained with continuous intravenous infusion of penicillin G sodium at various doses, and the organisms susceptible at these levels. The latter relationships vary considerably, even within a given species.

Intrathecal Administration.   Penicillin does not appreciably penetrate the subarachnoid space; therefore, in meningitis, 10,000 units in a concentration not exceeding 1000 units per milliliter may be injected intrathecally. This method is usually avoided, as penicillin is irritating to the tissues of the central nervous system.

Oral and Sublingual Administration.   Oral administration of penicillin requires from five to six times the dose recommended for parenteral administration. It should be given between meals, buffered with an antacid or in the form of aluminum penicillin G or benzathine penicillin G. This method of administration has recently gained much favor, since the drug is rapidly absorbed and very large doses may be taken readily. Soluble tablets of penicillin G without excipient or binders are available for use as aerosols. They may also be used in pediatrics to be mixed with the children's formulas and may be administered sublingually to patients who cannot swallow the larger tablets.

Local Administration.   "The use of penicillin topically in troches, lozenges, ointments, and aerosols should be abandoned completely because of the frequency with which sensitization is produced. All necessary penicillin medications should be given orally whenever possible."[1]

Advantages of the Use of Penicillin.   Penicillin is one of our most

---

[1] Hewitt, W. L.: "The Penicillins," *J.A.M.A.*, **185**:264, 1963.

━━━━━━━━━━━━━━━ **Table 8** ━━━━━━━━━━━━━━━

The Relationship Between the Amount of Penicillin Administered Daily by Continuous Intravenous Infusion, the Resulting Level of the Antibiotic in the Blood, and the Organisms Likely to Be Poisoned at Various Levels *

Total Dose of Penicillin in Units per Day by Continuous Intravenous Infusion	Amount of Penicillin in Units per Milliliter of Blood Serum	Some Organisms Likely to Be Poisoned at the Blood Level Achieved
200,000	0.2	Neisseria gonorrhoeae and N. meningitidis, Streptococcus pyogenes, Staphylococcus aureus, Bacillus anthracis, Clostridium tetani, Cl. welchii
1,000,000	0.9	The above + Corynebacterium diphtheriae, Streptococcus pneumoniae, Str. viridans
10,000,000	9.2	All the above + Proteus vulgaris, Salmonella typhi, Brucella abortus

* Modified from Collier, H. O. J.: *Chemotherapy of Infections.* Chapman & Hall, Ltd., London, 1954; John Wiley & Sons, Inc., New York, 1954.

important antibiotics. Since it is bactericidal it may eradicate infections in certain diseases when our defense mechanisms are not operating efficiently. It is 1000 times more potent than the sulfonamides and thus the dose can be 1000 times smaller. It is nontoxic, its efficiency is high, and the injectable forms are now quite inexpensive to the physician and the hospital. Oral forms are available for many types of infections. The newer penicillins, sodium methicillin and sodium oxacillin, are useful in the treatment of penicillin G-resistant staphylococcal infections, while ampicillin is effective against both gram-negative and gram-positive microorganisms.

Penicillin Preparations

Potassium Penicillin G, U.S.P. This is the form most widely used in clinical medicine. A number of salts and preparations having different solubilities and rates of absorption and duration of action are available.

Potassium Penicillin G (Sterile), U.S.P. Aqueous solution of potassium or sodium penicillin G (sterile) may be administered intramuscularly or intravenously. The drug is rapidly absorbed and produces high levels which fall rapidly. Doses should be repeated every three to four hours to maintain therapeutic levels in the blood and tissues.

The intramuscular dose is 400,000 U.S.P. Units (300,000 to 2,000,000 units) four times a day. The intravenous dose is 10 million U.S.P. Units (6 to 40 million units) daily. In severe infections as much as 50 to 100 million units may be administered by intravenous drip or by injection of divided doses every three or four hours. This amount may be necessary for patients with overwhelming infections such as meningitis, bacterial endocarditis caused by enterococci or resistant streptococci, and gram-negative bacillary bacteremias resistant to other drugs. Streptomycin should be used with penicillin in endocarditis.

Preparations

Potassium Penicillin G, U.S.P. Sodium Penicillin G, N.F.	Vials containing 100,000, 300,000, 400,000, 500,000, and 1 million U.S.P. Units
Buffered Potassium Penicillin G for Injection, U.S.P (buffered with Sodium Citrate)	Vials containing 500,000, 1, and 5 million units
Benzylpenicillin Injection, B.P.	150 mg. in 1 ml.

The U.S.P. gives the doses for penicillin G in units. The B.P. expresses the dose in milligrams. The approximate equivalents are as follows: 300,000 units—200 mg.; 400,000 units—250 mg.; and 1 million units—600 mg.

The usual oral or sublingual dose of penicillin G is 400,000 U.S.P. Units (200,000 to 2 million units) four times a day.

Preparations

Potassium Penicillin G Tablets, U.S.P.	50,000, 100,000, 200,000, 250,000, and 500,000 U.S.P. Units
Benzylpenicillin Tablets, B.P.	

Trade names: Cilloral; Confets, Orapen; Pentids; Penioral

Soluble Tablets Penicillin G	50,000 and 100,000 units

Trade names: Hyabsorb; Jacilin; Nebutabs; Penalev; PSL; R.D. Dis-Pen-Tabs; R.D. Pentabs; Solutabs; Til-Pen

PROLONGED-ACTING PENICILLIN G SALTS OR REPOSITORY FORMS

Penicillin is more slowly absorbed when its sparingly soluble salts, such as procaine penicillin G in aqueous suspension or oil, and benzathine penicillin G, are administered intramuscularly. A depot is formed in the tissues from which penicillin is slowly liberated. Therapeutic concentrations are obtained in the blood and tissues in one to three hours after injection and are maintained for 20 to 240 hours with these depot (repository) preparations. Dosage forms containing a combination of crystalline penicillin G with either procaine penicillin G or benzathine penicillin G are available if both rapid and prolonged effects are desirable.

Procaine Penicillin G, U.S.P., B.P.   Procaine penicillin G is a combination of procaine and penicillin which is quite insoluble in water. It is suspended usually in water and sometimes in oil. When the suspensions are injected intramuscularly, the absorption of penicillin into the blood is prolonged so that injections every 12 to 24 hours are adequate. The addition of 2 per cent aluminum monostearate to the oil suspension of procaine penicillin prolongs its activity to 60 hours.

The intramuscular dose of procaine penicillin G is 300,000 U.S.P. Units (300,000 to 1,200,000 units) once or twice a day.

Preparations

Sterile Procaine Penicillin G Suspension, U.S.P.

300,000 and 600,000 U.S.P. Units in 1 ml. and 3 million units in 10 ml.

Procaine Penicillin Injection, B.P.

Trade names: Abbocillin DC; Aquacillin; Aquasuspension G; Crysticillin; Diurnal; Dorsallin "AR"; Duracillin; Flo-Cillin; Hypercillin; Parencillin; Plasmacillin; Premocillin; Sharcillin; Til-Cillin; Wycillin

Sterile Procaine Penicillin G, with Aluminum Stearate Suspension, U.S.P.

300,000 U.S.P. Units in 1 ml. and 3 million units in 10 ml.

Trade names: Depo-Penicillin; Duracillin in Oil; Flo-Cillin "96"; Hypercillin Prolonged; Ledercillin; Lentopen; Millicillin; Monocillin; Pazillin

Sterile Procaine Penicillin G and Buffered Penicillin G for Suspension, N.F.

400,000, 2 and 4 million U.S.P. Units in 1-, 5-, and 10-dose vials

Fortified Procaine Penicillin Injection, B.P.

Trade names: Abbocillin 800; Aquapropen; Bi-Pen; Crystifor 400; Crystifor 800; Crystifor 1200; Diurnal Fortified 400M; Dorsallin-400; Eldi-Pen; Flo-Cillin "96" Fortified; Forticillin; Homocillin; Ledercillin; Magnacillin; Myropen; Parencillin Fortified; Pen Aqua Fortified; Sharcillin Fortified; Wycillin Fortified; Penicillin S-R

Procaine Penicillin in Oil Injection, N.F.   I.M. 300,000 units

Trade names: Readicillin; Til-Cillin in Oil

Benzathine Penicillin G, U.S.P., B.P. (Bicillin).   Benzathine penicillin G is a modified form with prolonged activity. It consists of two molecules of penicillin combined with dibenzylethylenediamine (an antihistaminic). The compound has no odor or taste. It is stable in aqueous suspension at room temperature and produces a prolonged action when injected intramuscularly or ingested orally. One injection (600,000 units) maintains a detectable blood concentration for several days to two weeks. One injection of 2.4 million units produces cures in syphilis and other infectious diseases. Like procaine penicillin, it has a local anesthetic effect. The incidence of hypersensitivity is low.

High blood levels are not obtained with these aqueous preparations because of the low solubility of benzathine penicillin G in water, but low concentrations may be provided over long periods of time. It is therefore useful as a prophylactic agent against streptococcal infections in rheumatic fever patients and in the treatment of syphilis. This long-acting penicillin may be fortified by the addition of procaine penicillin G and/or potassium penicillin G if higher concentrations are desired.

The intramuscular dose is 600,000 U.S.P. Units (300,000 to 3,000,000 units), repeated as necessary.

Preparations

Sterile Benzathine Penicillin G Suspension, U.S.P.	600,000 U.S.P. Units in 1 ml.; 900,000 units in 1.5 ml.; 1.2 million units in 2 ml., 2.4 million units in 4 ml., and
Benzathine Penicillin G (Sterile), B.P.	3 million units in 10 ml.

Trade names: Bicillin; Duapen; Neolin; Penadur; Permapen

Procaine Penicillin G and Benzathine Penicillin G

Trade names: Permopen Fortified in Aqueous Suspension

Procaine Penicillin B, Benzathine Penicillin G and Potassium Penicillin G

Trade names: Bicillin All-Purpose, Panbiotic, Pronapen Plus

Phenoxymethyl Penicillin (Penicillin V) N.F., B.P. This antibiotic is acid resistant and therefore passes through the stomach unchanged. It is insoluble in acid solution but soluble in alkaline medium and hence dissolves in the alkaline medium of the small intestine and is well absorbed. As a result, higher blood levels are obtained with the oral administration of phenoxymethyl penicillin than with comparable amounts of penicillin G administered orally. Unless it is administered in higher doses, phenoxymethyl penicillin is not so effective as parenterally administered penicillin G. The antibacterial spectrum, therapeutic uses, and untoward effects are the same as those for penicillin G. Oral doses of 125 to 250 mg. are administered four times a day.

Preparations

Phenoxymethyl Penicillin Capsules, N.F.	125 and 250 mg.
For Oral Suspension, N.F.	1 Gm. in 40-ml., 2 Gm. in 80-ml., 3 Gm. in 60-ml. containers
Tablets, N.F., B.P.	125 and 250 mg.

Trade names: Penicillin V; Pen-Vee, Dural; Icipen; V-Cillin

Potassium Phenoxymethyl Penicillin, U.S.P. This preparation, when administered orally, is effective more rapidly and produces higher blood levels than the free acid. It is available as tablets containing 125 and 250 mg.

SEMISYNTHETIC PENICILLINS

Potassium Phenethicillin, N.F. (Alpen; Broxil, Chemipen; Darcil, Maxipen, Penicillin B, Syncillin). This penicillin is active upon oral administration against strains of staphylococci that are resistant to other penicillins. The oral dose is 125 or 250 mg. (up to 500 mg.) three times a day. Tablets of 125 and 250 mg. are available.

Sodium Methicillin, U.S.P., Methicillin Sodium, B.P. (Staphcillin, Celbenin, Dimocillin), is effective against staphylococci regardless of the amount of penicillinase produced by these organisms. In contrast, phenethicillin is inactivated slowly by penicillinase. Methicillin appears to have no advantages over the older penicillins in the treatment of infections other than those caused by penicillinase-producing staphylococci. Therefore, it should be reserved for hospital use for severe penicillin G–resistant staphylococcal infections. Methicillin should not be used for routine bacterial infections for which older oral or parenteral penicillins are effective. The intramuscular or intravenous dose is 1 Gm. every four to six hours.

Preparation

Sodium Methicillin for Injection, U.S.P.   Vials containing 1, 4, and 6 Gm.

Trade names: Celbenin, Dimocillin, Staphcillin

Sodium Nafcillin (Unipen) is recommended mainly for the treatment of severe infections caused by staphylococci resistant to penicillin G. It is readily soluble and is administered orally or parenterally. Untoward reactions such as skin rash, pruritus, and possibly drug fever have been infrequent and mild in nature. In severe infections the intravenous dose is 500 mg. to 1 Gm. every four hours. The calculated dose may be dissolved in 15 to 30 ml. of sterile distilled water or sterile normal saline and injected over a 5- to 10-minute period through the tubing of an intravenous infusion fluid, or the drug may be dissolved in 100 to 150 ml. and given by intravenous drip at the rate of 100 to 150 drops per minute for no longer than 24 to 48 hours because of the possible occurrence of thrombophlebitis, particularly in the elderly. The intramuscular dose is 500 mg. every four to six hours. The oral dose in mild to moderate infections is 250 to 500 mg. every four to six hours; in severe infections, 1 Gm. every four to six hours, preferably one to two hours before meals.

Preparations

Nafcillin Capsules   250 mg.
Nafcillin Injection   Vials containing 500 mg.

Trade name: Unipen

Sodium Oxacillin, U.S.P. (Prostaphlin, Resistopen) is effective upon oral administration in the treatment of infections caused by resistant staphylococci. It is stable to acid hydrolysis and rapidly absorbed from the gastrointestinal tract. It is well tolerated, although allergic reactions such as those observed with other penicillins may occur occasionally. Its use should be limited to the treatment of staphylococcal infections resistant to penicillin G. The oral dose is 500 mg. every four to six hours for mild to moderate infections of the skin and soft tissues or upper respiratory tract. For septicemias or other severe infections, 1 Gm. every four to six hours may be necessary. The intramuscular dose is one-half of the oral dose.

Preparations

Sodium Oxacillin Capsules, U.S.P.	125, 250, and 500 mg.
Sodium Oxacillin Tablets	250 mg.
Sodium Oxacillin Injection	

Trade names: Prostaphlin, Resistopen

Cloxacillin (Orbenin) is the penicillin of choice in the treatment of infections caused by staphylococci resistant to penicillin G. It is more active than methicillin and oxacillin and is better absorbed. The oral dose is 500 mg. every six hours one hour before meals. If the oral dose is inadequate, it may be given intramuscularly. The intramuscular dose is 250 mg. every four to six hours.

Ampicillin (Penbritin, Polycillin), a new broad-spectrum penicillin, is active against gram-positive organisms but is destroyed by penicillinase and so is not effective against penicillin G–resistant staphylococci. However, it is effective against gram-negative organisms, particularly the *Salmonella, Escherichia coli, Shigella,* and *Hemophilus influenzae.* Some strains of *Proteus* are sensitive, while others prove resistant. Ampicillin and other penicillins are bactericidal in contrast to the other broad-spectrum antibiotics, which are bacteriostatic. Urticarial rashes, loose stools, and *Candida* superinfections have been observed in a few cases.

Therapeutic Uses and Dosage. Ampicillin is used in infections caused by both gram-positive and gram-negative organisms. The most important uses are in the treatment of tetracycline-resistant coliform bacteria or strains of *Proteus,* especially *Proteus mirabilis,* diarrheal conditions due to *Salmonella* (including typhoid fever) and *Shigella,* and meningitis caused by *Hemophilis influenzae.*

The dose, which is administered orally, depends upon the severity of the infection. For gram-positive infections, 250 mg. are given every six hours; for gram-negative infections, 1.5 and 2.25 Gm. in divided doses are recommended over a period of 24 hours. Since the drug is highly concentrated in the urine, 250 mg. every six hours should be sufficient in urinary infections. It is relatively ineffective in gastrointestinal infections.

Preparation

Ampicillin Capsules	250 mg.

Trade names: Penbritin, Polycillin

Cephalosporins

The cephalosporins are a fermentation product of fungi, the *cephalosporium*.

1. Cephalosporin N, identical with Synnematin B, is active mainly against gram-negative organisms. It has been used successfully in the treatment of typhoid fever (see pp. 145, 146).

2. Cephalosporin P has a steroid structure and is related to fucidin.

3. Cephalosporin C, useful in the treatment of resistant staphylococcic and coliform infections, is closely related to the penicillins. Its nucleus, 7-amino-cephalosporanic acid (7-ACA), is similar to although larger than that of 6-aminopenicillanic acid. It contains a 6-membered sulfur ring in contrast to the 5-membered ring of penicillanic acid. By addition of side chains to this nucleus by synthetic manipulation similar to that applied to the penicillin nucleus, about 600 derivatives have been prepared. In this manner improved yields and compounds with greater activity have been obtained. Cephalothin is an alternative to penicillins for resistant staphylococci and a rival to ampicillin and other antibiotics for coliform infections.

Cephalothin (Keflin), a semisynthetic antibiotic, is prepared by adding a side chain to the nucleus of cephalosporin C. It is bactericidal against some gram-positive and gram-negative bacilli; streptococci, pneumococci, and all strains of *staphylococcus aureus,* including those producing penicillinase, are highly susceptible and develop resistance very slowly. A majority of the strains of *Klebsiella, H. influenza, E. coli, Aerobacter, Proteus, Salmonella,* and *Shigella* are sensitive to concentrations of cephalothin that can be attained in either the serum or the urine.

Bactericidal activity against gram-positive and gram-negative organisms is seen in concentrations slightly greater than required for bacteriostatic action. It, like penicillin, selectively inhibits bacterial cell wall synthesis leading to morphological changes in the bacteria. The mechanism of this action is unknown.

Cephalothin is not absorbed upon oral administration and is injected intramuscularly or intravenously. Peak levels are attained within one-half hour following intramuscular injection, and the action lasts for six hours. The drug is rapidly excreted in the urine in which antibacterial concentrations are high.

Side Effects.   Untoward reactions such as neutropenia, allergy, maculopapular rash, and hives occur infrequently. Superinfections have not been noted. In patients with allergy, particularly drug allergy, the drug should be used only when absolutely necessary and then only with extreme caution.

Therapeutic Uses.   The drug is indicated in infections of the respiratory, urinary, or gastrointestinal tracts, and of soft tissue and skin, and in osteomyelitis and septicemia caused by coagulase-positive staphylococci and gram-negative bacteremias due to colon bacillus and *Proteus. Pseudomonas* and enterococci (*Strep. faecalis*) are said to be resistant. It is of particular value in treating infections in patients with impaired renal function, a condition in which many other antibiotics would be undesirable.

Methods of Administration and Dosage. Cephalothin is injected deeply in a large muscle, in doses no greater than 500 mg., to minimize pain and induration. The usual intramuscular dosage range is 500 mg. to 1 Gm. every four to six hours. A dosage of 500 mg. every six hours is adequate for uncomplicated pneumonia, furunculosis with cellulitis, and most urinary infections. In severe infections the dosage may be increased by giving the drug every four hours or raising the dose to 1 Gm. The intravenous dose is the same as the intramuscular dose, i.e., 2 to 6 Gm. daily. This method of administration is necessary when patients with bacteremia or septicemia are poor risks because of lowered resistance (resulting from debilitating conditions, such as malnutrition, trauma, surgery, diabetes, heart failure, or malignancy, particularly if shock is present or impending). It may be given by intermittent or continuous infusion. The drug is dissolved in 5 per cent dextrose or normal salt solution and injected directly into the veins or through tubing when the patient is receiving parenteral fluids.

Preparation of Solution. Each gram is diluted with 4 ml. of Sterile Water for Injection. The reconstituted material will provide two 500-mg. doses of 2.2 ml. each. Solutions should be stored in the refrigerator and should not be used after 48 hours. A precipitate which may form can be redissolved with warming. During storage color may change from pale straw to brown without significant loss of potency.

Preparation

Cephalothin as sodium salt   1 Gm. in rubber-stoppered ampul
Trade name: Keflin

SYPHILOTHERAPY

Prior to the introduction of penicillin in the treatment of syphilis, the chemotherapy of this disease consisted of prolonged administration of organic arsenicals, such as arsphenamine, neoarsphenamine, oxophenarsine, and sulfarsphenamine, in alternating combinations with a preparation of bismuth. Since antibiotics have proved to be of such great value in syphilotherapy, all other methods of therapy have been discontinued.

SYPHILIS

Syphilis is a chronic relapsing disease caused by *Treponema pallidum*, a spirochete. It is always a systemic infection and, if untreated, may cause involvement of the brain, heart, or bones, or destructive lesions in the skin. Early diagnosis and treatment are essential. With the introduction of antibiotics in the management of this systemic disease, its incidence was greatly reduced, almost to the point of eradication, by 1954. However, treatment of the syphilitic patient in the early stages without examining his or her contacts does little to control the disease. Since 1957, there has been an alarming increase in the occurrence of infectious syphilis. Conservative estimates place the total number of new infectious cases annually at 100,000.[2] Early reporting of such cases with interviews and investigation of contacts by trained persons to afford these infected contacts early treatment is necessary if the present increase in syphilis is to be reduced and controlled.

Penicillin, tetracycline, chloramphenicol, and erythromycin are spirocheticidal drugs. Penicillin is the antibiotic of choice because of its potency against the *Treponema,* ease of administration, and lower cost. In patients sensitive to penicillin two alternate antibiotics, erythromycin and tetracycline, are recommended.[3]

PENICILLIN FOR SYPHILIS

Dosage Schedules for Penicillin. There are three dosage forms of penicillin G used in the treatment of primary and secondary syphilis:

1. Benzathine penicillin G: 2.4 million units total (1.2 million units in each buttock) intramuscularly or

2. Procaine penicillin G in oil with 2 per cent aluminum monostearate (PAM): 4.8 million units usually given 2.4 million units at first session as above and 1.2 million units at each of two subsequent injections three days apart or

3. Aqueous procaine penicillin G: 600,000 units daily for eight days to a total of 4.8 million units or

Alternate antibiotics, if penicillin sensitivity precludes its use, are 20 to 30 Gm. of erythromycin or 30 to 40 Gm. of tetracycline given orally over a period of 10 to 15 days.

Somewhat higher doses and longer periods of treatment are required in (1) some later complications of the disease, especially neurosyphilis; (2) syphilis during the last three months of pregnancy; and (3) congenital syphilis.

Prophylactic (Abortive) Use of Penicillin. After sexual contact with cases known to have infectious early syphilis, a single intramuscular injection of 2.4 million units of benzathine penicillin G or PAM is adequate to abort infection in most individuals who would otherwise contract the disease.

A large majority of the patients receive enough penicillin to render them noninfectious for long periods of time or perhaps permanently, if reinfection does not occur.

---

[2] *Social Health News,* November, 1963.
[3] *Notes on Modern Management of VD.* Public Health Service Publication No. 859, p. 3, reprinted 1962.

GONORRHEA AND ITS TREATMENT

Gonorrhea, another communicable and infectious disease, is transmitted almost exclusively by sexual intercourse. It occurs about ten times more frequently than syphilis. Conservative estimates place the total number of new cases at 1 million annually. The most essential factor in its management and control is the simultaneous treatment of marital partners and/or regular sexual contacts.

The drug of choice for the treatment of gonorrhea is penicillin. Aqueous procaine penicillin G, procaine penicillin G in oil with 2 per cent aluminum monostearate (PAM), or benzathine penicillin G is given in doses of 1.2 million units intramuscularly for prophylactic treatment or for uncomplicated gonorrhea in men. For women or in patients with severe complications larger doses are required.

Some strains of gonococci have shown decreased susceptibility to penicillin but not absolute resistance. Gonorrhea patients sensitive to penicillin may be treated effectively with streptomycin, one of the tetracyclines, chloramphenicol, erythromycin, or oleandomycin.

PENICILLIN SUBSTITUTES

Erythromycin and a number of antibiotics produced by *Streptomyces* closely resemble the action of penicillin on various microorganisms. They are less potent but are important clinically because they may be used as alternates to penicillin in infections resistant to penicillin or in patients who are sensitive to that antibiotic. Erythromycin is the most widely used of this group.

Erythromycin, U.S.P., B.P. (Erythrocin, Ilotycin, Ilosone)

Erythromycin is an antibiotic obtained from a strain of *Streptomyces erythreus*. It forms salts with organic acids that are slightly soluble in water. It is stable in the dry form.

Antibiotic Spectrum. Erythromycin is active against gram-positive bacteria, gonococci, spirochetes, the rickettsiae, the organism causing whooping cough, and some larger viruses. It has little or no action against gram-negative organisms. Its activity closely resembles that of penicillin. It is useful in infections in which the organisms have become resistant to penicillin and in persons allergic to penicillin.

Some strains of bacteria, particularly staphylococci, develop resistance to erythromycin, but as a rule resistance to this drug is rare. No cross-resistance exists between erythromycin and penicillin on the one hand and the broad-spectrum antibiotics on the other, a fortunate situation. Among antibiotics, erythromycin has the advantage that it will be effective after others have failed. Thus it has been urged that this agent be reserved for severe cases.[4]

Absorption, Distribution, and Excretion. Erythromycin is readily absorbed from the gastrointestinal tract. It is distributed in the tissues of the body but is concentrated in the liver and bile. It is also found in the adrenals, lungs, kidneys, muscle, and spleen. It circulates freely in the fetal blood and passes into the pleural and abdomial (ascitic) fluids but does not readily diffuse into the spinal fluid. It is excreted in the urine and the feces.

Side Actions Doses large than 500 mg. may cause nausea, vomiting, and diarrhea. Jaundice has been reported on rare occasions.

Dosage and Methods of Administration. Erythromycin is usually administered orally or intravenously. The usual oral dose of the base is 250 mg. every six hours. The intravenous dose is 250 mg. of the base as a 0.1 per cent solution every six hours. The usual dose range for oral or intravenous administration is 1 to 2 Gm.

Therapeutic Uses

1. Primarily in staphylococcal infections resistant to penicillin G.

2. In infections caused by streptococci, staphylococci, pneumococci, and enterococci.

3. In syphilis and gonorrhea.

4. In acute and chronic amebiasis.

Preparations

Erythromycin or several of its salts are used for preparing suspensions or tablets for oral administration. Erythromycin Estolate, B.P. (Ilosone), is more stable in acid than the other oral forms and can be given with food. It produces more rapid, higher, and more prolonged blood levels. It may produce hepatitis. Since this form is tasteless it is prepared for pediatric use.

Erythromycin Estolate, B.P.	5 mg. in 1 drop in 10-ml. dropping bottles
Erythromycin Estolate Oral Suspension	125 mg. in 1 ml.
Erythromycin Estolate Tablets	125 and 250 mg.

Trade name: Ilosone

Erythromycin Oral Suspension, U.S.P.	200 mg. in 5 ml.; 2.4 Gm. (dry) in 60-ml. container
Erythromycin Tablets, U.S.P., B.P.	100 and 250 mg.
Erythromycin Ethylcarbonate, U.S.P.	1 Gm. in dry flavored mixture; when mixed in suspension, 100 mg. in 1 ml.
Erythromycin Propionate Capsules	125 and 250 mg.
Erythromycin Stearate, U.S.P.	

Trade names: Erythrocin; Ilotycin

---

[4] "Restriction of Antibiotics" (editorial), *Lancet,* **2**:193, 1956.

Erythromycin for Injection, U.S.P., is a sterile dry mixture of the gluceptate, the lactobionate, or other suitable salt or ester such as the propionate and a suitable buffer from which solutions may be prepared for parenteral administration.

Erythromycin for Injection, U.S.P.	250, 300, 500 mg., and 1 Gm.
Erythromycin Gluceptate, U.S.P. ⎫ Erythromycin Lactobionate, U.S.P. ⎭	Ampuls containing 250 or 500 mg. or 1 Gm. of the base

Oleandomycin (Matromycin)

Oleandomycin, isolated from cultures of *Streptomyces antibioticus,* is chemically related to erythromycin. It has now been replaced in medicine by triacetyloleandomycin.

Triacetyloleandomycin, N.F., is rapidly absorbed upon oral administration and produces high levels in the blood stream and urine. It is effective against a wide variety of gram-positive and gram-negative organisms, the rickettsiae, large viruses, and amebae. Many strains of staphylococci resistant to streptomycin, penicillin, erythromycin, and the tetracyclines are susceptible to this antibiotic. Resistance does not readily occur.

Allergic reactions are infrequent and seldom severe although those of the anaphylactoid type have occurred on rare occasions. The use of this drug may result in overgrowth of nonsusceptible organisms, particularly monilia. Abnormalities in liver function have been reported following two weeks or more of continuous therapy. Jaundice has been observed infrequently.

The drug is used primarily in staphylococcal infections resistant to penicillin. The oral adult dose is 250 to 500 mg. four times a day depending upon the severity of the infection. The dose for children is 125 to 250 mg. four times a day.

Preparations

Triacetyloleandomycin Capsules, N.F.	125 and 250 mg.
Triacetyloleandomycin Suspension	125 mg. in 5 ml.

Trade names: Cyclamycin, TAO

Novobiocin (Albamycin, Cathomycin)

Novobiocin is obtained form cultures of *Streptomyces spheroides.* It is absorbed rapidly by mouth and is widely distributed in the body. It is excreted in the urine and the bile. The toxic reactions are skin rashes, urticaria, fever, and leukopenia. It is moderately effective against penicillin-resistant infections. Novobiocin is available as the calcium and sodium salts. The usual oral dose of these salts is the equivalent of 250 mg. novobiocin acid every six hours. The usual dose range is 1 to 2 Gm. of the acid daily. This drug was formerly used in the treatment of resistant staphylococcal infections but is now largely replaced by vancomycin.

Preparations

Calcium Novobiocin Oral Suspension, N.F.	Approximately 2.5 Gm. of the free acid in 100 ml.
Sodium Novobiocin Tablets, N.F.	250 mg.

Trade names: Albamycin, Cathomycin

ANTIBIOTICS EFFECTIVE IN COMBATING STAPHYLOCOCCI RESISTANT TO OTHER ANTIBIOTICS

In recent years medical centers throughout the world have reported a marked increase in the incidence and spread of pathogenic penicillinase-producing and penicillin-resistant strains of staphylococci and other bacteria. A temporary solution to this problem was achieved with the introduction of streptomycin, chloramphenicol, the tetracyclines, erythromycin, and other antibiotics; however, resistance to these drugs has also occurred after extensive hospital use.

Three new antibiotics—vancomycin, ristocetin, and kanamycin—have proved effective in combating staphylococci resistant to other commonly used drugs. They are especially valuable in the treatment of severe infections in children.

Vancomycin, B.P. (Vancocin)

Vancomycin is elaborated by growing cultures of *Streptomyces orientalis*. It is bactericidal at low concentrations and is active primarily against gram-positive bacteria, particularly staphylococci. Resistance is slow to develop. The clinical material now available is better tolerated and produces very few side effects.

There is little absorption of the antibiotic from the gastrointestinal tract, but relatively high and prolonged serum concentrations are attained after intravenous administration. For systemic infections caused by vancomycin-susceptible organisms, it is administered intravenously. The intravenous dose is 500 mg. at six-hour intervals.

Therapeutic Uses. Vancomycin is probably the best drug available for severe staphylococcal infections caused by penicillin-resistant organisms. It it especially useful in severe infections occurring in children.

Preparation

Vancomycin Hydrochloride (Sterile), U.S.P.	500 mg.

Trade name: Vancocin

Ristocetin, U.S.P. (Spontin)

Ristocetin is obtained from the fermentation of *Nocardia lurida*, a species in the family *Actinomycetaceae*. The antibiotic is a mixture of two components, ristocetins A and B. It is effective against pathological gram-positive cocci and is bactericidal in about the same concentrations at which it is bacteriostatic.

Side Effects. Leukopenia and neutropenia have been reported. Drug fever, skin eruptions, diarrhea, and local *phlebothrombosis* occur.

Therapeutic Uses. Ristocetin is useful in treating severe staphylococcal and enterococcal infections. Resistance to ristocetin may develop.

The intravenous dose is 1 Gm. twice a day. This drug is rarely used now.

Preparation

Sterile Ristocetin, U.S.P.   500 mg.

Trade name: Spontin

Kanamycin, U.S.P. (Kantrex, Kannasyn)

Kanamycin, an antibiotic that is related chemically to neomycin, is obtained from *Streptomyces kanamyceticus*. It is active against a wide variety of gram-positive, gram-negative, and acid-fast organisms. Resistance appears to develop slowly with the staphylococcus but rapidly with the tubercle bacillus.

Kanamycin is not absorbed from the gastrointestinal tract. However, it is readily absorbed when injected intramuscularly, and high concentrations appear in the blood in one hour and peak concentrations in two hours.

Side Effects. Oral administration is well tolerated, even when large doses are employed. Diarrhea has been observed infrequently. With intramuscular injection the side effects observed thus far have been mild or moderate. Sensitization, drug fever, and rashes rarely occur. The major toxic effects are on the kidney and the eighth cranial nerve.

Dosage and Methods of Administration. The oral dose is 3 to 4 Gm. daily, in divided amounts. The daily intramuscular dose for adults is 1 to 2 Gm.; the daily intramuscular dose for children is 15 to 30 mg. per kilogram of body weight, administered in two to four equally divided amounts.

Therapeutic Uses. Kanamycin is of particular value in the treatment of staphylococcal infections, including severe cases and those resistant to other antiboitics (especially penicillin, streptomycin, and the tetracyclines). It is effective in combating male gonorrhea, severe anthrax infections, and acute and chronic infections of the urinary tract. It is one of the most effective intestinal antiseptics available. Some favorable results have been attained in severe chronic and resistant cases of tuberculosis, but tolerance to kanamycin is rapidly acquired by the offending organism.

Preparations

Kanamycin Capsules, U.S.P.	500 mg.
Kanamycin Injection, U.S.P.	500 mg. in 2 ml. and 1 Gm. in 3 ml.

Trade names: Kantrex; Kannasyn

REVIEW QUESTIONS

1. *Define antibiosis.*
2. *How are antibiotics prepared?*
3. *How is the potency of penicillin expressed?*
4. *How is penicillin assayed?*
5. *In what ways are penicillins administered?*
6. *Explain the need and use of repository penicillins.*
7. *What are some of the problems that have arisen from the administration of penicillin?*
8. *Explain the mechanism by which penicillin exerts its antibacterial effects.*
9. *Give some of the important therapeutic uses of pencillin.*
10. *When the doctor has ordered the administration of penicillin to a patient, why is it vital for the nurse to be punctual with each dose?*
11. *When administering penicillin in an oral form, the nurse notes that the amount ordered is considerably different from the usual intramuscular dose. Compare the recommended daily doses of oral penicillin G and aqueous solutions of sodium or potassium penicillin G for injection. What is the reason for this difference?*
12. *Name some of the serious disease conditions caused by antibiotic-resistant staphylococci.*
13. *Discuss the transmission of staphylococcal infections within the hospital.*
14. *Name some of the methods recommended to control the spread of these hospital infections.*
15. *What advantages have been obtained from the production of the new penicillins? Name two penicillins and give an important clinical use for each.*
16. *What drug is now available for the treatment of septicemias caused by certain gram-negative organisms? How is it administered?*
17. *What advantages were gained by the introduction of erythromycin in therapeutics?*
18. *Name three new antibiotics that are useful in treating infections caused by resistant strains of staphylococci. Give dosage and methods of administration for each antibiotic.*

REFERENCES

Anderson, D. G., and Keefer, C. S.: *The Therapeutic Value of Penicillin: A Study of 10,000 Cases.* J. W. Edwards, Publisher, Inc., Ann Arbor, Mich., 1948.

Collier, H. O. J.: *Chemotherapy of Infections.* Chapman & Hall, Ltd., London, 1954; John Wiley & Sons, Inc., New York, 1954.

Fleming, Sir A.: *Chemotherapy: Yesterday, Today and Tomorrow.* Cambridge University Press, London, 1946.

Fleming, Sir A.: *Penicillin: Its Practical Application.* C. V. Mosby Company, St. Louis, 1950.

Florey, Sir H. W. (ed.): *Antibiotics: A Survey of Penicillin, Streptomycin and Other Microbial Substances from Fungi, Actinomycetes, Bacteria and Other Plants.* Oxford University Press, London and New York, 1949.

————: "The Use of Microorganisms for Therapeutic Purposes," *Yale J. Biol. & Med.,* **19**:101, 1946.

Hewitt, W. L.: "The Penicillins," *J.A.M.A.,* **185**:264, 1963.

Hussar, A. E., and Holley, H. L.: *Antibiotics and Antibiotic Therapy.* The Macmillan Company, New York, 1954.

Longacre, A. B.: "A Report of Very Low Reactions Rate in Therapy with a New Penicillin Salt" (Compenamine), *Antibiotics & Chemother.,* **1**:223, 1951.

Marriott, H. J. L.: *Medical Milestones.* William & Wilkins Company, Baltimore, 1952.

Pratt, R., and Dufrenoy, J.: *Antibiotics,* 2nd ed. J. B. Lippincott Company, Philadelphia, 1953.

Smith, L. W., and Walker, A. D.: *Penicillin Decade, 1941–1951.* Arundel Press. Inc., Washington, D.C., 1951.

Sullivan, N. P.; Symmes, A. T.; Miller, H. C.; and Rhodehamel, H. W., Jr.: "A New Penicillin for Prolonged Blood Levels," *Science,* **107**:169, 1948.

Szabo, J. L.; Edwards, C. D.; and Bruce, W. F.: "N,N'-dibenzylethylenediamine Penicillin: Preparation and Properties," *Antibiotics & Chemother.,* **1**:499, 1951.

Welch, H.: "The Antibiotic Resistant Staphylococci" (editorial), *Antibiotics & Chemother.,* **3**:561, 1953.

————: "The Newest Addition to the Repository Penicillins (Dibenzylethylenediamine Dipenicillin)," *Antibiotics & Chemother.,* **3**:347, 1953.

————: "Phenoxymethyl Penicillin (Penicillin V)," *Antibiotic Med.,* **2**:11, 1956,

Welch, H., and Lewis, C. N.: *Antibiotic Therapy.* Arundel Press, Inc., Washington, D.C., 1951.

SEMISYNTHETIC PENICILLINS

Annotation: "The Penicillin Nucleus," *Brit. M. J.,* **1**:701, 1959.

Barber, Mary, and Chain, E. B.: "Antibacterial Chemotherapy; Semisynthetic Penicillins," *Ann. Rev. Pharmacol.,* **4**:115, 1964.

Barber, Mary, and Waterworth, P. M.: "Penicillinase-Resistant Penicillins and Cephalosporins," *Brit. M. J.,* **2**:344, 1964.

Batchelor, F. R.; Doyle, F. B.; Naylor, J. H. C.; and Rolinson, G. N.: "Synthesis of Penicillin; 6-Aminopenicillanic Acid in Penicillin Fermentations," *Nature,* **183**:257, 1959.

Dowling, Harry F.: "The Newer Penicillins," *Clin. Pharm. and Ther.,* **2**:572, 1961.

"New Penicillins," *Brit. M. J.,* **2**:323, 1964.

Sheehan, J. C., and Henery-Logan, K. R.: "The Total Synthesis of Penicillin V," *J. Am. Chem. Soc.,* **79**:1262, 1957.

PHENETHICILLIN

Knudsen, E. I., and Rolinson, G. N.: "6(α-Phenoxypropionamido) Penicillanic Acid," *Lancet,* **2**:1105, 1959.

Morigi, E. M. E.; Wheatley, W. B.; and Albright, H.: "Clinical and Laboratory Studies with Potassium Penicillin-152 (Potassium α-Phenoxyethyl Penicillin):

A New Synthetic Penicillin (Syncillin)," *Antibiotics Annual, 1959–1960.* Medical Encyclopedia, Inc., New York, 1960.

METHICILLIN

Brown, D. M., and Acred P.: "Chemotherapeutic Studies on a New Antibiotic—BRL 1241," *Lancet,* **2**:568, 1960.

Douthwaite, A. H., and Trafford, J. A. P.: "A New Synthetic Penicillin," *Brit. M. J.,* **2**:687, 1960.

Elek, S. D., and Fleming, P. C.: "A New Technique for the Control of Hospital Cross-Infection, Experience with BRL 1241 in a Maternity Unit," *Lancet,* **2**:569, 1960.

———: "Relative Antibacterial Activity of Three Penicillins," *Brit. M. J.,* **1**:527, 1960.

Garrod, L. P.: "The Relative Antibacterial Activity of Four Penicillins," *Brit. M. J.,* **2**:1695, 1960.

OXACILLIN

Kirby, W. M. M., Rosenfeld, L. S.; and Brodie, J.: "Oxacillin: Laboratory and Clinical Evaluation," *J.A.M.A.,* **181**:739, 1962.

CLOXACILLIN

Sidell, Sheldon, *et al.*: "Cloxacillin, A New Oral Synthetic Penicillin. Comparisons with Oxacillin," *Clin. Pharmacol. Ther.,* **5**:26, 1964.

AMPICILLIN

Brown, D. M., and Acred, P.: "Penbritin—A New Broad-spectrum Antibiotic," *Brit. M. J.,* **2**:197, 1961.

Rolinson, G. N., and Stevens, S.: "Microbiological Studies on a New Broad-spectrum Antibiotic," *Brit. M. J.,* **2**:191, 1961.

Stewart, G. T., *et al.*: "Penbritin: An Oral Penicillin with Broad-spectrum Activity," *Brit. M.J.,* **2**:200, 1961.

"Today's Drugs," *Brit. M.J.,* **2**:1145, 1961.

CEPHALOSPORINS

Barber, Mary, and Waterworth, P. M.: "Penicillinase-Resistant Penicillins and Cephalosporins," *Ann. Rev. Pharmacol.,* **4**:115, 1964.

Griffith, Richard S., and Black, H. B.: "Cephalothin—A New Antibiotic," *J.A.M.A.,* **189**:823, 1964.

Weinstein, Louis, *et al.*: "Treatment of Infections in Man with Cephalothin," *J.A.M.A.,* **189**:829, 1964.

ANTIBIOTIC-RESISTANT BACTERIA

"Conference on Staphylococcic Infections in the Hospital and Community," *J.A.M.A.,* **166**:1177, 1958.

Gillespie, W. A.; Simpson, K.; and Tozier, R.: "Staphylococcal Infection in a Maternity Hospital," *Lancet,* **2**:1075, 1958.

Gosling, W. R. O., and Büchli, K.: "Nasal Carrier Rate of Antibiotic Resistant Staphylococci," *A.M.A. Arch. Int. Med.,* **102**:691, 1958.

Jawetz, E.: "Patient, Doctor and Bug," *Antibiotics Annual, 1957–1958*. Medical Encyclopedia, Inc., New York, 1958, p. 287.

Lawrence, C. A.: "The Effects of Disinfectants on Antibiotic Resistant and Antibiotic Sensitive Strains of *Micrococcus pyogenes,* var. *aureus,*" *Surg., Gynec. & Obst.,* **107**:679, 1958.

Levin, M.: "Staphylococcal Hospital Infections," *New England J. Med.,* **256**:155, 1957.

Newton, G. G. F., and Abraham, E. P.: "Some Chemical and Medical Aspects of the Antibiotics," *J. Pharm. & Pharmacol.,* **10**:401, 1958.

Wise, R. I.: "Principles of Management of Staphylococcic Infections," *J.A.M.A.,* **166**:1178, 1958.

Syphilis and Gonorrhea

Kampmeir, R. H.: "Responsibility of a Physician in a Program for the Eradication of Syphilis," *J.A.M.A.,* **183**:102, 1963.

Manson, R. C., and Trice, E. R.: "The Changing Pattern of Syphilis," *South Med. J.,* **56**:705, 1963.

Notes on Modern Management of VD. Public Health Publication No. 859, reprinted 1962.

Shapiro, L. H.: "Gonorrhea in Females," *GP,* **28**:78, 1963.

Social Health News, **38**:1, 1963.

Erythromycin

Finland, M. (moderator, panel discussion) : "The Current Status of Erythromycin, Kanamycin, Novobiocin, Oleandomycin, Ristocetin and Vancomycin, with Particular Use in Staphylococcal Disease," *Antibiotics Annual, 1958–1959*. Medical Encyclopedia, Inc., New York, 1959, p. 1051.

Haight, T. H., and Finland, M.: "The Antibacterial Action of Erythromycin," *Proc. Soc. Exper. Biol. & Med.,* **81**:175, 1952.

————: "Laboratory and Clinical Studies on Erythromycin," *New England J. Med.,* **247**:227, 1952.

————: "Resistance of Bacteria to Erythromycin," *Proc. Soc. Exper. Biol. & Med.,* **81**:183, 1952.

Heilman, F. R.; Herrell, W. E.; Wellman, W. E.; and Geraci, J. E.: "Some Laboratory and Clinical Observations on a New Antibiotic, Erythromycin (Ilotycin)," *Proc. Staff Meet., Mayo Clin.,* **27**:285, 1952.

Herrell, W. E.: "Erythromycin in Infectious Diseases," *M. Clin. North America,* **38**:569, 1954.

"Restriction of Antibiotics" (editorial), *Lancet,* **2**:193, 1956.

Neomycin

Waksman, S. A.: *Neomycin, Nature, Formation, Isolation and Practical Application*. Rutgers University Press, New Brunswick, N.J., 1953.

Waksman, S. A.; Katz, E.; and Lechevalier, H. A.: "Antimicrobial Properties of Neomycin," *J. Lab. & Clin. Med.,* **36**:93, 1950.

Waksman, S. A., and Lechevalier, H. A.: "Neomycin, a New Antibiotic Active Against Streptomycin Resistant Bacteria Including Tuberculosis Organisms," *Science,* **109**:305, 1949.

Novobiocin

David, A. N., and Burgner, P. R.: "Clinical Effectiveness and Safety of Novobiocin," *Antibiotic Med.*, **2**:219, 1956.
Martin, W. J., *et al.*: "Streptonivicin (Albamycin), a New Antibiotic," *Proc. Staff Meet., Mayo Clin.*, **30**:540, 1955.
Mullins, J. F., and Wilson, C. J.: "Novobiocin Treatment of Pyodermas," *Antibiotic Med.*, **2**:201, 1956.
Simon, H. J., *et al.*: "Studies on Novobiocin, a New Antimicrobial Agent," *Antibiotic Med.*, **2**:205, 1956.
Smith, C. G., *et al.*: "Streptonivicin, a New Antibiotic: Discovery and Biological Studies," *Antibiotics & Chemother.*, **6**:135, 1956.
Taylor, R. M., *et al.*: "Streptonivicin, a New Antibiotic: Absorption, Distribution and Excretion," *Antibiotics & Chemother.*, **6**:162, 1956.
Welch, H., and Wright, W. W.: "The Common Identity of Cathomycin and Streptonivicin," *Antibiotics & Chemother.*, **5**:670, 1955.

Vancomycin

Ehrenkranz, N. J.: "The Clinical Evaluation of Vancomycin in the Treatment of Multi-antibiotic Refractory Staphylococcal Infections," *Antibiotics Annual, 1958–1959*. Medical Encyclopedia, Inc., New York, 1959, p. 587.
Kirby, W. M. M., and Divelbiss, C. L.: "Vancomycin: Clinical and Laboratory Studies," *Antibiotics Annual, 1956–1957*. Medical Encyclopedia, Inc., New York, 1957, p. 107.
Kirby, W. M. M.; Perry, D. M.; and Lane, J. L.: "Present Status of Vancomycin Therapy of Staphylococcal and Streptococcal Infections," *Antibiotics Annual, 1958–1959*. Medical Encyclopedia, Inc., New York, 1959, p. 580.

Ristocetin

Busch, L. F.: "Use of Ristocetin (Spontin) in Staphylococcal Infections," *Antibiotics Annual, 1958–1959*. Medical Encyclopedia, Inc., New York, 1959, p. 456.
Calvy, G. L.: "Ristocetin and the Staphylococcus," *J.A.M.A.*, **167**:1585, 1958.
Schneierson, S. S.; Amsterdam, D.; and Bryer, M. S.: "Bacterial Sensitivity to Ristocetin," *Antibiotics & Chemother.*, **8**:204, 1958.
Schumacher, L. R.: "Experience with Ristocetin in Staphylococcal Infections," *Antibiotics Annual,* 1958–1959. Medical Encyclopedia, Inc., New York, 1959, p. 464.
Terry, R. B., and Bradley, L. F.: "Ristocetin in Adults and Children," *Antibiotics Annual, 1958–1959*. Medical Encyclopedia, Inc., New York, 1959, p. 458.

Kanamycin

Duke, C. J., *et al.*: "A Critical-Evaluation of Kanamycin in Severe Infections," *Antibiotics Annual, 1958–1959*. Medical Encyclopedia, Inc., New York, 1959, p. 595.
Finland, M.: "Kanamycin," *Lancet*, **2**:209, 1958.
Symposium, *Ann. New York Acad. Sc.*, **76**:17, 1958.

8

Streptomycin, Dihydrostreptomycin, Viomycin, and Cycloserine. Drugs Used in the Treatment of Tuberculosis and Leprosy

Streptomycin

Streptomycin is a purified antibiotic principle produced by certain strains of *Streptomyces griseus* when grown on certain media. *Streptomyces* is an aerobic genus of fungus whose species are found in the soil. Such useful drugs as streptomycin, erythromycin, chloramphenicol, neomycin, chlortetracycline, and many others are elaborated by these microorganisms. Streptomycin was first isolated by Dr. Selman Waksman and his associates in 1944 as a result of years of research to find such an extract, and was the first antibiotic of practical significance isolated from the actinomycetes. It is a white crystalline substance which may be prepared as several salts, including the hydrochloride, the sulfate, and the calcium chloride–complex double salt.

Antibacterial Spectrum. Streptomycin is active against a variety of gram-negative organisms, including *Escherichia coli, Pseudomonas aeruginosa, Pasteurella tularensis* and *pertussis, Hemophilus influenzae, Salmonella typhi,* and the *Brucella* species. It is active also against a few gram-positive organisms and the tubercle bacillus. The tubercle bacillus and other streptomycin-sensitive organisms develop very rapidly a resistance to this drug; therefore, careful bacteriological studies should be made before and during treatment with streptomycin to ascertain that the organisms are still sensitive to the drug. (See Table 7, pp. 108, 109.)

Mechanism of Action. Streptomycin interferes with the carbohydrate metabolism in the susceptible organisms. It prevents the formation of oxalacetic acid from pyruvic acid.

Absorption, Distribution, and Excretion. Streptomycin is poorly absorbed from the gastrointestinal tract, and most of the drug administered orally is excreted in the feces. Therefore, oral administration is of no value in systemic infections; however, it is useful in preparing surgical patients for operations on the large intestine where it is desirable to reduce the

130

number of organisms present. Streptomycin is readily absorbed from intramuscular administration and is well distributed in the body fluids except the spinal fluid. Maximum blood levels are obtained in one to two hours and usually remain fairly steady for four hours with a gradual falling off in the next eight hours. Forty to eighty per cent of the total dose is excreted in the urine in 24 hours. Small amounts are elminated in the bile, milk, saliva, sweat, and tears.

Toxicity.   When streptomycin is given for a few days, the toxic effects are negligible. However, with prolonged administration, numerous toxic reactions occur. The most serious symptoms are those related to the involvement of the vestibular and sometimes the cochlear branch of the eighth cranial nerve. These include dizziness, ringing in the ears, disturbances in equilibrium, and diminished auditory acuity. Deafness may result. Other toxic symptoms include severe headache, anorexia, nausea, abdominal pain, skin rash, generalized arthralgia, fever, and pain at the site of injection. There have been several cases of agranulocytosis.

Therapeutic Uses.   The most important use for streptomycin is in the treatment of tuberculosis, which is discussed on pages 135–37. It is also employed in the treatment of tularemia and brucellosis, in bacteremias, meningitis, endocarditis, pneumonias, and intestinal infections caused by organisms that are streptomycin susceptible, and in infantile gastroenteritis, and it is useful in treating urinary tract infections when the organisms are penicillin and sulfonamide resistant. Development of resistance on the part of the organism is a serious limiting factor in the use of this drug, and its administration should be limited to the treatment of infections produced by bacteria which have been shown by laboratory tests to be susceptible to it.

Dosage and Methods of Administration.   For nontuberculous systemic infections streptomycin is administered intramuscularly, and the dose is determined by the susceptibility of the organism and the severity of the infection. In acute infections 1 to 2 Gm. daily are given intramuscularly in divided doses every six hours. In less severe infections 0.5 to 1 Gm. daily may be adequate. Drug fastness is always possible; hence it is necessary to bring the infection under control as quickly as possible. To prepare a solution for intramuscular injection, the powder is dissolved in water for injection or isotonic salt solution to give 100 to 200 mg. per milliliter. Solutions for injection are available in ampuls.

Streptomycin may be administered also by nebulizer. It may be used alone or in combination with penicillin in nontuberculous bronchial and pulmonary infections. The solution in purified water contains 50 to 100 mg. per milliliter. Orally, 2 to 3 Gm. of streptomycin daily in divided doses are administered in gastrointestinal infections prior to surgery. It is given in water. The drug is no longer used intrathecally, and there is doubt as to its value intrapleurally. Intravenous administration is rarely used because of the danger of the severe fall in blood pressure. The dose and method of administration in tuberculosis are discussed on page 135.

Streptomycin Sulfate, U.S.P., I.P. (B.P.). This salt is marketed as a sterile powder in airtight vials and also in solution, which for all practical purposes is reasonably stable without refrigeration. The solution, although less stable and slightly more expensive, is more practical and easier to administer because it eliminates the necessity of preparing solutions from the powder and the consequent possibility of contamination. Skin rashes may occur on the hands of personnel who frequently administer streptomycin. For this reason, many nurses wear gloves when preparing and administering the drug. All preparations of this drug are labeled with an expiration date.

Preparations

Streptomycin Sulfate Injection, U.S.P., I.P.; Streptomycin Sulphate Injection, B.P.	The equivalent of 1 Gm. in 2 and 2.5 ml.; 5 Gm. in 10 and 12.5 ml. B.P. 0.33 Gm. of the base in 1 ml.
Streptomycin Sulfate, U.S.P., I.P. (B.P.)	Vials containing 1 and 5 Gm. of the base
Streptomycin-Calcium Chloride, I.P. (Streptomycin Calcium Chloride Complex)	Vials containing the equivalent of 1 and 5 Gm. of the base

Dihydrostreptomycin

Dihydrostreptomycin is prepared by the hydrogenation of streptomycin. The bacterial spectra of the two substances are similar. Dihydrostreptomycin is better tolerated by some patients than streptomycin. At first it was believed to have less neurotoxicity. Its action is less acute and more subtle. For short treatment it has less effect on the vestibular nerve, but with prolonged treatment there may be impairment in hearing and deafness may result. It is administered mainly in the treatment of tuberculosis and is given intramuscularly only. The intramuscular dose is 500 mg. (500 mg. to 3 Gm.) of the base daily. Because of its toxicity its use is restricted to patients who are sensitive to streptomycin.

Preparations

Dihydrostreptomycin Sulfate (B.P., I.P.)	Vials containing the equivalent of 1 Gm. or 5 Gm. of the base
Dihydrostreptomycin Sulfate Injection	The equivalent of 1 Gm. in 2 and in 2.5 ml., 5 Gm. in 10 and in 12.5 ml.

Viomycin

Viomycin is an antibiotic obtained from a culture of *Streptomyces puniceus*. It has a marked ability to inhibit the growth of the tubercle bacillus, but its toxicity to the eighth nerve and the kidney limits its use. It is not so effective and its cost is much greater than that of streptomycin. It is used only in tuberculosis where the tubercle bacillus has become resistant to streptomycin, or in persons allergic to streptomycin. It may be administered alone or in combination with sodium aminosalicylic acid or isoniazid. One gram of the base is injected intramuscularly every third day. The dose is divided into equal parts and injected at 12-hour intervals. The dry powder is stable for 12 months. A solution is prepared for injection by dissolving 1 Gm. of the drug in 2 ml. of either water for injection or isotonic sodium chloride solution. The solution may be stored at refrigerator temperature for a week without loss of potency.

Preparation

Viomycin Sulfate   Vials containing 1 Gm. of the base

Trade names: Vinactane Sulfate; Viocin Sulfate

Cycloserine, B.P. (Seromycin)

Cycloserine is an antibiotic obtained from *Streptomyces orchidaceus* and *Streptomyces garyphalus*. It inhibits both gram-positive and gram-negative organisms, particularly in chronic infections of the urinary tract and the *tubercle bacilli*.

Absorption, Distribution, and Excretion. On oral administration cycloserine is readily absorbed and is well distributed in the various tissue fluids, bile, and sputum, and in the lungs, central nervous system, and other tissues. It is excreted in the urine, and the concentration there from ordinary clinical doses reaches levels as high as 1 mg. per milliliter.

Untoward Effects. Drowsiness, dizziness, and headache occur but may subside within a day or two despite continuation of treatment. The drug is neurotoxic and may produce convulsions in large doses.

Therapeutic Uses. Cycloserine is used in the treatment of tuberculosis accompanied by PAS or isoniazid and in urinary tract infections.

Dosage and Method of Administration. The usual oral daily dose is 250 mg. two or four times daily.

Preparation

Cycloserine Capsules, B.P.   250 mg.

Trade names: Seromycin; Oxamycin

Neomycin Sulfate, U.S.P., B.P. (Mycifradin)

Neomycin is an antibiotic elaborated by *Streptomyces fradiae* when the organism is grown on suitable culture media. It is an extremely stable substance and is active against both gram-positive and gram-negative organisms. It appears to be more active against the staphylococci than the streptococci. It is sometimes effective against *Pseudomonas* and *Proteus* infections.

Neomycin is applied topically as a solution or ointment in the treatment or prevention of infections of the skin and eye, including pyogenic or secondarily infected stasis dermatoses, impetigo, wounds, burns, ulcers, conjunctivitis, blepharitis, and sty. In severe or extensive infections, local therapy with neomycin should be supplemented with the oral administration of the sulfonamides or penicillin. Neomycin is also administered orally as an intestinal antiseptic to reduce the usual bacterial flora of the colon in operations on the large intestine or anus. Since it is poorly absorbed from the gastrointestinal tract, it rarely causes toxic reactions. However, prolonged therapy may cause an overgrowth of yeasts and *Aerobacter aerogenes*. It has a mild laxative effect. It is too toxic to be injected.

Dosage and Method of Administration.   The usual oral dose is 1 Gm. of the base every four hours (4 to 12 Gm. daily). Topically, 0.5 per cent ointments or solutions are used. The solutions are used as wet dressings, packs, irrigations, or instillations.

Preparations

Neomycin Sulfate, U.S.P.	Vials containing 0.5 Gm.
Neomycin Sulfate Ointment, U.S.P.	5 mg. in each gram (not less than 3.5 mg.)
Neomycin Sulfate Tablets, U.S.P.	500 mg.

Trade names: Mycifradin sulfate; Myciguent

DRUGS USED IN THE TREATMENT OF TUBERCULOSIS

Tuberculosis is an infectious disease caused by the *tubercle bacillus*. This organism, discovered by Robert Koch in 1882, most commonly first invades the lung by inhalation of droplet nuclei or air-borne material containing the infecting agent. The disease may spread to almost any part of the body—lymph nodes, central nervous system, bones, joints, genitourinary and gastrointestinal tracts. Miliary tuberculosis, one of the most serious tuberculous infections, is characterized by small lesions scattered throughout the body. The tubercle bacillus, *Mycobacterium tuberculosis*, has a high lipid content which makes the organism impervious to many drugs. It causes tubercles, specific lesions in this disease, to form in animal tissues. The organism can often be recovered from these tubercles. When the sputum analysis reveals no tubercle bacilli (so-called negative sputum), aspiration of gastric contents may demonstrate them, since they are being swallowed in "open" cases.

The death rate from tuberculosis in the United States has dropped to 5.8 in 100,000. However, approximately 55,000 new cases are reported each year.

The number of persons requiring treatment in the world is increasing. This includes inactive, active, and potentially active cases; some are persons who have been discharged from the hospital and others who refuse hospitalization or treatment in the home. The infectiousness of the disease tends to increase its incidence. Eradication of tuberculosis will require the cooperation and support of the community, the nation, and indeed the whole world.

Isoniazid, streptomycin, and PAS (para-aminosalicylic acid) remain the three best antitubercular drugs. The administration of any one of these drugs for any length of time, even in adequate dosage, leads to the development of resistant organisms. Two of the above-mentioned drugs should be given together in long-term therapy. The administration of three is not superior to the administration of two. Any regimen containing isoniazid is superior to all others in sputum conversion and x-ray improvement.[1] Streptomycin is given in doses of 1 Gm. daily (in some cases twice weekly) with 300 mg. of isoniazid daily. The Veterans Administration and the armed forces of the United States obtain very satisfactory results with the combination of 300 mg. of isoniazid and 10 to 12 Gm. of PAS in most cases in the primary treatment of patients with sensitive organisms. This regimen also simplifies home treatment as no injection is necessary. Long-term uninterrupted therapy for a minimum of two years is necessary.

The success of drug therapy has been responsible for the liberalization of bed rest programs and shorter periods of hospitalizations. After an initial few months of hospitalization most patients are able to continue drug treatment at home under the supervision of a private physician or the health department clinics. As a result, nursing responsibilities for teaching and public health follow-up of patients and their families have increased considerably. Patients must understand the importance of prolonged administration of the antituberculosis drugs, frequent sputum and x-ray examinations, and good health habits. Intermittent or interrupted drug therapy before the disease process is controlled can lead to the development of drug-resistant organisms and/or treatment failures.

Aminosalicylic Acid, U.S.P. (PAS, Para-aminosalicylic Acid); Sodium Aminosalicylate, U.S.P., B.P.

Aminosalicylic acid (PAS) is a very valuable drug in the treatment of tuberculosis because in addition to its bacteriostatic action it delays the development of resistance of the *tubercle bacilli* to other tuberculostatic drugs. It is less effective than streptomycin and must be given in very large doses. Upon oral administration it is rapidly absorbed and rapidly excreted after partial acetylation. Within seven hours 85 per cent may be excreted in the urine in

[1] Badger, T. L.: "Tuberculosis," *New England Med. J.*, **261**:30, 74, and 131, 1959.

the free and acetylated form. PAS acetylates more readily than isoniazid and thus reduces the acetyl groups available to acetylate and inactivate isoniazid. The side effects noted are gastrointestinal irritation with nausea, vomiting, and diarrhea. Sodium PAS is less irritating and is the drug of choice. It is used to supplement streptomycin, isoniazid, and other antitubercular drugs in the treatment of tuberculosis.

When a patient responds to streptomycin and PAS or isoniazid and PAS administration, there is an improvement in the appetite, cough is diminished, fever is reduced, lesions are improved (as shown in x-rays), the mental outlook improves, and there are fewer bacilla in the sputum or they may disappear entirely. These drugs are not a substitute for other therapeutic measures, but when combined with bed rest, fresh air, good nursing and good food, they are an important factor in the many cases that can be arrested or cured.

The usual oral dose of PAS or sodium PAS is 4 Gm. three times a day with meals. The most undesirable feature of the use of these drugs is the large number of tablets that a patient must take over a long period of time. When therapy is initiated, PAS may be given in graduated doses until the maximum dose of 12 Gm. daily is reached. This prevents the development of the severe gastrointestinal side effects.

Preparations

Aminosalicylic Acid Tablets, U.S.P. 500 mg.
(PAS)

Trade names: Pamisyl; Para-Aminosalicylic Acid; Para-Pas; Parasal; Propasa

Sodium Aminosalicylate Tablets, U.S.P., 500 mg. and 1 Gm.
B.P. (Sodium PAS)

Trade names: Pamisyl Sodium; Para-Pas Sodium; Parasal Sodium; Pasara Sodium; Pasem Sodium; Pasmed Sodium; Sodium Para-Aminosalicylate

Isoniazid, U.S.P., B.P. (Isonicotinylhydrazine, INH)

Isoniazid is another drug now being used in combination with streptomycin or PAS to combat tuberculosis. It is very potent against the *tubercle bacilli*. It is a colorless, odorless, tasteless, stable powder, which is rapidly absorbed from the gastrointestinal tract. Peak levels appear in the plasma one to three hours after oral administration. It is inactivated by acetylation. PAS prolongs its action by competing with the acetylation mechanism. From three fourths to one half of the dose is excreted in the urine within 24 hours. It is uniformly distributed in the blood plasma, spinal fluid, and such tissues as the brain, lungs, liver, and spleen. INH is effective against intracellular as well as extracellular organisms. Samples of body fluids such as sputum, urine, cerebrospinal fluids, plasma, and pleural exudates exhibit antituberculosis activity after the administration of isoniazid, but resistant strains appear in a few weeks when the drug is administered alone. It is administered simultaneously with PAS or streptomycin to delay this effect. Oral administration is preferred, but the drug may be given intramuscularly. Most patients tolerate the drug well and gain prodigious amounts of weight.

The toxic effects are visual disturbances, dizziness, postural hypotension, peripheral neuritis, excitability, hyperreflexia, convulsions, and coma. Pyridoxine is given simultaneously in doses of 50 mg. daily to offset neurotoxicity only when large doses of INH (500 to 600 mg.) are given.

The advantages of isoniazid are that the side effects are negligible, the dose is small, and it can be given orally. In comparing a large series of cases, the combinations of streptomycin and sodium PAS and streptomycin and isoniazid are practically the same as far as therapeutic results are concerned. The combination of PAS and INH seems to be preferred because of the ease of administration.

The usual oral or intramuscular dose is 100 mg. three times a day with meals (300 mg. daily).

Recent studies conducted by the Public Health Service have shown that isoniazid is an effective prophylactic drug when given to children and adults who have been recently exposed to tuberculosis. Isoniazid, taken daily for a period of one year, prevented many serious extrapulmonary complications of primary tuberculosis in children and reduced the incidence of active disease among household contacts of newly diagnosed cases of tuberculosis.[2,3]

Preparations

Isoniazid Tablets, U.S.P.   50 and 100 mg.

Isoniazid Injection, U.S.P.   10-ml. vials containing 100 mg. in 1 ml.

Trade names: Armazide; Cotinazin; Dinacrin; Ditubin; INH; Isolyn; Niadrin; Nicozide; Nydrazid; Pyrizidin; Rimifon; Tisin; Tyvid; Zinadon; Zuiadon

Pyrazinamide (Pyrazinoic Acid Amide)

Pyrazinamide is a new and potent tuberculostatic drug that may be used for short-term therapy with selected patients. With pyrazinamide alone the organisms develop a resistance to the drug in about six or seven weeks, and after that time subsequent use of the drug is ineffective. Combined with isoniazid, the total tuberculostatic effect appears to be greater than that of any known agent or combination of agents.

---

[2] Mount, Frank, and Ferebee, S. H.; "Preventive Effects of Isoniazid in the Treatment of Primary Tuberculosis in Children," *New England J. Med.*, **265**:713, 1961.
[3] Ferebee, S. H., and Mount, F. W.: "Tuberculosis Morbidity in a Controlled Trial of the Prophylactic Use of Isoniazid Among Household Contacts," *Am. Rev. Resp. Dis.*, **85**: 490, 1962.

Toxicity. Pyrazinamide may produce severe and even fatal liver damage. It should be used only when it is possible to have reliable liver function tests performed before treatment is started and at regular intervals thereafter. Bacteriological determinations should also be made for the presence of resistant strains of *M. tuberculosis*. Treatment should be discontinued if the patient shows signs of jaundice or significantly impaired liver function, or the presence of resistant strains of the infecting organism.

Therapeutic Uses. Pyrazinamide is used with isoniazid for short-term protection of patients (resistant to other forms of antimicrobial therapy) about to undergo chest surgery in order to prevent or minimize the spread of infection. It is also used in hospitalized patients seriously ill with tuberculosis when other drugs are ineffective or contraindicated (allergic sensitivity, resistant organisms, etc.).

The oral dose is 20 to 40 mg. per kilogram of body weight daily with a maximum of 3 Gm. daily in divided doses.

Preparation

Pyrazinamide Tablets   500 mg.

Trade names: Aldinamide; PZA

Ethioniamide (Trecator)

Ethioniamide (Trecator) is active against strains of *tubercle bacilli* resistant to streptomycin, PAS, and isoniazid. Rapid devolpment of resistant strains of organisms is also a problem. For this reason, ethioniamide is administered in combination with other drugs.

The oral dose is 500 mg. to 1 Gm. daily.

Preparation

Ethioniamide Tablets   250 mg.

Trade name: Trecator

DRUGS USED IN THE TREATMENT OF LEPROSY

Leprosy (Hansen's disease) is a chronic disease caused by *Mycobacterium leprae*, which is an acid-fast bacillus related to the tubercle bacillus. It is probable that the organism penetrates the skin and enters the nerves by way of the nerve terminals there. Later the organisms may "burst" out of the nerves into the corium of the skin. The pathological lesions produced consist of red patches on the skin followed by scar tissue and atrophy. Nodules and tubercles may develop in the mouth, nose, pharynx, larynx, conjunctiva, and viscera. Leprosy is a deforming and multilating disease. However, early treatment will prevent these unsightly deformities. Leprosy affects at least 12 million persons throughout the world. Of these, not more than 100,000 can receive treatment in the hospitals. About 1,500,000 lepers live at home with their families. It is now believed that it is no longer necessary to segregate them. Resistance to leprosy can be acquired, so that persons who have this resistance and who then contract the disease have it only in a mild form.[4]

THE SULFONES

Domagk discovered that sulfathiazole was active, to a limited degree, against the tubercle bacillus. Compounds related to the sulfonamides—the sulfone drugs, dapsone (DDS) and sodium glucosulfone (Promin)—seemed to be effective; but they now have been supplanted by newer drugs except in the treatment of leprosy where they are very effective chemotherapeutic agents. With these drugs clinical improvement, which is noted in almost every patient, is slow but progressive. Lesions of the mucous membrane of the mouth, nose, and throat, etc., heal first, and later there is improvement in the skin lesions. Sometimes the nodules may become smaller and are resorbed; at other times there may be necrosis of the nodules, which is followed by ulceration and rapid healing. With these drugs used wisely, it is possible to control endemic leprosy and prevent deformity and other sequelae if the disease is treated in the early stages.

The sulfones are synthetic drugs derived from dapsone diaminodiphenylsulfone (DDS), which is often called the *parent* substance. They are bacteriostatic, not bactericidal to both *tubercle* and *leprae* bacilli and depend upon the cooperation of the host to bring about a cure when this occurs. It is believed that they may act by depriving the bacillus of one of the essential amino acids. (PABA).[5] The disease does not progress under treatment, but improvement is slow and relapses may occur; consequently the drugs must be given over long periods of time with rest periods, when the drug is not given, at periodic intervals.

Toxic Effects. The toxic effects are nausea, hematuria, rashes, mental confusion, leukopenia, and normocytic or hemolytic anemia.

Dapsone, U.S.P., B.P. (Diaminodiphenylsulfone, DDS)

Cochrane, in 1949, administered this drug orally. It is now considered the standard treatment of leprosy because of its effectiveness, ease of administration, and low cost. It is completely absorbed upon oral administration and is distributed to all body tissues. The drug is excreted slowly in the urine over a period of two weeks. The side reactions are excitement, dermatitis, and, in some cases, hemolytic anemia.

[4] "Segregation of Lepers," *J.A.M.A.*, **166**:186, 1960.
[5] Cochrane, R. G.: "The Treatment of Leprosy," *A.M.A., Arch. Int. Med.*, **97**:208, 1956.

The intial oral dose is 25 to 50 mg. twice weekly, increasing by 50 to 100 mg. every month to a maximum of 200 to 400 mg. weekly. The widespread use of this drug has greatly reduced the number of patients with diffuse lepromatous leprosy.

Preparations

Dapsone Tables, U.S.P., B.P.   100 mg.

    Trade names: Alvosulfon; DAPS; DDS; Disulone; Sulphonemere

Sodium Glucosulfone (Promin)

The intravenous dose of glucosulfone sodium in the treatment of leprosy is 2 to 5 Gm. administered daily for six consecutive days, omitted on the seventh day, and then administered for the next six days. Treatment may be interrupted for a week at the conclusion of each two-week period. This treatment may be continued for a long time, depending on the patient's response.

Preparation

Sodium Glucosulfone Injection, U.S.P.   Ampuls containing 2 Gm. in 5 ml. and 5 Gm. in 12.5 ml.

Glucosulfone Sodium Jelly

    Trade names: Promin Sodium; Aceprosol; Promanide

New Drugs For Leprosy

In order to reduce the long period of treatment necessary in leprosy the search continues for more active drugs and ones that may be used in patients who are hypersensitive to the ones now available.

Etisul (Dithiolisophthalate).   This oily yellow liquid is a derivative of ethyl mercaptan. When applied to the skin lesions as a cream by inunction, the drug is absorbed rapidly and completely. The clincial responses are rapid and definitely greater than those observed with dapsone during the first few months of treatment. After that time there is evidence of increasing resistance of the organisms to the drug. A more rapid and effective control of leprosy is obtained by giving Etisul and dapsone together for 8 to 12 weeks and then continuing the standard treatment with dapsone alone. The dosage for Etisul is 3 to 6 ml. by inunction weekly for two to three months. No toxic effects have been noted. The disadvantages of the use of this drug are (1) its unpleasant and persistent odor, which may be masked somewhat by perfume; and (2) the development of resistance.

Preparations

Etisul cream, 75 per cent   Tubes, 5 and 7 Gm.

Chloroquine.   This drug has been found useful in providing symptomatic relief for lepra reactions. There is a disappearance of fever with subsidence of inflammatory skin lesions and arthritis.[6] The recommended oral dose is 250 mg. three times a day for one week and 250 mg. twice a day for another two weeks.

Hydnocarpus Oil, I.P. (Chaulmoogra Oil); Ethyl Ester of Hydnocarpus Oil, I.P. (Ethyl Chaulmoograte)

Hydnocarpus and chaulmoogra oils and their ethyl esters have been used for years in the treatment of leprosy. In fact they were the only remedies until the introduction of the sulfones, which have supplanted them to a large extent. The esters of these oils are sometimes administered intradermally in combination with sulfone therapy. These are the only drugs available in many places where leprosy is endemic.

Preparations

Injection of Hydnocarpus Oil, I.P.

Injection of Ethyl Esters of Hydnocarpus Oil, I.P.

Chaulmoogra oil and its preparations are no longer official in the United States or in Great Britain.

REVIEW QUESTIONS

1. List the important clinical uses for streptomycin. How is the drug administered?
2. Compare the antibacterial spectra of streptomycin and penicillin.
3. What are some of the toxic effects produced by streptomycin?
4. Name several drugs used in the treatment of tuberculosis and explain why it is good practice to use two or more drugs at the same time in treating this disease.
5. What nursing observations are important when patients are receiving streptomycin? INH? Pyrizinamide?
6. What are the points that should be emphasized when the nurse is preparing a patient for antituberculosis treatment in the home?
7. What are the advantages and disadvantages of viomycin as an antituberculosis drug?
8. What times during the day are considered to be best for administering sodium PAS to the patients on a tuberculosis ward? Why?
9. A patient receiving daily dosages of isoniazid and PAS reports a tingling sensation in his fingers. What is the significance of his complaint?
10. When teaching patients about the drugs commonly used in the treatment of tuberculosis, what drugs would you discuss? What are some of the points you would stress in your discussion?
11. Name several drugs useful in the treatment of leprosy. What clinical improvement may be anticipated by their administration?

---

[6] "Chloroquine for Lepra Reactions," *J.A.M.A.*, **171**: 1861, 1959.

REFERENCES

STREPTOMYCIN

Waksman, S.: *Microbial Antagonisms and Antibiotic Substances.* The Commonwealth Fund, New York, 1947.

———: "Streptomycin: Background, Isolation, Properties and Utilization," *Science,* **118**:259, 1953.

——— (ed.): *Streptomycin, Nature and Practical Applications.* Williams & Wilkins Company, Baltimore, 1949.

Waksman, S., and Lechevalier, H. A.: *Actinomycetes and Their Antibiotics.* Williams & Wilkins Company, Baltimore, 1953.

DRUGS USED IN THE TREATMENT OF TUBERCULOSIS

Badger, T. L.: "Tuberculosis," *New England J. Med.,* **261**:30, 74, 131, 1959.

Barclay, W. R.; Ebert, R. H.; and Koch-Weser, D.: "Mode of Action of Isoniazid," *Am. Rev. Tuberc.,* **67**:490, 1953.

Bartz, Q. R.; Ehrlich, J.; Mold, J. D.; Penner, M. A.; and Smith, R. M.: "Viomycin, a New Tuberculostatic Antibiotic," *Am. Rev. Tuberc.,* **63**:4, 1951.

Bogen, E.; Loomis, R. N.; and Will, D. W.: "Para-aminosalicylic Acid Treatment of Tuberculosis, a Review," *Am. Rev. Tuberc.,* **61**:226, 1950.

Cohen, S. S.; Johnson, L.; Lichtenstein, M. R.; and Lynch, W. J.: "A Comparative Study of Streptomycin and Dihydrostreptomycin in the Treatment of Pulmonary Tuberculosis," *Am. Rev. Tuberc.,* **68**:229, 1953.

Ferebee, S. H., and Mount, F. W.: "Tuberculosis Morbidity in a Controlled Trial of the Prophylactic Use of Isoniazid Among Household Contacts," *Am. Rev. Resp. Dis.,* **85**:490, 1962.

Mount, F. W., and Ferebee, S. H.: "Preventive Effects of Isoniazid in the Treatment of Primary Tuberculosis in Children," *New Eng. J. Med.,* **265**:713, 1961.

Poole, G., and Stradling, P.: "Chemotherapeutic Pitfalls in the Treatment of Tuberculosis," *Brit. M. J.,* **1**:161, 1960.

Report of the Council on Pharmacy and Chemistry: "Chemotherapy of Tuberculosis in Man," *J.A.M.A.,* **154**:52, 1954.

Reported Tuberculosis Data. U.S. Department of Health, Education and Welfare, Public Health Service, Washington, D.C., 1962 Edition.

Riley, Richard L., and O'Grady, Francis: *Airborne Infection.* The Macmillan Company, New York, 1961.

Tucker, W. B.: "Evaluation of Streptomycin Regimens in the Treatment of Tuberculosis," *Am. Rev. Tuberc.,* **60**:715, 1949.

Waksman, S., *et al.: Neomycin: Nature, Formation and Practical Application.* Rutgers University Press, New Brunswick, N.J., 1953.

Waksman, S., and Lechevalier, H. A.: "Neomycin, a New Antibiotic Active against Streptomycin Resistant Bacteria Including Tuberculosis Organisms," *Science,* **109**:305, 1949.

Weiss, Moe: "Chemotherapy and Tuberculosis," *Am. J. Nursing,* **59**:1711–14, 1959.

DRUGS USED IN THE TREATMENT OF LEPROSY

"Chloroquine for Lepra Reactions," *J.A.M.A.,* **171**:1861, 1959.

Cochrane, R. G.: "The Treatment of Leprosy," *A.M.A. Arch. Int. Med.,* **97**:208, 1956.

Cochrane, R. G.; Ramanujam, K.; Paul, H.; and Russell, D.: "Sulfone Group of Drugs in Leprosy," *Leprosy Rev.*, **20**:4, 1949.

INDIA, "Segregation of Lepers," *J.A.M.A.*, **172**:186, 1960.

Reports of Societies, "Chemotherapy of Leprosy," *Brit. M. J.*, **1**:796, 1960. Paper by Dr. T. F. Davey, "Some Recent Chemotherapeutic Work in Leprosy."

Symposium: "Leprosy," *Ann. New York Acad. Sc.*, **54**:1, 1951.

Today's Drugs, "Etisul," *Brit. M. J.*, **2**:238, 1959.

9

Broad-Spectrum Antibiotics: Chloramphenicol, the Tetracyclines, and Other Antibiotics. Antifungal Antibiotics. Antibiotics from Bacteria

BROAD-SPECTRUM ANTIBIOTICS

Chloramphenicol (Chloromycetin) and the tetracyclines, chlortetracycline (Aureomycin), oxytetracycline (Terramycin), tetracycline (Achromycin, Tetracyn), and demethylchlortetracycline (Declomycin), are grouped together because they have a similar antibacterial spectrum which includes gram-positive and gram-negative bacteria, the rickettsiae, and some of the larger viruses. They are effective against many more types of infections than penicillin, which is mainly effective against gram-positive organisms, with the exception of ampicillin and streptomycin, which are primarily effective against gram-negative organisms.

For a number of diseases there is no choice among them as to their therapeutic efficacy; for others, one drug or group of drugs may be more effective. All are active upon oral administration and are relatively nontoxic.

Chloramphenicol, U.S.P., B.P., I.P. (Chloromycetin)

Chloramphenicol is an antibiotic isolated by Dr. P. R. Burkholder from *Streptomyces venezuela*, a mold found in the soil near Caracas, Venezuela. It was soon isolated in the pure form and was the first antibiotic synthesized. It is now produced commercially by synthesis rather than by extraction.

Absorption, Distribution, and Excretion. Chloramphenicol is readily absorbed from the intestinal tract. When 1 Gm. is administered, the drug appears in the blood in about 30 minutes; concentrations are maximal in about two hours and gradually diminish over a period of several hours. With single larger doses low concentration may be detected for 24 hours. Effective therapeutic levels may usually be maintained if the dose is administered at four- to eight-hour intervals. It is well distributed in the tissues of the body and passes into the cerebrospinal and pleural fluids and penetrates all parts of

144

the eye; appreciable amounts are found in the bile. Chloramphenicol is inactivated in the body by both degradation of the molecule and conjugation of the drug with glucuronic acid. About 75 to 90 per cent of the drug ingested is excreted in the urine within 24 hours. About 10 per cent is excreted unchanged and the remainder as degradation products or as the conjugate with glucuronic acid.[1]

Rickettsial Diseases.   These diseases are classified together because the organisms causing them, the rickettsiae, which are intermediate between bacteria and viruses, possess many similar characteristics. The principal diseases of this group are (1) louse-borne epidemic typhus; (2) flea-borne endemic typhus; and (3) Rocky Mountain spotted fever, transmitted by the wood and dog ticks. The latter two diseases are important in the United States. Chloramphenicol was the first drug found to be effective in epidemic, endemic, and scrub typhus. Later the tetracyclines were found to be equally as effective.

Mechanism of Action.   Sensitive bacteria and rickettsiae are inactivated by chloramphenicol, which produces a prompt and selective inhibition of bacterial protein synthesis.

Toxicity.   Chloramphenicol may produce nausea, vomiting, and diarrhea, but it does so less often than the other broad-spectrum antibiotics. At first it was thought to be almost nontoxic. However, a few cases of depression of bone marrow, resulting in aplastic anemia and agranulocytosis, have been reported. Because of this potential danger, chloramphenicol is used mainly in the treatment of typhoid fever and other serious infectious diseases caused by organisms sensitive to chloramphenicol but resistant to other antibiotics or other forms of treatment.

A small percentage of premature and newborn infants are particularly susceptible to the toxic effects of chloramphenicol. They develop a symptom complex called the "gray syndrome." The first symptoms which may occur after three or four days of therapy are vomiting or regurgitation of feedings and abdominal distention. Later, respiratory depression, flaccidity, and an ash-gray color may develop. In seriously poisoned infants, death may occur in 24 to 48 hours after the first symptoms. In others, symptoms may disappear 24 to 36 hours after discontinuance of the drug. It is believed that the immature liver of newborn infants is unable to form the glucuronide, causing a progressive increase in active chloramphenicol in the blood after repeated doses. These toxic effects in infants may be prevented by reducing the dose of the drug.

Typhoid Fever.   Chloramphenicol is superior to any other drug in the treatment of typhoid fever. Although penicillin in large doses and Synnematin B (identical with cephalosporin N, see p. 117) have been used successfully, in

---

[1] Woodward, T. E., and Wissman, C. L., Jr.: *Chloromycetin (Chloramphenicol), Antibiotics Monographs No. 8.* Medical Encyclopedia, Inc., New York, 1958.

the treatment of this infection, chloramphenicol is the only drug that is uniformly effective. It is now recommended that the drug be given for five days and, following an eight-day rest period, a second course should be given for five days. It has been impossible to prevent relapses of typhoid fever in all patients no matter how vigorous or prolonged the treatment with chloramphenicol. The development of the patient's resistance is presumably aided by allowing the regrowth of the typhoid organisms in the body during the rest periods between drug courses. Second rest periods and third courses of drug therapy are being evaluated. The periods of drug administration are timed simultaneously with the expected relapses of the disease. With this method, the patient is kept out of danger and yet allowed to develop the immunity that will allow his recovery. The drug is only bacteriostatic; it alone cannot abolish all the organisms.

In the therapy of typhoid fever, Dr. T. E. Woodward and co-workers[2] administer an initial dose of 50 mg. per kilogram of body weight, followed by a maintenance dose of this amount daily in three equal doses at eight-hour intervals. A therapeutic blood level may thereby be maintained.

Summary of Therapeutic Uses

1. Typhoid fever.
2. Typhus fevers.
3. Tularemia.
4. Urinary infections, particularly mixed infections.
5. Acute and chronic brucellosis.
6. Atypical pneumonia (a virus infection).
7. Influenzal meningitis.
8. Resistant staphylococcal infections.
9. Severe *Salmonella* infections.

Dosage and Method of Administration.   In acute and chronic systemic infections, the usual oral dose is 500 mg. to 1 Gm. every six hours. In acute infections some clinicians use a loading dose of 2 Gm. The usual dose range is 2 to 4 Gm. For topical application a 1 per cent ointment or solution is used.

In typhoid fever and other serious infections chloramphenicol sodium succinate may be injected intramuscularly. The usual intramuscular dose is 1 Gm. every eight hours. The usual daily dose range is 1.5 to 3 Gm. daily. A new ester, chloramphenicol succinate, is highly soluble and nonirritating. It is available for subcutaneous, intramuscular, or intravenous administration. One gram of this substance may be dissolved in 2 to 3 ml. of physiological

---

[2] Woodward, T. E.; Smadel, J. E.; and Parker, R. T.: "The Therapy of Typhoid Fever," *M. Clin. North America*, **38**:577, 1954.

salt or glucose solution and injected intravenously. In children, smaller daily doses based on body weight are given in three or four divided doses. In premature infants or infants under two weeks of age the dose should not exceed 25 mg. per kilogram daily.

Preparation of Chloramphenicol Succinate Solution. To ensure the withdrawal of 1 Gm. chloramphenicol equivalent in 2.5 ml. (40 per cent solution), an intentional excess of approximately 20 per cent has been provided. The powder in the vial adds a constant volume of 1 ml. to the final solution regardless of the amount of diluent added. In summary, the following table is presented to aid in preparing the solution.

Table 9

Preparation of Chloramphenicol Solutions

Strength of Solution %	mg. per ml.	Volume of Diluent Required, ml.	Volume Contributed by Dried Material, ml.	Total Volume, ml.	Volume Containing 1 Gm. Chloramphenicol Equivalent, ml.
40	400	2.0	1	3.0	2.5
25	250	3.8	1	4.8	4.0
10	100	11.0	1	12.0	10.0

The above technique provides sufficient solution to accommodate vial-wall drainage and an excess for withdrawal of solution containing 1 Gm. of chloramphenicol equivalent at all concentrations. Sterile water, saline, or glucose solution may be used as the diluent.

Preparations

Chloramphenicol Capsules, U.S.P., B.P.	50, 100, and 250 mg.
Chloramphenicol Ophthalmic Ointment, U.S.P.	1 per cent
Chloramphenicol for Ophthalmic Solution, U.S.P.	25 mg.
Sterile Chloramphenicol for Suspension, N.F.	1 and 2 Gm.
Chloramphenicol Palmitate Oral Suspension, U.S.P.	1.875 Gm. of the base in 60 ml.
Chloramphenicol Sodium Succinate (Sterile), U.S.P.	Steri-vial 1 Gm.

Trade name: Chloromycetin

THE TETRACYCLINES

Chlortetracycline (Chlortetracycline Hydrochloride, N.F., B.P.; Aureomycin Hydrochloride, I.P.) was isolated from the actinomycete *Streptomyces aureofaciens* by Dr. B. M. Duggar in 1947. Later, in 1950, a similar substance,

Oxytetracycline, N.F., B.P. (Terramycin), was obtained from *Streptomyces rimosis* by Dr. A. C. Finlay and associates. In 1953, a third substance, Tetracycline, U.S.P. (Achromycin, Tetracyn), was introduced into medicine. Demethylchlortetracycline, B.P., produced by a mutant of Dr. Duggar's original strain, was available for clinical use in 1959. Tetracycline is a semisynthetic substance obtained from chlortetracycline by the removal of chlorine. It is also prepared biosynthetically by one of the streptomycetes (still unnamed) obtained from the soil of Texas. It is more stable than chlortetracycline and more soluble than either chlortetracycline or oxytetracycline, and there is a lower incidence of side reactions. These drugs resemble each other very closely chemically and in their therapeutic activity and are therefore discussed together as a group.

All of these compounds are yellow crystalline substances which are amphoteric and therefore readily form acid or basic salts that are freely soluble in water. In the dry crystalline state, the salts are stable at room temperature. Aqueous solutions are not stable and should be freshly prepared.

Antibiotic Spectrum. The antibiotic spectrum for the tetracyclines is the same as that from chloramphenicol. However, they appear to be more effective in infections caused by the gram-positive organisms and the rickettsiae and are, as a rule, less active against gram-negative organisms. They are useful in combating the psittacosis, lymphogranuloma, and trachoma group of viruses and for infections caused by *Endamoeba histolytica*. The tetracyclines are bacteriostatic in therapeutic concentrations. They suppress the multiplication of organisms and depend upon the defense mechanisms of the patient to eradicate the remaining organisms. (See Table 7, pp. 108, 109.)

Microorganisms may develop a resistance to these drugs, and when this occurs, they are resistant to all the broad-spectrum antibiotics. This is noted most often with the staphylococci.

Mechanism of Action. The mechanism of the antibacterial action of the tetracyclines is not well understood, but there is some evidence that they may interfere with protein synthesis.

Absorption, Distribution, and Excretion. All these antibiotics are readily absorbed from the gastrointestinal tract. However, they are not completely absorbed and rather large amounts are excreted in the feces. This may cause changes in the fecal flora and irritation of the anus. They are widely distributed in the fluids and tissues of the body, and diffuse into the pleural and cerebrospinal fluids when infection is present.

An appreciable amount of the drugs is secreted from the liver with the bile and excreted in the feces. The remainder is partially metabolized and eliminated in the urine. The maximum concentration in the urine occurs in four to eight hours, but the drugs may be found in the urine several days after the last dose.

Side Reactions. These drugs are all relatively nontoxic. However, some patients experience nausea, vomiting, diarrhea, and itching of the anus. These gastrointestinal symptoms are less likely to occur with tetracycline. Because the tetracyclines kill or inhibit some of the bacteria normally present in the mouth, vagina, and gastrointestinal tract, superimposed infections with yeast-like organisms (monilia) may occur in the skin and mucous surfaces of the vagina and rectum.

Summary of Therapeutic Uses of the Tetracyclines

1. Pneumonia, both typical (bacterial) and atypical (virus).
2. Tularemia.
3. Brucellosis.
4. Whooping cough.
5. Rickettsial diseases, including typhus fevers and Rocky Mountain spotted fever.
6. Urinary infections.
7. Syphilis.
8. Gonorrhea.
9. Amebiasis.
10. Various streptococcal and staphylococcal infections which are resistant to penicillin.
11. Eye infections.

Dosage and Methods of Administration. The tetracyclines are available for oral, intravenous, and topical administration. They are usually prescribed orally, but they may be administered intravenously in critically ill patients who are in a moribund condition, unconscious, or unable to swallow. As soon as possible, intravenous administration is discontinued and the drugs are given orally.

The usual oral dose of chlortetracycline or oxtetracycline is 250 mg. four times a day. The usual oral dose for tetracycline is 500 mg. four times a day. The usual dose range is 1 to 4 Gm. daily. The oral adult dose of demethyl-chlortetracycline is 150 mg. q.i.d. or 300 mg. b.i.d. The daily oral dose for children is 3 to 6 mg. per pound of body weight, administered in four equally divided amounts. The drugs are available for oral administration as capsules and tablets, and as flavored powders and soluble salts for the preparation of oral suspensions. The usual intravenous dose for tetracycline is 500 mg. two times a day with a range of 1 to 3 Gm. daily. Topically, 0.1 to 0.2 ml. of a 0.5 per cent solution is applied to the eyelid or conjunctiva. For topical administration, ointments, ophthalmic ointments, troches, and drugs for the preparation of solutions are available.

Preparation of Solutions. The sterile dry mixture of the drug with a suitable buffer, usually an amino acid, is available in 10-ml. rubber-stoppered vials. For intravenous injection the drug is diluted with 10 ml. of Water for Injection, U.S.P., Sodium Chloride Injection, U.S.P., or 5 per cent Dextrose Injection, U.S.P. Oxytetracycline and tetracycline may be administered by intravenous infusion. For intravenous infusion the above solution is withdrawn from the vial and diluted to a final volume of at least 100 ml. This solution is administered slowly, not more than 100 ml. in five minutes. Solutions not used may be stored in the refrigerator but must be discarded after four or five days.

Ophthalmic solutions are prepared by adding 5 ml. of freshly boiled purified water to the rubber-stoppered vial containing 25 mg. of a sterile mixture of the crystalline drug with a suitable buffer. Solutions not used may be stored in the refrigerator for 24 to 48 hours.

Rolitetracycline (Syntetrin, Velacycline)

This synthetic derivative of tetracycline is more soluble and has more than twice the antibiotic activity of the tetracycline phosphate. Its antibacterial potency is well sustained during treatment and is increased with repeated administration. The intramuscular preparation is available in two amounts (150 and 350 mg.) of sterile powder in a single-dose vial. The vials also contain 40 mg. of lidocaine and 300 mg. of ascorbic acid; they are reconstituted with 1.7 ml. of sterile distilled water before injection. The intravenous preparation is available as 700 mg. of sterile powder in a vial with 500 mg. of ascorbic acid; this vial is reconstituted with 10 ml. of sterile distilled water before use. The usual adult intramuscular dose is 350 mg. every four hours. The dose for children is 15 to 20 mg. per kilogram of body weight. The usual dose for intravenous infusion is 350 to 700 mg. every 12 hours. The infusion is prepared by adding 5 ml. (350 mg.) or 10 ml. of reconstituted solution to 300 to 500 ml. of sterile dextrose injection or physiological saline. The rate of infusion should not exceed 100 ml. every five minutes.

Tetracycline Compounds.   The addition of certain substances such as phosphates or glucosamine to tetracycline for oral administration enhances the absorption and increases the blood levels of the antibiotic.

Tetracycline Phosphate Complex.   This product, which is marketed as both a mixture and a compound or complex, produces initial blood levels of tetracycline which are almost twice those obtained when the hydrochloride is administered. The minimum adult oral dose is 250 mg. four times a day.

Tetracycline and Glucosamine   (Tetracyn).

Tetracycline, Glucosamine, and Nystatin (Tetrastatin).   Nystatin acts as a prophylactic against fungal infections that may occur during tetracycline therapy.

Preparations

Chlortetracycline Hydrochloride, N.F., B.P.; Aureomycin Hydrochloride, I. P.

Chlortetracycline Hydrochloride Capsules, N.F., B. P.	50, 100, or 250 mg.
Chlortetracycline Hydrochloride for Injection, N.F., B. P.	Vials containing 100 or 500 mg.
Ophthalmic Chlortetracycline, Hydrochloride, N.F.	25 mg.

Trade name: Aureomycin Hydrochloride

Oxytetracycline, N.F.

Oxytetracycline for Oral Suspension, N.F.	250 mg. per 5 ml.

Oxytetracycline Hydrochloride, N.F., B.P.

Oxytetracycline Hydrochloride Capsules, N.F.	50, 100, and 250 mg.
Oxytetracycline Hydrochloride for Injection, N.F.	100, 250, and 500 mg.
Ophthalmic Oxytetracycline Hydrochloride, N.F.	25 mg.
Oxytetracycline Injection, B.P. Oxytetracycline and Procaine Injection, B.P.	

Oxytetracycline Dihydrate, B.P.

Oxytetracycline Tablets, B.P.	250 mg.

Trade name: Terramycin

Tetracycline, U.S.P.

Tetracycline Oral Suspension, U.S.P.	125 and 250 mg. in 5 ml., 1.5 Gm. in 30- and 60-ml. containers

Trade names: Achromycin; Panmycin; Polycycline; Tetracyn

Tetracycline Hydrochloride, U.S.P., B.P.

Tetracycline Hydrochloride Capsules, U.S.P., B.P.	50, 100 and 250 mg.
Tetracycline Hydrochloride for Injection, U.S.P., Tetracycline Injection, B.P.	100, 250, 500 mg.
Tetracycline HCl for Ophthalmic Solution, U.S.P.	25 mg. in 5-ml. container
Tetracycline and Procaine Injection, B.P.	
Tetracycline Hydrochloride Tablets, N.F., B.P.	50, 100, and 250 mg.

Trade names: Achromycin Hydrochloride; Panmycin Hydrochloride; Polycycline Hydrochloride; Steclin Hydrochloride; Tetracyn Hydrochloride

Demethylchlortetracycline, N.F., B.P.

Capsules, N.F., B.P.	150 mg.
Pediatric Drops	60 mg. in 1 ml.
Oral Suspension, N.F.	75 mg. in 5 ml.

Trade name: Declomycin

Rolitetracycline

Rolitetracycline	I.M. vials containing 150 and 350 mg.
Rolitetracycline	I.V. vials containing 700 mg.

Trade names: Syntetrin Velacycline

Tetracycline Phosphate

Tetracycline Phosphate Capsules	250 mg.

Trade names: Achromycin V; Panmycin Phosphate; Sumycin; Tetrex

Tetracycline and Glucosamine

Tetracycline and Glucosamine Capsules	125 and 250 mg.
Tetracycline and Glucosamine Suspension	125 mg. in 5 ml.
Tetracycline and Glucosamine Drops (Pediatric)	100 mg. in 1 ml.

Trade name: Tetracyn

Tetracycline, Glucosamine, and Nystatin

Tetracycline, Glucosamine and Nystatin Capsules	250 mg. tetracycline and glucosamine and 250,000 units of nystatin
Tetracycline, Glucosamine and Nystatin Suspension	125 mg. of tetracycline and glucosamine and 250,000 units of nystatin

Trade name: Tetrastatin

ANTIFUNGAL ANTIBIOTICS

Nystatin is useful in the treatment of infections caused by the monilial organism, *Candida albicans*. There are also two new systemic antifungal agents: (1) amphotericin B, which has proved useful in deep-seated mycotic infections; and (2) griseofulvin, which produces cures in ringworm infections.

Nystatin, U.S.P., B.P. (Mycostatin)

This antifungal antibiotic is obtained from *Streptomyces noursei*. It is effective in suppressing intestinal fungi either by inhibiting their growth or by destroying the actively growing fungi, especially yeast and yeastlike fungi. It is used (1) in the prevention and treatment of intestinal moniliasis; (2) in combination with tetracycline, as Mysteclin, for therapy or prophylaxis of fungal infections allowed to develop during the administration of antibiotics effective against intestinal bacteria; and (3) in monilial infections of the mouth, vagina, and skin as well as systemic moniliasis.

Dosage and Method of Administration. The usual oral dose as an aqueous suspension or tablets is 500,000 U.S.P. units three times a day with a usual dose range of 1,500,000 to 3,000,000 units daily. Topically, it is applied one to four times a day as required. The intravaginal dose is 100,000 units twice a day.

Preparations

Nystatin for Oral Suspension, U.S.P.	2,400,000 U.S.P. units in 24-ml. container
Nystatin Ointment, U.S.P.	100,000 U.S.P. units per Gm.
Nystatin Tablets (intravaginal)	100,000 U.S.P. units
Nystatin Tablets, U.S.P. (oral)	500,000 U.S.P. units
Mysteclin Capsules	250 mg. of tetracycline and 250,000 units of nystatin

Trade names: Fungicidin; Mycostatin

Amphotericin B, U.S.P. (Fungizone)

Amphotericin B is an antifungal antibiotic produced by a species of *Streptomyces*. It is useful clinically in a wide variety of disseminated mycotic infections.

Side Effects. Nausea, vomiting, marked anorexia, chills, fever, and a mild to moderate elevation of blood urea nitrogen have been observed. The elevation of blood urea nitrogen is reversible upon discontinuance of the drug.

Dosage and Method of Administration. Amphotericin B is administered by slow intravenous infusion. It is dissolved in 10 ml. of 5 per cent dextrose injection, to provide a concentration of 5 mg. in 1 ml. The recommended concentration of 0.1 mg. in 1 ml. is obtained by further dilution with 5 per cent dextrose injection. Therapy is started with 0.25 mg. per kilogram of body weight and gradually increased until the optimum level is attained. The total daily dose is usually 1 mg. per kilogram of body weight. Seriously ill patients may be given the maximum dose of 1.5 mg. per kilogram. The drug is excreted slowly by the kidneys; accordingly, it is administered on alternate days. Therapy is continued for four to eight weeks.

Therapeutic Uses. Clinical improvement and sometimes cures have been reported in histoplasmosis, blastomycosis, cryptococcal meningitis, musculoskeletal coccidioidomycosis, and cryptococcosis (torulosis), heretofore usually fatal.

Preparation

Amphotericin B for Injection, U.S.P.   50 mg. in 15-ml. vials

Trade name: Fungizone

Griseofulvin, U.S.P., B.P. (Fulvicin, Grifulvin, Grisovin)

Griseofulvin, an oral fungistatic, is an antibiotic isolated from *Penicillium griseofulvin*. It is absorbed from the gastrointestinal tract and permeates the keratin of the skin, hair, or nails in fungistatic amounts. The fungi in the keratin remain viable, but they do not migrate into the newly formed cells. As the skin, hair, or nails grow and the old cells are shed or removed, they are replaced by new cells or structures free of fungi. Symptomatic relief of itching and inflammation occurs in a few days. Ringworm of the scalp or body often clears in two to five weeks; ringworm of the feet, in three to six weeks. Ringworm of the nails usually requires three to four months of treatment. Griseofulvin is not effective against bacteria and yeasts or in the treatment of deep-seated mycotic infections.

Side Effects.   No serious side reactions have been observed. Symptoms transient in nature include nausea, mild diarrhea, headache, and occasionally urticaria or other skin rashes. Patients receiving the drug over prolonged periods should be under careful supervision and peripheral blood counts should be made periodically.

Dosage and Method of Administration.   The oral dose is 1 Gm. daily in divided doses (250 mg. q.i.d.). In severe cases, up to 2 Gm. may be given. The dose for children over 50 lb. is 750 mg. daily (250 mg. t.i.d.); for children weighing 30 to 50 lb., 500 mg. daily (250 mg. b.i.d.).

Therapeutic Uses.   Griseofulvin is used in the treatment of ringworm of the skin, hair, and nails.

Preparation

Griseofulvin Tablets, U.S.P., B.P.   125, 250, and 500 mg.
Trade names: Grifulvin; Grisovin

ANTIBIOTICS FROM BACTERIA

All the antibiotics discussed so far have been obtained from fungi, and all but one have been isolated from a species of *Streptomyces*. There are three antibiotics used clinically that are obtained from bacteria. They are all bactericidal. These antibiotics are tyrothricin, bacitracin, and polymixin.

Tyrothricin, N.F.

Tyrothricin is an antibiotic isolated from an extract of the cultures of a soil bacillus, *Bacillus brevis*. It contains two substances, tyrocidin and gramicidin. Tyrocidin inhibits cell respiration and disrupts the cell wall of bacteria. Gramicidin inhibits growth but does not lyse bacteria (destroy their cell membrane). It is administered topically as a 0.5 per cent solution.

Antibiotic Spectrum. The organisms susceptible to the bactericidal action of tyrothricin are gram-positive bacteria such as pneumococci, streptococci, and staphylococci.

Method of Administration. Tyrothricin is administered locally, in isotonic solutions containing 0.5 mg. per milliliter, for instillation, irrigation, or wet dressings. It causes hemolysis of the red blood cells if it is injected in amounts adequate to control infectious processes.

Therapeutic Uses. Tyrothricin is effective in the treatment of indolent ulcers, mastoiditis, empyema, sinusitis, osteomyelitis, and eye infections.

Preparations

Tyrothricin Spray, N.F.	0.05 per cent
Tyrothricin Solution, N.F.	Manufacturers select own concentration
Tyrothricin Solutions	2 and 4 per cent
Tyrothricin Troches	1 and 2 mg.
Gramicidin, N.F.	0.05 per cent solution

Trade name: Soluthricin

Bacitracin, U.S.P., B.P.

Bacitracin is an antibiotic isolated from a strain of *Bacillus subtilus,* obtained from a culture of contaminated tissue removed at operation from a compound fracture of the tibia. Patients seldom are sensitive or develop a sensitivity to bacitracin, and bacteria are slow to develop resistance to this antibiotic.

Antibacterial Spectrum. Bacitracin is active against pneumococci, hemolytic and nonhemolytic streptococci, staphylococci, meningococci, and several spirochetes. It is ineffective against most gram-negative organisms; but since it is not destroyed by them, as is penicillin, it may be used to control gram-positive organisms in mixed infections.

Bacitracin is not absorbed from the gastrointestinal tract, but it is readily absorbed upon intramuscular injection and is eliminated slowly. Appreciable amounts may be detected in the blood for six to eight hours.

Toxicity. Bacitracin is practically nontoxic on local administration or upon intraneural injection. However, toxic effects may be noted after intramuscular injection. Renal injury, particularly tubule damage, has been observed. Other untoward effects include pain at the site of injection, induration, rash, loss of appetite, nausea, and vomiting.

Dosage and Methods of Administration. Bacitracin is administered mainly by topical administration or local infiltration. It is also administered orally, intramuscularly, and intraneurally (intrathecal, intraventricular, intracisternal, or intracerebral injection). For topical administration to the skin, eye, nose, and mouth, ointments containing 500 units per gram or solutions having 500 to 1000 units per milliliter are used. For respiratory tract infections the drug is combined with vasoconstrictors and other anti-biotics, or is used alone, as an aerosol or as nasal drops. Solutions containing 20,000 units per 20 ml. may be instilled intraperitoneally to prevent or treat peritonitis or may be sprayed over the site of operation in resection of the bowel. Solutions containing 500 to 1000 units per milliliter are injected directly into areas of infection, such as carbuncles or abscesses. The average oral adult dose is 20,000 U.S.P. units every four hours. The usual intramuscular dose is 20,000 units every eight hours with a dose range of 30,000 to 100,000 units daily. The drug is dissolved in 2 per cent procaine hydrochloride solution. The intraneural dose for adults is 10,000 units, whereas that for infants and children is 250 to 5000 units, depending upon the age and route of administration. The powdered drug is dissolved in sodium chloride solution to prepare a solution containing 1000 units per milliliter. Procaine is never used to prepare the solution for extraneural injections.

Therapeutic Uses

1. Locally in infections of the eye, nose, throat, mouth, and respiratory tract.

2. In carbuncles, superficial and deep abscesses, infected traumatic and surgical wounds, infected ulcers.

3. In systemic infections such as pneumonia, subacute bacterial endocarditis, meningitis, chronic suppurative osteomyelitis, and many other conditions caused by sensitive organisms.

4. In neurosurgery and infections of the central nervous system, such as osteomyelitis of the skull and brain abscess. (It may be applied intraneurally directly to the brain tissue without producing untoward effects.)

Preparations

Bacitracin Ointment, U.S.P.	500 units per gram
Bacitracin Ophthalmic Ointment	500 units per gram
Bacitracin Powder, U.S.P. (Topical)	Vials containing 2000, 10,000 and 50,000 units
Bacitracin (Sterile), U.S.P.	Vials containing 10,000 and 50,000 units

Trade names: Baciguent, Topitracin

Polymixin

Polymixin is a mixture of antibiotics obtained from *Bacillus polymyxa.* Various polymixins have been isolated, of which polymixin B is the least toxic.

Polymixin B Sulfate, U.S.P., B.P.   This salt is rather stable in solution.

Antibiotic Spectrum.   Polymixin is a most effective drug against gram-negative organisms, such as *E. coli, A aerogenes, K. pneumoniae, H. influenzae, Shigella* organisms, and most strains of *Pseudomonas. Proteus* is more resistant. Polymixin is bactericidal.

Toxicity. Polymixin B is toxic to the kidney and nervous system. It causes dizziness, tingling in the face and scalp, and muscular weakness.

Therapeutic Uses

1. Bacteremias and urinary tract infections that do not respond to other antibiotics.
2. Meningitis caused by gram-negative organisms, particularly *E. coli, A. aerogenes, K. pneumoniae,* and *H. influenzae.*
3. Gastrointestinal infections caused by *Shigella or Pseudomonas* organisms.
4. Skin infections.

Dosage and Method of Administration. Polymixin B is administered intramuscularly, intrathecally, orally, and topically. In urinary infections with gram-negative organisms it is administered intramuscularly. The usual daily intramuscular dose is 10,000 to 20,000 units per kilogram body weight. The usual dose range is up to 1,500,000 units daily. The usual oral adult dose is 750,000 U.S.P. units four times a day with a usual dose range of 500,000 to 6,000,000 units daily. For topical administration an ointment containing 17,000 U.S.P. units in 1 Gm. is used.

Preparations

Polymixin B Sulfate Tablets, U.S.P.	250,000 and 500,000 U.S.P. units
Sterile Polymixin B Sulfate, U.S.P.; Polymixin B Sulphate, B.P.	Each vial contains 500,000 U.S.P. units
Sterile Polymixin B Sulfate Powder (Topical)	Each vial contains 200,000 U.S.P. units
Polymixin B Sulfate Ointment, U.S.P.	10,000 units in each gram

Trade name: Aerosporin Sulfate

Colimycin (Colistin)

Colimycin is an antibiotic produced by *Bacillus* (aerobacillus) *colistinus.* It has been studied and used in Japan, Italy, and France for several years and in the United States since 1957. It is similar in structure and antibacterial action to polymixin B. The drug is both bacteriostatic and bactericidal but is more effective against gram-negative microorganisms than against gram-positive bacteria and fungi. No bacterial resistance to colimycin has been observed.

Oral Administration. Colimycin is poorly absorbed upon oral administration and therefore is useful as an intestinal antiseptic. The drug has been especially valuable in the treatment of acute diarrhea in infants (from birth to one year of age). It is administered as the sulfate in daily doses of 3 to 5 mg. per kilogram of body weight, divided in four equal amounts. Cures have been noted in three to four days. Relapses have not occurred when treatment was discontinued, nor have toxic effects been noted. Colimycin sulfate tablets are available for oral use.

Sodium Colistimethate, U.S.P. (Coly-Mycin Injectable) is a modification of colimycin. Colistimethate is well absorbed upon intramuscular injection. High blood levels are observed in 30 minutes, with a peak in two to four hours; but the drug may be detected in the blood for 12 to 24 hours. It is excreted in the urine over a period of 24 hours. Intramuscularly administered colimycin is used in the treatment of severe and chronic urinary tract, respiratory tract, surgical, wound, and burn infections, and in septicemias caused by certain strains of *Pseudomonas, Aerobacter, E. coli, Klebsiella,* and other gram-negative organisms resistant to streptomycin, sulfonamides, and broad-spectrum antibiotics. It is the drug of choice in urinary infections caused by *Pseudomonas.*

Side Effects.   Occasional rashes and mild azotemia with slight to moderate fever have been noted, particularly in infants. The most serious toxic effect is impairment of urinary function.

Dosage and Method of Administration.   Colistimethate sodium is administered intramuscularly only in two to four divided doses totaling 1.5 to 5 mg. per kilogram daily. In adults a 150-mg. injection may be given once or twice daily.

Preparation

Sodium Colistimethate for Injection, U.S.P.   Vials containing 150 mg.

Trade names: Coly-Mycin Injectable, Colomycin

REVIEW QUESTIONS

1. *What are some of the important advancements achieved by the introduction of the broad-spectrum antibiotics?*
2. *What are the tetracyclines? Why are they discussed as a group? How are these drugs administered?*
3. *A patient with pneumonia is receiving oxytetracycline (Terramycin). What symptoms would the patient be most likely to describe to the nurse if he were experiencing a side reaction to the drug?*
4. *In preparing an intramuscular injection of tetracycline, the nurse must inject a fluid as sterile water into the vial. If the drug is not used, what should the nurse do with the prepared vial?*
5. *What advantages are obtained in the treatment of systemic bacterial infections with demethylchlortetracycline?*
6. *What is Syntetrin? How is it administered?*
7. *What new antibiotic is useful in the treatment of systemic fungus infections? How is the drug administered?*
8. *What new antibiotic is useful in the treatment of ringworm infections? How is the drug administered?*

9. *Discuss the therapeutic uses of colimycin. How is the drug administered?*
10. *How is colistimethate administered? Name three types of infection treated with this agent.*
11. *Give two therapeutic uses for nystatin. Why is it given in combination with tetracycline?*
12. *What antibiotics are obtained from bacteria?*
13. *Explain the advantages to be gained by the use of bacitracin in certain cases.*
14. *What drugs are especially useful in the following diseases?*

    Typhoid fever _____
    Brucillosis _____
    Typhus fever _____
    Meningitis _____
    Pyogenic infections _____

REFERENCES

CHLORAMPHENICOL

Bartz, Q. R.: "Isolation and Characterization of Chloramphenicol," *J. Biol. Chem.*, **172**:445, 1948.

Council on Pharmacy and Chemistry, Report of Council: "Chloramphenicol," *J.A.M.A.*, **154**:44, 1954.

Ehrlich, J.; Bartz, Q. R.; Smith, R. M.; Joslyn, D. A.; and Burkholder, P. R.: "Chloromycetin, a New Antibiotic from a Soil Actinomycete," *Science*, **106**:417, 1947.

Smadel, J. E.: "Chloramphenicol (Chloromycetin) in the Treatment of Infectious Diseases," *Am. J. Med.*, **7**:671, 1949.

———: "Clinical Use of the Antibiotic Chloramphenicol (Chloromycetin)," *J.A.M.A.*, **142**:315, 1950.

Woodward, T. E.; Smadel, J. E.; and Parker, R. T.: "The Therapy of Typhoid Fever," *M. Clin. North America*, **38**:577, 1954.

Woodward, T. E., and Wissman, C. L., Jr.: *Chloromycetin (Chloramphenicol)*, Antibiotics Monographs No. 8. Medical Encyclopedia, Inc., New York, 1958.

TETRACYCLINES

English, A. R.; P'An, S. Y.; McBride, T. J.; Gardocki, J. F.; Van Halsema, G.; and Wright, W. A.: "Tetracycline—Microbiologic, Pharmacologic and Clinical Evaluation," *Antibiotics & Chemother.*, **4**:411, 1954.

Finland, M.; Grigsby, M. E.; and Haight, T. H.: "Efficacy and Toxicity of Oxytetracycline (Terramycin) and Chlortetracycline (Aureomycin) with Special Reference to Use of Doses of 250 mg. Every Four to Six Hours," *Arch. Int. Med.*, **93**:23, 1945.

Finland, M.; Purcell, E. M.; Wright, S. S.; Lovw, B. D., Jr.; Mou, T. W.; and Kass, E. H.: "Clinical Observations of a New Antibiotic, Tetracycline," *J.A.M.A.*, **154**:561, 1954.

Finlay, A. C.; Hobby, G. L.; P'An, S. Y.; Regna, P. P.; Routien, J. B.; Seeley, D. B.; Shull, G. M.; Sobin, B. A.; Solomons, I. A.; Vinson, J. W.; and Kane, J. H.: "Terramycin, a New Antibiotic," *Science*, **111**:85, 1950.

Love, B. D., Jr.; Wright, S. S.; Purcell, E. M.; Mou, T. W.; and Finland, M.:
"Antibacterial Action of Tetracycline: Comparison with Oxytetracycline and
Chlortetracycline," *Proc. Soc. Exper. Biol. & Med.*, **85**:25, 1954.
Symposium: *Antibiotics Annual, 1953–1954*. Medical Encyclopedia, Inc., New
York, 1953.
Symposium: "Aureomycin—A New Antibiotic," *Ann. New York Acad. Sc.*, **51**:175,
1948.
Symposium: "Terramycin," *Ann. New York Acad. Sc.*, **53**:221, 1950.

DEMETHYLCHLORTETRACYCLINE (DECLOMYCIN)

Hirsch, H. A., and Finland, M.: "Antibacterial Activity of Serum of Normal
Subjects after Oral Doses of Demethylchlortetracycline, Chlortetracycline and
Oxychlortetracycline," *New England J. Med.*, **260**:1099, 1959.
Kunin, C. M., and Finland, M.: "Demethylchlortetracycline: New Tetracycline
Antibiotic That Yields Greater and More Sustained Antibacterial Capacity,"
New England J. Med., **259**:999, 1958.
Sweeney, W. M.; Hardy, S. M.; Dornbush, A. C.; and Ruegsegger, J. M.:
"Demethylchlortetracycline: A Clinical Comparison of a New Antibiotic with
Chlortetracycline and Tetracycline," *Antibiotics & Chemother.*, **9**:13, 1959.

ROLITETRACYCLINE (SYNTETRIN, VELACYCLINE)

Dimmling, T.: "Experimental and Clinical Investigations with Pyrrolidinomethyl
Tetracycline," *Antibiotics Annual, 1959–1960*. Medical Encyclopedia, Inc.,
New York, 1960, p. 350.

NYSTATIN

"The Place of Nystatin in Chemotherapy" (editorial), *Antibiotic Med.*, **2**:79, 1956.
Robinson, R. C. V.: "Candida Albicans Infection of Skin and Mucous Membrane
Treated with Nystatin," *Antibiotics Annual, 1955–1956*. Medical Encyclopedia,
Inc., New York, 1955, p. 851.
Wright, E. T., *et al.*: "The Use of Nystatin in the Treatment of Moniliasis,"
Antibiotics Annual, 1955–1956. Medical Encyclopedia, Inc., New York, 1955, p.
846.

AMPHOTERICIN B

Klapper, M. S.; Smith, D. T.; and Conant, N. F.: "Disseminated Coccidioido-
mycosis Apparently Cured with Amphotericin B," *J.A.M.A.*, **167**:463, 1958.
Rubin, H., *et al.*: "Amphotericin B in the Treatment of Cryptococcal Meningitis,"
Antibiotics Annual, 1957–1958. Medical Encyclopedia, Inc., New York, 1958, p.
71.
Stough, A. R.: "Prophylaxis of Antibiotic-Induced Moniliasis," *Antibiotic Med.
and Clin. Therap.*, **6**:11, 1959.
Stough, A. R.; Groel, T. J.; and Kraeger, W. H.: "Amphotericin B, a New
Antifungal Agent for the Prophylaxis of Antibiotic Induced Moniliasis,"
Antibiotic Med. and Clin. Med., **6**:653, 1959.
Utz, J. P., *et al.*: "Amphotericin B: Intravenous Use in 21 Patients with Systemic
Fungus Disease," *Antibiotics Annual, 1958–1959*. Medical Encyclopedia, Inc.,
New York, 1959, p. 628.

————: "A Report of Clinical Studies on the Use of Amphotericin in Patients with Systemic Fungal Diseases," *Antibiotics Annual, 1957–1958*. Medical Encyclopedia, Inc., New York, 1958, p. 65.

GRISEOFULVIN

Blank, H., and Roth, F. J.: "The Treatment of Dermatomycoses with Orally Administered Griseofulvin," *A.M.A. Arch. Dermat.*, **79**:259, 1959.

Robinson, H. M., Jr.; Robinson, R. C.; Bereston, E. S.; Manchey, L. L.; and Bell, F. K.: "Griseofulvin: Clinical and Experimental Studies," *A.M.A. Arch. Dermat.*, **81**:66, 1960.

Sternberg, T. H., *et al.*: "The Treatment of Superficial Fungus Infections in Man with Orally Administered Griseofulvin," *Current Ther. Res.*, **1**:1, 1959.

BACITRACIN

Johnson, B. A.; Anker, H.; and Meleney, F. L.: "Bacitracin, a New Antibiotic Produced by a Member of the *B. subtilis* Group," *Science*, **102**:376, 1945.

Longacre, A. B., and Waters, R.: "Parenteral Bacitracin in Surgical Infections," *Am. J. Surg.*, **81**:599, 1951.

Teng, P.; Cohen, I.; and Meleny, F. L.: "Bacitracin in Neurosurgical Infections," *Surg., Gynec., & Obst.*, **92**:53, 1951.

POLYMIXIN

Brownlee, G.; Bushby, S. R. M.; and Short, E. I.: "The Chemotherapy and Pharmacology of the Polymixins," *Brit. J. Pharmacol.*, **7**:170, 1952.

Stansly, P. G.: "The Polymixins, a Review and Assessment," *Am. J. Med.*, **7**:807, 1949.

COLIMYCIN

Greengard, J., and Aliseda, A. F.: "Treatment of Acute Diarrheas of Infancy with Colistin Sulfate," *Antibiotics Annual, 1959–1960*. Medical Encylopedia, Inc., New York, 1960, p. 101.

McCabe, W. R.; Jackson, G. G.; and Kozii, V. M.: "Clinical and Laboratory Observations on the Use of Colistin in Infections by Gram-Negative Bacilli," *Antibiotics Annual, 1959–1960*. Medical Encyclopedia, Inc., New York, 1960, p. 80.

COLISTIMETHATE SODIUM

McCabe, W. R., *et al.*: "Clinical and Laboratory Observations on the Use of Colistin in Infections by Gram Negative Bacilli," *Antibiotics Annual 1959–1960*. Antibiotica, Inc., New York, 1960, p. 80.

Schwarz, B. S., *et al.*: "Microbiological and Pharmacological Studies of Colistin Sulfate and Sodium Colistimethate," *Antibiotics Annual 1959–1960*. Antibiotica, Inc., New York, 1960, p. 41.

10

The Sulfonamides

The clinical use of sulfanilamide in the treatment of various bacterial septicemias resulted from the work of Gerhardt Domagk. In 1932, while working in the German dye industry, he found that an azo dye, which he called Prontosil, was effective in curing mice infected experimentally with several times the lethal dose of *Streptococcus hemolyticus*. A search for a more soluble dye resulted in the introduction into medicine of Neoprontosil.

Early clinical trials established the therapeutic usefulness of Prontosil in hemolytic streptococcal septicemias. The drug was used by physicians in Queen Charlotte's Hospital in London. Dr. Perrin Long went to London to observe its use and brought some of the dye back to the United States.

Experimental work by the Tréfouëls, Nitti, and Bovet in Fourneau's laboratory in Paris showed that the complex dye molecule was metabolized in the body to a simple substance, which was not a dye. The metabolite (*p*-aminobenzenesulfonamide), which proved to be the active part of the molecule, was called *sulfanilamide*. The pharmacology and a test for the identification of sulfonamides in body fluids were worked out by Dr. E. K. Marshall and associates in the United States. The discovery of the anti-infective action of sulfanilamide led to intensive researches; consequently, over 5000 related compounds have been prepared. Ten or fifteen of these have had extensive clinical use.

$$H_2N-\langle \bigcirc \rangle -SO_2NH_2$$

Sulfanilamide

With the introduction of these drugs, new advantages have been attained. In some cases increased antibacterial activity, better diffusion into the cerebrospinal fluid, or decreased toxicity occurs. With sulfisoxazole, sulfisomidine (sulphasomidine), and the triple sulfonamides, there is a low degree of acetylation with high solubility in the urine, which eliminates renal complications that are a hazard in the use of the older sulfonamides. Recent research activity in this field has developed three new sulfonamides (sulphaphenazole, sulfadimethoxine, and sulfamethoxypyridazine) which have the additional advantages of greater potency (smaller dose) and a more

162

prolonged action in the body. Therapeutic levels may be maintained by administering these drugs every 24 hours.

Antibacterial Spectrum. The sulfonamides are effective against gram-positive organisms, especially streptococci, staphylococci, and pneumococci, and many gram-negative organisms, including gonococci, meningococci, *Shigella, Proteus, Pseudomonas, E. coli,* and *Hemophilus influenzae.* The *Actinomyces* and the large viruses, trachoma, and lymphogranuloma are also susceptible.

Absorption, Distribution, and Excretion. The degree and rate of absorption of the sulfonamides from the gastrointestinal tract are variable. Some are rapidly and almost completely absorbed (sulfanilamide and sulfathiazole), some are more slowly and less completely absorbed (sulfamerazine and sulfadiazine), while others are so poorly absorbed (phthalylsulfathiazole and succinylsulfathiazole) that they are used for their local antiseptic effect in the intestinal tract.

The sulfonamides are, as a rule, evenly distributed in the tissues and fluids of the body. Certain ones are found in the cerebrospinal fluid in therapeutic concentrations. The concentrations vary with the particular drug. With adequate doses of the various types of sulfonamides available, many types of infections in all parts of the body may be treated.

After absorption, the sulfonamides are partially and temporarily bound in the plasma protein. The bound sulfonamide is inactive but is released slowly and becomes free drug in the plasma. It is then able to leave the blood stream and pervade all intercellular spaces in the various tissues and organs.

These drugs are partially *acetylated* in the body and hence are found in the body fluids in the free, and thus conjugated, or acetylated form. The acetylated compounds are no longer therapeutically active, but they may still produce toxic effects. Both the free and acetylated forms are excreted in the urine, and several of the conjugated forms are less soluble than the free sulfonamides in the urine. The former crystallize out during the concentration of the urine in the kidneys and produce bleeding and even obstruction in the kidney tubules. Anuria (cessation of urinary flow) may result, which may prove fatal.

Sodium bicarbonate is administered with these substances in order to prevent or minimize this danger. The bicarbonate is capable of changing the urine from an acidic fluid to an alkaline one, in which the drugs are more soluble. Increasing the urinary output by maintaining a high fluid consumption will prevent crystalluria by keeping the concentration below the saturation point. Both the use of sodium bicarbonate and increased fluid intake lead to an increase in the amount of active drug being excreted. This in turn makes it more difficult to maintain a satisfactory blood level of the drug. Combinations of smaller doses of two or three sulfonamides decrease the danger of precipitation of crystals in the urinary tract. The saturation concentration of each is not approached and each remains in solution. A mixture of these sulfonamides is known as "triple sulfonamides."

Mechanism of Action. Long and Bliss demonstrated that the sulfonamides are *bacteriostatic* in therapeutic concentrations. They act directly on susceptible bacteria and inhibit their growth and multiplication and reduce their production of toxic substances. After the organisms are weakened or attenuated, the white blood cells (polymorphonuclear leukocytes) and the reticuloendothelial system eventually eradicate the infection. The sulfonamides thus require the cooperation of the host in eliminating the infection. In high concentrations, as occur in the urine, the sulfonamides may become bactericidal; they may kill bacteria without this cooperation.

Woods and Fildes advanced the theory of *competitive inhibition* to explain the mode of action of sulfonamides. The sulfonamides, which are closely related structurally to the vitamin p-aminobenzoic acid (PABA), prevent the incorporation of PABA into the folic acid molecule by substrate competition. Since folic acid is essential for the normal metabolic processes of bacteria, these drugs interfere with their growth and reproduction. Susceptible bacteria which are impermeable to folic acid require PABA for its synthesis. Nonsusceptible organisms are likely to be permeable to preformed folic acid and may acquire the necessary amount from the surrounding media. Folic acid is an essential metabolite for the cells of the patient's own tissues. They are unable to synthesize it but obtain an adequate supply of this vitamin in the patient's diet. Therefore, sulfonamides can selectively inhibit the growth of bacterial cells without causing similar injury to the tissues of the host.

Bacterial Resistance to Sulfonamides. As a result of repeated exposure to sulfonamides, some of the organisms become resistant to them; hence it is important to provide as quickly as possible an adequate concentration of the drug to prevent further multiplication of the organisms present. The bacteria may develop alternate pathways for their own biochemical processes and thus become capable of living and of multiplying in the presence of the sulfonamides. Other resistant *variants* (offspring of bacteria with new biochemical characteristics and capabilities) may actually grow better in the presence of these drugs. Although the antibiotics have replaced the sulfonamides in the treatment of many infectious diseases, the latter are still widely used either alone or in combination with the antibiotics. Their lower cost and convenience of use largely account for their continued use.

Toxicity. The toxic manifestations are unpredictable. They may be mild or they may even cause death. Hypersensitivity usually occurs as a dermatitis or drug fever. It may not appear until the drug has been administered for some time (several days to weeks). Nausea and vomiting are the most common untoward effects and may occur even with the newer sulfonamides. Other undesirable actions, which are seen less frequently, are headache, dizziness, mental disturbances, toxic psychoses, and peripheral neuritis. The most serious effects are cyanosis, granulocytopenia, agranulocytosis, hemolytic anemia, hematuria, and severe kidney damage. With the newer drugs available today, these severe reactions are rare. The use of less toxic drugs, such as sulfisoxazole, sulfisomidine, sulfadimethoxine, sulfamethoxypyridazine, and the triple sulfonamides, has greatly decreased these untoward effects.

SUMMARY OF UNTOWARD SIDE EFFECTS

1. Hypersensitivity (allergic response)
   a. Dermatitis
   b. Drug fever

2. Gastrointestinal distress
   a. Nausea, vomiting, and epigastric awareness

3. Central nervous system
   a. Vertigo
   b. Mental disturbances
   c. Depression

4. Genitourinary tract
   a. Crystalluria (seldom encountered now)

5. Hematopoietic system (infrequent)
   a. Leukopenia, granulocytopenia
   b. Granulocytosis and hemolytic anemia

Therapeutic Uses. The sulfonamides are effective in many types of infections. It is desirable to identify the organism responsible for the infection and to determine if it is sulfonamide susceptible.

1. Genitourinary infections with gram-negative organisms. The sulfonamides are widely used in bacterial infections of the urinary tract. They are valuable in many cases of infection with species of *Proteus* and *Pseudomonas*. Here, the triple sulfonamides and the more soluble ones, sulfisoxazole (Gantrisin), sulfamethoxazole (Gantanol), sulfisomidine (Elkosin), sulfamethoxypyridazine (Kynex, Lederkyn, Midicel), and sulfadimethoxine (Madribon), are very useful.

2. Upper respiratory tract infections such as tonsillitis, pharyngitis, pneumonia, otitis media, and bronchitis. Sulfadimethoxine and sulfamethoxazole are very effective.

3. Prophylactically against meningococcal and streptococcal infections,

rheumatic fever recurrences, and secondary invaders in virus infections. Sulfamethoxypyridazine and sulfadimethoxine are uniquely applicable to prophylactic therapy.

4. Meningitis. Sulfisoxazole and sulfadiazine are very useful because they are distributed in the cerebrospinal fluid.

5. Ulcerative colitis, bacillary dysentery, and preoperatively and postoperatively to surgery of the intestinal tract. Succinylsulfathiazole (Sulfasuxidine) and phthalylsulfathiazole (Sulfathalidine) are often used. Vitamin K may be administered concomitantly as these drugs inhibit intestinal bacteria necessary for its synthesis.

6. Conjunctival infections. The sodium salt of sulfacetamide is used for chronic infections of the conjunctiva in 30 per cent solution and 10 per cent ointment. A 4 per cent solution of sulfisoxazole diethanolamine is used in acute and subacute conjunctivitis.

Dosage and Method of Administration. The sulfonamides are generally administered orally. For the adult, a large initial dose of 4 Gm. is given orally, followed by 1 Gm. every four hours. This dosage is continued for 72 hours after the temperature and pulse rate are normal. In critically ill patients, where it is desirable to obtain a therapeutic level quickly, or where patients cannot retain the drug by mouth, 5 per cent solutions of the sodium salts are administered intravenously. The dose is calculated on the basis of 100 mg. per kilogram of body weight, and the maximum dose is 5 Gm. The criterion of dosage is the concentration in the blood and body fluids, which can be determined by chemical analysis. For most infections, 5 to 10 mg. per cent in the blood is sufficient; in acute infections, 10 to 15 mg. per cent is necessary. The dry crystalline salts are available in ampuls and the solutions are freshly prepared.

Local application of the crystalline sulfonamides and sulfonamide ointments, creams, and lotions has been disappointing in the treatment of wound infections or infections of the skin and mucous membranes. They are not recommended in the treatment of burns and superficial infections. The sodium salt of sulfacetamide has been used for chronic infections of the conjunctiva in 30 per cent solution and 10 per cent ointment. A 4 per cent solution of sulfisoxazole diethanolamine is used in acute and subacute conjunctivitis.

Individual Sulfonamides

Sulfanilamide, Sulphanilamide, B.P. In 1937, sulfanilamide was administered orally, intravenously, and intrathecally in the treatment of various infectious diseases. Doctors had such confidence in this new drug that it was often given before a diagnosis was made. It was effective in streptococcal, staphylococcal, and gonococcal infections, but it was not useful in the treatment of pneumonia. There were numerous toxic manifestations. The search for a less toxic substance resulted in the introduction of sulfapyridine.

Sulfapyridine, U.S.P. This compound was made available in 1939. The bacterial spectrum of sulfapyridine was broadened to include pneumonias. The hospital deaths from this disease were greatly reduced by its administration. However, the drug was poorly and irregularly absorbed and caused such untoward effects as nausea, vomiting, anorexia, and avitaminosis. It was soon replaced for systemic infections by newer sulfonamides. It is now used only in the treatment of certain dermatoses.

Sulfathiazole. The high incidence of untoward reactions and the availability of less toxic sulfonamides caused the deletion of this drug from the United States Pharmacopeia. However, it is still used in medical practice.

Sulfadiazine, U.S.P. This drug was synthesized in 1940. It is slowly absorbed from the gastrointestinal tract, and adequate blood concentrations are not reached for several hours. It is not readily distributed to the tissues of the body; therefore, relatively high blood concentrations are easily obtained. It is found in the cerebrospinal fluid following oral administration. Sulfadiazine is less toxic than sulfanilamide or sulfathiazole.

Sulfamerazine, U.S.P. Sulfamerazine is absorbed more rapidly than sulfadiazine. Comparable blood levels may be obtained with half the dose, and it is more completely absorbed and more slowly excreted than sulfadiazine. This permits smaller doses and less frequent administration. Sulfamerazine and its acetylated derivatives are more soluble in neutral or acid urine. There appears to be little danger of crystalluria. Sulfamerazine is found in the spinal fluid.

Sulfamethazine, U.S.P.; Sulphadimidine, B.P. Sulfamethazine appears to be comparable to sulfamerazine in antibacterial properties. Its absorption from the gastrointestinal tract is more rapid and it also appears in the cerebrospinal fluid. The drug is readily acetylated and excreted by the kidneys and is less likely to produce crystalluria and kidney damage than sulfadiazine or sulfamerazine. It is given in sulfonamide mixtures containing sulfadiazine and sulfamerazine.

Sulfacetamide, N.F. Sulfacetamide is a soluble compound useful in the treatment of urinary infections. The sodium salt is nonirritating, and 30 per cent solutions may be instilled in the eye in conjunctivitis.

Sulfisoxazole, U.S.P. (Gantrisin). Sulfisoxazole is very soluble in the body fluids; hence there is no danger of crystalluria. It has a broad bacterial spectrum and is one of the best genitourinary antiseptics. It is administered orally. The diethanolamine salt of sulfisoxazole is water soluble and is available for intravenous or intramuscular injection and for the preparation of ophthalmic solutions and ointments.

Acetyl Sulfisoxazole, N.F. (Gantrisin Acetyl). Acetyl sulfisoxazole is a tasteless substance suitable for oral administration, especially in liquid preparations. It is likely split into sulfisoxazole in the gastrointestinal tract; therefore, its absorption, excretion, solubility in the body fluids, and toxicity are the same as for sulfisoxazole.

Sulfamethoxazole (Gantanol) is closely related chemically to sulfisoxazole. It is used in the treatment of acute and chronic urinary tract and respiratory and soft-tissue infections.

Sulfisomidine, Sulphasomidine (Sulfadimetine, Elkosin). Sulfisomidine is readily absorbed from the gastrointestinal tract, and high blood levels may be obtained with moderately small doses. It readily diffuses into the cerebrospinal, pleural, and ascitic fluids. The drug is rapidly excreted in the urine and is acetylated to a low degree. It is generally used for urinary tract infections.

Sulfamethizole, N.F. (Thiosulfil, Urolucosil). This highly soluble sulfonamide is useful in the treatment of urinary tract infections. It is administered in pyelonephritis, ureteritis, prostatitis, cystitis, and urethritis caused by bacteria that are susceptible to the sulfonamides.

Sulfamethoxypyridazine, U.S.P. (Kynex, Lederkyn, Midicel). This sulfonamide is well absorbed upon oral administration. It is very slowly excreted in the urine, in which it is readily soluble. Considerable amounts of the drug may be detected in the blood for several days after a single dose. The "half-life" (time required to excrete half the dose in the urine) is at least 60 hours. Because of its prolonged sojourn in the body fluids, one daily dose is sufficient. This is a decided advantage in the treatment of infections in children. One dose a week is adequate for the prophylaxis of rheumatic fever. Sulfamethoxypyridazine is widely used in the treatment of urinary and respiratory infections.

Sulfadimethoxine, N.F. (Madribon). This is a new long-acting sulfonamide with a wide antibacterial spectrum which includes both gram-positive and gram-negative organisms. Its activity against some species of bacteria probably exceeds that of the other sulfonamides. Sulfadimethoxine is readily absorbed from the gastrointestinal tract and therefore is administered orally. It is slowly excreted in the urine in a very soluble form. Because of its effective and prolonged therapeutic levels in the blood and tissues, the drug is administered once a day. Nausea and vomiting, when they have occurred, have been mild and transient. Sulfadimethoxine is especially useful in the treatment of upper respiratory, urinary tract, and soft tissue infections; it may also be used to prevent meningitis and rheumatic fever. The microcrystalline suspension is a safe and effective drug in pediatric practice.

Sulphaphenazole (Orisulf). This is another new long-acting sulfonamide. It is effective in the treatment of infections of some bacteria that are resistant to other sulfonamides and in such conditions as chronic cholangitis (inflammation of the biliary ducts) and diverticulitis.

Sulfaethidole (Sul-Spansion, Sul-Span-Tab). Sulfaethidole is prepared in a sustained-release form so that therapeutic blood levels may be
maintained for 12 hours. It is used in the treatment of systemic and urinary
infections caused by organisms that are sensitive to the sulfonamides. It is
available as a suspension and in tablet form.

Sulfonamides in Combination with Pyridium. A number of preparations containing Pyridium in combination with one of the sulfonamides
are available for the treatment of urinary infections. Pyridium, a urogenital
analgesic, helps relieve pain and discomfort in these conditions. Combinations
of this type are Azo-Gantrisin, Urosulfin, Thiosulfil A, and Suladyne.

Salicylazosulfapyridine (Azulfidine). Salicylazosulfapyridine is
broken down in the body to aminosalicylic acid and sulfapyridine, and shares
the toxic effects of sulfapyridine. It is administered orally only and is used
in the treatment of chronic ulcerative colitis. The usual oral adult dose is 1
Gm. four to six times a day. Larger doses may be used in severe cases.

SULFONAMIDES POORLY ABSORBED FROM THE GASTROINTESTINAL TRACT

The sulfonamides that are absorbed from the gastrointestinal tract to only
a limited degree are used in intestinal disorders.

Succinylsulfathiazole, U.S.P. (Sulfasuxidine). This drug is used in
the treatment of bacillary dysentery and carriers of this disease.

Phthalylsulfathiazole, B.P. (Sulfathalidine). This drug is used in
the treatment of ulcerative colitis and preoperatively and postoperatively in
patients undergoing surgery of the intestines. It is sometimes used in amebiasis
and paratyphoid fever.

Sulfaguanidine; Sulphaguanidine, B.P. Sulfaguanidine tends to stay
in the colon and exert its bacteriostatic action there. It is administered orally
prior to and after surgery of the colon.

Phthalylsulfacetamide, N.F. (Talsutin). Upon oral administration,
phthalylsulfacetamide diffuses into the intestinal wall. It is useful in enteric
infections such as mild and early bacillary dysentery, paradysentery, and
ulcerative colitis.

SUMMARY OF THE THERAPEUTIC USES OF THE SULFONAMIDES

There are many therapeutic advantages and disadvantages of sulfonamide
chemotherapy. It is difficult to decide at times whether to use the sulfonamides
or the antibiotics. The newer and less toxic sulfonamides do not produce
crystalluria, and there are few allergic reactions. The antibiotics have become
less expensive and are readily available.

The triple-sulfonamide dosage forms containing a mixture of sulfadiazine,

[*Text continued on page 172*]

Table 10

Average Doses of Sulfonamides

Sulfonamide	Initial Dose	Maintenance Dose
AVERAGE DOSES OF SULFONAMIDES FOR SYSTEMIC INFECTIONS		
Sulfacetamide, N.F.	4 Gm.	1 Gm. (500 mg. to 4 Gm.) every four hours
Sulfadiazine, U.S.P.	4 Gm.	1 Gm. (500 mg. to 4 Gm.) every four hours
Sulphadiazine, B.P., I.P.	3 Gm.	1 to 1.5 Gm. every four to six hours
Sulfadimethoxine, N.F.	2 Gm.	1 Gm. every 24 hours
Sulfaethidole	—	1.3 Gm. every 24 hours
Sulfamerazine, N.F.	4 Gm.	1 Gm. (500 mg. to 4 Gm.) every six hours
Sulphamerazine, B.P.	3 Gm.	1 to 1.5 Gm. every eight hours
Sulfamethizole, N.F.	500 mg.	500 mg. four to six times daily
Sulphadimidine, B.P.	3 Gm.	1 to 1.5 Gm. every four to six hours
Sulfamethoxazole	2 Gm.	1 Gm. every 12 hours
Sulfamethoxypyridazine, U.S.P., B.P.	1 Gm.	500 mg. daily
Sulfanilamide	2 Gm.	
Sulfapyridine, U.S.P.	500 mg.	500 mg. (500 mg. to 1 Gm.) three times a day
Sulfathiazole	2 Gm.	
Sulfisomidine Sulphasomidine, B.P.	2 Gm.	1 Gm. every four hours
Sulfisoxazole, U.S.P. Sulphafurazole, B.P.	4 Gm.	1 Gm. (500 mg. to 4 Gm.) every six hours
Acetyl Sulfisoxazole, N.F.	4 Gm. (base)	1 Gm. (of the base) every four to six hours
Trisulfapyrimidines, U.S.P.	4 Gm.	1 Gm. (500 mg. to 4 Gm.) every four hours
Trisulfapyrimidines Suspension, U.S.P.	40 ml. 4 Gm.	10 ml. (5 to 40 ml.) every four hours

Table 10 *(Continued)*

Average Doses of Sulfonamides

Sulfonamide	Initial Dose	Maintenance Dose
PARENTERAL DOSES OF SULFONAMIDES		
Sodium Sulfadiazine, U.S.P.	4 Gm. in 5 per cent solution	May be repeated in eight hours
Sulfamerazine Sodium, N.F.	2 Gm. in 6 or 25 per cent solution	May be repeated in eight hours
Sulfathiazole Sodium	2 Gm. in 25 per cent solution	
Sulfisoxazole Diethanol-amine Injection	4 Gm. (500 mg. to 4 Gm.) of the base in 40 per cent solution	May be repeated in eight hours
AVERAGE ORAL DOSES OF ALIMENTARY TRACT INFECTIVES		
Phythalylsulfacet-amide, N.F.	2 Gm.	
Phthalylsulphathiazole, B.P.	10 to 15 Gm. daily in divided doses	
Succinylsulfathiazole; Succinylsulphathiazole, B.P.	2 Gm. every four hours	
Sulfaguanidine, I.P.; Sulphaguanidine, B.P.	10 to 20 Gm. daily in divided doses	
Salicylazosulfapyridine	1 Gm. four to six times a day	
RECTAL DOSE OF A SULFONAMIDE		
Para-Nitrosulfathiazole, N.F.	100 mg. (10 ml. of a 10 per cent suspension)	

━━━━━━━━━━━━━━━━━━━ **Table 10** *(Continued)* ━━━━━━━━━━━

Average Doses of Sulfonamides

Sulfonamide	Initial Dose	Maintenance Dose
TOPICAL ADMINISTRATION IN THE EYE		
Sulfacetamide Sodium, U.S.P., B.P.	6 and 10 per cent ophthalmic (eye) ointments and 30 per cent solutions	
Sulfisoxazole Diethanol-amine, U.S.P.	4 per cent ophthalmic ointments and solutions	

sulfamerazine, and sulfamethazine or sulfacetamide are very satisfactory. The clinical experience with the more soluble sulfonamides, such as sulfisoxazole, sulfamethoxypyridazine, sulfisomidine, and sulfadimethoxine, indicates that these drugs may be the sulfonamides of choice.

There are special cases where combined sulfonamide and antibiotic therapy is indicated. For example, sulfonamides are combined with penicillin in the treatment of meningitis, with streptomycin in plague and brucellosis, and with the tetracyclines in *H. influenzae* meningitis. These combinations are available in suitable dosage forms.

Preparations

Sulfacetamide, N.F.
  Sulfacetamide Tablets, N.F.   500 mg.
                  Trade name: Sulamyd

Sodium Sulfacetamide, U.S.P.; Sulphacetamide Sodium, B.P.
  Sodium Sulfacetamide Ophthalmic
  Ointment, U.S.P.   10 per cent
  Sulphacetamide Eye Ointment, B.P.   6 per cent
  Sodium Sulfacetamide Ophthalmic
  Solution, U.S.P.   30 per cent
       Trade names: Albucid; Sulamyd Sodium; Steramide; Sulphasil

Sulfadiazine, U.S.P.; Sulphadiazine, B.P.
  Sulfadiazine Tablets, U.S.P.; Sulphadiazine Tablets, B.P., I.P.   300 and 500 mg.
          Trade names: Debenal; Pyrimal

Sodium Sulfadiazine, U.S.P.
   Sulfadiazine Sodium Injection, U.S.P.,
   I.P.   2.5 Gm. in 10 and 50 ml.
Sodium Sulfadiazine, U.S.P.   Vials containing 1 and 5 Gm.
Sulfadimethoxine, N.F.
   Sulfadimethoxine Suspension, N.F.   250 mg. in 5 ml.
   Sulfadimethoxine Tablets, N.F.   500 mg.

                Trade name: Madribon

Sulfaethidole
   Sulfaethidole Suspension   130 mg. in 1 ml.
   Sulfaethidole Tablets   650 mg.

       Trade names: Sul-Spansion; Sul-Span-Tab; Sethadil

Sulfamerazine, U.S.P.
   Sulfamerazine Tablets, N.F.   500 mg.
Sulfamerazine Sodium
   Sodium Sulfamerazine Injection, N.F.
   (I.P.)   2.5 Gm. in 10 ml. and 3 Gm. in 50 ml.

Sulfamethazine, U.S.P.; Sulphadimi-
dine, B.P.
   Sulphadimidine Tablets, B.P.   500 mg.
Sulphadimidine Sodium, B.P.
   Sulphadimidine Sodium Injection,
   B.P.

       Trade names: Diazil; Pirmazin; Sulphamethazine

Sulfamethoxazole Tablets   500 mg.

             Trade name: Gantanol

Sulfamethoxypyridazine, U.S.P.
   Sulfamethoxypyridazine Tablets,
   U.S.P.   500 mg.
   Sulfamethoxypyridazine Syrup   250 mg. in 5 ml.

        Trade names: Kynex; Lederkyn; Midicel

Sulfamethizole, N.F.
   Sulfamethizole Suspension, N.F.   250 mg. in 5 ml.
   Sulfamethizole Tablets, N.F.   250 mg.

        Trade names: Thiosulfil; Urolucosil

Sulfanilamide
   Sulfanilamide Tablets   300 and 500 mg.
Sulfapyridine, U.S.P.
   Sulfapyridine Tablets, U.S.P.   500 mg.
Sulfathiazole
   Sulfathiazole Tablets   300 and 500 mg.
Sulfathiazole Sodium
   Sulfathiazole Sodium Injection   2.5 Gm. in 10 ml.
Salicylazosulfapyridine
   Salicylazosulfapyridine Tablets   500 mg.

            Trade name: Azulfidine

Sulfisomidine, Sulphasomidine
   Sulfisomidine Syrup   250 mg. in 4 ml.
   Sulfisomidine Tablets   500 mg.

             Trade name: Elkosin

Sulfisoxazole, U.S.P., Sulphafurazole, B.P.
  Sulfisoxazole Tablets, U.S.P.   500 mg.
                  Trade name: Gantrisin
Acetyl Sulfisoxazole, N.F.
  Acetyl Sulfisoxazole Oral Suspension,   100 mg. in 1 ml.
  N.F.
  Acetyl Sulfisoxazole Syrup   100 mg. in 1 ml.
              Trade name: Gantrisin Acetyl
Sulfisoxazole Diethanolamine
  Sulfisoxazole Diethanolamine Injec-
  tion   2 Gm. in 5 ml.; 4 Gm. in 10 ml.
  Ophthalmic Ointment   4 per cent
  Ophthalmic Solution   4 per cent
          Trade name: Gantrisin Diethanolamine

Sulfonamide Mixtures

Trisulfapyrimidines
  Sulfonamide mixture containing equal
  parts of sulfadiazine, sulfamerazine,
  and sulfamethazine
  Oral Trisulfapyrimidines Suspension,   100 mg. (33 mg. of each of the drugs
  U.S.P.   in the mixture in each milliliter)
  Trisulfapyrimidines Tablets, U.S.P.   500 mg. (167 mg. each of sulfadiazine,
                        sulfamerazine, and sulfamethazine)
Trade names: Metha-Merdiazine; Multazine; Ray-Tri-Mides; Sulfaloid; Sulfa-tri-
azine; Sulfatryl; Terfonyl; Tersulfas; Trifonamide; Trionamide; Tripazine Tri-
          Sulfazine Tri-Sulfmeth Truozine

Sulfacetamine, Sulfadiazine and Sulfamerazine Suspension, N.F. (Acet-
Dia-Mer-Sulfonamides)   167 mg. of each sulfonamide in each
                        4 ml.
      Trade names: Buffonamide; Dorsulfas; Incorposil; Tricombisul

Sulfacetamide, Sulfadiazine, and Sulfamerazine Tablets, N.F. (Acet-Dia-Mer-
Sulfonamides)   500 mg.
      Trade names: Cetazine; Dorsulfas; Incorposul; Tricombisul

Sulfadiazine and Sulfamerazine Tablets,
N.F. (Dia-Mer Sulfonamides)   500 mg. total sulfonamides
Trade names: Bi-Sulfazine; Bisulfon; Diamerazine; Disulfyn; Duo-Sulfanyl; Duo-
zine; Mer-Diazine; Merdisul; Sul-Di-Mill; Sulfadimer; Sulfonamides Duplex;
                  Sulmeradine

Gastrointestinal Tract Anti-infectives

Phthalylsulfacetamide, N.F.
  Phthalylsulfacetamide Tablets,
  N.F.   500 mg.
             Trade name: Thalamyd

Phthalylsulfathiazole, U.S.P.;
Phthalylsulphathiazole, B.P.
  Phthalylsulfathiazole Tablets,   500 mg.
  U.S.P.
  Phthalylsulphathiazole Tablets,
  B.P.
            Trade name: Sulfathalidine

Succinylsulfathiazole; Succinylsulphathiazole, B.P.
   Succinylsulfathiazole Tablets; Tablets
   of Succinylsulphathiazole, B.P.   300 and 500 mg.
           Trade name: Sulfasuxidine

Sulfaguanidine, I.P.
Sulphaguanidine
   Sulfaguanidine Tablets   300 and 500 mg.
Para-Nitrosulfathiazole, N.F.
   Para-Nitrosulfathiazole Suspen-
   sion, N.F.   10 per cent

REVIEW QUESTIONS

1. Explain the importance of the introduction of sulfonamides into clinical medicine.
2. Compare the sulfonamides and the antibiotics with regard to (a) therapeutic usefulness, (b) toxicity, and (c) cost of treatment.
3. Explain the mechanism of action of the sulfonamides.
4. What are the main therapeutic uses for the sulfonamides?
5. What is the usual dose and method of administration?
6. Outline some of the toxic effects.
7. What advantages are gained by the use of the triple sulfonamides? By the use of sulfisoxazole (Gantrisin)?
8. Why are fluids usually "forced" when a patient is placed on sulfonamide therapy? Plan a schedule of oral fluid administration for this patient.
9. A patient is on Gantrisin—1 Gm. q. 4 h. Should she be awakened during the night for the administration of this medication? If so, why; if not, why not?
10. Why are patients who are to have intestinal surgery sometimes put on a regimen of sulfonamides pre- and postoperatively? Why might vitamin K be administered in conjunction with these drugs?

REFERENCES

Brickhouse, R. L.; Lepper, M. H.; Stone, T. E.; and Dowling, H. F.: "The Treatment of Pneumonia and Other Infections with a Soluble Sulfonamide, Gantrisin," Am. J. M. Sc., **218**:133, 1949.

Davis, B. D.: "The Binding of Sulfonamide Drugs by Plasma Proteins. A Factor in Determining the Distribution of Drugs in the Body," J. Clin. Investigation, **22**:753, 1943.

Domagk, G.: "Ein Beitrag zur Chemotherapie der Bakterieller Infektionen," Deutsche med. Wchnschr., **61**:250, 1935.

———: "Eine neue Klasse von Disinfektionsmitteln," Deutsche med. Wchnschr., **61**:829, 1935.

Fildes, P. A.: "A Rational Approach to Research in Chemotherapy," Lancet, **1**:955, 1940.

Hawking, F., and Lawrence, J. F.: The Sulfonamides. Grune & Stratton, Inc., New York, 1951.

Jawetz, E., and Gunnison, J. B.: "Antibiotic Synergism and Antagonism," Pharmacol. Rev., **5**:175, 1953.

Kutscher, A. H.; Lane, S. L.; and Segall, R.: "The Clinical Toxicity of Antibiotics and Sulfonamides," *J. Allergy*, **25**:135, 1954.

Lehr, D.: "Choice of Sulphonamides for Mixture Therapy," *Brit. M. J.*, **2**:601, 1950.

————: "Comparative Merits of 3,4-Dimethyl-sulfanilamido-isoxazole (Gantrisin) and a Sulfapyrimidine Triple Mixture," *Antibiotics & Chemother.*, **3**:71, 1953.

————: "Lowered Incidence of Sensitization Through Use of Sulphonamide Combinations: A New Concept," *Brit. M. J.*, **2**:543, 1948.

————: "Prevention of Renal Damage by the Use of Mixtures of Sulphonamides," *Brit. M. J.*, **2**:943, 1947.

Long, P. H., and Bliss, E. A.: *The Clinical and Experimental Use of Sulfanilamide, Sulfapyridine and Allied Compounds.* The Macmillan Company, New York, 1939.

Marshall, E. K., Jr.: "Experimental Basis of Chemotherapy in the Treatment of Bacterial Infections," *Bull. New York Acad. Med.*, **16**:722, 1940.

Northey, E. H.: *The Sulfonamides and Allied Compounds.* Reinhold, New York, 1948.

Prior, J. A., and Saslow, S.: "Observations on Absorption, Distribution and Excretion of Elkosin in Man," *J. Lab. & Clin. Med.*, **38**:420, 1951.

Rutenburg, A. M.; Schweinburg, F. B.; and Sears, B.: "Sulfadimetine, A New Sulfonamide for the Treatment of Urinary Infections," *Surgery*, **32**:980, 1949.

Tréfouël, J.; Tréfouël, Mme. J.; Nitti, F.; and Bovet, D.: "Activité du *p*-amino-phenyl-sulfamide sur les infections streptococciques expérimentales de la souris et du lapin," *Compt. rend. Soc. de biol.*, **120**:756, 1935.

Woods, D. D.: "Relations of *p*-Aminobenzoic Acid to Mechanism of Action of Sulphanilamide," *Brit. J. Exper. Path.*, **21**:74, 1940.

Work, T. S., and Work, E.: *The Basis of Chemotherapy.* Interscience Publishers, New York, 1948.

SULFAETHIDOLE

Council on Drugs: "Sulfaethidole," *J.A.M.A.*, **167**:1937, 1958.

SULFONAMIDES

Annotations: "New Sulphonamides," *Brit. M. J.*, **2**:482, 1959.

SULFAMETHOXYPYRIDAZINE

Jones, W. F., and Finland, M.: "Sulfamethoxypyridazine and Sulfachlorpyridazine," *Ann. N. Y. Acad. Sci.*, **69**:473, 1957.

Lepper, M. H.; Simon, A. J.; and Marienfeld, C. J.: "Use of Sulfamethoxypyridazine in the Prevention of Streptococcal Infections in Rheumatic Patients," *Ann. N. Y. Acad. Sci.*, **69**:485, 1957.

Nichols, R. L., and Finland, M.: "Absorption and Excretion of Sulfamethoxypyridazine, a New Long-acting Antibacterial Sulfonamide," *J. Lab. & Clin. Med.*, **49**:410, 1957.

Smith, G. F., *et al.*: "Blood and Cerebrospinal Fluid Levels of Sulfamethoxypyridazine After Intravenous Administration in Children," *Antibiotics Annual, 1958–1959.* Medical Encyclopedia, Inc., New York, 1959, p. 69.

SULFADIMETHOXINE

Daeschner, C. W.: "Modern Sulfonamides in Pediatric Practice," *Ann. N. Y. Acad. Sci.*, **82**:64, 1959.

DeLorenzo, W. F., and Schnitzer, R. J.: "Comparative Chemotherapeutic Studies with the Newer Sulfonamides," *Ann. N. Y. Acad. Sci.*, **82**:10, 1959.

Kiser, W. S.; Beyer, O. C.; and Young, J. D.: "Sulfadimethoxine in Urinary Tract Infections," *Ann. N. Y. Acad. Sci.*, **82**:105, 1959.

Moore, G. A.: "The Treatment of Respiratory, Urinary Tract, and Soft Tissue Infections with Madribon," *Ann. N. Y. Acad. Sci.*, **82**:61, 1959.

Ross, S.; Puig, J. R.; and Zarema, E. A.: "Sulfadimethoxine, A New Long-Acting Sulfonamide," *Antibiotics Annual, 1958–1959.* Medical Encyclopedia, Inc., New York, 1959, p. 56.

Townsend, E. H., Jr., and Borgstet, A.: "Newer Sulfonamides in Pediatric Practice," *Ann. N. Y. Acad. Sci.*, **82**:71, 1959.

SULFAPHENAZOL

Boger, W. P.: "Sulfaphenazol 'Orisul' a Long Acting Antibacterial Sulfonamide," *J. Am. Geriat. Soc.*, **7**:314, 1959.

METHENAMINE MANDELATE (MANDELAMINE)

Knight, V.; Draper, J. W.; Brady, E. A.; and Altmore, C. A.: "Methenamine Mandelate: Antimicrobial Activity, Absorption, and Excretion," *Antibiotics & Chemother.*, **2**:615, 1952.

SULFAMETHOXAZOLE

Pena, E. E.: "Clinical Results with a New Sulfonamide (RO-4-2130) in the Treatment of Urinary Tract Infections," *Antibiotics & Chemother.*, **11**:620, 1961.

11

Therapy of Neoplastic Diseases

The term "neoplasm" (meaning "new growth") is applied to all tumors, benign and malignant. Malignant growths are formed from cells which grow rapidly without restraint, are irreversible and self-perpetuating, and invade other tissues of the body where they exert pressure or cut off the blood supply of other tissues which then become necrotic and die. Certain cells may separate off from the primary growth and be carried by the circulation and lymphatics to the bones and soft tissues, where they promote secondary growths or metastases. The type of cell varies with the tissue in which growth originated and may be partially differentiated from, but often closely resembles, the normal cells with which it is associated in biochemical characteristics and enzymatic composition. Other types of neoplastic disease include those of the blood-forming organs, the bone marrow and the lymph nodes. Such diseases are polycythemia vera, the leukemias, and the lymphomas.

Research has been directed toward discovering qualitative or quantitative differences between normal and malignant cells in order to find substances that can inhibit the growth or destroy tumors with minimum damage to normal cells of the patient. As a result, radioactive isotopes, alkylating or radiomimetic drugs, enzyme inhibitors, antimetabolites, and hormones which alter the metabolism of cells have been found useful in bringing about temporary remissions of certain neoplastic diseases, particularly those of the blood-forming organs. Remissions are periods of considerable improvement in the course of the disease which, at times, resemble cures.

Since the differences between neoplastic and normal cells are slight, there is a narrow margin of safety between the dose necessary to affect the malignant cells and that which produces harmful effects on the normal cells of the patient, especially those which are rapidly growing and dividing such as cells of the hematopoietic system and the mucosal cells of the gastrointestinal tract. Often it is necessary to produce definite toxicity in order to obtain a clinical response. The available drugs cause only temporary remissions as the malignant cells ultimately develop resistance to them and continue to proliferate despite further treatment.

Polycythemia Vera. Polycythemia vera is a rare disease characterized by a marked increase in the number of red blood cells. The number of white blood cells and platelets may also be increased. The disease comes on spon-

178

taneously in middle or later life, and the symptoms are lassitude, weakness, headache, vertigo, and cyanosis. The decreased velocity of the circulation of the blood, resulting from the increased number of blood cells, increases the work load of the heart and a vascular catastrophe of some nature is eventually imminent unless the disease is checked.

Formerly, treatment consisted of venesection, or bleeding, and later administration of benzene and phenylhydrazene, which are substances that depress the bone marrow and thus reduce the number of red and white blood cells. Now, radioactive phosphorus is the drug of choice and successful remissions have been obtained, in some cases up to five years.

The Leukemias.   The primary characteristic of the leukemias is an excessive production of certain white blood cells, many of which fail to mature and are unable to protect the body against infection; at times, however, the number of leukocytes may be normal or, in certain stages, lower than normal, even as low as 200 per cubic millimeter. The type of cell present in the blood determines the disease. There are two types of leukemias: (1) *myelocytic,* in which the number of granulocytes and their precursors is greatly increased (100,000 to 500,000 per cubic millimeter) ; and (2) *lymphocytic,* in which the lymphocytes and their precursors are usually present in very large numbers (40,000 to 500,000 per cubic millimeter) although, at times, the white blood cell count may be low. Either of these two forms may be chronic or acute. The acute form occurs chiefly in children and almost always in persons under 25 years of age. It is rapidly fatal in a few days or weeks unless therapy is instituted.

In leukemia there is enlargement of the spleen and lymph nodes with tenderness of the sternum and shins. The patient is pale and there is persistent fever without infection. Progressive anemia and complete exhaustion may occur. The patients die from hemorrhage, infection, or leukocytic infiltration.

Radioactive phosphorus and x-ray treatment have been used with success in some cases. The other drugs used are nitrogen mustards, urethan, folic acid antagonists, and mercaptopurine. After prolonged use, the effectiveness of all these drugs diminishes as the malignant cells become resistant to their action. However, it is possible to change from one drug to another for additional remissions.

Lymphomas.   Lymphomas are tumors of the lymph nodes. Hodgkin's disease (malignant lymphoma) is characterized by enlargement of the lymph nodes and spleen, often of the liver and kidney, and by lymphoid infiltration along the vessels. There is no pronounced increase in the white blood cells. This disease, which has also been called *pseudoleukemia* and *lymphoadenoma,* is usually fatal in two or three years. Lymphosarcoma is another malignancy in this category. X-ray treatment, radioactive phosphorus, and nitrogen mustards are used in the treatment of various lymphomas.

CHORIOCARCINOMA

Choriocarcinoma, a relatively rare disease in women, is caused by a highly malignant tumor that usually arises from placental tissue. Although surgical cures have been reported, the usual course is early metastasis, rapid growth of the tumor, and death of the patient within a year of diagnosis. Spontaneous remissions are rare. These tumors secrete chorionic gonadotropin, which may be detected in the urine and serum. The level of urinary excretion provides a quantitative guide for the initial activity of the tumor and the therapeutic response to chemotherapeutic agents.

Methotrexate and vinblastine sulfate have been shown to cause remissions of varying duration and, in some cases, cures of this disease.

AGENTS USED IN THE TREATMENT OF NEOPLASTIC DISEASES

The agents used in the treatment of neoplastic diseases may be divided into three groups.

1. X-rays and radioactive isotopes, such as P^{32}, I^{131}, and Au^{198}, whose ionizing radiations destroy both normal and neoplastic cells by a direct action
2. Chemotherapeutic agents, which are also somewhat toxic to all cells
    a. Alkylating or radiomimetic agents
        (1) Mechlormethamine (nitrogen mustard, HN_2)
        (2) Mannomustine
        (3) Chlorambucil (Leukeran)
        (4) Uracil mustard
        (5) Triethylenemelamine (TEM)
        (6) Triethylenethiophosphoramide (Thio-TEPA)
        (7) Busulfan (Myleran)
        (8) Cyclophosphoramide (Cytoxan)
    b. Antimetabolites
        (1) Folic acid
            (a) Aminopterin
            (b) Methotrexate (Amethopterin)
        (2) Purines and pyrimidine
            (a) Mercaptopurine (Purinethol)
            (b) 5-Fluorouracil
            (c) Fluorodeoxyuridine
    c. Alkaloids
        (1) Vinblastine (Velban)

(2) Vincristine (Oncevin)
d. Urethan
e. Antibiotics
  (1) Asaserine (Serynl)
  (2) Mitomycin C
  (3) Actinomycins
f. Hormones
  (1) Estrogens and androgens
  (2) Corticosteroids and synthetic derivatives
  (3) Corticotrophin (ACTH)
3. Narcotics and supportive measures

Table 13 (see pp. 196–97) summarizes the specific agents used in cancer chemotherapy, and Table 14 (see pp. 200–202) summarizes the neoplastic diseases responding to chemotherapy.

RADIOACTIVE ISOTOPES

The introduction of radioactive materials into medicine shortly after the discovery of radium by the Curies in 1898 followed the observation that emissions from these materials were destructive to cells. It is known that in order for atoms to maintain a state of stability a delicate balance must exist within the nucleus. When in nature this balance is not present, spontaneous emissions occur as the nucleus attempts to reach a state of stability. All naturally occurring elements having an atomic number which is greater than 83 and a mass greater than 209 are unstable and are termed radioactive. This includes two elements frequently used in medicine: radium (atomic number 88, atomic weight 226.05) and radon.

When the nucleus of a stable element is subjected to neutron bombardment, the balance within the atom is disturbed and radioactive isotopes are formed. Isotopes are forms of an element which are alike in chemical reaction and atomic number but differ in atomic weight. They are termed radioactive when they are unstable and emit alpha particles, beta particles, and/or gamma rays as do the natural radioactive elements. These emissions or radiations all interfere with the ability of the cell to reproduce. They are all capable of some range of movement and of penetrating solid material.

Alpha particles, having the structure of helium nuclei, are rarely used in medical treatment. They have a very short range and a low penetration, and may be blocked by a single sheet of paper.

The activity of beta particles is confined to the immediate vicinity of their emanation. Their range in tissue varies from a few millimeters to about 1 cm. They are blocked by the patient's body when within it or by thin containers when being handled.

Gamma rays are not particles of matter but electromagnetic waves similar to x-rays but of shorter wave length. They are very penetrating, and a centimeter or more of a heavy metal or several feet of concrete is required to block them. Being the most dangerous type of radioactive emission, gamma rays must be used in medicine with great care.

Half-Life. As was stated previously, an unstable (radioactive) isotope emits radiation in order to attain stability. This emission proceeds continuously until there is complete conversion to the more stable isotope. In this process the radioactive isotope is said to disintegrate or decay. The time required for 50 per cent of a given amount of a radioactive isotope to disintegrate is known as the physical half-life ($T\frac{1}{2}$). This time or decay curve remains constant for each isotope. With the exception of radium, most radioactive isotopes used in medicine are characterized by a short half-life. Thus, for radioactive iodine (I^{131}) the half-life is 8.08 days; for radioactive phosphorus (P^{32}), 14.3 days; for radioactive gold (AU^{198}), 64 hours.

Diagnostic Uses. At the present time radioactive isotopes are used in medicine more widely for diagnosis than for therapy. For diagnostic purposes a minute amount of an isotope (measured in microcuries) or a substance normally found in the body combined with an isotope (tagged) is given internally to obtain information concerning a particular function of the body. For example, a tracer dose of radioactive iodine (I^{131}) may be given for study of the thyroid gland or serum albumin may be tagged with I^{131} and used for study of circulation time, cardiac output, or blood or plasma volume.

Table 11 lists some of the more common diagnostic studies and the isotopes used today.

Therapeutic Uses. The isotopes that are commonly used therapeutically in medicine are radium, cobalt, iodine, phosphorus, and gold. They are frequently beneficial in the treatment of chronic leukemia, polycythemia vera, certain malignant tumors, hyperthyroidism, and metastatic effusions. Table 12 presents pertinent facts concerning each of these isotopes.

Precautions. Normally, when radioactive isotopes are used for diagnostic purposes, no special precautions need to be taken as the amounts used are quite minimal. In the use of therapeutic doses certain precautions become necessary in order to protect the patient, personnel, and visitors from overexposure. The precautions required in each situation are based on: the half-life of the isotope, the type of radiation emitted, the amount of isotope used, the method of administration, the method of excretion and other ways it can be lost from the body.

For example, the need for precautions when caring for a patient being treated with radioactive gold decreases after 64 hours—its physical half-life—whereas in the care of a patient with a radium implant, the need remains constant since the half-life of radium is 1600 years. Patients who receive radiation therapy from external sources do not require special precautions between treatments as they do not have any source of radioactivity within them. If a patient has been given radioactive phosphorus (orally or intravenously), no precautions are necessary as it emits only beta particles, which are blocked by the body tissues. However, if that patient vomits immediately after taking the phosphorus, then precautions need to be taken when handling the materials that have been contaminated by the vomitus. These precautions might include:

1. Wearing gloves and gown when handling contaminated materials.

2. Placing contaminated linens in a covered metal can until they are safe to handle.

3. Disposing of vomitus by radiation safety officer in a special sink.

4. Decontaminating patient by bathing, preferably in a shower rather than a tub.

5. Monitoring patient and area contaminated to determine if the material has been successfully removed.

When one is carrying out the above precautions or working with any person receiving therapeutic doses of radioactive materials, application of three basic facts concerning radioactivity will result in safety for the personnel and more effective care for the patient.

1. Time: Each radioactive isotope emits radiation constantly. The length of time a person is exposed to the radiation determines the amount received.

2. Distance: Radiation varies inversely as the square of the distance. Thus the amount of radiation received at 2 ft from the source is one fourth that received at 1 ft; the amount received at 7 ft is one forty-ninth of that at 1 ft.

3. Shielding: All radiation can be blocked. Since gamma rays are the most penetrating, they require more dense material to block them. Whenever radioactive material is used, it should be shielded.

These facts may be used in many ways, for instance:

The nurse who prepares and checks equipment to be used by the patient before bringing it into the room rather than carrying out these tasks at the bedside is utilizing her knowledge of the importance of distance and time. The wearing of rubber gloves and the use of lead bricks to surround the container in which urine from a patient receiving radioactive iodine (I^{131}) therapy is saved reflect knowledge of shielding. Since it is rather difficult to adequately shield a patient without isolating him completely, time and distance are more frequently utilized by nurses.

Toxic Effects.   The toxic effects of radioactive materials are known as

———————————————— **Table 11** ————————————————

Common Diagnostic Studies

Diagnostic Study	Radioisotope Used

THYROID FUNCTION STUDIES

Radio-iodine uptake and thyroid scintigram pattern	I^{131}

CARDIOVASCULAR FUNCTION STUDIES

Blood volume	IHSA (I^{131} serum albumin)
Plasma volume	IHSA
Red cell mass	Cr^{51}
Circulation time	Na^{24}, IHSA, I^{131} Hippuran
Cardiac output	I^{131} Hippuran, IHSA
Cardiac shunt studies	Kr^{85} (Krypton^{83} Gas)
Cardiac scintigram for pericardial fluid	I^{131} Cholografin, IHSA

RENAL FUNCTION STUDIES

Renogram	I^{131} Hippuran, Hg^{203} Neohydrin
Renal scintigram pattern	Hg^{197}, Hg^{203} Chlormerodrin

INTESTINAL ABSORPTION STUDIES

Fat absorption studies	I^{131} Triolein, I^{131} oleic acid
Vitamin B_{12} Absorption studies (Schilling test)	Cobalt^{57} or Cobalt^{60} labeled vitamin B_{12}
Radioiron absorption studies	Fe^{59} citrate

ERYTHROKINETIC STUDIES—Red Cell Production and Destruction

Red cell survival studies with external organ counting for splenic sequestration	Cr^{51}-tagged red cells
Red cell production studies with external counting over liver, spleen, and bone marrow, plasma-iron turnover	Fe^{59} citrate
Platelet production and/or destruction	DFP^{32}, Cr^{51}

ORGAN SCANNING AND LOCALIZATION STUDIES

Brain scanning	Hg^{197}, Hg^{203} Chlormerodrin, IHSA, As^{74}, Cu^{64}
Liver scanning	Au^{198}, I^{131} rose bengal
Spleen scanning	Cr^{51}-tagged red cells (heated)
Pancreatic scanning	Se^{75} Methionine
Bone scanning	Sr^{89}, Ca^{47}
Lung scanning	Heat-denatured IHSA

radiation sickness or radiation reaction. The symptoms depend upon the location of the radiation effect in the body. Tissues which are actively growing or regenerating such as hematopoietic, skin, intestinal, or germinal cells are more readily affected. However, all tissues may be affected if high enough doses are received. A skin reaction frequently occurs with the use of external and implanted sources. The skin becomes erythematous and temporary epilation occurs. The area should be kept dry and free from irritation. A mild pigmentation may occur. Symptoms of radiation of the gastrointestinal tract include vomiting, diarrhea, ulceration, and bleeding. Radiation of the blood-forming organs causes depression of the leukocytes, platelets, and erthocytes.

Radioactive Phosphorus (P^{32})

Radioactive phosphorus is prepared by the neutron bombardment of sulfur. The atoms of this substance undergo a nuclear transformation with the emission of electrons known as ionizing radiations. They then become stable sulfur atoms. It is the emission of beta rays that affects tissues and has proved useful in bringing about remission in polycythemia vera and leukemias, particularly in the chronic types. Radioactive phosphorus is not useful in solid tumors.

Sodium Phosphate (P32) Solution, U.S.P., is a clear solution (in saline) containing radioactive phosphate in the form of sodium phosphate. This preparation is depressant to neoplastic and polycythemic tissues. The oral or intravenous dose for diagnostic purposes is the equivalent of 250 microcuries to 1 millicurie. The therapeutic dose is the equivalent of 1 to 5 millicuries.[1] **Sodium Phosphate (^{32}P) Injection, B.P.,** is suitable for intravenous administration.

Radioactive phosphorus is carried to all parts of the body by the blood. The bone marrow, which is rich in phosphorus, is markedly affected, and the manufacture of red and white blood cells is slowed down. The half-life of radioactive phosphorus is 14.3 days, which is advantageous, for after two weeks much of the drug has undergone decay or has been excreted and the electron emission is nearly over. The initial dose of 3 to 7 millicuries is often sufficient. Subsequent doses may be administered, if required, but not more often than once every six or eight weeks. It requires about three months for the full effect to be manifested in the blood, and one dose will usually maintain the patient without symptoms for six months.

The initial intravenous dose in leukemia is 1 to 2 millicuries. Then four doses of 0.5 to 1 millicurie each are given over a period of two weeks, follow-

---

[1] A millicurie (mc) is the amount of radioactive subtance which undergoes 3.7 x 10^7 (37 million) disintegrations per second. A microcurie (μc) is 1/1000 of that amount, or 3.7 x 10^4.

Table 12

Isotopes Commonly Used Therapeutically

Radio-isotope	Half-life	Rays Emitted	Therapeutic Uses	Method of Administration	Contamination		Special Handling
					Excreted from Body	Ways Lost	
Iodine I^{131}	8.08 days	Beta Gamma	Thyroid malignancies, hyperthyroidism	Orally usually Intravenously	Urine primarily, stool, diarrhea, saliva, sweat	Vomiting immediately after ingestion	Urine, feces, vomitus, linens
Gold Au^{198}	64 hours	Beta Gamma	Malignant effusions	Intracavitarily	None	Leakage from injection site	Dressing, linens
Phosphorus P^{32}	14.22 days	Beta	Malignant effusions, chronic leukemia, polycythemia vera	Orally Intravenously Intracavitarily	Feces—if given orally, urine	Vomiting immediately after ingestion Leakage from injection site	Linens if soiled, dressings if leakage.
Cobalt Co^{60}	5.26 years	Gamma Beta	Localized malignant neoplasms	Externally Interstitially		Dislodgment of needles or seeds from site of insertion	Monitor linen and other equipment used before removing from area.
Radium Ra^{226}	1620 years	Gamma Beta Alpha	Localized malignant neoplasms	Externally Interstitially		Dislodgment of needles or seeds from site of insertion	Monitor linen and other equipment used before removing from area.

ing which the intervals between the doses are extended to one week. This regimen is continued until the white blood count falls to 30,000.

The chief disadvantage in the use of radioactive phosphorus is the danger of excessive depression of bone marrow. Large doses may actually induce neoplasms. The advantages of its use are ease of administration, absence of radiation sickness, longer remission, and reduced incidence of thrombosis and hemorrhage. It is not necessary to hospitalize the patient. As radioactive phosphorus emits only beta particles, which are totally absorbed by the patient's tissues, no special precautions, other than careful disposal of body wastes, are necessary.

Chromic Radio-Phosphate (Cr $P^{32}O_4$)

Chromic radio-phosphate is used in the treatment of pleural effusions and ascites. The usual dose by intracavitary instillation is 5 to 7 millicuries. If the effusion recurs, the instillation may be repeated. The isotope is also used in the diagnosis of tumors of the eye. The intravenous dose for this purpose is 500 microcuries. If a malignant tumor is present, the involved eye will take up more of the isotope.

Radioactive Gold (Aurcoloid[198])

Radioactive gold is used in the palliative management of ascites and pleural effusions associated with metastatic malignancies in closed serous cavities and as a palliative prophylactic agent against dissemination of tumor cells after surgical removal of tumors from these cavities. As a side effect, mild radiation sickness may occur after three or four days. Pronounced fibrosis and hypoplasia of the bone marrow have been noted in a few cases.

The intracavitary doses vary from 35 to 150 millicuries. A clinical effect may not be noted for three or four weeks. *Dosage should not be repeated at intervals of less than four weeks, and then only if the rate of fluid accumulation necessitates it.* Radioactive gold is available in 10- and 20-ml. multiple-dose vials containing 20, 50, 100, 200, 300, 400, 600, or 800 millicuries.

Alkylating or Radiomimetic Agents

Nitrogen mustards are related to mustard gas, which was used in World War I. They contain two or more alkyl groups which react with many of the constituents of cells. Deoxyribonucleic acid (DNA) in the nucleus appears to be the most susceptible. Their action, which is nucleotoxic, is somewhat different from other known chemical agents and resembles in some ways the action of x-rays on cells. They are local vesicants causing blistering of the skin and severe damage to the eyes and cells of the respiratory tract. They are especially injurious to the rapidly proliferating cells in the lymphatic and hematopoietic systems and the epithelial lining of the gastrointestinal tract and the testes. They do not selectively damage malignant cells but also have a toxic action on normal cells. The action is due to the formation of cyclic ethyleneimmonium derivatives which are unstable and highly reactive and combine with chemical groupings found in proteins and nucleic acids. Systemic toxic effects are nausea and vomiting due to their destructive action on the gastrointestinal tract, reduction in the number of white and red blood cells, and hemorrhagic diathesis.

Mechlorethamine Hydrochloride, U.S.P. (Nitrogen Mustard); Mustine Hydrochloride, B.P.; Mustargen, HN₂

Procytox Mechlorethamine hydrochloride is a nitrogen mustard. It is used in the treatment of Hodgkin's disease, lymphatic and myeloid leukemia, and certain other neoplastic diseases. A total intravenous dose of 0.4 mg. per kilogram is usually administered. It may be given at one time or once daily in doses of 0.1 mg. per kilogram for four consecutive days.

A saline solution of the drug is freshly prepared by adding 10 ml. of water for injection to the vial, which contains 10 mg. mechlorethamine and 90 mg. of sodium chloride to increase the bulk. The treatment may be repeated in four weeks. The drug is usually injected into the tubing of a rapidly running infusion of 5 per cent dextrose in water in order to decrease the possibility of chemical thrombi and local extravasation causing induration and slough at the site of injection. Nitrogen mustard is very irritating to the skin, causing blistering on contact (vesication). For this reason, precautions such as wearing gloves should be taken when handling it, and the skin surrounding the injection site should be protected.

Side Actions. Patients receiving nitrogen mustard usually experience loss of appetite, nausea, vomiting, and sometimes diarrhea within eight hours after taking the drug. Sedatives and antiemetics such as prochlorperazine are helpful in decreasing the severity of these symptoms.

Other delayed toxic effects are headache, severe abdominal pain, fever, anemia, alopecia, great weakness, and shock. Salivation, bradycardia, low blood pressure, and hyperpnea may occur due to the stimulant effect of the drug on the parasympathetic system. Hemoconcentration and loss of intra- and extracellular fluid may be caused by changes in electrolyte and fluid balance of the tissues. Thrombophlebitis may result because of the irritating effect on the blood vessels.

Therapeutic Uses. Nitrogen mustard is used in Hodgkin's disease, lymphosarcoma, choriocarcinoma, chronic myelocytic leukemia, polycythemia vera, and miscellaneous carcinomas and sarcomas. It is the drug of choice in Hodgkin's disease. It does not cure the disease but it does cause periods of remission up to two months which become progressively shorter until the disease becomes resistant to the drug. There is only a slight increase in life expectancy but there is relief from pain, fever, and pruritus and the patient feels much more comfortable. It is useful as an adjunct to radiotherapy only when the disease is generalized. Life is not prolonged, but the amount of radiation required is decreased and the patient is without symptoms for longer periods of time.

Preparation

Mechlorethamine Hydrochloride for Injection, U.S.P.	20-ml. rubber-stoppered vials containing 10 mg. and 90 mg. of sodium chloride
Mustine Injection, B.P.	

Trade name: Mustargen Hydrochloride

Mannomustine

Mannomustine is a cytotoxic compound used in the treatment of leukemia, polycythemia, reticulosis, and malignant disease. The drug is administered intravenously or intrapleurally in doses of 100 mg. daily or on alternate days. It is available as a dry crystalline substance in ampuls containing 50 mg. Before use, the contents of the ampul or ampuls are dissolved in physiological saline or ascorbic acid solution so that the solution contains 10 to 20 mg. in 1 ml.

Side effects such as nausea and vomiting may occur. Severe toxic effects, particularly on the bone marrow, have been reported. Thrombophlebitis may occur in the vein in which the injection is made.

Uracil Mustard

Uracil mustard is administered orally in the palliative treatment of neoplasms of the reticuloendothelial system such as chronic leukemia, malignant lymphomas including Hodgkin's disease, polycythemia vera, and carcinoma of the lung and ovary. The side effects noted are nausea, vomiting, diarrhea, irritability or depression, nervousness, various skin reactions, and loss of hair. The more serious toxic effects are thrombocytopenia, and granulocytic and lymphocytic leukopenia. Blood counts, including platelet counts, should be done once or twice weekly. The drug is administered orally in doses of 1 to 2 mg. daily for three weeks. After the drug is omitted for a week, the dosage schedule is repeated. In some cases, 3 to 5 mg. is given daily for seven days. This is followed by a maintenance dose of 1 mg. daily. Uracil mustard is available in capsules containing 1 mg.

Chlorambucil, U.S.P., B.P. (Leukeran)

Chlorambucil is related to the nitrogen mustards. It is well absorbed upon oral administration. Few side effects are noted in therapeutic dosage; with large doses, anorexia, nausea, and vomiting occur. Toxicity is related to bone marrow depression and therefore blood examinations should be made at least once a week. Chlorambucil is used in the treatment of chronic lymphocytic leukemia and malignant lymphomas. It is administered orally in doses of 0.1 to 0.2 mg. per kilogram of body weight for three to six weeks.

Preparation
Chlorambucil Tablets, U.S.P.   2 mg.
Trade name: Leukeran

The fact that nitrogen mustards undergo conversion into ethyleneimmonium compounds which are very unstable and highly reactive led to the synthesis of a number of these derivatives.

Triethylenemelamine, N.F. (TEM)

Triethylenemelamine is related to the nitrogen mustards and produces the same toxic reactions. It is administered orally and intravenously and is used in the treatment of Hodgkin's disease, chronic lymphocytic and myelocytic leukemias, lymphosarcoma, and carcinoma of the ovary. When it is taken orally, there is less action on the gastrointestinal tract with less nausea and vomiting than with mechlorethamine. It has no vesicant action. The initial dose is 2.5 mg. daily for two or three days. Continued administration is determined on the basis of weekly blood counts. Treatment is interrupted if there is a rapid fall in leukocytes, but if the count remains high, 5 mg. may be given. The drug is given in the morning with water and 2 Gm. of sodium bicarbonate to prevent its inactivation by gastric acidity. When it is desirable to decrease the leukocytes rapidly, it is given intravenously. The intravenous dose is 0.04 mg. per kilogram body weight daily for three or four days. The drug is injected into the tubing of a rapidly flowing saline infusion.

The advantages in its use are that it can be administered orally and can be used in ambulatory patients. It causes less nausea and vomiting. The delayed onset of action is the main disadvantage.

Great care should be used in its administration because it may produce severe bone marrow depression. And the rapid dissolution of leukemic cells may cause uricemia and kidney damage.

Preparation
Triethylenemelamine Tablets   5 mg.
Trade name: TEM

Thiotepa, U.S.P. (Triethylene Thiophosphoramide, Thio-TEPA)

This is another compound related to mustard. It is used in the treatment of Hodgkin's disease, lymphosarcoma, and chronic leukemias, but it is contraindicated in acute leukemia. It may also be used in the treatment of mammary and ovarian tumors. In advanced cases of breast cancer it may relieve dyspnea resulting from pulmonary metastases and neurological symptoms due to cerebral metastases. Triethylene thiophosphoramide is administered intravenously, intra-arterially, intramuscularly, by pleural or peritoneal infusions, or by direct injection into the tumor. The dose is 0.2 mg. per kilogram of body weight daily for three to five days. The drug is dissolved in distilled water so that a concentration of 10 mg. in 1 ml. is available. Clinical improvement of varying degrees has been obtained in about 80 per cent of the patients treated.

Preparation

Thiotepa for Injection, U.S.P.   Vials containing 15 mg.

Trade name: Thio-TEPA

Busulfan, U.S.P., B.P. (Myleran)

Busulfan is unrelated chemically to nitrogen mustards, but it does produce the same type of alkylating action on tissues. Its action is limited to the bone marrow. It is indicated only in chronic granulocytic leukemia. The oral dose is 2 mg. (1 to 6 mg.) daily. The dose is continued until clinical improvement is evident, unless toxic effects such as an abrupt drop in the leukocyte count or bleeding tendencies are noted. Treatment may be necessary for three to four weeks or perhaps several months. During remissions maintenance doses of 1 to 3 mg. daily may be given.

Preparation

Busulfan Tablets, U.S.P., B.P.   2 mg.

Trade name: Myleran

Cyclophosphoramide, N.F. (Cytoxan)

Cyclophosphoramide is a new potent cytotoxic agent that has a palliative effect on malignant tumors. It is less toxic than nitrogen mustard. Nausea, vomiting, dizziness, and alopecia, which is not permanent, occur. Leukopenia and thrombocytopenia have been reported with large doses. Cyclophosphoramide is used in the treatment of Hodgkin's disease, lymphomas, leukemias, and for certain tumors. It is administered intravenously, intramuscularly, intraperitoneally, or directly into the tumor. The intravenous dose is 2 to 3 mg. per kilogram of body weight daily for six days or until a loading dose of 2 to 8 Gm. has been given. Then an oral maintenance dose of 50 to 200 mg. daily is given.

Preparations

Cyclophosphoramide for Injection	Vials containing 100 mg. with 45 mg. sodium chloride
Cyclophosphoramide Tablets, N.F.	50 mg.

Trade name: Cytoxan

REGIONAL PERFUSION BY USING EXTRACORPOREAL CIRCULATION

The circulation of areas of the body or of organs containing tumors has been isolated and perfused with nitrogen mustards under high arterial oxygen tension, using the heart-lung apparatus. By this method limbs and parts of the intestines, liver, pelvis, and lungs, etc., containing tumors may be isolated from the general circulation and perfused for periods up to 30 minutes or longer. This permits much larger doses of the alkylating agents to come in contact with the tumors than could be tolerated by intravenous or intramuscular medication. This method may prove valuable as adjunctive therapy for localized tumors and for palliation of far-advanced tumors.

One of the major drawbacks of this technique is leakage into the circulation with subsequent serious depression of the bone marrow. Therefore, care must be taken not to prolong the procedure. A promising method of overcoming this problem is to remove bone marrow from the patient before treatment and preserve and reinject it after treatment.

Define ## ANTIMETABOLITES

These compounds resemble substances essential for the metabolism and growth of cells but differ slightly in chemical structure and are antagonistic to them. They may inhibit the normal activity of enzymes or coenzymes in the cells by competing with the normal substrate or be incorporated into the molecule to form an abnormal substance in the cell. They prevent the proliferation of both normal and neoplastic cells by interfering with the synthesis of deoxyribonucleic acid (DNA) and ribonucleic acid (RNA) by either altering the rates of synthesis of purines, pyrimidines, and nucleic acids or by substituting abnormal constituents. Since there is a constant need for these substances, decreased or altered synthesis will affect the functions, multiplication, and integrity of the cells.

Define ## FOLIC ACID ANTAGONISTS

Folic acid deficiency is accompanied by leukopenia (decrease in the normal leukocytes in the blood). This observation led to the synthesis of folic acid antagonists or antimetabolites to inhibit the growth of neoplasms in the white blood cell-forming organs. These antagonists have been used successfully in some cases of leukemia. It has been observed that human neoplasms contain a higher concentration of folic acid than normal tissues, and substances that deprive these tumors of their essential supply of this vitamin interfere with the conversion of folic acid to its active form, folinic acid (citrovorum factor) and block several steps in the formation of purines and a pyrimidine. Many folic acid antagonists have been prepared. Of this group methotrexate (amethopterin) seems to be the most successful.

Aminopterin Sodium

Aminopterin does not appear to be useful in chronic leukemia but causes remission of symptoms in some cases of acute leukemia. The remission rates are higher in children than in adults. The oral or intramuscular dose is 0.25 to 0.5 mg. three to six times weekly over a period of three weeks or more until remission occurs. It is indicated only in acute leukemia in children. The toxic effects are loss of appetite, ulcerative stomatitis, anemia, alopecia, abdominal pain, bloody diarrhea, leukopenia, depression, and coma.

Preparation

Aminopterin Tablets   0.5 mg.

Methotrexate, U.S.P.; Amethopterin

Methotrexate is another folic acid antagonist that elicits a response similar to that of aminopterin. The toxic effects which are the same may be less severe. It is the drug of choice for acute leukemia in children. Remission of symptoms usually lasts for about seven months during which time the blood picture may return to normal. There is less bone pain and the patient feels better. It is far less effective in adults, and chronic cases are resistant to the drug. The daily oral dose of methotrexate is 5 mg. (5 to 10 mg.). Methotrexate is administered intrathecally in doses of 0.25 mg. per kilogram of body weight every second or third day or 0.5 mg. per kilogram of body weight every fourth or fifth day when there is central nervous system involvement with leukemia.

Methotrexate has been used in the treatment of choriocarcinoma and related trophoblastic tumors in women. Remissions of varying duration have been reported, some for as long as five years. The drug is usually given intramuscularly in doses of 10 to 30 mg. daily for five days. In some cases it was given orally or intravenously. The course of treatment is repeated 10 to 14 days after the last dose if all toxic effects related to the drug have decreased. Several courses of treatment may prove necessary. Development of drug resistance after the initial response to methotrexate has been observed.

Preparations

Methotrexate Injection   Vials containing 5 mg.
Methotrexate Tablets   2.5 and 5 mg.

Calcium Leucovorin, U.S.P.

Calcium leucovorin is an antidote to lessen the toxicity of aminopterin sodium and other folic acid antagonists. It is given intramuscularly in doses of 3 mg. once or twice daily. It is available as Calcium Leucovorin Injection, U.S.P., which contains 3 mg. in 1 ml.

Mercaptopurine, U.S.P., B.P.; 6-Mercaptopurine, Purinethol

Mercaptopurine (a derivative of natural purines) is a purine antagonist. It interferes with the incorporation of essential purines in nucleic acid. It is rapidly abosorbed from the gastrointestinal tract and some is rapidly excreted unchanged. It is well tolerated and produces no immediate toxic manifestations. After prolonged administration, nausea and abdominal discomfort may occur, more often in adults than in children. Its main actions are on the bone marrow and the epithelium of the gastrointestinal tract. Excessive doses cause leukopenia, thrombocytopenia, and anemia.

Therapeutic Uses.   Mercaptopurine is used in the treatment of acute leukemia and produces remissions, particularly in children, which last three to four months or longer. It is the drug of choice in myelocytic leukemia. The drug is indicated in patients who have become refractory to alkylating agents and radiation and may provide an additional period of improvement.

Dosage and Method of Administration.   The initial daily oral dose of 2.5 mg. per kilogram of body weight may be tolerated for a long time. Resistance develops rapidly if therapy is interrupted; so a maintenance dose of 1.5 to 2.5 mg. per kilogram of body weight is given orally once a day. Blood counts should be taken weekly.

Preparation

Mercaptopurine Tablets, U.S.P., B.P.   50 mg. (scored)

Trade name: Purinethol

6-Thioguanine

This drug is effective and well tolerated but has no apparent advantage over mercaptopurine. The oral daily dose is 2.5 mg. per kilogram of body weight.

5-Fluorouracil (5-FU)

5-Fluorouracil, a pyrimidine antagonist, acts in three ways: (1) it blocks the formation of a pyrimidine, thymidine; (2) it directly inhibits the synthesis of RNA; and (3) it is itself incorporated in RNA. Since it affects normal as well as malignant tissues, the therapeutic dose is close to that which produces toxic effects. The main action of the drug is on the hematopoietic and gastrointestinal systems. The earliest toxic effects are anorexia, nausea, and occasionally vomiting. The patient should be warned that temporary alopecia may occur. Ulceration of the mouth is a more serious side effect, and when this occurs, therapy should be discontinued to prevent further serious symptoms such as diarrhea, ulceration, and bleeding of the gastrointestinal tract and depression of the bone marrow, which may occur in 10 to 14 days. Diarrhea may be serious enough to require fluid replacement.

Therapeutic Uses.   5-Fluorouracil is used in the treatment of cancer of the colon, thyroid, ovary, liver, and bladder and in metastatic breast tumor. It is also of some value in leukemias.

Dosage and Method of Administration.   The drug is given intravenously in doses of 15 mg. per kilogram for three to five days. Treatment is stopped for one day and then one half of the above dose is given every second day until a mild stomatitis develops. Once the patient has responded, the course may be repeated but only once every four to six weeks to avoid severe toxicity. The drug is also available for oral administration. The oral effective dose is up to twice the amount required for the intravenous dose.

Preparations

5-Fluorouracil Injection	10-ml. vials containing 50 mg. in 1 ml.
5-Fluorouracil Tablets	50 mg.

5-Fluorodeoxyuridine (5-FUDR)

This drug is also a pyrimidine antagonist and has the same therapeutic uses as 5-fluorouracil. However, it is more potent and more toxic. Toxic effects may be lessened by the administration of thymidine, but efficacy of 5-fluorodeoxyuriline is then decreased. The intravenous dose is 30 mg. per kilogram for three to five days. 5-Fluorouracil is cheaper and more readily available.

Alkaloids

Vinblastine Sulfate (Velban, Velbe)

Vinblastine (vincaleukoblastine) is an alkaloid derived from the periwinkle plant (*Vinca rosea*). It has antitumor activity in women with metastatic trophoblastic disease who have become resistant to methotrexate and other chemical agents. It has been used with some success in Hodgkin's disease refractory to irradiation and alkylating agents. It has also been shown to be effective in some solid tumors as well as against monocytic leukemia.

Table 13

Specific Agents Used in Cancer Chemotherapy*.

Agents	Usual Dose and Method of Administration	Acute Toxic Signs	Major Late Toxic Manifestations
	RADIOACTIVE ISOTOPES		
Iodine (I^{131})	Oral, i.v. 100-200 mc.	None	Myxedema, bone marrow depression, renal damage
Phosphorus (P^{32})	Oral, i.v. 3.7 mc.	None	Bone marrow depression
P^{32} as chromic phosphate	Intracavitary, 5-10 mc.	None	
Gold (Au^{198})	Intracavitary, 75-150 mc.		
	POLYFUNCTIONAL ALKYLATING AGENTS		
Mechlorethamine (HN$_2$, nitrogen mustard)	I.v. 0.4 mg./kg. single or divided doses	Nausea and vomiting	Therapeutic doses produce moderate depression of peripheral blood cell count; excessive doses cause severe bone marrow depression with leukopenia, thrombocytopenia, and bleeding. Maximum toxicity may occur two or three weeks after last dose. Dosage must therefore be carefully controlled. Alopecia and hemorrhagic cystitis occur occasionally with cyclophosphoramide
Chlorambucil (Leukeran)	Oral, 0.1-0.2 mg./kg./day 6-12 mg./day	None	
l-Sarcolysin (Alkeran, Mephalan)	Oral, 6-10 mg./day initially; 2-4 mg./day maintenance	None	
Cyclophosphoramide (Cytoxan, Endoxan)	I.v. 3.5-5 mg./kg./day x 10 40-60 mg./kg. single dose Oral, 50-300 mg./day	Nausea and vomiting	
Triethylenethiophosphoramide (Thio-TEPA)	I.v. 0.2 mg./kg. x 5	None	
Busulfan (Myleran)	Oral, 2.8 mg./day 150-250 mg./course	None	
	ANTIMETABOLITES		
Methotrexate	Oral, 2.5-5.0 mg./day	None	Oral and digestive tract ulcerations; bone marrow depression with leukopenia, thrombocytopenia, and bleeding

Drug	Dose	Acute toxic reactions	Chronic toxic reactions
Mercaptopurine (Purinethol)	Oral, 2.5 mg./kg./day	None	Therapeutic doses usually well tolerated; excessive doses cause bone marrow depression
6-Thioguanine	Oral, 2.5 mg./kg./day	None	
5-Fluorouracil (5-FU)	I.v. 15 mg./kg./day 3 to 5 times	None	Stomatitis, nausea, gastrointestinal injury, bone marrow depression

ALKALOIDS

Drug	Dose	Acute toxic reactions	Chronic toxic reactions
Vinblastine (Velban)	I.v. 0.1-0.15 mg./kg. weekly	Nausea and vomiting	Alopecia, muscular weakness, areflexia, bone marrow depression
Vincristine (Oncovin)	I.v. 0.03-0.075 mg./kg. weekly	None	Areflexia, peripheral neuritis, paralytic ileus, mild bone marrow depression
Demecoline (Colcemide)	Oral, 5-8 mg./day	None	Alopecia, bone marrow depression

MISCELLANEOUS

Drug	Dose	Acute toxic reactions	Chronic toxic reactions
Urethan	Oral, 2-4 Gm./day	Nausea and vomiting	Bone marrow depression
Quinacrine (Atabrine)	Intracavitary, 100-200 mg./day 5 x	Local pain, fever, hemolytic anemia	

ANTIBIOTIC

Drug	Dose	Acute toxic reactions	Chronic toxic reactions
Actinomycin D (Cosmegan)	I.v. 15 mcg./kg./day 5 x or 50 mcg./kg. weekly	Nausea and vomiting	Stomatitis, gastrointestinal disturbances, alopecia, bone marrow depression

HORMONES

Drug	Dose	Acute toxic reactions	Chronic toxic reactions
Androgen			
Testosterone Propionate	I.m. 50-100 mg. 3 x weekly	None	Fluid retention, masculinization
Fluoxymesterone (Halotestin)	Oral, 10-20 mg./day		
Estrogen			
Diethylstilbestrol	Oral, 1-5 mg. 3/day	Occasional nausea and vomiting	Fluid retention, feminization, uterine bleeding
Ethinyl estradiol (Estradiol)	Oral, 0.1-1.0 mg. 3/day		
Progestin			
Hydroxyprogesterone (Delalutin)	I.m. 1 Gm. twice weekly	None	
Corticosteroids			
Cortisone Acetate	Oral, 50-300 mg./day	None	Fluid retention, hypertension, diabetes, increased susceptibility to infection, ulcer formation
Hydrocortisone Acetate	Oral, 50-200 mg./day		
Prednisone (Meticorten)	Oral, 20-100 mg./day		

* From Karnofsky, D. A.: "Cancer Chemotherapeutic Agents," *CA*, **14**:67, 1964.

The amount of vinblastine to be injected is dissolved in 10 to 20 ml. of saline just prior to use and injected into tubing of rapidly running infusion of normal saline. The drug is irritating locally, and extravasation is painful. Vinblastine is given only intravenously. The dose depends upon the age of the patient and the white blood count, but the usual initial dose is 0.1 to 0.15 mg. per kilogram of body weight. The dose may be repeated after one week if the blood picture has returned to normal. Further doses may be given at intervals of 7 to 14 days according to the response, if necessary.

Toxic Effects. Vinblastine causes a suppression of the bone marrow and leukopenia. Complete recovery of all bone marrow elements is manifested by peripheral blood examination within three weeks. Other side effects observed are numbness and parathesias of the fingers, constipation, urinary retention, dry mouth, increased hair loss, even alopecia (reversible). Mental depression occurs during the height of systemic reaction but quickly disappears. Fever that may occur is prevented or treated with antibiotics.

Preparation

Vinblastine Sulfate   Ampuls containing 10 mg.
Trade names: Velban, Velbe

Vincristine Sulfate (Oncovin)

Vincristine (Oncovin), another alkaloid obtained from *Vinca rosea*, has produced partial or complete remissions in 50 per cent of children with acute leukemia resistant to other forms of treatment. The remissions are brief and associated with considerable toxicity. After one injection nausea and weakness which disappear in a few days are noted. After three of four injections certain toxic symptoms such as paresthesias, disturbance in equilibrium, peripheral neuritis, muscle pain, constipation with distention, and ileus may occur. Other toxic effects observed less frequently are ulcerations in the mouth, depression and headache. At this time the dosage should be decreased or terminated. Only mild depression of the bone marrow occurs.

The usual intravenous dose is 0.03 to 0.075 mg. per kilogram at weekly intervals. Extravasation of the drug causes a severe local reaction.

Preparation

Vincristine Sulfate   Ampuls containing I and 5 mg.
Trade name: Oncovin

Demecoline (Colcemid)

Demecoline, an analog of colchicine (see p. 695) is used in the treatment of chronic myelocytic leukemia. It is well tolerated and causes a decrease in the white blood cell count and clinical improvement. The daily oral dose is 5 to 10 mg.

Urethan, N.F., Urethane, B.P. (Ethyl Carbamate)

Urethan was used for many years as a sedative and hypnotic. It is a neo-plastic depressant similar to nitrogen mustards, but it is less potent. It is used in the treatment of leukemia and is more effective in chronic myelogenous leukemia than in the lymphatic variety. The usual oral dose is 3 Gm. daily (2 to 6 Gm.). It is given in enteric-coated tablets or flavored syrup to lessen irritation.

Toxicity. Urethan produces depression of the bone marrow, nausea, vomiting, and sedation, which may prove dangerous to persons doing hazard-ous work. In hypersensitive persons, severe leukopenia and aplasia of the bone marrow may occur.

Preparation

Urethan Tablets, N.F.   300 mg.

Quinacrine, U.S.P. (Atabrine)

Quinacrine is administered by intracavitary injection into the appropriate cavity to control pleural and ascitic effusions. It probably produces its clinical effect by a fibrolytic reaction. It is also used as an anthelmintic (see p. 235) and in antimalarial therapy (see p. 213).

ANTIBIOTICS

Azaserine (Serynl)

Azaserine is obtained from the fermentation cultures of *Streptomyces fragi-lis*. It has little or no action against microorganisms, but Dr. C. C. Stock and associates have reported that it inhibits the growth of mouse sarcoma, Dr. R. R. Ellison and her associates have suggested its possible use in leukemia. When given alone, it has little value in this disease; but when given with Purinethol, Dr. David A. Karnofsky found that the remissions were increased to 72 per cent. Under Purinethol alone the remissions were only 44 per cent. The oral dosage with Purinethol is 2.5 mg. per kilogram of body weight. The success with this combination is much greater with children than with adults. The only untoward effect of the administration of azaserine is an inflamed, sore tongue.

Mitomycin C

Mitomycin C is a new antitumor antibiotic that is now available in crystal-line form. It has been used clinically in Japan in the treatment of patients with advanced malignancies and has caused regression of tumors in about

Table 14

Neoplastic Diseases Responding to Chemotherapy*

Diagnosis	Polyfunctional Alkylating Agents	Antimetabolites	Radioactive Isotopes	Hormones	Miscellaneous Drugs	Results
Leukemia Acute, children	Cyclophosphamide	Mercaptopurine Methotrexate		Adrenocorticosteroids	Vincristine	70% bone marrow improvement; 50% patients live one year or longer
Acute, adults		Mercaptopurine		Adrenocorticosteroids		15-25% improved for several months or longer
Chronic myelocytic	Busulfan Nitrogen mustard	Mercaptopurine	P^{32}		Demecolcine	Patients maintained in good condition during major portion of disease; life occasionally prolonged
Chronic lymphatic	Chlorambucil Thio-TEPA		P^{32}	Adrenocorticosteroids		Patients maintained in good condition during major portion of disease; life occasionally prolonged
Hodgkin's disease	Chlorambucil Nitrogen mustard Thio-TEPA			Adrenocorticosteroids	Vinblastine	Occasional favorable response but no definite prolongation of life
Lymphosarcoma	Chlorambucil Nitrogen mustard Thio-TEPA			Adrenocorticosteroids	Vinblastine	Occasional favorable response but no definite prolongation of life
Multiple myeloma	Alkeran Cyclophosphamide		P^{32}	Adrenocorticosteroids	Urethan	Symptomatic relief in about 50% of cases and objective improvement in 20-30%
Polycythemia vera	Busulfan Chlorambucil Nitrogen mustard		P^{32}			Prolonged clinical remissions, particularly with P^{32}

* From Karnofsky, D. A.: "Cancer Chemotherapeutic Agents," *CA*, 14:67, 1964.

Table 14. (Continued)

Diagnosis	Polyfunctional Alkylating Agents	Antimetabolites	Radioactive Isotopes	Hormones	Miscellaneous Drugs	Results
Carcinoma of lung	Nitrogen mustard Cyclophosphamide					Brief improvement in about 30% of cases
Carcinoma of ovary	Thio-TEPA Chlorambucil	5-FU				30 to 50% of cases improved for one to three months, sometimes longer
Carcinoma of thyroid			I^{131}			Frequently marked improvement in properly selected cases
Carcinoma of breast	Thio-TEPA	5-FU		Estrogens, androgens, adrenocorticosteroids		20 to 50% improved by hormonal therapy; life may be prolonged in some cases
Carcinoma of endometrium				Delalutin		25% respond, chiefly pulmonary metastases
Carcinoma of prostate				Estrogens		80% of cases respond to hormonal therapy; definite prolongation of life
Wilms's tumor, children	Nitrogen mustard Cyclophosphamide				Actinomycin D	Temporary regression; 50% pulmonary metastases respond with long survivors
Choriocarcinoma, female	Nitrogen mustard Chlorambucil	Methotrexate			Actinomycin D Vinblastine	50% respond of whom 40% show "permanent" regression
Carcinoma of colon		5-FU				15% respond for several months or longer
Carcinoma of testis	Chlorambucil	Methotrexate			Actinomycin D	35% of patients show favorable and sometimes prolonged response

Table 14 (Continued)

Neoplastic Diseases Responding to Chemotherapy

REGIONAL CANCER CHEMOTHERAPY

Diagnosis	Polyfunctional Alkylating Agents	Antimetabolites	Radioactive Isotopes	Hormones	Miscellaneous Drugs	Results
Pleural, pericardial, and abdominal effusions (instillation into appropriate cavity)	Nitrogen mustard		Au^{198} $CrP^{32}O_4$		Quinacrine	About 25 to 50% of patients respond
Carcinoma in facial area		Methotrexate plus citrovorum factor (intra-arterial infusion)				Favorable response of tumors supplied by external carotid artery in selected cases
Tumors of the extremities	Nitrogen mustard (extracorporeal perfusion)					Response in selected cases
Leukemic involvement, central nervous system		Methotrexate (intrathecal injection)				About 80% of children with CNS involvement respond temporarily

one fourth of the cases treated. Investigators in the United States have failed to confirm this; however, extensive research is continuing.

Actinomycins

The actinomycins are a group of antibiotics isolated from *Streptomyces antibioticus*. They have a slight but definite effect in causing tumor regression. The ones most widely used are actinomycin C (Sanamycin) and actinomycin D. The toxic effects are bone marrow depression, gastrointestinal tract lesions, alopecia, and skin eruptions. The intravenous dose for actinomycin C is 0.1 to 0.4 mg. per kilogram body weight daily for two to three weeks; the intravenous dose for actinomycin D is 0.015 mg. per kilogram body weight for five days. The oral maintenance dose for actinomycin D is 3 to 10 mg. daily in divided doses. Better responses are observed with Wilms's tumor and lymphomas than with other tumors.

HORMONES

Cortisone and Corticotropin (ACTH, Adrenocorticotropic Hormone)

The pharmacology and other therapeutic actions of these drugs are discussed on pages 681–90. Prednisone and prednisolone are also used in acute leukemia, and the remission of symptoms is more rapid than with the folic acid antagonists or mercaptopurine. Asymptomatic periods may last from two weeks to several months, but relapses often occur and then the tumors become more resistant. These drugs are rarely effective in adult acute leukemia.

Cortisone and corticotropin are also used in malignant lymphoma. It is not likely that they destroy the tumor cells, but they provide symptomatic relief and improve the patient's general well-being. They alter the response of tissues to injury.

Estrogens and Androgens

The use of estrogens and androgens in cancer of the breast and prostate gland is discussed on pages 610, 618.

Progesterone

Hydroxyprogesterone Caproate (Delalutin) is effective in the treatment of metastatic carcinoma of the endometrium. The response is greater in patients with pulmonary metastases than in those with massive intra-abdominal disease. The drug does not appear to have any androgenic or estrogenic activity but fluid retention may occur.

The intramuscular dose is 1 Gm. twice a week. If regression is not noted in four weeks, the dose may be doubled. The patients do not respond immediately. Usually two to three months' treatment is required.

For other uses see page 614.

Preparation

Hydroxyprogesterone Caproate Injection   Vials containing 125 and 250 mg.

Trade name: Delalutin

REVIEW QUESTIONS

1. *How do antimetabolites affect malignant cells? Normal cells? Why are they effective in some malignancies?*
2. *Compare and contrast the action and side and toxic effects of antimetabolites, alkylating agents, and radioactive drugs.*
3. *Discuss the nursing responsibilities in the care of a patient receiving nitrogen mustard.*
4. *How would you teach a nurse's aide about radioactivity and the care of a patient receiving intra-abdominal radioactive gold therapy?*
5. *The orderly states that he will not care for a patient being treated with radioactive phosphorus because he does not want to expose his children to radiation. How would you handle the problem?*
6. *What benefits may be anticipated from the administration of the drugs in leukemia?*
7. *How do alkylating agents produce their effects in neoplastic disease? Name three.*

REFERENCES

Arnold, Patricia: "Total-body Irradiation and Marrow Transplantations," *Am. J. Nursing,* **63**:83, 1963.

Blatz, H. (ed.): *Radiation Hygiene Handbook.* McGraw-Hill Book, Co., New York, 1959.

Burchenal, J. H.: "Chemotherapy of Cancer," *Mod. Med.,* April, 1960, p. 145.

Ellison, R. R.:" Treating Cancer with Antimetabolites," *Am. J. Nursing,* **62**:79, 1962.

Karnofsky, D. A.: "Cancer Chemotherapeutic Agents," *CA,* **14**:67, 1964.

————: "Chemotherapy of Cancer," *Mod. Med.,* Dec. 1, 1958.

————: "Drugs for Cancer and Allied Diseases," in Modell, W. (ed.): *Drugs of Choice 1964–1965.* The C. V. Mosby Co., St. Louis, 1964.

Kautz, H. D.; Storey, R. H., and Zimmermann, A. J.: "Radioactive Drugs," *Am. J. Nursing,* **64**:24, 1964.

Lyman, M. S., and Burchenal, J. H.: "Acute Leukemia," *Am. J. Nursing,* **63**:82, 1963.

Murphy, M. L.: "Leukemia and Lymphoma in Children," *Ped. Clin. North America,* **6**:611, 1959.

Radioisotopes in Medicine. Abbott Laboratories, North Chicago, Ill., 1962.

Tahern, D. L., and Gleason, G. I.,: "What Nurses Should Know About Isotopes," *Modern Hospitals*, **8**:67, Aug. 1955.
Zaino, Costantino: "Eliminating the Hazards from Radiation," *Am. J. Nursing*, **62**:60, 1962.

RADIOACTIVE PHOSPHORUS

Craver, L. F.: "Treatment of Leukemia by Radioactive Phosphorus," *Bull. New York Acad. Med.* **18**:254, 1942.
Doan, C. A.; Wiseman, B. K.; Wright, C.; Geyer, J. H.; Meyers, W.; and Meyers, J. W.: "Radioactive Phosphorus P³². 6 Year Clinical Evaluation of Internal Radiation Therapy," *J. Lab. & Clin. Med.*, **32**:943, 1947.
Marinelli, L. D.: "Symposium on Radioactive Isotopes; Dosage Determination in Use of Radioactive Isotopes," *J. Clin. Investigation*, **28**:1271, 1949.
Quimby, E. H.: *Safe Handling of Radioisotopes in Medical Practice*. The Macmillian Company, New York, 1960.
Reinhard, E. H.; Moore, C. V.; Bierbaum, O. S.; and Moore, S.: "Radioactive Phosphorus as a Therapeutic Agent," *J. Lab. & Clin. Med.*, **31**:107, 1946.
Stroebel, C. F.; Hall, B. E.; and Pease, G. L.: "Evaluation of Radiophosphorus Therapy in Primary Polycythemia Vera," *J. Lab. & Clin. Med.*, **146**:1301, 1951.

NITROGEN MUSTARDS

Alpert, L. K.; Greenspan, E. M.; and Paterson S. S.: "The Treatment of Lymphomas and Other Neoplastic Diseases with Nitrogen Mustard," *Ann. Int. Med.*, **32**:393, 1950.
Bauer, B. D., and Eef, L. A.: "The Clinical Effect of Nitrogen Mustard on Neoplastic Diseases," *Am. J. M. Sc.*, **219**:16, 1950.
Burchenal, J. H.; Myers, W. P. L.; Craver, L. F.; and Karnofsky, D. A.: "The Nitrogen Mustards in the Treatment of Leukemia," *Cancer*, **2**:1, 1949.
Gellhorn, A., and Collins, V. P.: "A Quantitative Evaluation of the Contribution of Nitrogen Mustard to the Therapeutic Management of Hodgkin's Disease," *Ann. Int. Med.*, **35**:1250, 1951.
Kennedy, B. J., and Aub, J. C.: "The Therapeutic Indications for Nitrogen Mustards in Lymphoma," *M. Clin. North America*, **33**:1301, 1949.
Molander, D. W.: "The Management of Lymphomas," *Am. J. Nursing*, **63**:110, 1963.

MANNOMUSTINE

Barlow, A. M.; Leeming, J. T.; and Wilkinson, J. F.: "Mannomustine in the Treatment of Leukaemias, Polycythaemia and Malignant Disorders," *Brit. Med. J.*, **2**:208, Aug. 22, 1959.

URACIL-MUSTARD

Shanbrom, E.; Miller, S.; and Haar, H.: "Uracil-Mustard, A New Chemotherapeutic Agent: Preliminary Clinical Evaluation in Hematologic Disorders," *Clin. Res.*, **7**:57, 1959.
————: "Uracil-Mustard, A New Oral Anti-Tumor Drug," *J.A.M.A.*, **174**:1702, 1960.

CHLORAMBUCIL

Ultmann, J. E.; Hyman, G. A.; and Gellhorn, A.: "Chlorambucil in the Treatment of Chronic Lymphocytic Leukemia and Certain Lymphomas," *J.A.M.A.*, **162**:178, 1956.

TRIETHYLENE MELAMINE

Gellhorn, A.; Klingerman, M.M.; and Jaffe, I.: "Triethylene Melamine in Clinical Cancer Chemotherapy," *Am. J. Med.*, **13**:428, 1952.

Karnofsky, D. A.; Burchenal, J. H.; Armistead, G. C., Jr.; Southam, C. M.; Bernstein, J. L.; Craver, L. F.; and Rhoads, C. P.: "Triethylene Melamine in the Treatment of Neoplastic Disease," *A.M.A. Arch. Int. Med.*, **87**:477, 1951.

Paterson, E., and Kunkler, P. B.: "Triethylene Melamine in Human Malignant Disease," *Brit. M. J.*, **1**:59, 1953.

TRIETHYLENE PHOSPHORAMIDE

Bateman, J. C.: "Chemotherapy of Solid Tumors with Triethylene Thiophosphoramide," *New England J. Med.*, **252**:879, May 26, 1955.

Farber, S., *et al.*: "Clinical Studies on the Carcinolytic Action of Triethylene Phosphoramide," *Cancer*, **6**:135, 1953.

Smith, N. J., *et al.*: "The Effect of Triethylene Phosphoramide in the Treatment of Leukemias and Certain Lymphomas in Infants and Children," *J. Ped.*, **46**:493, 1955.

BUSULFAN (MYLERAN)

Galton, D. A. G.: "Myleran in Chronic Myeloid Leukemia," *Lancet*, **1**:208, 1953.

Haddon, A., and Timmis, G. M.: "Myleran in Chronic Myeloid Leukemia," *Lancet*, **1**:207, 1953.

Petrakis, N. L., *et al.*: "Effect of Myleran upon Leukemia," *Cancer*, **7**:383, 1954.

CYCLOPHOSPHAMIDE (CYTOXAN)

Ravdin, R. G., *et al.*: *Proc. Am. Assoc. for Cancer Res.*, **3**:55, 1959.

REGIONAL PERFUSION

Abel, A. L.: "Chemotherapy for Cancer by Perfusion," *Brit. M. J.*, **1**:952, March 26, 1960.

Creech, O., Jr., *et al.*: "Chemotherapy of Cancer: Regional Perfusion Utilizing an Extracorporeal Circuit," *Ann. Surg.*, **148**:616, 1958.

Levine, L. A.: "Intra-arterial chemotherapy for the Cancer Patient," *Am. J. Nursing*, **64**:108, 1964.

Stehlin, J. S., *et al.*: "Malignant Melanoma of the Extremities: Experiences with Conventional Therapy: A New Surgical and Chemotherapeutic Approach with Regional Perfusion," *Cancer*, **13**:55, 1960.

AMINOPTERIN

Farber, S.; Diamond, L. K.; Mercer, R. D.; Sylvester, R. F., Jr.; and Wolff, J. A.: "Temporary Remissions in Acute Leukemia in Children Produced by Folic Acid

Antagonist, 4-Aminopteroylglutamic Acid (Aminopterin)," *New England J. Med.*, **238**:787, 1948.

Amethopterin (Methotrexate)

Hertz, R., *et al.*: "Chemotherapy of Choriocarcinoma and Related Trophoblastic Tumors in Women," *J.A.M.A.*, **168**:845, 1958.
Holland, J. F.: "Chemical Control of Cancer," *Pub. Health Rep.*, **69**:1151, 1954.
———: "Symposium on the Experimental Pharmacology and Clinical Use of Antimetabolites. Part VIII. Folic Acid Metabolites," *Clin. Pharm. and Ther.*, **2**:374, 1961.
Whiteside, J. H.; Philips, F. S.; Dargeon, H. W.; and Burchenal, J. H.: "Intrathecal Amethopterin in Neurological Manifestations of Leukemia," *A.M.A. Arch. Int. Med.*, **101**:279, 1958.

Mercaptopurine

Burchenal, J. H.; Murphy, M. L.; Ellison, R. R.; Sykes, M. P.; Tan, T. C.; Leon, L. A.; Karnofsky, D. A.; Craver, L. F.; Dargeon, H. W.; and Rhoads, C. P.: "Clinical Evaluation of a New Antimetabolite, 6-Mercaptopurine, in the Treatment of Leukemia and Allied Diseases," *Blood*, **8**:965, 1953.

Pyrimidine Antagonists

Burchenal, J. H., and Ellison, Ruth: "Symposium on the Experimental Pharmacology and Clinical Use of Antimetabolites, Part IX. The Pyrimidine and Purine Antagonists," *Clin. Pharm. and Ther.*, **2**:523, 1961.

Vinblastine Sulfate

Hertz, R., *et al.*: "Effect of Vincaleukoblastine on Metastatic Choriocarcinoma and Related Trophoblastic Tumors in Women," *Cancer Res.*, **20**:1050, 1960.

Urethan

Hirschboeck, J. A., *et al.*: "Effects of Urethane in the Treatment of Leukemia and Metastatic Malignant Tumors," *J.A.M.A.*, **136**:90, 1948.

Antibiotics

Ellison, R. R., *et al.*: "Clinical Trials of o-Diazoacetyl-L-serine (Azaserine) in Neoplastic Diseases," *Cancer*, **7**:801, 1954.
Karnofsky, D. A.: "Management of Leukemia," *New York M. J.*, **54**:3225, 1954.
Stock, C. C., *et al.*: "Azaserine, a New Tumor Inhibitory Substance," *Nature*, **173**:71, 1954.

Mytomycin C

Shiraha, Y.; Sakan, K.; and Teranaka, T.: "Clinical Trials of Mitomycin C, a New Antitumor Antibiotic," *Antibiotics Annual, 1958–1959*. Medical Encyclopedia, Inc., New York, 1959, p. 533.

Actinomycin

Tau, C. T. C.; Murphy, M. L.; Dargeon, H. W.; and Burchenal, J. H.: "Clinical Effects of Actinomycin D," *Proc. Am. Cancer Research*, **2**:254, 1957.

12

Chemotherapy of Malaria, Amebiasis, and Tropical Infections

CHEMOTHERAPY OF MALARIA

Malaria is a febrile disease caused by one or more species of plasmodia, protozoal organisms that are transmitted to man by the bite of certain species of the *Anopheles* mosquito. It is one of the oldest diseases known to man and is the most prevalent of all human infections, being widely distributed over the world, particularly in underdeveloped countries in temperate or tropical climates. It is estimated that three hundred million cases occur annually and that three million are fatal. There is a very low incidence in the United States at the present time. However, many of our military men and women are in areas of the world where malaria is endemic, and since they may suffer relapses on their return home, it is important to know the new advances that have been made in the treatment of this disease.

All three species of the causative organism responsible for human malaria belong to the genus *Plasmodium* (abbreviated *P.* when used with specific names). The most prevalent species is *P. vivax*, the cause of *benign tertian malaria*, which may be incapacitating but does not usually cause death unless complicated with other diseases. This organism has a tendency to persist for a long time in the host, even in the absence of clinical symptoms, and is responsible for the relapses that often occur. The species *P. malariae* causes quartan malaria, which is very rare and is found in sharply localized areas. The species *P. falciparum* causes *malignant tertian malaria*, which is the most severe form and will cause death unless treated early. The acute infection responds well to treatment, and in most cases a cure results with no relapses, as in *vivax malaria*. This disease is particularly dangerous because the *P. falciparum*–infected red blood cells have a tendency to clump and adhere to the walls of the capillaries, obstructing the circulation to the vital organs.

To diagnose malaria clinically, it is important to find and identify the parasite by an examination of blood smears. However, the clinical course is usually so characteristic as to be diagnosed without blood smears.

Life Cycle of the Malarial Parasite. This complex life cycle is divided into three phases, one in the mosquito and two, the pre-erythrocytic and

208

erythrocytic phases, in man. The parasites multiply in the mosquito sexually and in man asexually. The mosquito bites a patient with malaria and ingests some of the asexual forms (schizonts) and the sexual forms (gametocytes). In the mosquito the asexual forms are destroyed, but the female gametocyte is fertilized by the male gametocyte and the development of the asexual forms takes place in the stomach of the mosquito. These organisms are secreted in the saliva of the mosquito and are transferred to another person by the bite of that mosquito.

The forms of the organism injected into man are known as sporozoites. They do not cause fever until after approximately two weeks. During this "incubation period" the organisms multiply profusely in liver cells and a certain type of body cells called *reticuloendothelial (R-E) cells*. These cells are widely distributed in the body and are present in the spleen, lymph glands, liver, and are scattered elsewhere. Their function is one of scavenging or engulfing foreign material, such as bacteria, for our protection. In malaria, however, and in other infections, these erstwhile protective cells serve as victim-host cells to the invading parasite.

After extensive multiplication through many generations, the sporozoites burst the cells of the R-E system, and myriads of parasites (merozoites) are liberated. Large numbers are swept along in the blood in the capillaries near the R-E cells, then enter the red blood cells, one parasite per erythrocyte. This phase is know as the *erythrocytic* phase; the organisms multiply in the red cells as they circulate in the blood stream. After approximately two days in *P. vivax* or benign tertian malaria, one merozoite has multiplied into 16 (rarely 32) merozoites. They burst the red cell and are liberated in the plasma. A large number of red blood corpuscles rupture at nearly the same time, freeing 15 to 20 times that number of parasites, malarial pigment and waste products, and red cell debris. The toxic action causes an abrupt rise in temperature. While these are floating freely in the plasma, the fever rises sharply, followed by a state of shock (the chill). The new merozoites enter more red cells. Their maturation in erythrocytes is complete in another 48 hours; and massive liberation as these cells break up, as before, causes another bout of fever, chills, and prostration. These recurring episodes are called *paroxysms*. In the case of *P. falciparum* malaria alone, the tissue phase is pre-erythrocytic only. It disappears when the red blood cycle is established; it does not cause relapses.

Development or multiplication of the parasites in the R-E and other so-called "fixed-tissue cells" (i.e., not circulating as the red corpuscles) is called the *exoerythrocytic* phase of the disease in man. It is this phase, with the parasites often lying dormant after partial treatment, that causes relapses of malaria months after arrest of the clinical attacks by eradicating all parasites in the blood.

Control of Malaria.   It is possible to control malaria in some areas by eliminating the mosquitoes with insecticides such as chlorophenothane (DDT) and benzene hexachloride (Gammexane). Sometimes the use of insecticides augments antimalarial therapy.

Treatment with Antimalarials.   Some of the important antimalarial drugs are quinine, chloroquine, hydroxychloroquine (Plaquenil), amodiaquine (Camoquin), quinacrine (Atabrine), primaquine, chlorguanide (Paludrine) and pyrimethamine (Daraprim).

These drugs relieve symptoms but seldom achieve a complete cure in vivax malaria unless used in effective combinations. Relapses are frequent when the person's resistance is lowered. Some of the drugs produce a complete cure in malignant tertian malaria (falciparum).

Antimalarials are used for suppression, to protect the individual against the acute manifestation of malarial infection and also in the acute attack, whether it is the first attack or a relapse. In the acute attack, it is important to give the maximum dose of the drug as soon as possible. In the grave or complicated attack of malignant tertian malaria when the patient is vomiting or is unconscious, parenteral treatment is necessary. Quinine dihydrochloride or chloroquine phosphate or sulfate may then be given by intravenous drip. Chloroquine is also effective by intramuscular injection. As soon as possible chloroquine orally should follow the parenteral administration of quinine or chloroquine. Control of the febrile attacks is achieved by a suppressive drug that provides symptomatic relief. Relapses may occur following discontinuance of the drug. Real cure is complete eradication of the secondary parasite. This type of cure is desirable if the patient is moving to a place where malaria is not endemic, and thus not likely to be acquired again from mosquitoes.

In recent years there have been radical changes in the treatment of malaria due to the introduction of new antimalarials, which have replaced, to a large extent, the older drugs.

SPECIFIC DRUGS USED IN THE TREATMENT OF MALARIA

The first real success in chemotherapy was the treatment of malaria with the powdered bark of the cinchona tree in Lima, Peru, three hundred years ago. Pelletier and Caventou isolated the alkaloid quinine from the bark in 1820, and since that time quinine has replaced the powdered bark in the treatment of the disease.

Quinine

Quinine is one of a number of alkaloids isolated from the bark of the cinchona tree. It is described first because of its long use and its great importance in malaria. Quinine, in malaria, and quinidine, in atrial fibrillation, are the only alkaloids of this group that are widely used in medicine. Quinine was made synthetically in 1944 by Drs. R. B. Woodward and W. E. Doering. It has a bitter taste and was formerly used in bitters, tonics, and cordials to stimulate the appetite.

Pharmacological Action.   Quinine is a general protoplasmic poison and interferes with the nutrition, activity, and reproduction of practically all cells if its concentration is great enough. It reduces surface tension and penetrates the cell membrane causing coagulation. It is mildly bactericidal. Its action in malaria depends on a more specific action on the plasmodia of malaria than on the red blood cells.

Quinine is an antipyretic (fever-reducing drug) and produces vasodilatation in the periphery. It is an analgesic (pain-relieving drug). It also stimulates uterine contractions.

Absorption, Fate, and Excretion.   When quinine sulfate is administered orally, 80 to 90 per cent is absorbed from the gastrointestinal tract. Seventy-five per cent is rapidly metabolized, and the remainder, which passes through the body unchanged, is excreted unchanged or conjugated with glycuronic acid in the urine along with the products of metabolism.

Therapeutic Uses.   The principal use of quinine is in the treatment of malaria. It suppresses the clinical attacks and kills the asexual forms (schizonts) of all forms of parasites. The gametocytes are not killed, but it is believed that they are so altered that they do not multiply in the mosquito. Quinine is not active against the exoerythrocytic forms of the parasites; hence relapses usually occur when the drug is discontinued in the treatment of benign tertian and quartan malaria.

Dosage and Method of Administration.   The usual oral dose of quinine sulfate administered to abort the acute attack is 1 Gm. daily for two days and then 600 mg. for five days. The suppressive dose is 600 mg. daily. The intravenous dose of quinine dihydrochloride is 1 Gm. The intravenous dose of the hydrochloride is 600 mg.

Toxicity.   Large therapeutic doses may produce dimness of vision, ringing in the ears, mental confusion, and severe headache. This is known as *cinchonism.* Nausea, vomiting, and skin eruptions may occur. Very large doses produce major toxic symptoms such as delirium, fever, and apprehension, followed by loss of consciousness. The respiration is first stimulated and then depressed. Cyanosis may develop, the body temperature falls, the pulse becomes weak, and death results from respiratory paralysis.

Preparations

Quinine Dihydrochloride Injection, B.P.	250 mg. and 300 mg. in 1 ml.; 500 mg. in 1 ml. and 1.5 ml.; 1 Gm. in 2 ml.
Quinine Hydrochloride Injection	600 mg.
Quinine Hydrochloride Tablets, B.P.	300 mg.
Quinine Sulfate Capsules, N.F.	120, 200, and 300 mg.
Quinine Sulfate Tablets, N.F., B.P.	120, 200, and 300 mg.

SYNTHETIC ANTIMALARIALS

Chloroquine Phosphate, U.S.P., B.P., I.P. (Aralen); Chloroquine Sulphate, B.P.

Chloroquine is the preferred antimalarial drug. It is three to four times as potent as quinacrine against *P. vivax* and *P. falciparum*. Chloroquine is rapidly and completely absorbed from the gastrointestinal tract, and it may be found in the spleen, liver, kidney, and lungs. Eighty per cent of the drug is slowly metabolized, whereas the remainder is slowly excreted in the urine. Chloroquine does not prevent infection or relapses in vivax malaria because it does not eradicate the exoerythrocytic phase in this type. However, the drug is useful in this infection as a suppressive agent and rapidly terminates the acute attack. Chloroquine produces a complete or radical cure in malignant tertian malaria. The drug does kill the parasites in the exoerythrocytic phase of this type. Chloroquine is well tolerated and produces neither yellow pigmentation of the skin nor symptoms of cinchonism. Personnel in the armed forces in malarious zones receive chloroquine to prevent illness. It is given once weekly as long as the individual is in such an area.

Untoward Effects. The untoward effects, such as headache, gastrointestinal distress, and visual disturbances, are not serious and disappear with the discontinuance of the drug.

Dosage and Method of Administration. The usual oral dose to suppress symptoms is 500 mg. weekly. The oral dose for the acute attack is 1 Gm. immediately, followed by 500 mg. in six hours and on the second and third days. The adult intravenous or intramuscular dose is 200 to 300 mg. of the base; for children the dose is 5 mg. of the base per kilogram of body weight. (For use in amebiasis, see p. 216).

Preparations

Chloroquine Phosphate Tablets, U.S.P., B.P., I.P.	125 and 250 mg.
Chloroquine Phosphate Injection, B.P.	40 mg. of the base in 1 ml.
Chloroquine Sulphate Injection, B.P.	40 mg. of the base in 1 ml.
Chloroquine Sulphate Tablets, B.P.	200 mg.

Trade name: Aralen

Amodiaquine (Camoquin); Amodiaquine Hydrochloride, N.F., B.P., I.P.

Amodiaquine is closely related to chloroquine, and its effectiveness in malaria is similar. It is rapidly absorbed from the gastrointestinal tract and and is excreted slowly. Like chloroquine, the drug causes a rapid suppression and cure of falciparum malaria. It suppresses, but does not cure, vivax malaria and controls the clinical attacks rapidly. The toxicity of the drug is low.

Dosage and Method of Administration.   Amodiaquine is administered orally, and the dosage is expressed in terms of the base. The suppressive dose for endemic malaria is 400 mg. of the base once every two weeks. In the acute attack the single adult dose is 600 mg. of the base. The usual dose range is 100 to 600 mg. of the base.

Preparation

Amodiaquine, N.F., B.P., Hydrochloride   200 mg.
Tablets

Trade name: Camoquin

Quinacrine Hydrochloride, U.S.P.; Mepacrine Hydrochloride, B.P., I.P. (Atabrine)

Quinacrine is quickly absorbed from the gastrointestinal tract and is slowly excreted in the urine and feces. It controls the symptoms of vivax malaria, but it does not prevent infection or relapses. It is thus called a *suppressant* drug. An adequate dosage will terminate the acute attack rapidly. The exo-erythrocytic forms of *P. vivax* are not affected, for relapses occur when the drug is discontinued. Quinacrine will bring about a cure in falciparum malaria. It was extensively used in World War II and after, but it has now been replaced, to a large extent, by chloroquine and amodiaquine.

Dosage and Method of Administration.   To suppress symptoms, the usual oral dose is 100 mg. daily. In the acute attack, 200 mg. is administered every six hours for five doses and then 100 mg. three times a day for six days. For the dose as an anthelmintic, see page 239.

Untoward Effects.   The disadvantages of the use of quinacrine for prolonged suppression are yellow coloration of the skin, vomiting, and diarrhea.

Preparation

Quinacrine Hydrochloride Tablets,   100 mg.
U.S.P.; Mepacrine Tablets, B.P.

Trade names: Atabrine; Atebrin; Chinacrin; Chinacrine Hydrochloride

Primaquine Phosphate, U.S.P., B.P.

Primaquine is a potent antimalarial which destroys the parasites in the reticuloenthelial cells and is thus effective in curing vivax malaria and preventing infection. Primaquine is recommended for the prevention of relapses. It may be given with chloroquine. Primaquine, given to troops for a 14-day course after departing from a malarious theater of duty, has been found to ensure against latent relapses in most cases. It may be classified as a curative drug.

Dosage and Method of Administration.   The oral dose of primaquine given simultaneously with chloroquine is 15 mg. daily for 14 days. The usual dose is 10 to 15 mg. of the base.

The only great disadvantage of primaquine is a rapid hemolysis, with a reduction in the red blood count, in the Negro race in a few cases.

Preparation

Primaquine Phosphate Tablets, U.S.P., B.P.   26.5 mg (15 mg of the base) B.P., 7.5 mg. of the base

Proguanil Hydrochloride, B.P., I.P. (Chloroguanide, Paludrine, Guanatol)

Proguanil is slow in controlling symptoms; hence it is dangerous in malignant tertian malaria. *Plasmodium falciparum* develops resistance to chloroguanide. The drug is used for the suppression, prophylaxis, and cure of malignant tertian malaria and for the suppression and treatment of benign tertian malaria. Chloroquine and quinacrine are preferable in the treatment of vivax malaria.

Dosage and Method of Administration.   The suppressive dose for both types of disease is 300 mg. weekly. For prophylaxis of falciparum malaria, 100 mg. may be given twice weekly. A dose of 100 mg. three times a day for ten days will usually cure falciparum malaria. This dose is usually only partially effective against vivax malaria.

Preparation

Proguanil Hydrochloride Tablets, B.P.   100 mg.
Trade names: Chloroguanide; Guanatol; Paludrine

Chlorproguanil (Lapudrine)

Chlorproguanil is a new antimalarial. It has a more persistent action than proguanil. It is effective against the erythrocytic forms of all malarial parasites and acts as a causal prophylactic against the primary exoerythrocytic form of *P. falciparum*. The recommended dose upon entering a malarial area is 20 mg. weekly. At least one dose should be taken upon leaving the area. Chlorproguanil is well tolerated and side effects are rare. It is a useful and inexpensive malarial prophylactic. Tablets containing 20 mg. are available.

Pyrimethamine, U.S.P., B.P. (Daraprim)

Pyrimethamine is a suppressive antimalarial drug effective in small oral doses administered at weekly intervals. It may slowly sterilize the fixed tissue forms of *P. vivax*, producing suppressive cures, when the drug is administered eight weeks or longer. Pyrimethamine is effective in all types of malaria. It is slow in action and resistance develops.

Dosage and Method of Administration.   For suppressive prophylaxis, the oral dose for adults is 25 mg. weekly; for children under 15, the oral

dose is 12.5 mg. weekly. For the acute attacks, the oral dose is 25 mg. daily
for two days. The dose for a child is one half the adult dose. Weekly doses
of 25 mg. for at least ten weeks are continued where malaria is present.

Preparation

Pyrimethamine Tablets, U.S.P., B.P.   25 mg.

Trade name: Daraprim

Cycloguanil Pamoate (Camolar), a metabolite of chloroguanide and
perhaps the active form, is a causal prophylactic against human vivax malaria
and a Southern Rhodesian strain of *P. falciparum*. On intramuscular injection
this insoluble salt is released slowly from tissue depots over a period of many
months. Its systemic toxicity is low. The intramuscular dose is 2 to 5 mg. per
kilogram body weight once or twice a year.

SUMMARY

All antimalarial drugs have potential toxic effects. The group discussed has
less toxicity than hundreds of other antimalarials that have been found and
discarded. When the drugs are properly used, the dangers are not great. We
are now able to treat successfully the vast majority of malaria victims. Progress
in the worldwide eradication of malaria has been rapid and spectacular. However, within the past ten or fifteen years the development of resistant malarial
strains (*P. falciparum*) to chloroguanide and pyrimethamine has been frequently reported in southeast Asia, Africa, and South America. More recently
resistance to chloroquine and amodiaquine has also been observed. Quinine
alone is effective in treating these recently discovered resistant cases.

AMEBIASIS

Amebiasis is an infectious disease caused by the presence of the protozoa
Endamoeba histolytica in the intestinal tract or tissues of man. The disease
is quite prevalent in the tropics but is also found in many other areas of
the world. It is estimated that about 10 per cent of the population in the
United States pass the organisms in their stools, and there have been several
epidemics here in the past few years.

The parasite occurs in two forms: the active or motile form, the trophozoite,
and the more resistant form, the cyst. The cysts enter the human intestinal
tract with food and water contaminated by carriers or convalescents. The
amebae may burrow their way into the intestinal mucosa, where they may
produce ulcerations of varying degrees.

The active forms live and multiply at the expense of the tissues of the host.
They feed upon the mucosal cells, causing lysis and inflammation. Often the

host may repair much of the damage to his tissues without apparent impairment to his health, and there are no symptoms of diarrhea. Most of the active forms pass into the cyst stage and many are eliminated in the formed stools. This gives rise to the "carrier" or "cyst passer." The cysts, which may survive for some time outside the body, are the source of infection and are transmitted by flies, drinking water, and food.

The primary infection in the intestine is called *intestinal amebiasis*. The lesions may be small and produce transient diarrhea. When large areas of the mucosa are destroyed, liquid stools containing mucus, blood, and a large number of active amebae (these are not infective) are passed. The infection, which is confined largely to the lumen of the colon, is called *ulcerative colitis* or *amebic dysentery*. *Secondary amebiasis* occurs when the active forms enter the blood stream and go to other parts of the body. *Hepatic amebiasis* occurs when the amebae invade the liver. This may result in *amebic abscess* of the liver. The parasites may also produce abscesses in the lung, brain, and spleen.

The symptoms of *amebic dysentery* are malaise, lassitude, flatulence, griping, and constipation alternating with diarrhea. The purpose of treatment is to prevent growth and invasion of the tissues by the active forms and to eradicate the cysts in the bowel to prevent reinfection and transmission of the disease.

The oral amebicides, which are active against both motile and cyst forms in the intestinal tract, include the organic arsenicals, such as carbarsone, the thioarsenites, and glycobiarsol; the iodohydroxyquinolines, such as chiniofon, iodochlorhydroxyquin, and diiodohydroxyquin; and the antibiotics, such as fumagillin, oxytetracycline, carbomycin, and others. For hepatic amebiasis and amebic abscess of the liver, the antimalarial chloroquine phosphate is the drug of choice. It is given orally, and since it has no effect on the intestinal amebae, it should be given in combination with a "lumen" amebicide, such as carbarsone or glycobiarsol. Emetine hydrochloride, administered subcutaneously, is also useful in the treatment of hepatic amebiasis and other tissue forms and in acute amebic dysentery; it is not effective against cysts in doses that can be tolerated. This drug should also be given with a "lumen" amebicide.

Chloroquine Phosphate, U.S.P., B.P.; Chloroquine Sulphate, B.P.

Chloroquine phosphate is almost completely absorbed from the intestinal tract upon oral administration, and some is slowly excreted in the urine. Rather large amounts are concentrated in the various cells of the body, especially the liver cells. It is slowly metabolized and may remain in the tissues some time after treatment has been stopped. It is relatively nontoxic. The oral adult antiamebic dose is 500 mg. three times a day for two weeks, and then 750 mg. twice weekly for several months. The B.P. dose is 0.5 to 1 Gm. daily.

Preparations

Chloroquine Phosphate Tablets, U.S.P.,   125 and 250 mg.
B.P.
Chloroquine Sulphate Tablets, B.P.   200 mg.
Trade name: Aralen Phosphate

Emetine Hydrochloride, U.S.P., B.P., I.P.

Emetine is an alkaloid obtained from the root of *Cephaelus ipecacuanha,* a shrub that grows in Brazil. It is readily absorbed upon oral administration but is irritating to the gastric mucosa and will usually produce nausea and vomiting. In amebiasis, it is administered subcutaneously. Emetine, after injection, is carried to the liver and is excreted in the bile and into the intestinal tract, where it kills the motile forms as a contact poison. It is not effective against cysts; therefore, persons who are apparently cured may be carriers of the disease. It must be given in combination with a good "lumen" amebicide, such as carbarsone, iodochlorhydroxyquin, or glycobiarsol, in order to remove the cysts. Emetine is detoxified and slowly excreted.

Emetine hydrochloride relieves the symptoms of amebic dysentery very quickly. It is second only to chloroquine in the treatment of patients with amebic hepatitis and amebic abscess of the liver. The dose of emetine hydrochloride is 60 mg. (30 to 60 mg.), administered subcutaneously once a day for a maximum of five to ten days. It is a toxic drug, and prolonged administration produces harmful effects on heart muscle. It should not be repeated in less than three months. Emetine is contraindicated in heart disease and hypotension.

Preparation

Emetine Hydrochloride Injection, U.S.P.,   30 and 60 mg. in 1 ml.
B.P., I.P.

Glaucarubin (Glarubin)

Glaucarubin is a crystalline glycoside obtained from the fruit of *Simarouba glauca,* a tropical plant found in Central America and northern South America. It is used in the treatment of intestinal amebiasis. The oral daily dose is 3 mg. per kilogram of body weight. The dose is divided and given two or three times daily for five to ten days. The maximum daily adult dose is 200 mg. The side effects are anorexia, nausea, and vomiting. More serious effects are abdominal pain, bloody stools, giddiness, and difficulty in urination. Tablets of 50 mg. are available.

ARSENICAL AMEBICIDES

Both the pentavalent arsenicals, such as acetarsone, carbarsone, and glyco-biarsol, and the trivalent preparations, such as the thioarsenites (thiocarbar-sone), are amebicidal. The thioarsenites are more effective against the tissue forms than are the other arsenicals.

Carbarsone, U.S.P., B.P., I.P.

Carbarsone is administered orally in the treatment of chronic amebiasis without hepatic involvement. It is used mainly as a "lumen" amebicide and is often used with chloroquine or emetine. The drug is absorbed slowly from the gastrointestinal tract and is excreted by the kidney. Serious untoward effects are rare, but a skin rash, diarrhea, abdominal pain, and loss of weight may occur. It is contraindicated in liver or kidney disease.

The adult dose of carbarsone is 250 mg. two or three times a day for ten days. The usual dose range is 100 to 250 mg. A second course of treatment may be repeated after an interval of at least ten days. In acute amebiasis, a retention enema containing 2 Gm. of carbarsone in 200 ml. of warm 2 per cent sodium bicarbonate solution is often administered. The vaginal dose is 130 mg. (up to 130 mg.) for trichomonal vaginitis.

Preparations

Carbarsone Tablets, U.S.P., B.P. (I.P.)	250 mg.
Carbarsone Capsules, N.F.	250 mg.
Carbarsone Suppositories, N.F.	130 mg.

Arsthinol (Balarsen)

Arsthinol is a thioarsenite that produces effects similar to those of carbar-sone, but it appears to be less toxic than that drug. The daily oral dose of 10 mg. per kilogram of body weight is usually given once a day for five days in the treatment of intestinal amebiasis and yaws.

Preparation

Arsthinol Tablets	100 mg.

Trade name: Balarsen

Glycobiarsol, N.F. (Milibis)

Glycobiarsol is a pentavalent arsenical combined with bismuth. It is not acutely toxic and is said to have more than ten times the margin of safety of carbarsone. It is a very useful intestinal amebicide and is most effective in the treatment of asymptomatic carriers and in chronic intestinal amebiasis. The usual adult oral dose is 500 mg. three to four times a day for seven to ten days or longer, if necessary.

Preparation

Glycobiarsol Tablets, N.F.   500 mg.
                          Trade name: Milibis

IODOHYDROXYQUINOLINES

Chiniofon, I.P.

Chiniofon is used only for organisms in the intestinal tract. It is active against both the motile and cyst forms. The oral adult dose for either form is 250 mg. and is administered three times a day for seven to eight days. Chiniofon is used in mild cases of amebiasis and in the treatment of carriers. It is not toxic in therapeutic doses, but it should not be administered to patients with liver damage and should be given cautiously to patients with thyroid disease or known iodine sensitivity. One to five grams may be given rectally.

Preparations

Chiniofon Tablets   250 mg.
                  Trade names: Anayodin; Quinoxyl; Yatren

Iodochlorhydroxyquin, N.F. (Vioform)

Iodochlorhydroxyquin appears to be superior to chiniofon as an intestinal amebicide. The oral adult dose is 250 mg. (250 to 500 mg.) three times a day for ten days. Gastrointestinal irritation may occur. It should be used with caution in liver disease.

Preparation

Iodochlorhydroxyquin Tablets, N.F.   250 mg.
                          Trade name: Vioform

Diiodohydroxyquin, U.S.P.; Di-iodohydroxyquinoline, B.P. (Diodoquin)

Diiodohydroxyquin is a relatively nontoxic compound, and when given with emetine, it is effective in the treatment of amebiasis. It is administered orally in doses of 650 mg. (650 mg. to 1 Gm.) three times a day for 20 days. The B.P. dose is 1 to 2 Gm. daily.

Preparations

Diiodohydroxyquin Tablets, U.S.P.   200 and 650 mg.
Di-iodohydroxyquinoline Tablets, B.P.   300 mg.
                  Trade names: Diodoquin; Yodoxin

ANTIBIOTICS IN AMEBIASIS

During the past several years a number of antibiotics, such as chlortetracycline, oxytetracycline, tetracycline, erythromycin, carbomycin, bacitracin, and puromycin, have been used successfully in controlling intestinal amebiasis. These antibiotics have no amebicidal action, but they alter the intestinal flora and eliminate the intestinal bacteria that are essential for the survival of the ameba. In the hands of a large number of investigators, oxytetracycline appears to be the most effective in eliminating the ameba from the tissues and lumen of the intestines. Of the broad-spectrum antibiotics it is the drug of choice. The dose is 500 mg. four times a day for ten days. Fumagillin and paromomycin (Humatin) are amebicidal.

Antibiotics have no apparent effect on extraintestinal amebiasis. In fact, liver abscesses may develop while the patient is taking antibiotics. Therefore, it is advisable to administer at the same time chloroquine, which is the drug of choice in liver abscess.

Fumagillin (Fumidil)

Fumagillin, a crystalline antibiotic obtained from a strain of *Aspergillis fumigatus*, is a specific drug used in intestinal amebiasis. It acts directly on the amebae, but it is not active against bacteria. There should be no danger of overgrowth of yeasts and fungi because the normal flora of the gastrointestinal tract is not changed following its administration. The adult oral dose is 30 to 60 mg. daily in divided doses, three or four times a day, for 10 to 14 days.

Preparation

Fumagillin Capsules   10 mg.

Paromomycin (Humatin)

Paromomycin is an antibiotic obtained from a culture of *Streptomyces*. It has a direct and marked amebicidal action. It is also effective against many enteric bacteria. This antibiotic is only slightly absorbed from the gastrointestinal tract and therefore is not toxic upon oral administration. The only side effect is an increase in the number of stools. Excellent results have been obtained by its use in intestinal amebiasis and enteric bacterial diarrheas. It has been used alone and with chloramphenicol in diarrheas of infants and children. In amebiasis the oral dose is 15 to 20 mg. per kilogram of body weight for five days. For enteric bacterial infections the dose is 25 to 50 mg. (up to 100 mg. in severe infections) in divided doses daily for six to seven days.

Preparation

Paromomycin Sulfate Capsules   250 mg. of the base
Trade name: Humatin

Puromycin (Stylomycin)

This antibiotic is effective in asymptomatic and acute carrier cases. The daily oral dose is 500 mg. for six days. There are no side effects noted when this antibiotic is administered.

Oxytetracycline and Erythromycin

These antibiotics (see pp. 121 and 148) are effective in intestinal amebiasis in doses of 500 mg. four times daily for ten days.

TROPICAL INFECTIONS

Trypanosomiasis (African Sleeping Sickness)

Trypanosomiasis, a nonvenereal disease similar to syphilis, is caused by the trypanosome, a protozoan parasitic organism. There are two species that cause the disease in man: *Trypanosoma gambiense* (jungle), which produces a less virulent type, and *T. rhodesiense* (desert), which produces a more virulent form. The suspected intermediate hosts are the antelope, other wild game, and domestic animals. The tsetse fly carries the infection from the intermediate hosts to man. The symptoms of the disease are lassitude, progressive weakness, enlarged glands, prolonged lethargy, emotional and neurological disturbances, and anemia. The organisms increase in the blood stream and circulation is slowed, resulting in circulatory failure, coma, and death.

The drugs used in the treatment of this disease are suramin sodium, pentamidine, and tryparsamide. Both suramin and pentamidine may be administered prophylactically and will prevent the infection for a period of three months. Both drugs are useful in the early infection. They are given in combination with tryparsamide, which is especially valuable in the treatment of the later stages of trypanosomiasis because of its ability to penetrate the central nervous system. Tryparsamide is given in doses of 3 Gm. (1 to 3 Gm.) once a week for 12 or more injections. It is an organic arsenical and is discussed on page 223.

South American trypanosomiasis (Chagas' disease) occurs in Panama, Mexico, and South America. It is caused by the *T. cruzi* and is transmitted by the bite of the reduviid bugs. There is no known drug for the treatment of this disease. Spraying the houses or huts with benzene hexachloride is a good prophylactic measure.

Leishmaniasis

Leishmaniasis is a tropical disease caused by a group of protozoans of the genus *Leishmania*. This disease occurs in a number of forms: (1) visceral

(Indian kala-azar), caused by *L. donovani,* which spreads by the blood to all tissues of the body except the central nervous system; (2) cutaneous (Oriental sore), caused by *L. tropica,* which, as a rule, does not enter the blood; (3) mucocutaneous (South American), caused by *L. brasiliensis,* which starts from a primary lesion in the skin, which heals, and then spreads to the nasal, mouth, and pharyngeal mucous membranes; and (4) dermal, which may occur with or following kala-azar. The disease is believed to be transmitted by the sandfly. The symptoms of kala-azar are fever, loss of weight, weakness, diarrhea, pigmentation of the skin, and bleeding from the gums. Organic antimonials and aromatic diamides are useful in this disease. Recently the usefulness of amphotericin B has been reported.

Schistosomiasis (Bilharziasis)

Schistosomiasis is a disease caused by blood flukes, which burrow their way through the skin and mucous membranes of persons bathing in contaminated waters. The intermediate hosts are snails. The symptoms of the disease are enlargement of the spleen and liver, diarrhea and often bloody stools, cystitis, and hematuria. The disease is endemic in Egypt, Africa, and certain parts of China and Japan. The drugs used in this disease are tartar emetic, stibophen (Fuadin), and lucanthone (Miracil-D, Nilodin).

Granuloma Inguinale

Granuloma inguinale is a venereal disease caused by a filtrable virus, which enters the body through the skin and mucous membrane of the external genitalia. Ulcerative lesions may appear in the groin and may persist for years. This disease is present in all parts of the world. Tartar emetic, stibophen, antimony lithium thiomalate, and the antibiotics chlortetracycline, oxytetracycline, and chloramphenicol have been used in the treatment of this condition with satisfactory results.

Yaws (Frambesia)

Yaws, a chronic contagious disease resembling syphilis, is caused by the protozoa *Treponema pertenue.* The disease is not venereal, and infection in man usually occurs through abrasions in the skin, by direct contact with an infected person. Flies are generally considered potent factors in the spread of the disease. The disease is benign and the mortality low. The symptoms are fever, rheumatic pains, and a skin eruption. Arsenicals and antimonials have been used in the treatment, and recently penicillin has been used with satisfactory results.

DRUGS USED IN THE TREATMENT OF TROPICAL INFECTIONS

Organic arsenicals and antimonials have been used for years in the treatment of tropical diseases. New synthetic compounds have been found effective in some cases, and recently antibiotics have brought about cures in diseases formerly chronic or acutely fatal.

PENTAVALENT ORGANIC ARSENICAL

Tryparsamide, U.S.P., B.P.

Tryparsamide penetrates the central nervous system and is especially useful in the treatment of the intermediate and later stages of trypanosomiasis. The intravenous dose is 3 Gm. (1 to 3 Gm.) weekly. The B.P. dose by subcutaneous, intramuscular, or intravenous injection is 1 to 2 Gm.

Preparations

Tryparsamide, U.S.P.; Tryparsamide Injection, B.P. (Sterile)   In vials containing 1, 2, and 3 Gm.

TRIVALENT ORGANIC ANTIMONIALS

Antimony Potassium Tartrate, U.S.P., B.P. (I.P.) (Tartar Emetic)

This drug is antischistosomal. It is administered intravenously in doses of 40 mg. (40 to 140 mg.) as a 0.5 per cent solution. The initial dose is 40 mg. It is then given every two days, each dose increased by 20 mg. until 140 mg. is reached; then 140 mg. every two days for a total of 14 to 18 doses. The usual dose range is 40 to 140 mg. The B.P. dose by intravenous administration of either the sodium or potassium salt is an initial dose of 30 mg. increased by 30 mg. every 48 hours to a maximum of 120 mg. The total quantity administered is not less than 1.5 Gm.

Preparations

Antimony Potassium Tartrate Injection, B.P.   30 mg. in 1 ml.
Antimony Sodium Tartrate Injection, B.P.   60 mg. in 1 ml.

Trade name: Tartar Emetic

Stibophen, U.S.P., B.P., I.P. (Fuadin)

Stibophen is antischistosomal and antileishmanial. It is given intramuscularly in doses of 100 mg., increasing to 300 mg. on alternate days, for two weeks up to a total dose of 2.5 Gm.

Preparation

Stibophen Injection, U.S.P., B.P., I.P.   300 mg. in 5 ml.
Trade names: Fantorin; Fouadin; Fuadin; Neoantimosan

PENTAVALENT ORGANIC ANTIMONIALS

Pentavalent antimony is not used in *trypanosomiasis* because of its transient action. These drugs are used in *kala-azar, schistosomiasis,* and *filariasis.* They are administered intravenously or intramuscularly.

Stibamine Glucoside (Neostam Stibamine Glucoside)

Stibamine glucoside is administered intravenously or intramuscularly as a freshly prepared 4 per cent solution. The average dose is 100 mg. per 100 lb. of body weight. The injections are made on alternate days until a maximum of 3 Gm. per 100 lb. of body weight is given. This is usually sufficient to eradicate the infection.

The toxic effects are nausea, vomiting, skin rash, and in some cases collapse. The drug is contraindicated in pneumonia, nephritis, or jaundice.

Preparation

Stibamine Glucoside   Vials containing 100 mg.
Trade name: Neostam Stibamine Glucoside

Ethylstibamine (Neostibosan)

A 5 per cent solution (freshly prepared) is administered intravenously (slowly) or intramuscularly. The initial adult dose is 200 mg.; this may be increased to 300 mg. The total dose may be 3.5 to 5 Gm. over a period of three or four weeks.

The untoward reactions are fever, cough, nausea, vomiting, diarrhea, skin rash, nephritis, and convulsions. The drug is contraindicated in nephritis, heart disease, and diarrhea. Ampuls or vials containing 300 mg. of the dry powder are available.

Trade name: Neostam Stibamine Glucoside

Sodium Stibogluconate, B.P. (Pentostam)

Sodium stibogluconate is more stable in solution than ethylstibamine and is less irritating. Sodium Stibogluconate Injection, B.P., contains 2 Gm. in 6 ml. The intravenous or intramuscular dose is 2 to 6 ml. daily.

Ureastibamine (Stiburea)

This is a mixture of different antimony compounds combined with urea. The adult dose is 200 mg. every other day intravenously. The toxic reactions are the same as with the other antimony compounds.

Antimony Lithium Thiomalate (Anthiomaline)

This is a lithium-antimony-thiomalate compound. The adult dose is usually 0.5 to 5 ml. of a 16 per cent solution (1 ml. represents 10 mg. of antimony) intramuscularly. Twelve to twenty injections are given at the rate of two or three injections a week. Its low toxicity makes it a very useful drug.

Trade name: Anthiomaline

NONMETALLIC ORGANIC COMPOUNDS

Suramin Sodium, U.S.P.; Suramin, B.P. (Antrypol, Naphuride, Bayer 205)

Suramin is a nonmetallic dye. It is used prophylactically in the prevention of trypanosomiasis and in the treatment of the acute stages of *T. rhodesiense* infection and *T. gambiense* infection. It is slowly eliminated; hence the drug remains in the tissues for some time. Two intravenous weekly doses of 1 Gm. each will usually prevent the infection for a period of three months. The adult intravenous dose for the treatment of the infection is 1 Gm. (1 to 2 Gm.) weekly until 5 to 10 Gm. have been administered. A freshly prepared solution is used.

The untoward reactions are irritation of the kidney, albuminuria, headache, nausea, itching, and skin rashes. It is contraindicated in kidney disease.

Preparation

Suramin Sodium, Sterile, U.S.P.; Sur-   Ampuls containing 1 Gm.
amin Injection, B.P.

Trade names: Antrypol; Bayer 205; Germanin; Naganal; Naphuride; Noranyl

Lucanthone Hydrochloride, U.S.P., B.P.; Miracil-D (Nilodin)

This drug belongs to a new class of compounds. It is administered orally, in doses of 500 mg. to 1 Gm. twice a day for three days. The rate of cures in schistosomiasis is high.

Untoward reactions such as nausea, vomiting, and pain in the stomach limit its use.

Preparation

Lucanthone Tablets, U.S.P., B.P.   200 and 500 mg.
Trade names: Miracil-D; Miracol; Nilodin

AROMATIC DIAMIDINES

The drugs in this group are stilbamidine, propamidine, phenamidine, and pentamidine.

Stilbamidine Isethionate

This drug is useful in the treatment of certain protozoal and systemic fungal infections (actinomycosis). The adult dose of 150 mg., dissolved in 200 ml. of 5 per cent dextrose or isotonic salt solution, is administered by intravenous drip. This is repeated every 24 or 48 hours for a course of 15 injections. Therapy may be started with 50 mg. The dose is increased to 100 mg. on the second administration and to 150 on the third administration.

The side actions are a fall in blood pressure, rapid pulse, flushing, dizziness, sweating, nausea, vomiting, and fainting. These are usually temporary and disappear in about one-half hour.

Preparation

Stilbamidine Isethionate Powder   Ampuls containing 150 mg.

Hydroxystilbamidine Isethionate, U.S.P.

This derivative is less toxic than stilbamidine isethionate. It is antileishmanial and antiblastomycosal. The usual intravenous dose is 150 mg. (150 to 225 mg.) every one or two days. It is available in ampuls containing 225 mg.

Pentamidine Isethionate, B.P.

Pentamidine is very useful in the earlier stages of trypanosomiasis. It has a prolonged prophylactic action. A single dose will prevent infection for three months. The adult dose, intravenously or intramuscularly, is 150 to 300 mg. daily or every second day for about ten days. Doses are given daily or every other day until a total of 1.0 to 1.5 Gm. has been administered. It is occasionally given intramuscularly in a 10 per cent solution. Pentamidine is also useful in kala-azar and against antimony-resistant strains of leishmania. It is the least toxic drug of this group.

The untoward effects are flushing of the face, headache, sweating, a fall in blood pressure, and fainting.

Preparation

Pentamidine Injection, B.P. (Sterile)
              Trade names: Lomidine; M and B 800

ANTIBIOTIC

The complete healing of cutaneous lesions of leishmaniasis with the intravenous administration of amphotericin B has been reported. The maximum dose of 50 mg. daily was given by intravenous drip. This antibiotic is discussed on page 153.

REVIEW QUESTIONS

MALARIA

1. *Discuss the prevalence, transmission, and methods of control of malaria.*
2. *Name some of the drugs used in the treatment of malaria.*
3. *What are some of the advantages obtained by the administration of chloroquine?*
4. *What are some of the advantages of the use of primaquine?*

AMEBIASIS

1. *Define amebiasis and discuss the purpose of the treatment of the disease.*
2. *What drugs are important in the treatment of intestinal amebiasis?*
3. *What is the drug of choice in the treatment of liver abscess?*
4. *Explain why two types of amebicides are often given at the same time.*

REFERENCES

Adams, A. R. D.: "Drug Treatment of Malaria," *Brit. M. J.*, **2**:183, 1959.
Bruce-Chwatt, L. J.: "Changing Tides of Chemotherapy of Malaria," *Brit. M.J.*, **1**:581, 1964.
"Chemotherapy of Malaria," *Brit. M.J.*, **1**:1032, 1964.

CHLOROQUINE

Berberian, D. A., and Dennis, E. W.: "Field Experiments with Chloroquine Diphosphate," *Am. J. Trop. Med.*, **28**:755, 1948.
Coatney, G. R.; Ruhe, D. S.; Cooper, W. C.; Josephson, E. S.; and Young, M. D.: "Studies in Human Malaria. X. The Protective and Therapeutic Action of Chloroquine Against St. Elizabeth Strain Vivax Malaria," *Am. J. Hyg.*, **49**:49, 1949.
Most, H.; London, I. M.; Kane, C. A.; Lavietes, P. H.; Schroeder, E. F.; and Hayman, J. M., Jr.: "Chloroquine for Acute Attacks of Vivax Malaria," *J.A.M.A.*, **131**:963, 1946.

AMODIAQUINE

Coggeshall, L. T.: "The Treatment of Malaria," *Am. J. Trop. Med.*, **1**:124, 1952.
Love, J.; Fould, R.; Williams, R. G. W., Jr.; and Mitchell, R. B.: "Evaluation of Amodiaquin (Camoquin) in the Treatment of Relapsing Vivax Malaria," *Am. J. M. Sc.*, **225**:26, 1953.

QUINACRINE

Cooper, W. C.; Ruhe, D. S.; Coatney, G. R.; Josephson, E. S.; and Young, M. D.: "Studies in Human Malaria. VIII. The Protective and Therapeutic Action of Quinacrine Against St. Elizabeth Strain Vivax Malaria," *Am. J. Hyg.*, **49**:25, 1949.
Gordon, H. H., *et al.*: "A Comparison of Quinine and Quinacrine in the Treatment of Clinical Attacks of Vivax Malaria," *South. M. J.*, **39**:631, 1946.

PAMAQINE AND PRIMAQUINE

Alving, A. S.; Arnold, J.; and Robinson, D. H.: "Status of Primaquine. 1. Mass Therapy of Subclinical Vivax Malaria with Primaquine," *J.A.M.A.*, **149**:1558, 1952.
Alving, A. S.; Hankey, D. D.; Coatney, G. R.; Jones, R., Jr.; Coker, W. G.; Garrison, P. L.; and Donovan, W. N.: "Korean Vivax Malaria. II. Curative Treatment with Pamaquine and Primaquine," *Am. J. Trop. Med.*, **2**:970, 1953.
Archambeault, C. P.: "Mass Antimalarial Therapy in Veterans Returning from Korea," *J.A.M.A.*, **154**:1411, 1954.

PENTAQUINE

Alving, A. S.; Craig, B., Jr.; Jones, R., Jr.; Whorton, C. M.; Pullman, T. N.; and Eichelberger, E.: "Pentaquine, a Therapeutic Agent Effective in Reducing the Relapse Rate in Vivax Malaria," *J. Clin. Invest.*, **27**:25, 1948.

PYRIMETHAMINE (DARAPRIM)

Coatney, G. R., *et al.*: "Studies in Human Malaria. The Protective and Therapeutic Effects of Pyrimethamine (Daraprim) Against Chesson Strain Vivax Malaria," *Am. J. Trop. Med.*, **2**:777, 1953.
Goodwin, L. G.: "Daraprim, A New Antimalarial," *Brit. M. J.*, **2**:336, 1952.
"Symposium on Daraprim," *Tr. Roy. Soc. Trop. Med. & Hyg.*, **46**:467, 1952.

CYCLOGUANIL PAMOATE

Lunn, Joseph E., *et al.*: "Cycloguanil Pamoate (CI-501) as a Causal Prophylactic Against a Southern Rhodesian Strain of Falciparum Malaria," *Am. J. Trop. Med.*, **13**:783, 1964.

DRUGS FOR AMEBIASIS AND TROPICAL INFECTIONS

Adams, A. R. D.: "Amoebiasis and Amebic Dysentery," *Brit. M. J.*, **1**:956, 1960.
Anderson, H. H., *et al.*: "Fumagillin in Amebiasis," *Am. J. Trop. Med.*, **1**:552, 1952.
Berberian, D. A., *et al.*: "Drug Prophylaxis of Amebiasis," *J.A.M.A.*, **148**:700, 1952.
Chandler, A. C.: *Introduction to Parasitology*, 9th ed. John Wiley & Sons, Inc., New York, 1955.
Conan, N. J.: "Chloroquine in Amebiasis," *Am. J. Trop. Med.*, **28**:107, 1948.
del Pozo, E. C., and Alcarez, M.: "Clinical Treatment of Intestinal Amebiasis in Treatment of Amebiasis," *Am. J. Med.*, **20**:412, 1956.
Frye, W. W.: "The Pathogenesis and Therapy of Human Amebiasis," *Am. J. Gastroenterol.*, **25**:315, 1956.
McHardy, G.: "Amebiasis; Antibiotic Amebicides," *General Practitioner*, **13**:79, 1956.
Taylor, D. J., *et al.*: "Puromycin. I. Activity Against Experimental Amebiasis," *Antibiotics Annual, 1954-1955*. Medical Encyclopedia, Inc., New York, 1954, p. 745.
Wilmot, A. J.: "A Comparison of Puromycin and Tetracycline and Its Derivatives in Amebiasis," *Antibiotics Annual, 1955-1956*. Medical Encyclopedia, Inc., New York, 1955, p. 319.

PARAMOMYCIN

Courtney, K. O.; Thompson, P. E.; Hodgkinson, R.; and Fitzsimmons, J. R.: "Paromomycin as a Therapeutic Substance for Intestinal Amebiasis and Bacterial Enteritis," *Antibiotics Annual, 1959–1960*. Medical Encyclopedia, Inc., New York, 1960, p. 304.

Godenne, G. D.: "Paromomycin in Diarrheas of Infants and Children," *Antibiotics Annual, 1959–1960*. Medical Encyclopedia, Inc., New York, 1960, p. 310.

Shafer, A. Z.: "The Treatment of Amebic Dysentery with Paromomycin," *Antibiotic Med. and Clin. Therapy*, 7:273, 1960.

AMPHOTERICIN

Furtado, T. A.: "Clinical Results in the Treatment of American Leishmaniasis with Oral and Intravenous Amphotericin," *Antibiotics Annual, 1959–1960*. Medical Encyclopedia, Inc., New York, 1960, p. 631.

13

Chemotherapy of Helminthiasis. Anthelmintics

HELMINTHIASIS

Helminthiasis is a disease characterized by the presence of worms in the intestinal tract or tissues of man. This condition is widespread throughout the world, and well over 800 million persons harbor some type of parasitic worm. In many cases, multiple infestations occur.

The infestation does not necessarily cause clinical symptoms, but in many cases dangerous conditions may occur. The parasites may: (1) damage the intestinal mucosa and thus cause loss of blood and anemia; (2) produce toxic substances, which are absorbed by the patient; or (3) cause malnutrition by robbing the host of food. Large numbers of parasites may cause obstruction in the bile ducts, lymphatics, and intestines.

Diagnosis of the parasitic worms may be made by identifying either the ova or the mature forms in the stools. It is very important to identify the particular worms present and eradicate them as quickly as possible.

The worms may be divided into three groups: (1) the nematodes, (2) the cestodes, and (3) the trematodes.

NEMATODES

The nematodes are cylindrical, unsegmented worms which vary in size from $\frac{1}{12}$ in. to 5 or 15 in. in length. They develop in the small or large intestine and are susceptible to treatment with drugs.

Ancylostomiasis (Hookworm Disease). There are two species of hookworm: *Ancylostoma duodenale* and *Necator americanus.* These cylindrical worms have mouths containing hooks, with which they attach themselves to the intestinal mucosa, often producing small ulcers. They derive their nourishment by drawing blood from the blood vessels and gulping in food from the intestinal contents. The ova of these worms, passed in human stool, develop on warm, moist, shady ground. The larvae that hatch from the ova penetrate the skin of the feet and legs of children who run barefoot, and the arms and hands of adults. Inflammatory conditions ("ground itch") may be noted at the site of entry. The larvae enter blood vessels and are transported to the

230

lungs, where they leave the capillaries and enter the alveoli. From the alveoli they move up the respiratory tract to the pharynx and are then swallowed. They then attach to the mucosa of the bowel, develop into mature worms in 45 to 74 days, and reproduce in the intestinal tract. Sometimes the ova enter the intestinal tract with contaminated food and water.

Many persons harbor hookworms without clinical symptoms. Others manifest severe symptoms, such as chronic anemia due to blood loss and inadequate diet, loss of appetite, alternating constipation and diarrhea, mental and physical lethargy, and exhaustion. Dizziness, edema, dilatation of the heart, and even death may occur. In children, growth is retarded and puberty is delayed. The drugs used today in the treatment of hookworm infestation are tetrachloroethylene, bephenium, and dithiazanine. Carbon tetrachloride is also effective, but because of its greater toxicity it is rarely used. The anemia is treated with ferrous sulfate.

Ascariasis (Roundworm Infestation). Ascariasis, one of the most common worm diseases in man, is very prevalent in the United States. The causative parasite, *Ascaris lumbricoides,* is a worm about 6 to 14 in. long. The infestation occurs by ingesting food and water polluted with the fertilized ova passed in the excreta of infected human beings, or by eating with soiled hands contaminated with the ova. The larvae, which develop from the ova in the intestinal tract, penetrate its wall and enter the circulation and the lungs. Later, they reach the upper respiratory tract and are swallowed. In the intestinal tract the larvae develop into adult worms in two or three weeks. Often there are no symptoms as a result of the infestation. On the other hand, nausea, vomiting, and loss of appetite may be experienced. In the lungs the larvae may cause pneumonitis with fever, asthmatic dyspnea, and coughing. The adult worms rob the host of food, excrete toxic substances, and may cause intestinal or biliary blocking. They may also be regurgitated from the stomach and inhaled into the trachea, thereby causing suffocation. The drugs used most widely in the treatment of ascariasis are the piperazine, dithiazanine, and bephenium salts. Hexylresorcinol may also be used. The drug of choice is piperazine.

The prevention of ascariasis is based upon proper disposal of human excreta, treatment of infected persons, and personal cleanliness.

Enterobiasis (Oxyuriasis, Pinworm Infestation). *Enterobius vermicularis* is a small, glistening, white worm that varies in length from $\frac{1}{4}$ to $\frac{1}{2}$ in. The infestation, which is caused by the ingestion of the ova from contaminated fingers or contaminated objects placed in the mouth, is rather prevalent in the United States, particularly in children. The eggs hatch in the small intestine, and the worms mature in two to six weeks. The fertilized female migrates to the cecum and colon and deposits her eggs in the rectum and folds of the anus. Irritation and secretion of mucus result. The symptoms are itching of the anus, scratching, congestion, inflammation, insomnia, nervousness, loss of appetite, and anemia. Reinfestation may occur by way of contaminated fingers. Pinworm infestation may spread through an entire family and is prevalent in institutions. The drugs used are gentian violet and the piperazine and pyrvinium salts.

Strongyloidiasis. *Strongyloides stercoralis* is a small worm about $\frac{1}{12}$ in. long. The larvae penetrate the skin and migrate in the body in the same manner as hookworm. They may also be ingested with food. The eggs are hatched in the upper intestine, and the filariform larvae invade the mucosa and cause inflammation and diarrhea with mucus. Some of the larvae are passed in the feces and develop into skin-penetrating larvae. The drugs of choice are pyrvinium pamoate, gentian violet, and dithiazanine iodide. Gentian violet may be given in enteric-coated pills or in 1 per cent solution by duodenal tube.

Trichuriasis (Whipworm Infestation). Humans ingest the ova of *Trichuris trichiura* from polluted soil. These ova develop in the upper part of the duodenum, and the motile larvae that are hatched enter the cecum and attach themselves to the mucosa. Trichuriasis may be asymptomatic or there may be a skin rash, indigestion, mild anemia, and sleeplessness. The drug of choice is dithiazanine iodide.

Trichinosis. Trichinosis is caused by the presence of the larvae of *Trichinella spiralis* in the striated muscles. Although large portions of the world are free from this disease, one in six persons in the United States is infested. Hogs are the intermediate hosts. They eat garbage containing uncooked meat scraps infested with live trichinellae; the larvae which develop become encysted in their striated muscles. When these larvae are ingested by human beings in insufficiently cooked pork, they mature in the intestines of the host. The mature worms, in turn, produce larvae, which are carried in the lymph and blood to the striated muscles, where they become encysted. Their presence causes stiffness and swelling of the involved muscle, severe pain, edema, fever, and marked eosinophilia. There is no drug available to cure this infection. However, the disease may be prevented easily with adequate public health measures.

Thiabendazole (Thibenzole), an anthelmintic employed by veterinarians, was recently used clinically and produced what is believed to be the first cure of a proved case of trichinosis.[1]

Filariasis. This disease is caused by the presence of microfilariae (*Wuchereria bancrofti*) in the connective tissues, blood vessels, and body cavities. It occurs in Africa and India and other tropical and subtropical countries. The carrier is the mosquito *Culex fatigans*. The manifestations of

---

[1] "Texas Physicians Report a Triumph over Trichinosis," *Medical World News,* **5**:40, 1964.

the disease are inflammation of the lymph glands and hyperplasia of lymphatic tissue (elephantiasis). There is no known prophylactic drug; the best prophylactic measure is mosquito control. Diethylcarbamazine citrate (Hetrazan) is used in the treatment of the disease, since it destroys the microfilariae and prevents infection of the insect vector. Ethylstibamine (Neostibosan), which is also administered, is discussed on page 224. Another related disease is onchocerciasis, in which the filarial worms, the *Onchocerca volvulus*, migrate under the skin and into the eyeball and conjunctiva, producing blindness. Suramin is used in the treatment of this parasite.

CESTODES

The cestodes (tapeworms) are flattened, segmented worms with a head, or scolex, and a variable number of segments. There are four varieties: (1) *Taenia saginata* (beef tapeworm), (2) *Taenia solium* (pork tapeworm), (3) *Hymenolepis nana* (dwarf tapeworm), and (4) *Diphyllobothrium latum* (fish tapeworm).

Taeniasis (Tapeworm Infestation). Taeniasis is caused by the presence of *Taenia saginata* or *Taenia solium* in the bowel. These worms hold onto the intestinal mucosa with suckers in the head and take nourishment through the body wall. They are segmented and flat and may reach 6 to 30 ft. in length. Each worm may have several thousand segments, and each segment can produce hundreds of eggs. The head is small in comparison with the rest of the body. *Taenia saginata* (beef tapeworm) is acquired by eating raw or improperly cooked beef of cattle that have become infested by ingesting human feces containing tapeworm ova. *Taenia solium* (pork tapeworm) is acquired by eating improperly cooked pork infested with larvae. The adult worm is depicted in Figure 9. The ova hatch in the intestines of cattle, and the larvae penetrate the intestinal walls and finally become encysted in the muscles. These cysts may be killed with proper cooking of meat. However, after ingestion of the infested meat improperly cooked, the adult worms develop in man and attach themselves to the intestinal mucosa.

The life cycle of the beef and pork tapeworms and the symptoms of the diseases are the same for both organisms. These symptoms are abdominal pain, insatiable appetite, nausea, vomiting, anemia, leukocytosis, and mental depression. The drug of choice in the treatment of tapeworm infestation is quinacrine. Hexylresorcinol and aspidium oleoresin are sometimes used.

Cysticercosis is a serious condition which is unique to the pork tapeworm. After the ingestion of the living ova of this worm, the larval forms develop in the gastrointestinal tract. These larvae enter the blood stream and become encysted in the muscles and organs of the host, including the brain. The symptoms noted are muscular pain and weakness, loss of weight, and nervousness. In serious cases where the brain is invaded, paralysis, epileptic attacks, and convulsions may occur. There is no specific drug therapy for this disease.

The dwarf tapeworm is a small worm about 1½ in. in length. There is no intermediate host, and infestation results from eating food contaminated with living ova. These ova hatch in the stomach or small intestine. The larvae attach themselves to the mucosa of the intestinal tract. The patients

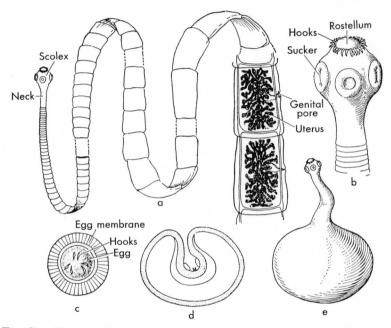

Fig. 9. *Taenia solium*, the pork tapeworm. *a.* Specimen about 8 ft. long consisting of about 900 proglottids, with four sections omitted; the uterus filled with eggs is shown in the last two proglottids; about four times natural size. *b.* Scolex, magnified about 35 times. *c.* Egg surrounded by a membrane and bearing six hooks. *d.* Bladderworm of cysticercus and scolex at bottom of invagination. *e.* Cysticercus with head evaginated and ready to become attached to the intestinal wall. (From Hegner, R. W., and Stiles, K. A.: *College Zoology*, 7th ed. The Macmillan Company, New York, 1959.)

may be asymptomatic; or abdominal pain, dizziness, and diarrhea may be experienced. The drugs used in this infestation are hexylresorcinol, either orally or by duodenal tube, and aspidium oleoresin.

The larvae of fish tapeworm are encysted in the muscles of fish, and man becomes infested by eating these fish raw or improperly cooked. Quinacrine is used to treat this infestation.

TREMATODES

Schistosomiasis, which is caused by blood flukes, is discussed on page 222.

ANTHELMINTICS

Anthelmintics are drugs used in the treatment of worm infestations. Vermifuges are drugs that narcotize or weaken the worms so that they can no longer attach themselves to the intestinal mucosa and thus can be expelled from the intestinal tract with a cathartic. Vermicides are drugs that paralyze or kill the parasites.

Sometimes the patient is fasted the evening before the administration of the drug. Sometimes a light, fat-free meal rich in carbohydrates is eaten to protect the liver from the toxic action of certain of these drugs. A saline cathartic is administered in the morning and then the drug is given. Several hours later another saline cathartic is given to expel the dead or paralyzed worms and the drug remaining in the intestinal tract. With some of the newer drugs fasting and purging are unnecessary.

In the case of tapeworm infestations, enemas may be indicated to remove the head. If the head is left behind, new segments will be formed. An examination of the stools of the patient at intervals for worms and ova will show if a cure has been effected.

Tetrachloroethylene, U.S.P., B.P., I.P.

This drug is used chiefly in the treatment of hookworm infestation. The usual adult oral dose is 3 ml. (2 to 4 ml.) in hard gelatin capsules. More recently an adult dose of 5 ml. which is not followed by a saline purge has been found to be more effective and less toxic. A single dose will eliminate about 92 per cent of *Necator americanus*. The dose for children is 0.2 ml. for each year up to 15 years of age. Fatty foods and alcohol are eliminated in the diet prior to the administration of the drug. In the absence of fats and alcohol, tetrachloroethylene is only very slightly absorbed from the intestinal tract. The drug should be fresh, and its administration should be preceded the night before by a saline purge, and another saline purge given two hours after the administration.

In therapeutic doses, tetrachloroethylene is nonirritating, relatively nontoxic, and inexpensive. Occasionally, upon absorption, it may cause dizziness, headache, and drowsiness. The drug is contraindicated in mixed infestation with ascaris, since it may stimulate the migration of the roundworms and cause intestinal obstruction or invasion of the bile ducts and liver; hexylresorcinol, which is also useful in hookworm infestation, should be administered first.

Preparation

Tetrachloroethylene Capsules, U.S.P., B.P.   0.2, 1, and 5 ml.

Hexylresorcinol, N.F., B.P. (Caprokol)

Hexylresorcinol is a safe and effective drug for the treatment of roundworm, hookworm, tapeworm, pinworm, and whipworm infestations. The usual oral adult dose of 1 Gm. is administered in gelatin-coated pills. The dose for children is 100 mg. for each year of age up to 10 years as a single dose. One dose has often proved effective; if not, treatment may be repeated in three days. One gram of hexylresorcinol and 1 Gm. of acacia may be dissolved in 30 ml. of water and administered by duodenal tube in tapeworm infestation. Retention enemas (500 to 700 ml.) of a 0.1 to 0.3 per cent solution are administered in trichuriasis.

Preparation

Hexylresorcinol Pills, N.F.   100 and 200 mg.
                    Trade name: "Crystoids" Anthelmintic
                    Synonym: Santokin

Diethylcarbamazine Citrate, U.S.P., B.P. (Hetrazan)

This drug is used in the treatment of filariasis. The dose for the treatment of filariasis is 2 mg. per kilogram of body weight three times daily after meals for 7 to 21 days.

Preparations

Diethylcarbamazine Citrate Tablets,   50 mg.
U.S.P.
Diethylcarbamazine Citrate Syrup,   125 mg. in 5 ml.
U.S.P.
          Trade names: Banocide; Carbilazine; Hetrazan; Notezine

Piperazine Salts

Piperazine hexahydrate is the drug of choice for the eradication of roundworms and pinworms. The citrate and tartrate, adipate and phosphate salts of piperazine and the chelated compound piperazine calcium edathamil are available for oral administration. They paralyze the ascaris, and normal intestinal peristalsis carries them out of the tract alive. The drug may be given in a single dose on one day. If it is given on two consecutive days, a cure will be produced in 95 per cent of the patients.

Preparations

Piperazine Citrate Syrup, U.S.P.   Syrup containing 100 mg. of pipera-
                                       zine hexahydrate in each milliliter
Piperazine Citrate Tablets, U.S.P.   250 and 500 mg.
          Trade names: Antepar, Multifuge, Parazine, Pipizan

Piperazine Adipate Tablets, B.P.   300 mg.
Piperazine Phosphate Tablets, B.P.   260 mg.
Piperazine Tartrate Solution   100 mg. in 1 ml.
Piperazine Tartrate Tablets   250 and 500 mg.

Trade name: Piperat

Piperazine Calcium Edathamil Syrup   100 mg. in 1 ml.
Piperazine Calcium Edathamil   500 mg.
Wafers

Trade name: Perin

Table 15

Dosage for One- and Two-Day Treatment with Piperazine*

Patient's Weight, lb.	Daily Dose as Citrate Syrup, ml.	Dose as Hexahydrate, Gm.
30–50	20	2.0
51–100	30	3.0
Over 101	35	3.5

In the treatment of pinworm the following doses are given over a period of six or seven days.

lb.	ml.	Gm.
Up to 15	2.5	0.25
6–30	5.0	0.50
31–60	10.0	1.00
Over 60	20.0	2.00

* Southworth, H., and Hofmann, E. G. (eds.): *Columbia-Presbyterian Therapeutic Talks.* The Macmillan Company, New York, 1963.

Gentian Violet, U.S.P.; Crystal Violet, B.P. (Methyl Violet)

This drug is used in strongyloidiasis and pinworm infestation. The usual adult oral dose is 60 mg. (10 to 60 mg.) three times a day before meals for one to two weeks. For children the dose is 10 mg. for each year of age, in divided doses (three times a day). Twenty-five milliliters of a 1 per cent solution may be administered by duodenal tube. The untoward effects are nausea, vomiting, diarrhea, and abdominal pain. The symptoms are temporary and disappear when the drug is discontinued. Gentian violet is contraindicated in mixed infestation with ascaris and in cardiac, hepatic, or renal disease.

Preparation
Gentian Violet Tablets, U.S.P.   10, 15, and 30 mg.

Dithiazanine Iodide, U.S.P. (Delvex)

Dithiazanine is an effective broad-spectrum anthelmintic. In clinical trials it has produced cures in single, multiple, light, and heavy infestations of whipworms (*Trichuris trichiura*), large roundworms (*Ascaris lumbricoides*), threadworms (*Strongyloides stercoralis*), and pinworms (*Enterobius vermicularis*). Dithiazanine is partially effective against hookworms (*Necator americanus*), but best results are achieved when the drug is given with subclinical doses of tetrachloroethylene. Preliminary studies suggest that dithiazanine is successful in combating beef tapeworms (*Taenia saginata*) and dwarf tapeworms (*Hymenolepis nana*). It is the drug of choice in whipworm and threadworm infestations.

Dosage and Method of Administration. The oral dose for adults varies from 100 to 200 mg., three times a day for five days. With threadworm infestation it is often necessary to continue treatment for 14 to 21 days. Children weighing between 20 and 60 lb. are given daily doses (in divided amounts) of 50 to 100 mg. per 10 lb. of body weight. Adjunctive measures, such as cathartics, are not required. Tablets should not be chewed.

Side Effects. The side effects are minimal. Nausea, vomiting, and diarrhea may occur and necessitate using smaller doses. Abdominal cramps and diarrhea have been observed. In the presence of a malabsorption syndrome the drug is quite toxic and several deaths have resulted; so great care should be exercised in its use.

Preparations

Dithiazanine Iodide Tablets (enteric coated)	100 mg.
Dithiazanine Suspension	20 mg. in 1 ml.

Trade names: Delvex; Abminthic; Amelmid; Partel; Telmid

Bephenium Hydroxynaphthoate (Alcopar, Alcopara)

Bephenium hydroxynaphthoate is a new British drug that is safe and effective against hookworms. It is especially useful in persons with heavy infestations and advanced anemia and diarrhea. No purge is necessary. It is also valuable in the treatment of roundworms when they occur simultaneously with hookworms. However, roundworm infestations occurring singly are best treated with piperazine salts. The only side effects reported are nausea and vomiting in a few patients. This may be accompanied by diarrhea. The drug has been given successfully to infants, pregnant women, and seriously ill patients with a hemoglobin level below 50 per cent.

The standard oral dose is 5 Gm. (2.5 Gm. of bephenium base) irrespective of age or weight. It is administered between breakfast and lunch. A single dose or multiple doses given on successive days or three times the same day are as effective as tetrachlorethylene in the treatment of hookworm.

Preparation

Bephenium Hydroxynaphthoate Sachets or Packets	5 Gm. (2.5 Gm. of the base)

Trade names: Alcopar, Alcopara

Pyrvinium Salts

Pyrvinium chloride (Vanquin) and the pamoate (Poquil, Povan) are complex salts of cyanine dyes. The chloride, the original compound, was very effective against pinworms when given for five to eight days. It caused considerable nausea and vomiting. Pyrvinium pamoate is more effective, and the incidence of vomiting is reduced. A single dose will produce a cure in 95 per cent of the patients. The oral dose for children is 1 teaspoon (5 ml.) as a suspension per 22 lb. (10 kg.) of body weight; the oral adult dose is four tablets. The whole family should be treated and given one dose before going to bed. The drug colors the stools red, and the solution will stain clothing and other materials.

Preparations

Pyrvinium Chloride Suspension 5 mg. in 1 ml.
Trade name: Vanquin

Pyrvinium Pamoate Suspension, U.S.P.   10 mg. of the base in 1 ml.
Pyrvinium Pamoate Tablets, U.S.P.   50 mg. of the base
Trade names: Poquil, Povan

Quinacrine Hydrochloride, U.S.P.; Mepacrine Hydrochloride, B.P. (Atabrine)

Quinacrine as an antimalarial is discussed on page 213. It is now the drug of choice for tapeworm infestation. It is given in doses of 500 mg. with 500 mg. of sodium bicarbonate. A saline cathartic one hour after the last dose is followed by a soapsuds enema. The same dose may be given in solution by duodenal tube.

Aspidium Oleoresin; Male Fern Extract, B.P. (I.P.) (Oleoresin of Male Fern)

Aspidium oleoresin is an ether extract prepared from the roots of *Dryopteris Filix-mas* (male fern), a perennial plant with a sword-shaped leaf. It is a dark-green liquid with a disagreeable taste. Filicin is the most important active constituent. Aspidium oleoresin is often also used in the treatment of pork tapeworm disease. It is very irritating to the intestinal mucosa; hence it is given in the form of an emulsion or capsules. An emulsion of 6 to 10 Gm. of aspidium oleoresin, 8 Gm. of acacia, and 30 Gm. of sodium sulfate in 100 ml. of water may be given by duodenal tube. One half the dose is given to children. The adult oral dose of 5 Gm. (3 to 5 Gm.) is given in gelatin capsules (0.5 Gm.) at half-hour intervals until the calculated dose is given. Children under ten are given 0.5 Gm. for each year of age. Two days prior to treament, fat should be excluded from the diet. A saline purgative is administered from one to two hours after the last dose.

OLDER ANTHELMINTICS

The older anthelmintics, santonin, oil of chenopodium thymol, and betanaphthol, were once widely used. They are toxic drugs and produce severe gastrointestinal irritation and very undesirable disturbances of the central nervous system. They are not discussed here because less toxic and more effective drugs are now available. It seems that their use in the treatment of these diseases is no longer justified.

REVIEW QUESTIONS

1. *Define helminthiasis.*
2. *How may helminthiasis be diagnosed?*
3. *Define anthelmintics.*
4. *Explain how anthelmintics produce their effects.*
5. *For what diseases is piperazine hexahydrate the drug of choice? How is this drug administered? How is it available? What are the advantages of using this drug?*
6. *What is the drug of choice in hookworm infestation? How is it administered and in what dosage form?*
7. *What drugs are used for the eradication of tapeworms?*
8. *What new broad-spectrum anthelmintic has been introduced recently? What are some of the advantages of its use?*
9. *What new drug may effect a cure of hookworm with one dose?*

REFERENCES

Bracken, E. C.: "Antihelminthic Therapy: A Simplified Approach," *South. Med. J.*, **57**:227, 1964.
Chandler, A. C.: *Introduction to Parasitology*, 9th ed. John Wiley & Sons, Inc., New York, 1955.

TETRACHLOROETHYLENE

Council on Pharmacy and Chemistry: "Tetrachloroethylene," *J.A.M.A.*, **107**:1132, 1936.

HEXYLRESORCINOL

Morales, H., and Stevenson, D. F.: "Treatment of Taenia Saginata with Hexylresorcinol Emulsion," *J.A.M.A.*, **142**:369, 1950.

DIETHYLCARBAMAZINE CITRATE

Etteldorf, J. N., and Crawford, L. V.: "Treatment of Ascariasis in Children; Use of Hetrazan," *J.A.M.A.*, **143**:797, 1950.
Hawking, F., and Laurie, W.: "Action of Hetrazan on Filariasis and Onchocerciasis," *Lancet*, **2**:146, 1949.

PIPERAZINE

Brown, H. W.: "The Treatment of *Ascaris lumbricoides* Infections with Pipera-
zine," *J. Pediat.*, **45**:419, 1954.
Brown, H. W., and Sterman, M. M.: "Treatment of *Ascaris lumbricoides* Infec-
tions with Piperazine Citrate," *Am. J. Trop. Med.*, **3**:750, 1954.
Bumbalo, T. S.; Gustina, F. J.; and Oleksiak, R. E.: "The Treatment of Pinworm
Infection (Enterobiasis)," *J. Pediat.*, **44**:386, 1954.
White, R. H. R.: "Ascariasis Treated with Piperazine Hydrate," *Lancet*, **2**:315,
1954.
White, R. H. R., and Standen, O. D.: "Piperazine in the Treatment of Thread-
worms in Children," *Brit. M. J.*, **2**:755, 1953.

PYRVINIUM

Beck, J. W., *et al.*: "Treatment of Pinworm Infections in Humans (Enterobiasis)
with Pyrvinium Chloride and Pyrvinium Pamoate," *Am. J. Trop. Med.*, **8**:349,
1959.
Southworth, H., and Hofman, F. G. (ed.): *Columbia Presbyterian Therapeutic
Talks*. The Macmillan Company, New York, 1963.

QUINACRINE HYDROCHLORIDE

Morales, H.: "Quinacrine in the Treatment of Taenia Saginata Infestation,"
J.A.M.A., **142**:368, 1950.
Sodeman, W. A., and Jung, R. C.: "Treatment of Taeniasis with Quinacrine
Hydrochloride," *J.A.M.A.*, **148**:285, 1952.

DITHIAZANINE IODIDE

Paine, D. H. D., and Lower, E. S.: "Treatment of Trichuriasis with Dithiazanine
in a Hospital for Mental Defectives," *Brit. M. J.*, **1**:770, 1960.
Swartzweider, J. C., *et al.*: "Dithiazanine, an Effective Broad Spectrum Anthel-
mintic," *J.A.M.A.*, **165**:2063, 1957.
———: "Therapy of Trichuriasis and Ascariasis with Dithiazanine," *Am. J. Trop.
Med. & Hyg.*, **7**:329, 1958.
Villarejos, V. M., and Saldaña, J.: "Mass Deparasitization Experiment with
Dithiazanine Iodide," *Antibiotic Med. & Clin. Therapy*, **6**:718, 1959.

BEPHENIUM HYDROXYNAPHTHOATE

Ahmad, N., and Rasool, G.: "Bephenium Hydroxynaphthoate Against Hookworm
in West Pakistan," *J. Trop. Med. and Hyg.*, **62**:284, 1959.
Goodwin, L. G., and Jayewardene, L. G.: "Clinical Trials with Bephenium
Hydroxynaphthoate Against Hookworm in Ceylon," *Brit. M. J.*, **2**:1572, 1958.
Nagaty, H. F., and Rifaat, M. A.: "Clinical Trials with Bephenium Hydroxynaphthoate Against Ancylostoma Duodenale and Other Helminthic Infestations," *J. Trop. Med. and Hyg.*, **62**:255, 1959.

III DRUGS ACTING ON THE CENTRAL NERVOUS SYSTEM

The central nervous system, together with the peripheral nerves, constitutes the body's equipment for rapid coordination of many of its activities. These activities must be set into play and governed to needs often in a fraction of a second. An example is the very rapid closing of the eyes when they are unexpectedly touched, as by a grain of sand, or when an object is seen menacing them. We move ourselves by sending at will electrical signals from the central nervous system to our skeletal muscles. These are so named because they move our bone structure. This nervous system is composed of the brain and the spinal cord. Together they coordinate many functions such as blood pressure, heart rate, salivary and gastric juice flow, sphincter function, and skin temperature. In addition, the brain serves to store knowledge and to cause, on the basis of past experience, conscious and unconscious reactions, physical and emotional, to stimuli and conditions. Our awareness of our environment, our satisfaction or dissatisfaction with it, happiness, love, and all emotions and moods are seated in our brain.

The brain can be depressed and stimulated. The use of alcoholic beverages and of plants having depressant effects had its beginnings in antiquity. The same is true of tea leaves, containing the stimulant caffeine. Anesthesia may be cited as one of the greatest boons to mankind, for it made possible life-saving surgery and painless childbirth. Depressants and stimulants of the brain, or specific parts thereof, and of the spinal cord have been developed with considerable precision.

Noteworthy advances in the effective treatment of the mentally ill with drugs have occurred within the past two decades. Much research has been in progress and more is now being done in exploitation of these and other findings. Efforts of surgeons, psychiatrists, biochemists, neurologists, electronic engineers, and other specialists are now being directed toward this field in hundreds of laboratories and centers. Progress should be made more rapidly now in understanding the causes of mental disease.

14

The Function of the Central Nervous System and Its Response to Drugs

The central nervous system, as we have noted, coordinates and directs the activities of the organs and tissues of the body. This achieves adjustment and adaptation to the environment of the organism. The *nerve endings* (receptors) in the sensory organs, skin, muscles, tendons, and joints, when stimulated by changes in the environment, initiate impulses to the central nervous system. These impulses are carried by the afferent nerve fibers to the spinal cord and brain. Efferent impulses (motor) are then carried by the efferent nerve fibers to the *effector cells* (muscle cells for contraction or glands for excretion).

THE BRAIN

The brain is mainly divided into five parts:

> Cerebrum
> Thalamus—hypothalamus
> Midbrain
> Cerebellum
> Medulla

Figure 10 may be referred to in studying the descriptions of these major divisions which follow.

The Cerebrum. The cerebrum, which is the largest part of the brain, is divided into two hemispheres. The gray surface layer, which is composed largely of nerve cell bodies, is called the *cerebral cortex*. Beneath the cortex are nerve fibers (white matter) that connect the lower centers of the brain and spinal cord and different areas of the cortex with each other. Deeper in the cerebrum there is more gray matter, the nuclei and synaptic connections between the nerves of the hemispheres and the brain stem. These are relay stations along the nerve pathways to the cortex. The cerebral cortex is the site of consciousness. It is divided into sensory, motor, and association areas. Sensations are received from the organs of special sense (for sight, hearing, smell, and taste) and from the skin, muscles, joints, and tendons (for touch, pain, and temperature) by the *sensory areas* via the important relay nuclei of the thalamus. The *association areas* of the cortex are concerned with storing,

244

interpreting, and integrating the separate sensations that are received from the various parts of the brain and transmitted by connecting fibers. They are responsible for the highest mental processes such as attention, memory, learning, reasoning, judgment, imagination, and will power. The mental activities control the intelligence and personality of the individual. The will power enables him to perform voluntary, purposeful, or inhibitory (restraining) acts. The motor impulses, which are sent out from the *motor areas* in response to

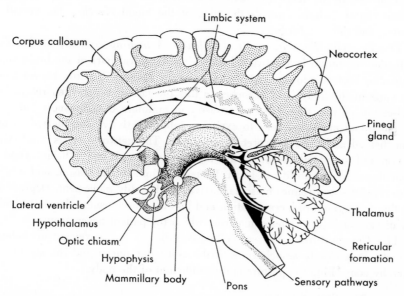

Fig. 10. Incoming stimuli along sensory pathways activate the reticular formation that alerts the brain and adds emotional awareness. (From Himwich, H. E.: "Tranquilizers and the Brain," *Med. World News,* June 17, 1960, p. 26. Redrawn after original by Mary Lorenc.)

the sensations received, are primarily for motion and speech. Impulses for muscular contraction cause well-integrated body movements, including reciprocal inhibition. Sensory elements are intermingled with some motor nerves to supply information about the state of tension or tone in the muscles and the position of the various parts of the body (proprioceptive sense).

The Thalami. The *thalamus,* which is a mass of gray matter composed of sensory nuclei, is a large sensory receptor center. It receives sensory impulses and relays them to and from the cerebral cortex. In lower animals, it is the highest sensory center. In man, it is the center for cruder forms of sensation. It gives rise to an undiscriminating type of consciousness and arouses a crude awareness of pain.

The *hypothalamus* lies ventral to the thalamus. It contains the higher centers for the autonomic nervous system, which is discussed on pages 240–46. It helps regulate body temperature, water balance, and the appetite. Centers for the regulation of sleep and wakefulness and of food and water intake are located here.

Midbrain, Pons, and Medulla.   These areas contain cranial nuclei, the ascending and descending pathways, and many important vital centers. The most important centers in the medulla are those controlling the respiration and the rate of the heart beat. Other centers in the same region are the vaso-motor center (which controls the tone of the blood vessels), the vomiting center, and the cough center.

The Reticular Formation, RF (Reticular Activating System, RAS).   The reticular formation is a network located in the central part of the brain stem extending from the lower medulla up to the tegmentum. Sensory nerves from all parts of the body send branches to this formation, which then relays im-pulses not only to the cortex to arouse and maintain consciousness but also to the spinal motor neurons to excite or inhibit activity. The alerted cortex can then identify and interpret these stimuli. The network exerts a selective action and may facilitate or inhibit the flow of stimuli to the brain. Thus it contributes to our ability to learn, focus attention, think, reason, and act. It also regulates and refines muscular activity and bodily movement. Depression of this formation produces sedation and loss of consciousness. Its destruction by disease or injury caues coma from which the patient never arouses.

The Cerebellum.   The cerebellum coordinates the movement of skeletal muscle. It is closely associated with the vestibular nuclei and the cerebrum, thereby controlling the posture and equilibrium of the body.

THE SPINAL CORD

The function of the spinal cord is to serve as a reflex center and to conduct impulses from the peripheral nerves to the brain and other centers, and from the brain and other centers to the peripheral nerves. The tracts of the spinal cord are bundles of nerve fibers, similar in origin, function, and termination. Reflex action is produced in an organ or tissue as the result of a stimulus or stimuli received by the centers in the spinal cord from an afferent nerve or nerves from the skin, mucous membranes, or other organs. These spinal reflexes may function independently but are normally controlled by inhibitory or facilitating impulses of the brain.

PERIPHERAL NERVES

The peripheral nerves, while not a part of the central nervous system, are briefly described for completeness. They originate or terminate in the skin, muscles, or various organs by means of microscopic bodies called *nerve end-ings* or *specialized end organs. Ganglia* are small groups of cells that relay impulses received from nerve fibers to other nerve fibers (pre- to postganglionic fibers). Impulses from higher centers (e.g., brain) reach the muscles by spinal tracts involving transmission along nerve fibers therein, across *synapses,* and then pass to the *neuromuscular junction* via the efferent nerves. The synapses are microscopic areas where nerve endings touch or make contact with other nerve structures in order to transmit their impulses to other nerves or to the spinal cord or the brain. The neuromuscular junction is the connection between the nerve ending and the muscle fiber. The receptors at the neuromuscular junction constitute the *motor end-plate.*

DRUGS ACTING ON THE CENTRAL NERVOUS SYSTEM

Depression of the central nervous system by drugs may be due either to the direct action of a depressant drug or to depression following over-stimulation with a stimulant. Mild depression of the brain causes loss of interest in an individual's surroundings as well as inability to concentrate. As depression continues, the pulse and respiration are slowed and the sensations of touch, heat, cold, sight, and pain, as well as motor and mental activities, are decreased. Thus, sedation, sleep, analgesia, and unconsciousness may be produced with drugs. Coma, respiratory and circulatory failure, and ultimately death may result owing to depression of the vital centers, particularly the respiratory center.

Some drugs have a selective action, for example, on the cough center or on the cerebrum, whereas others do not show this degree of selectivity. In addition, some drugs show a selective type of depression. They produce their effect on one area of the brain in the usual dose, and in larger doses the effects extend to other areas. The vital centers of the medulla are remarkably resistant to the action of most depressant drugs, which is indeed fortunate.

Anesthetics and sleep-inducing drugs block the flow of impulses in the reticular formation. They have little effect on the passage of nerve impulses along direct pathways from the sense organs to the cortex. As the effect of the drugs disappears, the passage of the nerve impulses through the network returns to normal. Stimulating drugs increase the conduction of impulses in the network.

Drugs Acting on the Brain.   *Phenobarbital* depresses both the sensory and the motor areas of the cerebral cortex and is used as a mild sedative and as an anticonvulsant in epilepsy. *Diphenylhydantoin sodium* (Dilantin) depresses only the motor areas of the cerebral cortex; therefore, it is useful in relieving convulsions without producing drowsiness. *Pentobarbital* depresses the sensory and motor areas more rapidly, and its action is less prolonged than that of phenobarbital. It is used to produce sleep.

Anesthetics like *ether* depress both motor and sensory areas of the cerebral cortex and also the cells of the spinal cord so that unconsciousness, analgesia, and muscular relaxation are produced. Muscular relaxation is also achieved by its action at the neuromuscular junction, causing blocking of the transmission of the impulse for contraction of skeletal muscle.

Morphine relieves severe visceral pain. It increases the threshold for pain by depressing the sensory areas in the cortex. The respiratory centers and the cough center are also depressed. The vomiting and the vagus centers, which are in the same medullary area, are stimulated.

Analgesic drugs, such as *aspirin* and *phenacetin,* relieve muscle and joint pains and headache without interfering with mental alacrity. They appear to produce their action in the thalamus by preventing the pain impulses, which reach the thalamus over the lateral spinothalamic tract, from being relayed to the cerebral cortex.

Antipyretic drugs, such as the *salicylates,* which reduce fever, produce their action by depressing the heat center in the hypothalamus.

Alcohol depresses the centers of inhibition in the cerebral cortex and permits freer play of emotional activity. It also lessens will power.

When the sensory areas of the brain are stimulated, the patient is brighter and more alert, and drowsiness is dispelled. When the mental functions are increased, the patient is better able to concentrate. Memory, reasoning, and judgment are improved. *Caffeine* and the *amphetamines,* in small doses, mildly stimulate the psychic centers.

During overstimulation, various sensory areas of the brain are overactive and certain stored memory patterns are revived. The patient then has many imaginary impressions called hallucinations. There may be hallucinations of sound, sight, touch, or hearing. When the areas of the motor cortex are overstimulated, the patient may move about a great deal or violent contractions of the muscles (convulsions) may result. This is caused by overdosage with convulsive drugs or by cerebral damage.

When the speech center is stimulated by drugs, fever, or infection, the patient becomes very talkative and delirium may occur.

Nalorphine hydrochloride (Nalline) stimulates the respiratory center in the medulla and increases the rate and depth of breathing, if these are depressed by a narcotic drug. It is used as an antidote in narcotic poisoning.

Drugs Acting on the Spinal Cord. *Strychnine,* in small doses, acts on the spinal cord and increases reflex action. In poisonous doses, convulsions are produced. *Morphine* also stimulates the spinal cord. However, its action on the cerebral cortex masks or conceals this action.

Drugs Acting on the Nerves and Nerve Endings. When the activity of the sensory nerves or nerve endings is depressed by local anesthetics such as *procaine* or *tetracaine,* the patient no longer experiences sensations such as touch, pain, and pressure in these areas. Numbness and tingling in the area supplied by the nerves and nerve endings are produced. When the activity of efferent nerves is blocked by drugs such as *curare* or *succinylcholine chloride* (Anectine), which act at the neuromuscular junction to block conduction of the impulse from the nerve to the muscle, skeletal muscle relaxation occurs. Excessive dosage of these drugs will produce muscle paralysis.

Spinal anesthesia is produced when local anesthetics are injected into the spinal canal. Both sensory and motor nerves are blocked at their point of entry into or exit from the intervertebral foramina.

CLASSIFICATION OF DRUGS ACTING ON THE CENTRAL NERVOUS SYSTEM

The drugs acting on the central nervous system may be divided into two groups: (1) those that depress and (2) those that stimulate its functions.

Central Nervous System Depressants. Drugs used as depressants of the central nervous system may be classified as follows:

1. *Analgesics.* Analgesics reduce or abolish suffering from pain without producing loss of consciousness. This is one of the most important uses of drugs.

a. THE MORE POTENT ANALGESICS, such as morphine and its derivatives and the newer synthetic drugs (meperidine [Demerol] and methadone), may produce tolerance and addiction. They are also called *narcotics* (fr. Gr. *narke*—numbness, torpor). They often produce sleep. Perhaps this name is closely associated with these drugs because of its use in the Harrison Narcotic Act, which has been discussed on page 28. The principal use of these drugs is to relieve or obtund severe visceral pain.

b. THE LESS POTENT ANALGESICS, such as the salicylates (aspirin and sodium salicylate) and the *p*-aminophenol derivatives (acetanilid and phenacetin), were first used as antipyretics and are sometimes called *analgesic* antipyretics. These drugs relieve tegumental pain without producing drowsiness or interfering with mental alacrity. They do not produce addiction.

2. *General Anesthetics.* The general anesthetics produce insensibility to pain and a readily reversible unconsciousness. They have a fairly wide safety margin.

3. *Hypnotics and Sedatives*

a. HYPNOTICS are drugs that produce sleep.

b. SEDATIVES quiet a patient without producing sleep. They reduce nervous tension and promote relaxation. With increased dosage, sedatives cause drowsiness and also produce sleep. They are also used to prevent or relieve convulsions in epilepsy.

4. *Alcohol and Alcoholic Beverages.* Alcohol and alcoholic beverages produce depression of the inhibitory centers of the cerebral cortex, which

causes an apparent stimulation or intoxication. In larger quantities, they may elicit sleep and stupor.

Central Nervous System Stimulants. Drugs used as stimulants of the central nervous system are classified as follows:

1. *Cerebral Stimulants.* Cerebral stimulants are drugs that increase the activity of the sensory and mental areas of the brain, such as the amphetamines and caffeine.

2. *Medullary or Emergency Stimulants.* Drugs such as nikethamide and pentylenetetrazol stimulate the respiratory center and improve the breathing of patients in whom this function (respiration) is depressed. Where respiratory depression has resulted from overdosage with narcotic drugs, nalorphine and levallorphan reverse the depression.

3. *Reflex Respiratory and Circulatory Stimulants.* Aromatic ammonia spirit and alcoholic beverages are examples of such drugs.

REVIEW QUESTIONS

1. *What are some of the effects produced by depressants of the central nervous system?*
2. *What are analgesics? Name two types and give examples of each. Discuss the kind of pain relieved by each type.*
3. *Discuss the therapeutic uses of hypnotics and sedatives.*
4. *What are the effects produced by the action of alcohol on the brain?*
5. *What causes the apparent stimulation observed after the ingestion of alcoholic beverages?*
6. *Classify the stimulants of the central nervous system. Discuss their actions and therapeutic uses in medicine.*
7. *What is the function of the reticular formation, RF (reticular activating system, RAS)?*

REFERENCES

Delafresnaye, J. F.: *Brain Mechanisms and Consciousness.* Blackwell Scientific Publications, Ltd., Oxford, 1954.

Feldberg, W.: "A Physiological Approach to the Problem of General Anesthesia and Loss of Consciousness," *Brit. M. J.,* **2**:771, 1959.

French, J. D.: "The Reticular Formation," *Scient. Am.* **196**:54, 1957.

Himwich, H. E.: "Tranquilizers and the Brain," *Med. World News,* June 17, 1960.

15

Opium Alkaloids. Morphine and Morphine Derivatives. Cough Suppressants. Synthetic Potent Analgesics. Marihuana. Addiction

The relief of pain has been, from earliest times, one of the greatest needs in the practice of medicine. The presence of pain, whether it arises from severe injury, disease, surgery, or childbirth, is of great and immediate importance to the patient and to the physician or nurse. Man found quite early that there is in nature a very potent material for the alleviation of pain.

OPIUM AND OPIUM DERIVATIVES

Opium is the hardened, dried juice (gum opium) obtained from the unripe capsules of the Oriental or white poppy, *Papaver somniferum*, which is cultivated in Turkey, Egypt, India, China, and Asia Minor. It is one of the oldest and most useful drugs, and was known to the Egyptians, Greeks, Romans, and Chinese before the Christian Era. Formerly the crude extracts of opium were used medicinally in the symptomatic control of diarrhea and dysentery. Since they produce addiction (see p. 270), opium, its alkaloids, and the synthetic narcotics to be discussed are under international control through the World Health Organization (WHO) of the United Nations and under national control in most civilized countries. In the United States they are under the regulation of the Harrison Narcotic Act (see p. 28).

The crude drug, gum opium, which is dark brown in color, contains more than 20 alkaloids. These alkaloids fall into two groups: (1) the phenanthrene derivatives, such as morphine and codeine; and (2) the isoquinoline group of drugs, which are, as a rule, antispasmodic alkaloids such as papaverine and narcotine. Morphine is the most important and represents from 10 to 10.5 per cent of the crude drug. Morphine, codeine and their derivatives, and the synthetic potent analgesics are known as narcotic drugs. They have a highly selective action in relieving pain, without causing drowsiness or sleep. They may be used also to produce sleep, relieve insomnia and restlessness, and preserve the patient's strength. These drugs may obtund or alleviate severe

251

visceral pain quickly and may prevent its recurrence. They also elevate the patient's mood and allay emotional distress and anxiety.

Morphine

In 1803, a German apothecary, Sertürner, isolated and described morphine, which was the first alkaloid obtained from any plant. Codeine was isolated in 1832 and papaverine in 1848. All morphine is obtained by extracting this alkaloid from opium. It is a white crystalline powder, which readily forms salts with acids. The salts are quite soluble in water, whereas the alkaloid itself, referred to as the base, is insoluble for all practical purposes. The salt most frequently employed is the sulfate.

Pharmacological Actions of Morphine. *On the Brain.* The depressant action of morphine (producing analgesia and sleep) is entirely central. It seems to lie in the thalamus or corticothalamic pathways and also in the sensory areas of the cerebral cortex. Morphine raises the threshold for the perception of pain so that moderate pain disappears and sharp, piercing pain is dulled and made more bearable. Besides elevating the pain threshold, morphine elevates the mood and alters the reaction to pain. Anxiety, fear, and panic give way to freedom from worry, relaxation, and a feeling of contentment or tranquillity. This is very important in the relief of recurring, excruciating pain, and also for use of the drug as a preanesthetic agent.

The action of morphine on the cerebral cortex causes some dulling of sensory perceptions and continuous attention may be impaired, but, as a rule there is not too much interference with mental work. Thomas De Quincey, a famous author, did his best work under the influence of the drug. Besides the analgesic effect, morphine may produce a hypnotic effect of varying degrees, depending on the dose and the susceptibility of the patient. However, in some few individuals, a form of excitement is observed.

Morphine has selective actions on the medullary centers. It depresses the respiratory and cough centers and stimulates the vomiting and vagus centers. While 2-mg. ($\frac{1}{30}$-grain) doses effectively depress the cough center, morphine is not commonly used for this purpose. The depressant action of morphine on the respiratory center may cause a slowing and deepening of the respiration, even in the usual therapeutic dose of 10 mg. (5 to 20 mg.) ($\frac{1}{6}$ grain; or $\frac{1}{12}$ to $\frac{1}{3}$ grain). With increased dosage, particularly in susceptible persons (the very young and the aged), the respiration may become irregular, shallow, slow, and periodical (Cheyne-Stokes respiration). The cause of death in morphine overdosage is usually respiratory standstill. The action of morphine on the chemoreceptor trigger zone (CTZ) (see p. 380) in the medulla may cause nausea and vomiting. Its action on the vagus center produces bradycardia.

On the Spinal Cord. The reflex centers of the spinal cord are stimulated by morphine. Small doses produce convulsive seizures in the decerebrate frog.

Apparently the depressant action of the drug on the higher centers of the brain antagonizes this action in man.

On the Pupil.   Morphine produces marked constriction of the pupil. This action is constant and is observed even in individuals who have developed a tolerance to other actions of morphine. Its action on the pupil is central in origin and is mediated through the oculomotor nerve, which innervates the sphincter muscle of the iris. Spasm of the sphincter muscle of the iris causes miosis (constriction of the pupil). This is an active contraction, which depends on an adequate supply of oxygen. Cerebral hypoxia causes the pupil to dilate. This miotic action is not observed when solutions of morphine are instilled in the eye.

On the Gastrointestinal Tract.   The over-all effect of morphine on the gastrointestinal tract is constipative. In general, the tone of the smooth muscle is increased and all of the sphincters are constricted. This is probably the result of a twofold action (1) directly on smooth muscle and (2) through the parasympathetic system which is evidenced by the fact that atropine partially relieves the induced spasm. The emptying time of the stomach is delayed as much as 12 hours or more. Gastric, biliary, and pancreatic secretions are reduced and the digestion of food is impaired. Propulsive peristaltic waves are diminished and the passage of the contents along the bowel is delayed. At the same time the increased tone of the musculature causes spasm of the muscles periodically. The nonpropulsive rhythmic contractions are increased. Gas pains and abdominal distention may occur.

Because of the delayed passage of the contents of the bowel, water is absorbed to a greater extent and this causes the feces to become dry and firm and slows their movement through the colon. The tone of the anal sphincter is increased, and failure to receive or react to the normal stimuli for the defecation reflex contributes to constipation. Atropine, which partially opposes the spasmogenic action of morphine, is sometimes used with morphine to relieve severe pain due to intestinal spasm.

Morphine is sometimes used in the treatment of diarrhea because of this action on the gastrointestinal tract. However, paregoric (see p. 262) is preferred.

On the Biliary Tract.   In man, morphine increases the tone of the smooth muscle of the bile ducts and constricts the sphincter of Oddi, which increases biliary pressure and may cause biliary spasm. The spasm is not antagonized by atropine. The relief of pain in biliary colic is due not to its action on the biliary tract but to its action on the pain centers and the resultant analgesia.

On the Urinary Tract.   Morphine increases the tone of the smooth muscle of the ureters and may cause spasm which would tend to increase pain. Its relief of pain in renal colic is due to a central action. Atropine, which antagonizes the spasm caused by morphine, may be used to relax the muscle.

Morphine increases the tone of the detrusor muscle of the urinary bladder and the vesicle sphincter. Spasm of the sphincter has a tendency to cause urinary retention. For this reason catheterization may be necessary, especially in morphine poisoning. Morphine also produces an antidiuretic effect by its action on the posterior lobe of the pituitary body.

On the Bronchioles. Therapeutic doses of morphine may cause constriction of the bronchioles which is insignificant. However, in asthma, constriction of the bronchioles in combination with respiratory depression may cause death. In status asthmaticus meperidine is preferred for the relief of pain.

On the Circulation. The effect of morphine on the circulation is not marked in therapeutic doses. For this reason it may be used to relieve pain of myocardial infarction and in acute pulmonary edema. The depressant action on the vasomotor center seems to play a minor role. The blood vessels in the coronaries, skin, and muscles dilate, whereas those in the abdomen constrict, under the influence of the drug. In larger doses dilatation of the capillaries due to histamine release may cause a fall in blood pressure. For this reason the drug should be used with caution in shock or severe trauma since in these conditions the arterioles and capillaries are already dilated. In general, patients receiving the drug should be discouraged from changing position rapidly (especially from supine to upright) as dizziness and fainting may occur.

On Metabolism. In full therapeutic doses, the basal metabolism is lowered 10 to 25 per cent. This decreases the utilization of oxygen. Morphine produces a transient hyperglycemia in man, which appears to be due to the mobilization of liver glycogen. The effect on the liver is probably brought about by the release of epinephrine through stimulation of the sympathetic glycogenolytic fibers. A pancreatic factor may be involved. There is no conclusive evidence that morphine produces an effect on protein fat or mineral metabolism in therapeutic doses.

On Body Temperature. The body temperature is lowered by morphine. This action is produced by (1) depression of the heat center in the hypothalamus, (2) increase of heat dissipation due to peripheral vasodilatation, (3) decrease of physical activity and the possible production of sleep, and (4) decrease of the metabolic rate.

On the Skin. As a result of peripheral vasodilatation the skin becomes flushed and warm particularly in the area of the face and neck. Sweating is also frequently observed. In some patients itching of the skin and nose is noted. Urticaria and other allergic reactions may be seen.

The following is a summary of the principal effects of morphine:

1. The relief of major pain
2. The production of sleep

3. The production of euphoria and addiction
4. The depression of respiratory rate and depth
5. The depression of movement of the intestines
6. The production of nausea or vomiting
7. Constriction of the pupils

Absorption, Fate, and Metabolism of Morphine.   Morphine is not readily absorbed from the gastrointestinal tract. After subcutaneous injection, if the circulation is adequate, the effects appear rapidly. In three to four minutes, the muscles of the arms, legs, neck, and back relax. This is followed quickly by a change in the mood and attitude. The effects may appear in 10 to 15 minutes, become maximum in 60 to 90 minutes, and last from three to five hours. Occasionally morphine is administered intravenously and will be effective in three to five minutes.

The normal person metabolizes 20 per cent of the morphine absorbed and excretes the remainder unchanged in the urine and feces. A large percentage of morphine excreted in the urine is in the conjugated form. Small amounts are excreted in the saliva and perspiration. The addict appears to metabolize morphine more readily.

Tolerance to Morphine.   Tolerance is produced to the analgesic effect of the drug; so it is necessary to increase the dose from time to time to relieve the same intensity of pain. However, no tolerance develops to its effect on the gastrointestinal tract or to pupillary constriction. Tolerance and physical dependence cause excessive use and addiction.

Morphine Poisoning.   Acute poisoning may result from clinical over-dosage or attempted suicide. Doses of morphine above 100 mg. (1½ grains) produce toxic effects that may prove fatal. Morphine, in quantities exceeding 200 mg. (3 grains), will usually be fatal unless restorative measures are instituted. The lethal dose varies with the susceptibility of the individual, the route of administration, and a possible existence of tolerance. The old and the young are very susceptible to this drug.

Symptoms.   The symptoms of poisoning are a progressive depression of the central nervous system, causing sleep and coma. The pupils are constricted. The drug causes peripheral dilatation of the blood vessels. This, coupled with the depression of respiration, causes extreme cyanosis. The pulse is slow, weak, and irregular, and the blood pressure falls. The progressive depression of the respiration causes Cheyne-Stokes (periodic) respiration, and respiratory paralysis may be the cause of death. However, in some cases, inadequate oxygenation of the blood due to respiratory depression may cause heart failure and death. Occasionally convulsions may occur prior to death owing to the action of the drug on the reflex centers of the spinal cord.

Treatment

1. Oxygen with artificial respiration is the means by which a patient may be kept alive until other restorative measures can be instituted.

2. Gastric lavage with chemical antidotes such as potassium permanganate (1:10,000) and strong tea or coffee should be instituted.

3. Nalorphine hydrochloride is the antidote that overcomes respiratory depression. The dose is 5 mg. (5 to 40 mg.) administered intravenously. The dose may be repeated in 10 to 15 minutes. Nalorphine is also an antidote for heroin, methadone, and meperidine poisoning.

4. Analeptics and respiratory stimulants such as caffeine with sodium benzoate, nikethamide, pentylenetetrazol, ephedrine, and amphetamine may be administered. Amphetamine phosphate is given intravenously in doses of 20 to 50 mg. to combat the fall in blood pressure and to keep the blood pressure elevated while the respiration is being restored.

5. Anti-infective and general supportive measures must be undertaken when needed.

Chronic poisoning and addiction are discussed on pages 270–73.

Therapeutic Uses

1. Relief of severe pain. It is indicated but often not instituted until other analgesics have failed.
   - a. The principal use is to relieve deep-seated visceral pain, especially that of biliary or renal colic.
   - b. It relieves pain in coronary insufficiency, angina pectoris, myocardial infarction, and cardiac dyspnea and allays the fear of impending death.
   - c. Acute pulmonary edema of cardiac origin.
   - d. Terminal carcinoma.
2. Treatment of diarrhea. The hazard of addiction must be considered.
3. Treatment of dry, nonproductive cough. Coughs that have failed to respond to codeine.
4. Premedication for surgical anesthesia. It is often given with atropine sulfate.
5. Shock. It relieves pain, controls restlessness, and produces sleep.
6. Hypnotic. It is seldom used for this purpose except when sleeplessness is due to severe pain or dyspnea.

Disadvantages and Contraindications to the Use of Morphine.
Morphine has the capacity to mask underlying causative factors in illness. This is particularly true in cases of acute abdominal distress in which morphine should be withheld until a positive diagnosis is made since, in visceral spasm, it reduces pain but may increase spasm. When first taken morphine

may stimulate the chemoreceptor trigger zone (CTZ) in the medulla and cause nausea and vomiting. It has been found that nausea and vomiting occur more frequently in ambulatory patients than in those who remain in bed after taking it.[1] For this reason patients should be encouraged to remain in bed for several hours after receiving morphine.

The degree of respiratory depression caused by the drug depends upon the dose given. The rapidity with which the respirations are affected is determined by the route of administration; e.g., intravenous morphine affects the respirations maximally within three to seven minutes, while with the intramuscular route the effect takes 30 to 60 minutes or longer.[2] When patients receive large doses of morphine, one of the antagonists should be readily available. Their respirations should be observed carefully especially during the period of maximal effect. Patients who have respiratory problems should be given morphine only with extreme caution and close observation.

The drug should not be given when patients have any condition which may cause increased intracranial pressure as it may increase the pressure of the cerebrospinal fluid and also because of its effect on respiration. Acute urinary retention may occur in patients with prostatic hypertrophy. Since morphine tends to decrease the metabolic rate, patients with hypothyroidism have an increased susceptibility to its effects. It should be used with care in patients with liver disease because the liver may be unable to detoxify it readily. Neurotic patients may be excited to the point of delirium with morphine. *The greatest drawback is its liability to cause addiction.*

Dosage and Methods of Administration. Subcutaneous injection is the most common method of administration. The oral and subcutaneous dose is 15 mg. (¼ grain), with a range of 8 to 20 mg. (⅛ to ⅓ grain), usually repeated every four hours but only when necessary. Although the increase in the pain threshold may last for only three hours, a form of complacency continues so that pain can be endured for six to seven hours. In shock, when the circulation is inadequate, subcutaneous morphine may appear not to relieve pain. Care must be taken in these circumstances not to overdose, since when the circulation is restored, as in the administration of plasma, the full impact of the drug may become evident. In such cases, it is advisable to use morphine intravenously in doses of one half the subcutaneous dose. In elderly individuals, all doses of morphine must be reduced, perhaps to one half, as they may be more sensitive to its action.

Morphine is not very effective in the relief of pain upon oral administration.

---

[1] Comroe, J. H., and Dripps, R. D.: "Reactions to Morphine in Ambulatory and Bed-Patients," *Surg., Gynec. & Obst.,* **87**:221, 1948.
[2] Dripps, R. D., and Comroe, J. H.: "Clinical Studies on Morphine. I. The Immediate Effect of Morphine Administered Intravenously and Intramuscularly upon the Respirations of Normal Man," *Anesthesiology,* **6**:462, 1945.

However, it is sometimes given orally for its antidiarrheic action. The official salts of morphine are: Morphine Hydrochloride, B.P., I.P.; Morphine Sulfate, U.S.P., I.P. (Morphine Sulphate, B.P.).

Preparations

Morphine Sulfate Tablets, U.S.P., B.P.	5, 8, 10, 15, and 30 mg. (1/12, 1/8, 1/6, 1/4, and 1/2 grain)
Morphine Injection, U.S.P. (I.P.); Morphine Sulphate Injection, BP.	1-ml. ampuls containing 10 and 15 mg. (1/6, 1/4 grain) of a suitable salt
Morphine and Atropine Sulfate Tablets, N.F.	15 mg. (1/4 grain) of morphine sulfate and 0.4 mg. (1/150 grain of atropine sulfate.

MORPHINE DERIVATIVES

Codeine Phosphate, U.S.P., B.P., I.P. (Methylmorphine)

Codeine occurs naturally in opium and is made from morphine. For many years codeine sulfate was used. Now codeine phosphate, which is more soluble, is preferred. The analgesic activity of codeine is about one sixth that of morphine. However, it is effective in the relief of moderate pain and is often used for that purpose. It is less narcotic, tolerance develops more slowly, and it is less likely to produce addiction. It depresses the cough center and raises the threshold for cough. In productive cough it is inadvisable to give codeine during the day because it interferes with the natural protective mechanisms for expectorating the secretions. However, codeine, perhaps with a sedative, may be given at night to produce sleep and relieve cough. In dry, irritating cough, codeine is administered day and night.

Therapeutic Uses

1. To check cough. This is the principal use of codeine. The dose to relieve cough is 8 to 15 mg. (1/8 to 1/4 grain).
2. Relief of minor pain.

Dosage and Methods of Administration. The usual oral or subcutaneous dose is 30 mg. (1/2 grain) with a range of 15 to 60 mg. (1/4 to 1 grain) every four hours.

Untoward Effects. Codeine produces constipation and dry mouth. It may cause convulsions, especially in children.

Preparations

Codeine Phosphate Injection, U.S.P.	30 and 60 mg. in 1 ml.; 600 mg. in 20 ml.; 1.8 Gm. in 30 ml.
Codeine Phosphate Tablets, U.S.P. (I.P.); B.P.	15, 30, and 60 mg. (1/4, 1/2, and 1 grain)
Codeine Sulfate Tablets, N.F.	15, 30, and 60 mg. (1/4, 1/2, 1 grain)
Terpin Hydrate and Codeine Elixir, N.F.	4 ml. contains 8 mg. (1/8 grain)

Hydrocodone Bitartrate, N.F. (I.P.) (Hycodan Bitartrate)

Hydrocodone bitartrate is made from codeine. It is similar to it in action and is used in the treatment of cough. It is said to be not constipative, but it may be more addicting than codeine. The usual oral dose is 10 mg. ($\frac{1}{6}$ grain). The maximum safe dose is 15 mg. ($\frac{1}{4}$ grain). The dose for children over two years of age is 2.5 mg. ($\frac{1}{25}$ grain); under two, the dose is 1.25 mg. ($\frac{1}{50}$ grain). It is available as tablets of 5 mg. and as a syrup containing 10 mg. in 5 ml.

Ethylmorphine Hydrochloride, N.F. (Dionin)

Ethylmorphine hydrochloride is closely related chemically to codeine and is intermediate between morphine and codeine in its capacity to relieve pain. It was formerly used in the treatment of cough. It is seldom, if ever, used as an analgesic.

The principal use today is in ophthalmology. The oculist instills a 1 to 5 per cent solution into the conjunctival sac. It produces irritation and hyperemia of the conjunctiva and stimulates healing of long-standing inflammatory processes.

Therapeutic Uses. Ethylmorphine hydrochloride is used in the treatment of ulcerations of the cornea and in indolent conditions in the eye. It is available as a powder in $\frac{1}{8}$- and 1-oz. bottles.

Heroin (Diacetylmorphine Hydrochloride)

Heroin is five to ten times more potent than morphine but many times more addictive. It cannot be made or imported into the United States legally. The Narcotic Act of 1956 requires that all heroin in the hands of pharmacists, physicians, veterinarians, hospitals, etc., be surrendered to the federal government. One exception is that small amounts may be available for research purposes. Heroin was removed from the market because its addiction liability and severity (p. 272) are significantly greater than those of morphine. It is the illegal traffic and use of heroin that produce the greatest problem of drug addiction in the United States, Canada, and many Western nations. It is the greater potency of the drug and the more vicious addiction pattern that account for its predominance. By converting morphine into heroin, which is not difficult for the chemist, many more doses are provided for the illicit sale, with correspondingly greater profit and demand.

Heroin has been used extensively since 1898 as an antitussive (cough suppressant) and is still used in some countries.

Hydromorphone Hydrochloride, U.S.P. (I.P.) (Dilaudid)

Hydromorphone is more potent than morphine in relieving pain; it is also more toxic. The usual oral and subcutaneous dose is 2 mg. (1 to 4 mg.) every four hours as necessary. It is used in the relief of pain and the treatment of cough.

Advantages of Hydromorphone over Morphine.   Hydromorphone is less constipative and there is less tendency to produce nausea. In the treatment of morphine addicts it is sometimes substituted for morphine, since the withdrawal symptoms associated with hydromorphone are less severe than those experienced with morphine. Hydromorphone does not produce miosis.

Preparations

Hydromorphone Hydrochloride Injection, U.S.P. (I.P.)	2 and 3 mg. in 1 ml.
Hydromorphone Hydrochloride Tablets, U.S.P.	2.5 mg.
Hydromorphone Hydrochloride Rectal Suppositories	2.5 mg. in cocoa butter

Trade names: Dilaudid Hydrochloride, Hymorphan

Metopon Hydrochloride, I.P.   (Methyldihydromorphinone Hydrochloride)

Metopon hydrochloride is a morphine derivative that is effective orally. It is slightly more analgesic than morphine and is less likely to produce drowsiness. It is devoid of emetic and respiratory effects in therapeutic doses. Tolerance and dependence develop less rapidly and disappear more quickly than with morphine. The usual oral dose is 3 mg. (3 to 9 mg.). It is used for the relief of pain in terminal carcinoma. It is available as tablets and capsules containing 3 mg.

Oxymorphone (Numorphan Hydrochloride)

Oxymorphone is a morphine derivative, used for the relief of severe pain. The side effects are similar to those of morphine, but there is less sedation, constipation, and other smooth-muscle spasm. Tolerance may develop more rapidly. It is doubtful whether this drug offers any therapeutic advantages over morphine. The subcutaneous and intramuscular dose is 1.5 mg. every four to six hours. Rectally, one suppository is administered every four to six hours. It is available in 1- and 2-ml. ampuls and 10-ml. vials containing 1.5 mg. in 1 ml. Suppositories containing 2 and 5 mg. are used.

Apomorphine Hydrochloride, N.F., B.P., I.P.

This drug, which is prepared from morphine, strongly but indirectly stimulates the chemoreceptor trigger zone (CTZ) and produces vomiting and retching that are quite severe. Apomorphine deteriorates on standing; if it is emerald green in color, do not use. It is administered only to produce vomiting and get rid of poison that has been ingested. It is not often used except perhaps in patients in a comatose condition. Care should be taken to prevent aspiration of the vomitus. The usually subcutaneous dose of 5 mg. may be repeated in one-half to one hour, if necessary.

Preparations

Apomorphine Hydrochloride Tablets,   5 mg.
N.F.
Apomorphine Hydrochloride Injection,   3 mg. in 1 ml.
B.P., I.P.

SYNTHETIC NONNARCOTIC ANTITUSSIVE DRUGS

Until 1952, the only specific and potent cough suppressants in extensive use were the narcotics, morphine, codeine, hydrocodone, and hydromorphone, which are also strong analgesics. Narcotine, a nonnarcotic, nonanalgesic, naturally occurring opium alkaloid, is also used, especially under its newer name, noscapine (p. 262).

——————————— Table 16 ———————————

Antitussive Drugs

Approved and Trade Names	Dosage and Methods of Administration	Preparations
Dextromethorphan Hydrobromide (Romilar)	Orally: 10 to 20 mg. q.i.d. Children under 4, 2.5 to 5 mg.	Syrup containing 15 mg. in 5 ml.
Caramiphen Ethanedisulfonate (Toryn)	Orally: 10 to 20 mg. q. 4h. Children: 5 to 10 mg.	Syrup containing 10 ml. in 5 ml. Tablets: 10 mg.
Benzonatate (Tessalon)	Orally: 100 mg. i.v. or i.m., 5 mg.	Injection: 5 mg. in 1 ml. Perles: 50 and 100 mg.
Dimethoxanate HCl (Cothera)	Orally: 25 mg. t.i.d.	Syrup: 25 mg. in 5 ml.
Chlophedianol HCl (Ulo)	Orally: 25 mg t.i.d. or q.i.d. Children, 2 to 6 yr., 12 mg.	Syrup: 25 mg. in 5 ml.
Levopropoxyphene (Novrad)	Orally: 50 to 100 mg. q. 4h. Children up to 50 lb., 25 mg.	Capsules: 50 mg. Suspension: 10 mg. in 1 ml.
Pipazethate (Theratuss)	Orally: 20 to 40 mg. t.i.d., q.i.d. Children, 50 mg. t.i.d., q.i.d.	Tablets: 10 and 20 mg.

The synthetic agents are, in general, similar in their effects. They exert a rather selective action against the medullary portion of the cough reflex, as do the narcotics. They are not habit-forming or addicting, have no analgesic activity, and do not usually produce drowsiness, constipation, or respiratory depression. Dry, irritative, repetitive coughing may be controlled by these drugs. Productive coughing that results in the expectoration of bronchial or pulmonary secretions should not be suppressed.

COUGH MIXTURES

Many cough mixtures are available which contain two or more of the following: (1) sedatives for depressing the cough reflex, (2) expectorants for stimulating and liquefying secretions, (3) antihistamines for antiallergic and antisecretory effects, (4) cholinergic blocking agents for antispasmodic and relaxant effects, and (5) adrenergic agents for decongestive and bronchodilating effects and demulcents (syrup) and local anesthetics for topical effects.

OTHER ALKALOIDS OF OPIUM

Papaverine is an alkaloid of opium of the isoquinoline type. It will be discussed with the antispasmodic drugs in Chapters 30 and 33.

Narcotine is also an alkaloid of opium of the isoquinoline type. It is not a narcotic or an analgesic. **Noscapine, U.S.P. (narcotine),** is used in various cough syrups for its antitussive (relief of cough) effects. The adult oral dose is 15 to 30 mg. three or four times a day. It is marketed under various trade names such as Nectadon, Coscopin, and Nicolane.

Pantopon (Omnipon)

Pantopon is a mixture of all the isolated alkaloids of opium in an injectable form. The average oral or parenteral dose is 20 mg. It is available as an injection containing 20 mg. in 1 ml. or as tablets containing 10 or 20 mg.

OPIUM PREPARATIONS

The therapeutically important actions of the opium preparations are provided mostly by their morphine content; hence they need not be discussed separately. Camphorated opium tincture (paregoric) is a widely used and valuable opium-containing preparation.

Paregoric, U.S.P.; Camphorated Opium Tincture, B.P. Paregoric contains opium, oil of anise, camphor, and benzoic acid. It is a valuable preparation to check diarrhea and is given to tranquilize the intestine after the irritating substance causing the diarrhea has been passed. The drug may be preferred over morphine in diarrhea, since the antispasmodic alkaloid papaverine is also present. The dose should be diluted with water before it is taken.

Preparations of Opium and Dosage

Opium Tincture, B.P. (I.P.) (Laudanum)	0.3 to 2 ml. containing 6 mg. (1/10 grain) of morphine in 1 ml.
Paregoric, U.S.P.; Camphorated Opium Tincture, B.P.	5 to 10 ml. q.i.d. containing 0.4 mg. (1/150 grain) of morphine in 1 ml.

SYNTHETIC POTENT ANALGESICS

The discovery of a drug with the pain-relieving property of morphine but lacking its addicting propensity has long been the goal of the chemist, pharmacologist, and physician. This ideal has not yet been achieved with any compound suitable for use. A great stride, however, was made in this direction with the discovery in Germany, in 1939, that a synthetic antispasmodic, known as meperidine, pethidine, dolantin, and by other names, was a potent analgesic in proper dosage. Here was the first time that a synthetic chemical agent could be used instead of morphine in the relief of severe pain. It has been used extensively and satisfactorily as a substitute for morphine and is still the most frequently used of the group of synthetic strong analgesics.

Meperidine Hydrochloride, N.F.; Pethidine Hydrochloride, B.P. (I.P.) (Demerol)

This synthetic analgesic drug is used as a substitute for morphine in the relief of pain. It is a less potent analgesic than morphine, with slight sedative effects. Meperidine relaxes some smooth muscle, like atropine and papaverine, and at the same time it is spasmogenic to other smooth muscle. It is not used to produce sleep, since it is not a powerful hypnotic. However, it will potentiate the activity of other hypnotics. The drug reduces the amount of most anesthetics required in surgery and is widely used during labor with or without nonnarcotic hypnotics. It is not useful in the treatment of cough.

Absorption and Fate in the Body.   Meperidine is well absorbed upon oral and intramuscular injection. It is rapidly metabolized in the body in the liver and also in other tissues.

Side Effects.   The side effects sometimes experienced with meperidine are dizziness (which occurs more often in ambulatory patients), nausea, vomiting, sweating, respiratory depression, and occasionally fainting. Because of the dizziness produced, it is dangerous to drive a motor vehicle after taking meperidine or any strong analgesic. Administration of this drug to relieve pain immediately postoperatively may cause a decrease in blood pressure. Tolerance develops with long-continued use. Meperidine produces euphoria, which may lead to habituation and addiction.

Toxic Effects.   Overdosage with meperidine may produce tachycardia, cerebral stimulation, disorientation, muscle twitchings, and convulsions followed by respiratory paralysis and death. Since this drug at high doses stimulates the central nervous system, the first signs of toxicity may be hyperexcitability and uncontrolled muscular movements. These symptoms are a warning to decrease the dose or discontinue the administration of the drug.

Therapeutic Uses

1. Severe pain of various diseases.
2. Premedication for surgical anesthesia to replace morphine.
3. Obstetrical amnesia. It is often used in combination with other sedatives (scopolamine, barbiturates, etc.).

Dose and Method of Administration.   The oral or parenteral dose is 100 mg. (25 to 200 mg.) every four hours as necessary. Intramuscular and even intravenous methods of administration are used for the rapid relief of severe pain. Oral administration is preferred for the relief of chronic pain. The analgesic effects last from three to four hours.

Preparations

Meperidine Hydrochloride Injection, N.F.; Pethidine Injection, B.P. (I.P.)	50 and 100 mg. in 1 ml., 100 mg. in 2 ml., 1.5 Gm. in 30 ml., and 2 Gm. in 20 ml.
Meperidine Hydrochloride Tablets, N.F.; Pethidine Tablets, B.P. (I.P.)	50 and 100 mg.

Trade names: Alodan; Centralgine; Demerol Hydrochloride; Dolantin; Dolantol; Isonipercaine; Lidol; Mefedina; Mephedine; Piridosal; Sauteralgyl

Alphaprodine Hydrochloride, N.F. (Nisentil Hydrochloride)

This synthetic narcotic analgesic is chemically similar to meperidine. Its analgesic potency is intermediate between those of morphine and meperidine, but its action is more prompt and of shorter duration. Analgesia usually occurs in five minutes and lasts about two hours. The untoward effects are similar to those occurring with morphine, but nausea, vomiting, and respiratory depression are less. Tolerance and addiction may develop. Alphaprodine is subject to the control of the federal narcotic law.

Therapeutic Uses.   Alphaprodine is used primarily in obstetrical analgesia. It produces amnesia in the mother and has no effect on the fetus. It is also used in certain minor surgical procedures. The drug may be administered with nerve block or inhalation anesthesia or with sedatives (barbiturates). When it is administered with barbiturates, the respiratory depression is more pronounced.

Dose and Method of Administration.   Alphaprodine is administered subcutaneously or intravenously. The usual subcutaneous dose is 40 mg. (20 to 80 mg.). In obstetrics, after the cervix begins to dilate, 20 to 30 mg.

may be injected intravenously. This produces analgesia in one or two minutes. Nalorphine is the antidote. The injection is available containing 40 or 60 mg. in 1 ml. and 600 mg. in 10 ml.

Anileridine Hydrochloride, N.F., and Phosphate (Leritine)

Anileridine is a synthetic analgesic closely related to meperidine in chemical structure and pharmacological activity. It is about two and one half times as potent. The side effects are similar except that the sedative and circulatory effects are less and the respiratory depression is of shorter duration.

Therapeutic Uses.   Anileridine is used for the relief of moderate to severe pain and as an adjunct in general anesthesia so that the amount of the anesthetic agent may be reduced. It is also administered in obstetrical analgesia alone or in combination with barbiturates or scopolamine.

Dosage and Methods of Administration.   The hydrochloride is administered orally. The usual oral dose is 25 mg., repeated every four to six hours. The phosphate is administered by subcutaneous, intramuscular, or intravenous injection. The subcutaneous or intramuscular adult dose is 25 to 50 mg. every four hours as required. The usual obstetrical analgesic dose is 50 mg., repeated in three to four hours. For intravenous use for anesthesia, the drug is well diluted and infused *slowly*. The adult dose of 50 to 100 mg. is diluted with 500 ml. of 5 per cent dextrose solution.

Preparations

Anileridine Hydrochloride Tablets, N.F.   25 mg.
Anileridine Phosphate Injection   25 mg. in 1 ml., 50 mg. in 2 ml.
Trade name: Leritine

Phenazocine (Narphen, Prinadol)

Phenazocine, a benzomorphan derivative, is reported to be approximately four times more potent than morphine in relieving pain. It seems to be somewhat less sedative than morphine in equieffective doses. The side effects are respiratory depression, fall in blood pressure, nausea, vomiting, dizziness, and addiction—the same as with morphine. It is used for the relief of moderate to severe pain when a strong analgesic narcotic is required.

Dosage and Methods of Administration.   The intramuscular dose is 1 to 4 mg., every four hours. An intravenous dose of 0.5 to 1 mg. is administered as an anesthetic adjunct. The injection contains 2 mg. in 1 ml.

Pentazocine, chemically related to phenazocine, is a potent analgesic which is apparently nonaddictive. Euphoria, hallucinations, and physical dependence have not been observed. It is also a weak narcotic antagonist. Analgesia, which occurs within 20 minutes after intramuscular injection, persists for three hours.

Side effects (observed infrequently) are drowsiness, mild respiratory depression, and moderate deviations in blood pressure. The incidence of nausea and vomiting is low.

Pentazocine is used to relieve or control postoperative pain. The intramuscular dose is 20 to 40 mg.

Piminodine Ethanesulfonate (Alvodine)

Piminodine is somewhat similar to meperidine but is much more potent, being equal to morphine as a pain-relieving agent. It produces much less sedative effect and respiratory depression than morphine, allowing more alertness. It also has fewer side effects than meperidine. Its uses include preoperative preparation and relief of postoperative pain, obstetrical pain, myocardial infarction, and other visceral and severe skeletal pain.

Dosage and Administration.   Adults may be given orally 25 to 50 mg. every four to six hours, or 10 to 20 mg. every four hours either subcutaneously or intramuscularly. Antidotes which may be used in overdosage are levallorphan and nalorphine.

Preparations

Piminodine Ethanesulfonate Tablets   50 mg.
Piminodine Ethanesulfonate Solution   1-ml. ampuls, containing 20 mg. in 1 ml.

Trade name: Alvodine

Diphenoxylate Hydrochloride

Diphenoxylate hydrochloride is a synthetic pain-relieving drug. Its addiction liability is less than that of morphine and probably less than that of codeine.[3] Although it requires a prescription form in other countries, it is an exempt narcotic in the United States. An oral mixture of diphenoxylate and atropine is useful for the symptomatic relief of acute and chronic diarrhea (see p. 594).

Methadone Hydrochloride, U.S.P., B.P., I.P. (Adanon)

Methadone is an analgesic that is perhaps somewhat more potent than morphine upon prolonged administration. It acts slowly and the effects are cumulative. The drug depresses the respiratory and cough centers and produces nausea, vomiting, constipation, and miosis. Methadone is readily absorbed from the gastrointestinal tract. The liver plays an important role in its metabolism. A small amount is excreted unchanged in the urine and feces.

Therapeutic Uses.   Methadone is used for the relief of postoperative

---

[3] Fraser, H. F., and Isbell, H.: "Human Pharmacology and Addictiveness of Ethyl 1-(3 Cyano-3-Phenylpropyl)-4-Phenyl-4-Piperidine Carboxylate Hydrochloride (R-1132, Diphenoxylate)," *Bull. on Narcotics,* **13**:29, 1961.

pain, pain of trauma, terminal carcinoma, renal colic, and for the relief of severe cough.

Dosage and Methods of Administration. Methadone is administered orally and by subcutaneous injection. It is more effective orally than morphine. The usual oral or subcutaneous dose for adults is 7.5 mg. (2.5 to 10 mg.) every four hours as necessary.

Untoward Effects. The untoward effects are nausea, vomiting, light-headedness, and dry mouth.

Addiction. The addiction hazard is as great as with morphine, but the withdrawal symptoms are not so severe and they do not last so long. Because of this, methadone may be substituted for morphine and then, in turn, withdrawn.

Preparations

Methadone Hydrochloride Tablets, 2.5, 5, 7.5, and 10 mg.
U.S.P., B.P.

Methadone Hydrochloride Injection, 10 mg. in 1 ml., 200 mg. in 20 ml.
U.S.P.

Trade names: Adanon Hydrochloride; Amidon Hydrochloride; Dolophine Hydrochloride; Physetone

Levorphanol Tartrate, N.F., B.P. (Levo-Dromoran)

Levorphanol is a potent synthetic analgesic that may be given orally or subcutaneously. Its properties are similar to those of morphine but it is less likely to produce constipation and nausea and vomiting. It relieves pain for longer periods of time than morphine or meperidine. The subcutaneous or oral dose is 2 to 3 mg.

Preparations

Levorphanol Tartrate Injection, N.F.   2 mg. in 1 ml. in 1-ml. ampuls and 10-ml. vials

Levorphanol Tablets, N.F., B.P.   2 mg.

Trade name: Levo-Dromoran

SPECIFIC ANTAGONISTS OF THE NARCOTIC ANALGESICS

The phenomenon of antagonism among drugs has been referred to on page 87. It has no greater specific meaning in any instance than in the case of the narcotics and their antagonists. By altering the chemical structure of morphine and a compound known as morphinan, the drugs nalorphine and levallorphan are produced. They have the ability to nullify or reverse the toxic effects of the narcotic analgesics. This action is prompt and dramatic and may be lifesaving in cases of overdosage. These antagonists do not reverse the deep hypnotic effects or the respiratory depression caused by overdosage with the barbiturates or other sedatives.

Nalorphine Hydrochloride, U.S.P.; Nalorphine Hydrobromide, B.P. (Nalline)

Nalorphine, a derivative of morphine, antagonizes most of the actions of the narcotic analgesics. Its administration to narcotic addicts precipitates the withdrawal syndrome which resembles the discontinuation of the narcotic itself. Nalorphine is used to abolish the respiratory and blood pressure depression, the nausea, vomiting, euphoria, drowsiness, muscular incoordination, bradycardia, and other side effects of morphine and its substitutes. It is sometimes useful in obstetrics just prior to delivery when the mother has received a synthetic analgesic. In this way the respiratory depressant effect of the drug circulating in the blood of the newborn can be prevented.

Both respiratory rate and minute volume are increased by nalorphine when they have been depressed by a narcotic analgesic. Combinations of nalorphine and a synthetic analgesic have been used for the purpose of lessening the respiratory depressant effects of the narcotic. Several clinics have reported good results with combinations of meperidine and nalorphine, or of meperidine and levallorphan.

Nalorphine reduces or abolishes the analgesic effect of the narcotic analgesics if given in sufficient dosage. Yet, given alone, it has certain analgesic effects. This activity would make nalorphine a useful analgesic agent except for the high incidence of mental symptoms, disorganized thinking, hallucinations, and other types of dysphoria. These effects may be compared with the euphoria produced by the narcotics. Nalorphine is a derivative of morphine and thus is subject to the control of the federal narcotic law.

Dosage and Methods of Administration. Nalorphine is administered subcutaneously, intramuscularly, or intravenously, depending upon the need for rapid action. The adult intravenous dose is 5 to 10 mg., repeated in 10 to 15 minutes if respiratory depression is not adequately reversed. The effects last two to three hours. The dose must be repeated if the narcotic effects responsible for respiratory depression last even longer. In cases of great overdosage of the narcotic analgesic, a total dose of 40 mg. may be required in divided amounts. The neonatal dose for infants exhibiting the depressant effects of maternally administered narcotics is 0.2 mg. (not above 0.5 mg.) in diluted solution (0.2 mg. in 1 ml.) injected into the umbilical vein. Several doses of 0.2 mg. to a total of 0.8 mg. are preferable.

Side Effects. Given alone, or in excessive amounts in the presence of narcotics, nalorphine may cause dysphoria, drowsiness, lethargy, sweating, miosis, drooping of the eyelids, nausea, pallor, and hot or cold flushes.

Therapeutic Uses. Nalorphine is used for the prevention and treatment of respiratory or blood pressure depression and other side reactions of the narcotic analgesics (1) in ordinary use in susceptible individuals; (2) following overdosage of narcotics; (3) in obstetrics, five to ten minutes prior to delivery, or for the newborn when narcotics have been employed in labor; (4) during surgery and postoperatively; and (5) as a diagnostic test to determine narcotic addiction.

Preparation

Nalorphine Hydrochloride Injection, 0.2 mg. in 1 ml., 5 mg. in 1 ml., 10 mg.
U.S.P., Nalorphine Injection, B.P. in 2 ml., and 50 mg. in 10 ml.
Trade names: Lethidrone, Nalline Hydrochloride

Levallorphan (Lorfan) Tartrate, N.F., B.P.

Levallorphan is an antagonist to the effects produced by the narcotic analgesics, with actions quite similar to those of nalorphine. It quickly abolishes or greatly reduces respiratory depression and the other side effects of narcotics. It is used in combination with meperidine in an optimal proportion of 80:1 (levallorphan present at one eightieth the amount of meperidine). This is said to produce analgesia without the occurrence of significant respiratory depression. Narcosis of the newborn may be diminished when this concentration is used in obstetrics.

The side effects and therapeutic uses are similar to those of nalorphine.

Dosage and Methods of Administration. Levallorphan may be given to adults subcutaneously, intramuscularly, or intravenously in average doses of 1 mg., with subsequent doses of 0.5 to 1 mg. as found necessary. The total dose should not exceed 5 mg. The newborn may receive 0.05 mg. by umbilical vein, repeated to a total of 0.5 mg. Package insert instructions should be followed for dosage determinations.

Preparation

Levallorphan Tartrate Injection, N.F. 1 mg. in 1 ml.; 10 mg. in 10 ml.
Trade name: Lorfan Tartrate

Marihuana (Cannabis Indica or Indian Hemp)

Marihuana (cannabis) has been used by the Orientals for over 2000 years. The active principle of the dried flowering tops of the plant is cannabinol. Recent use of marihuana is confined almost exclusively to the smoking of dried leaves in the form of cigarettes.

Pharmacological Actions of Marihuana. The effect of marihuana on the brain differs in various individuals. The main action is one of depression of the higher centers. It produces euphoria. There is no known valid medical use for marihuana. *It is not an antitussive agent.* It is included here because its illegal use and habit-forming properties place it more properly with the narcotics and the problems of drug addiction than elsewhere.

THE PROBLEM OF DRUG ADDICTION

The problem of drug addiction is a very serious one and offers a great challenge to both nurses and physicians. Drug addicts are sick, trapped persons and require medical treatment, sympathy, much aid, and encouragement. Their addiction is a symptom of (1) various sociologic or psychiatric disorders that are related to personality defects of neurotic, psychopathic, or psychotic individuals or (2) recurrence of intractable pain in individuals with normal personalities. It results from the abuse of some of the most effective therapeutic agents available to the medical profession.

The Expert Committee on Drugs Liable to Produce Addiction, a committee of the World Health Organization, has adopted the following definition:[4]

> Drug addiction is a state of periodic or chronic intoxication detrimental to the individual and to society, produced by the repeated consumption of a drug (natural or synthetic). Its characteristics include: (1) an overpowering desire or need (compulsion) to continue taking the drug and to obtain it by any means; (2) a tendency to increase the dose; (3) a psychic (psychological) and sometimes a physical dependence on the effects of the drug.

According to this definition the addicting drugs include: (1) opiates and synthetic analgesics (opium, opium tincture, camphorated opium tincture, morphine and morphine derivatives, methadone, and meperidine); (2) hypnotic and sedative drugs (barbiturates, chloral hydrate, paraldehyde, and bromides); (3) alcohol; (4) cocaine; (5) certain sympathomimetic amines (the amphetamines); (6) mescaline (peyote); and (7) marihuana.[5] Some of these drugs are stimulants, while others are depressants. Stimulants increase mental and physical ability and afford the person a sense of well-being, self-confidence, and power. The depressants relieve anxiety and pain and produce physical and mental relaxation which allows the unhappy persons to escape from unpleasant realities, tension, and frustrations of life caused by pain, disease, worry, overwork, a feeling of inadequacy or of an inability to adjust to his environment.

Causes of Addiction. A personality defect is the most important factor. Few individuals with normal personalities become addicted. Other contributing factors are: (1) proximity to drugs and their ease of attainment; (2) prolonged medical use to relieve pain and produce sedation during protracted illnesses; (3) unfavorable environments such as poor family and interpersonal

---

[4] *World Health Organization Technical Report,* Series No. 21, 1950, p. 7; Series No. 57, 1952, p. 9.
[5] Isbell, H., and White, W. M.: "Clinical Characteristics of Addiction," *Am. J. Med.,* **14:**558, 1953.

relationships; and (4) corruption by drug addicts and peddlers. Addiction to one drug predisposes to addiction to another. Thus marihuana addicts may change to morphine or heroin, and alcoholics to barbiturates or morphine. Sometimes mixed addictions may occur, and the barbiturates may be taken at the same time as morphine, alcohol, or one of the amphetamines.

Addiction to Morphine and Related Drugs.   Addiction to morphine and related drugs is very complex. It is composed of three characteristics: tolerance, habituation, and physical dependence. Physical dependence causes it to be continuous rather than periodic.

Tolerance.   Tolerance refers to the decreasing effect of the same dose of the drug upon its continued administration. Thus more and more of the drug must be taken to produce equivalent effects. The drug also loses its acute toxicity for the tolerant individual.

Habituation, or Emotional Dependence.   Habituation is a psychic type of phenomenon. Drugs are taken because the person desires the responses produced. The withdrawal symptoms are, as a rule, mainly psychic and not serious. Examples of substances that are habit forming are coffee, cigarettes, alcoholic beverages, and barbiturates.

Physical Dependence.   Physical dependence occurs as a result of the development of an altered physiological state which requires the continued administration of the drug to prevent withdrawal symptoms or the "abstinence syndrome." During this addiction there is a biological need for the drug, which is similar to the need for water or food to relieve thirst or hunger. When the drug is withheld, withdrawal symptoms are very severe and may result in death.

These withdrawal symptoms, which occur from 4 to 12 hours after the last dose, are extreme restlessness, chills, hot flushes, sneezing, sweating, salivation, running nose, and gastrointestinal disturbances such as nausea, vomiting, and diarrhea. There are severe cramps in the abdomen, legs, and back; the bones ache; and there is muscle irritability. Every symptom is in combat with another. The addict is hungry, but he cannot eat; he is sleepy, but he cannot sleep. These symptoms reach a peak in 12 hours and last from 5 to 14 days. Upon the administration of the drug the symptoms disappear.

In the beginning the drugs may be taken by mouth, as snuff (heroin), or subcutaneously, but later they are usually administered intravenously. The doses are increased and the intervals between injections become shorter. The need for the drugs becomes so great that the addict will do anything to obtain them. He will lie, cheat, or steal; consequently there is great loss of moral integrity.

Theory of Physical Dependence and Tolerance.   Homeostasis (condition of well-being) occurs as a result of the maintenance of *steady states* in man by the coordinated physiological processes which involve the brain (hypothalamus), nerves, lungs, kidney, and spleen. Dr. C. K. Himmelsbach believes that certain homeostatic responses that oppose some of the actions of morphine are increased by the repeated administration of the drug and that when morphine is withdrawn, these enhanced physiological counter-responses are still operative and therefore signs of abstinence appear.

Heroin, Metopon, and Dihydromorphinone Addiction. Addiction to all potent analgesics is similar to morphine addiction, but there are differences in potency and duration of action. Heroin, metopon, and dihydromorphinone are more potent than morphine; hence smaller amounts are required. Since the effects do not last so long, they are taken more often. The withdrawal symptoms appear and disappear more quickly.

Methadone Addiction. Methadone produces euphoria and marked dependence; consequently the addiction liability is almost as great as with morphine. However, the withdrawal symptoms are milder and do not last so long. The drug is more toxic and, in the doses used by addicts, causes even greater physical dependence and social loss.

Meperidine Addiction. The incidence of addiction to meperidine, which is rapidly increasing, is relatively high among physicians and nurses. This drug produces more dizziness and euphoria than morphine. The duration of action is relatively short, so that persons who are addicted usually inject the drug subcutaneously or intramuscularly every two or three hours day and night. Tolerance develops rapidly, and daily doses of 1 to 4 Gm. may be necessary. Meperidine is very toxic and dangerous when taken in the amounts necessary to satisfy an addict. Muscular twitchings, tremors, mental confusion, hallucinations, dilated pupils, and convulsions may occur. Abstinence symptoms resembling those of morphine occur in three or four hours and reach a peak in 8 to 12 hours after the last dose. These symptoms decrease quickly and disappear in four to five days.

Marihuana Addiction. Marihuana produces a euphoria that is keenly remembered and is responsible for the desire to take the drug again. It produces an excitation comparable to that of acute alcoholism. Periods of stimulation and hallucinations give way to calmness, contentment, and drowsiness which may last for hours. A majority of the marihuana addicts are from 15 to 25 years old. Insecure teenagers, who do not have the proper affection and understanding at home, are ready for a thrill, and so they drink alcoholic beverages or smoke marihuana cigarettes. Marihuana is habit forming, but it does not cause physical dependence. There are no withdrawal symptoms. Its prolonged use causes psychic, mental, and moral degenerative changes. The habit is a steppingstone to heroin addiction. The dope peddlers hope to graduate the boys and girls to heroin, since once they are "hooked" with that drug, they become constant customers.

Addiction to Cocaine, Mescaline (Active Principle of "Peyote"),

and the Amphetamines.   These are all stimulating addicting drugs. There are no true withdrawal symptoms when these drugs are withheld.

Barbiturate addiction is discussed on pages 319, 320.

Cocaine addiction is discussed on page 426.

TREATMENT OF ADDICTION

The treatment and cure of addiction to narcotic drugs are very difficult and prolonged and are best carried out in institutions. The United States Public Health Service hospitals at Lexington, Kentucky, and Fort Worth, Texas, are maintained for this purpose.

Treatment involves the withdrawal of the drug and a long period of rehabilitation and psychiatric therapy. Withdrawal is carried out by the administration of decreasing doses of morphine or an equivalent drug, such as methadone, over a period of seven to ten days. Additional treatment during withdrawal includes: (1) the use of sedatives and hypnotics to make the patient sleep and lessen the period of anxiety, (2) maintenance of fluid balance, (3) nutritious food, and (4) adequate psychotherapy. Occupational, recreational, and psychiatric therapy are all important factors in the rehabilitation of an addict. Many addicts receive benefit from belonging to a group such as Alcoholics Anonymous or the more recently organized Addicts Anonymous.

About 20 to 25 per cent of the patients treated and released from the Public Health Service hospitals have been cured. There have been about 40 per cent relapses, and the status of the remaining 40 per cent is unknown.[6]

REVIEW QUESTIONS

1. *What is opium? Where is it obtained? Name two preparations containing opium and give their dosage.*
2. *Outline and explain the various pharmacological responses of morphine in man.*
3. *List in two divisions the potent analgesics given in this chapter, those with greater and those with less addicting hazards.*
4. *List six therapeutic uses for morphine.*
5. *List the advantages and the disadvantages that morphine possesses in comparison with the synthetic potent analgesics as represented by meperidine.*
6. *Which of the narcotic analgesics presented in this chapter would you prefer in the following situations:*
   a. Immediate analgesic and antishock medication following a pedestrian accident with exceedingly painful leg fractures?

---

[6] Isbell, H., and Fraser, H. F.: "Addiction to Analgesics and Barbiturates," *Pharmacol. Rev.,* **2**:355, 1950.

b. *Severe toothache while awaiting a dental appointment 8 to 12 hours later?*
c. *Preoperative medication for use with nitrous oxide–oxygen inhalation anesthesia?*
d. *Severe, extensive, painful, third-degree burns requiring many weeks for healing?*
e. *Terminal (necessarily fatal, inoperable) metastatic carcinoma with chronic severe pain in an elderly bedridden patient?*

7. *What is the possible mechanism of action of morphine and its substitutes in relieving pain?*
8. *If a patient receiving a usual dose of morphine or meperidine on two or three successive occasions a few hours apart becomes somnolent, can scarcely be aroused, breathes slowly (eight respirations per minute) and shallowly, and appears bluish at the lips and fingernail beds, explain what has happened and outline all appropriate measures that could be taken to get the patient out of danger.*
9. *Name a moderately potent analgesic, with dosage, which is not under narcotic regulations in the United States.*
10. *What narcotics are popular antitussive agents?*
11. *Explain specific antagonism of narcotic analgesics by certain other drugs. Name these, give their dosage schedules, and list their uses.*
12. *Discuss some of the factors responsible for narcotic addiction and explain the phenomena of drug tolerance, habituation, and physical dependence.*
13. *Give the usual adult dose, methods of administration, principal therapeutic use, and another name for each of the following:*

Paregoric	*Methadone*
Codeine	*Phenazocine*
Dilaudid	*Nalline*
Demerol	

14. *The patient had a gastric resection yesterday. She has just told the nurse that she has some pain. Should the nurse administer the ordered dose of morphine sulfate now or wait until the pain has increased?*
15. *The patient has been receiving morphine sulfate q. 8 h. for pain for the past week. The nurse has noted that the patient's appetite has decreased and that she has not had a bowel movement for three days. What might be a possible explanation for this anorexia and constipation?*

REFERENCES

MORPHINE AND MORPHINE DERIVATIVES

Hanzlik, P. J.: "125th Anniversary of the Discovery of Morphine by Sertürner," *J. Am. Pharm. A.*, **18**:375, 1929.
Isbell, H., and Fraser, H. F.: "Addiction to Analgesics and Barbiturates," *Pharmacol. Rev.*, **2**:355, 1950.
Lasagna, L., and Beecher, H. K.: "The Optimal Dose of Morphine," *J.A.M.A.*, **156**:230, 1954.
Murphree, H. B.: "The Use of Potent Analgesics," *Am. J. Nursing*, **63**:104, 1963.

Numorphan

Samuels, M. L.; Stehlin, J. S.; Dale, S. C.; and Howe, C. D.: "A Critical Evaluation of Numorphan," *South. Med. J.*, **52**:207, 1959.

Synthetic Strong Analgesics

De Maio, F. J., and Wilson, W. L.: "The Old and the New; Morphine, Meperidine, and Anileridine," *Antibiotic Med.*, **7**:44, 1960.

Eddy, N. B.; Halbach, H.; and Braenden, O. J.: "Synthetic Substances with Morphine-Like Effect," *Bull. World Health Organization*, **17**:569–863, 1957.

Gordon, R. A., and Lunderville, C. W. P.: "The Analgesic Properties of Anileridine, Meperidine and Morphine; a Comparative Study," *Canad. Anaesthetists' Soc. J.*, **7**:32, 1960.

Meperidine

Batterman, R. C.: "Clinical Effectiveness and Safety of a New Synthetic Analgesic Drug, Demerol," *Arch. Int. Med.*, **71**:345, 1943.

———: "Demerol, a Substitute for Morphine in the Treatment of Postoperative Pain," *Arch. Surg.*, **46**:404, 1943.

Hartridge, V. B.: "Obstetric Analgesia and Anesthesia," *Anesth. & Analg.*, **38**: 243, 1959.

Noth, P. H.; Hecht, H. H.; and Yonkman, F. F.: "Demerol, a New Synthetic Analgesic, Spasmolytic and Sedative Agent. II. Clinical Observations," *Ann. Int. Med.*, **21**:17, 1944.

Ratelle, A. E., and Kim, M. K.: "Demerol as an Anesthetic Agent Used in 9,000 Surgical Cases," *Minnesota Med.*, **43**:22, 1960.

Rovenstine, E. A., and Batterman, R. C.: "The Utility of Demerol as a Substitute for Opiates in Preanesthetic Medication," *Anesthesiology*, **4**:126, 1943.

Yonkman, F. F.; Noth, P. H.; and Hecht, H. H.: "Demerol, A New Synthetic, Analgetic, Spasmolytic and Sedative Agent. I. Pharmacologic Studies," *Ann. Int. Med.*, **21**:7, 1944.

Anileridine

Therien, R. C.; Lee, L. W.; Malashock, E. M.; and Davis, N. B.: "Anileridine Hydrochloride—Its Clinical Use as an Analgesic and Sedative," *J.A.M.A.*, **168**: 2098, 1958.

Piminodine Ethanesulfonate

DeKornfeld, T. J., and Lasagna, L.: "Clinical Trial of Two Analgesics: WIN 14,098 (Alvodine) and Ethoheptazine," *Fed. Proc.*, **18**:382, 1959.

Cass, L. J., and Frederik, W. S.: "Clinical Comparison of the Analgesic Effects of Dextropropoxyphene and Other Analgesics," *Antibiotic Med.*, **6**:362, 1959.

Gruber, C. M.: "Codeine Phosphate, Propoxyphene Hydrochloride and Placebo," *J.A.M.A.*, **164**:966, 1957.

Phenazocine

David, N. A., and Porter, G. A.: "Phenazocine (Prinadol, SKF 6574): Oral Use in Chronic Pain," *Clin. Res.*, **9**:117, 1960.

DeKornfeld, T. J., and Lasagna, L.: "A Controlled Clinical Evaluation of Two New Analgesics," *Anesthesiology*, **21**:159, 1960.
Eckenhoff, J. E.: "Phenazocine, A New Benzomorphan Narcotic Analgesic," *Anesthesiology*, **20**:355, 1959.

PENTAZOCINE

Sadove, Max; Balagot, R. C.; and Pecora, F. N. "Pentazocine—A New Nonaddicting Analgesic," *J.A.M.A.*, **189**:199, 1964.

NALORPHINE

Isbell, H.: "The Search for a Non-addicting Analgesic," *J.A.M.A.*, **161**:1254, 1956.
Keats, A. S., and Telford, J.: "Nalorphine, a Potent Analgesic in Man," *J. Pharmacol. Exper. Therap.*, **117**:190, 1956.
Wikler, A.: *Opiates and Opiate Antagonists.* Public Health Monograph No. 52, U.S. Dept. of Health, Education, and Welfare, Washington, D.C., 1958.

LEVALLORPHAN

Megirian, R., and White, C. W., Jr.: "Effects of Levallorphan-Meperidine Combination on Respiration in Man," *Federation Proc.*, **16**:321, 1957.

DRUG ADDICTION

Fraser, H. F., and Grider, J. A., Jr.: "Treatment of Drug Addiction," *Am. J. Med.*, **14**:571, 1953.
Gelber, Ida: "The Addict and his Drugs," *Am. J. Nursing*, **63**:52, 1963.
Himmelsbach, C. K.: "Clinical Studies of Drug Addiction, Physical Dependence, Withdrawal and Recovery," *Arch. Int. Med.*, **69**:766, 1942.
———: "With Reference to Physical Dependence," *Fed. Proc.*, **2**:210, 1943.
Isbell, H., and Fraser, H. F.: "Addiction to Analgesics and Barbiturates," *Pharmacol. Rev.*, **2**:355, 1950.
Isbell, H., and White, W. M.: "Clinical Characteristics of Addiction," *Am. J. Med.*, **14**:558, 1953.
Johnson, O. W.: "The Problem of Narcotics as it Applies to Medical Practice," *North Carolina M. J.*, **20**:516, 1959.
Rohde, I. M.: "The Addict as an Inpatient," *Am. J. Nursing*, **63**:61, 1963.
Wikler, A.: *Opiate Addiction: Psychological and Neurophysiological Aspects in Relation to Clinical Problems.* Charles C Thomas, Publisher, Springfield, Ill., 1953.
Yost, O. R.: *The Bane of Drug Addiction.* The Macmillan Company, New York, 1954.

16

Less Potent Analgesics and Antipyretics

Analgesics are drugs that relieve pain. Antipyretics are drugs that reduce elevated body temperature. The two actions are combined in the salicylates— sodium salicylate, aspirin (acetylsalicylic acid), and salicylamide—and other synthetic drugs such as acetanilid, phenacetin, and aminopyrine. The analgesic action of these drugs is less potent than that of morphine and other narcotic drugs. However, they are useful in relieving pain of arthralgias, myalgias, neuralgias, headache, and tegumental pain.

Mechanism of Action. These drugs appear to reduce elevated body temperature by increasing heat elimination. It is believed that they act on the heat center in the hypothalamus, which controls body temperature through the transmission of sympathetic impulses to the skin vessels, the sweat glands, and the pilomotor muscles. Water is drawn from the tissues into the blood. The blood vessels in the periphery are dilated, and the volume of fluid passing through the heat-radiating system of the body is increased. Heat loss is also produced through sweating. Heat production is only slightly diminished.

Analgesia seems to result from the action of these drugs in the region of the thalamus. They appear to block or interfere with the pain impulses carried over the lateral spinothalamic tract and thus raise the threshold of pain stimuli relayed from the thalamus to the cerebral cortex. Their site of action is not the cerebral cortex because they do not generally interfere with mental alacrity and produce drowsiness or disturbance of memory. They do not reduce activity in skeletal muscle.

THE SALICYLATES

The salicylates occur as salicin and methyl salicylate in the leaves, bark, and fruit of many trees and plants.

Salicylic Acid, U.S.P. Salicylic acid was first prepared from salicin. It was later obtained from methyl salicylate (oil of winter green). It is now made synthetically from phenol. It has a corrosive or keratolytic action on the skin. The topical administration of salicylic acid produces a slow and painless destruction of the epithelium. It is used for the removal of warts and corns and in the treatment of fungous growth and certain skin diseases.

277

Methyl Salicylate, U.S.P., B.P. (Oil of Wintergreen). Methyl salicylate is made synthetically from phenol. It produces irritation to the skin and mucous membranes and is used locally as a counterirritant. Methyl salicylate, which is applied to the skin with rubbing, is rapidly absorbed and traces may be found in the urine in 15 minutes. It is more readily absorbed when it is dissolved in alcohol, oil, or lanolin. Poisoning, in children, has resulted from the application of this drug to large areas of the skin and also by its ingestion.

Sodium Salicylate, U.S.P., and Aspirin, U.S.P., Acetylsalicylic Acid, B.P. These are the two salicylates which are administered internally.

Pharmacological Action of the Salicylates. The principal action of the salicylates is on the central nervous system. They produce an analgesic action which is mild compared to that caused by morphine and other narcotic drugs. They do not produce sedation, euphoria, or addiction. They reduce elevated body temperature but do not have any effect on the temperature of the normal individual. The mechanism of the action of these drugs in reducing pain and body temperature is discussed above.

In the usual therapeutic doses, there is no effect on other parts of the central nervous system. Large doses stimulate the central nervous system and may produce hallucinations and delirium. They also stimulate and then depress the respiration. Death is generally due to respiratory arrest by action of these drugs on the respiratory center.

Ordinary doses of the salicylates have no effect on the blood vessels. Large doses relax the smooth muscle of the blood vessels and produce vasodilatation. The vasomotor centers may also be depressed. In therapeutic doses the salicylates are not known to produce harmful effects on the heart.

The sedimentation rate, which has been increased in disease, is reduced. The fibrinogen in the plasma is also reduced. The salicylates decrease the renal threshold to uric acid and increase the excretion of urates in the urine.

The salicylates have an anti-inflammatory action similar to that noted with the corticosteroids; in addition, the circulating corticoid levels are increased.

Absorption, Fate, and Excretion of the Salicylates. The salicylates are readily absorbed from the gastrointestinal tract. In some patients, they have an irritant action on the gastric mucosa. To reduce this effect, sodium salicylate particularly is administered with sodium bicarbonate. However, sodium bicarbonate also increases the excretion of salicylates, and its administration may reduce the drug level in the plasma, which may be undesirable. After absorption, the drug is carried to most of the tissues and organs of the body.

Excretion of the salicylates begins about one-half hour after administration. The entire dose is excreted in 24 hours. About 20 per cent is oxidized in the tissues. In patients with rheumatic fever, more may be metabolized.

It is almost entirely excreted in the urine as free salicylic acid and salicyluric acid conjugated with glucuronic acid. A small amount (about 1 per cent) is excreted as gentisic acid. A small amount is excreted in the sweat.

Tolerance to Salicylates.   Tolerance to salicylates has not been noted. Sometimes the dose to control pain must be increased, but this may be due to an increase in the intensity of pain resulting from progression of the disease.

Untoward Effects.   The safety range with these drugs is, as a rule, wide. However, they irritate the gastric mucosa and, with prolonged use, may cause gastrointestinal ulceration and activation of a pre-existing ulcer, and hemorrhage. The presence of occult blood in the stools and, at times, hematemesis (vomiting of blood) and melena (discharge of stools colored black by altered blood) have been observed. It has been suggested that anemia may have been caused in some patients taking aspirin over prolonged periods of time for the relief of severe headaches. A majority of persons consume aspirin without experiencing any side effects. However, patients should be advised not to take aspirin on an empty stomach but after meals so that the mucosa may be protected by food. Accidental poisoning after the ingestion of large numbers of pediatric tablets by children is common in both the United States and Great Britain and fatalities have occurred. Therefore, parents should be cautioned to keep this medication out of reach of children.

Extensive gastritis may occur without symptoms. Gastric symptoms, such as pain, nausea, and vomiting, experienced by some persons are believed to be due to a central rather than a local action. It has been shown that these symptoms are more likely to occur when sodium salicylate is given intravenously than when it is ingested orally.

Some persons are allergic to the salicylates and undesirable symptoms, such as skin rash, ringing in the ears, disturbances in hearing and vision, mental confusion, and dizziness, may occur. This is called *salicylism*. In more susceptible persons, small doses may produce a violent respiratory reaction similar to the asthmatic attack. Congestion of the nasal mucous membranes and edema of the eyelids, pharynx, larynx, and lips may occur. Deaths have resulted due to edema of the trachea.

Patients receiving large doses of the salicylates in rheumatic fever may develop low prothrombin levels, and thus the clotting time of blood is prolonged. Hemorrhagic tendencies, notably petechial hemorrhages, may occur following prolonged administration of large doses. To counteract this action, *menadione* is given with the salicylates to increase the clotting time of blood, when continued use is necessary. Patients receiving anticoagulants and salicylates need to have their prothrombin time checked frequently. The dose of anticoagulant may need to be reduced in order to prevent bleeding.

Vitamin C is frequently prescribed with these drugs because salicylates tend to lower the level of this vitamin in the blood.

Dangerous Symptoms of Poisoning. With large doses of the salicylates, hallucinations and delirium occur. The more dangerous symptoms of poisoning are depression, circulatory collapse, respiratory alkalosis, metabolic acidosis, and respiratory failure.

Treatment of Poisoning. The treatment of poisoning is largely symptomatic. The administration of the drug is discontinued immediately. Stimulants are given to combat the depression and sedatives are prescribed to counteract the hallucinations and delirium. Intravenous glucose or intravenous saline is administered to combat respiratory alkalosis. Sodium lactate or sodium bicarbonate may be given intravenously to combat metabolic acidosis. It is important to watch carefully the pH of the blood and the carbon dioxide–combining power of the plasma.

Therapeutic Uses

1. As an analgesic to relieve tegumental pain, pains of arthritis, bursitis, headache, etc., and to reduce fever. Many physicians look upon fever as a reaction to counteract infection, and hence its reduction is not always desirable.

2. The treatment of rheumatic fever.

Rheumatic Fever. Rheumatic fever is a febrile disease associated with streptococcal infections on a basis of hypersensitivity. It is a chronic disease with a marked tendency to recur. The sulfonamides or penicillin should be administered prophylactically to prevent recurrences. The symptoms manifested are inflammation, swelling and immobility of joints, fever, and carditis. Cardiac involvement is one of the most common features of rheumatic fever. The heart valves may become typically distorted, and lesions may occur in the heart muscle and pericardium.

Either sodium salicylate or aspirin is used in the treatment of this disease. The daily dose is 5 to 10 Gm. (75 grains to $2\frac{1}{2}$ drams). It is given orally in six divided doses every four hours, with equal amounts of sodium bicarbonate in the case of sodium salicylate. The drugs may also be given with crackers and milk to lessen gastric irritation. Therapy is continued for two weeks. Sodium salicylate may be administered intravenously when it is necessary to increase the blood level rapidly.

In the acute attack, rheumatic fever patients respond dramatically to the administration of the salicylates. The temperature falls in 24 to 48 hours. There is a rapid reduction in tenderness, redness, and swelling in the joints. Emotional strain and trauma are reduced as the symptoms decrease. Symptoms of salicylism, which were described above, may occur with this dose.

ACTH and particularly cortisone act in a manner similar to the salicylates in the treatment of rheumatic fever. It appears that the salicylates may possibly stimulate natural ACTH, which, in turn, may stimulate the production of cortisone; thus the salicylates may owe part of their efficacy to this mechanism. It has also been suggested (1) that the salicylates may act independently of the hormones by a common pathway or (2) that they may potentiate the action of naturally occurring hormones by blocking their destruction or increasing the sensitivity of local tissue.

Aspirin, U.S.P.; Acetylsalicylic Acid, B.P., I.P.

Acetylsalicylic acid, made by acetylating salicylic acid, is one of our most harmless analgesics. Its widespread use in the relief of headaches and muscular pains is an indication of its value. The drug is useful in pains of low intensity, not only when localized but also when widespread in origin. About 19 tons are used daily in the United States. Some 4000 million salicylate tablets are said to be consumed annually in Great Britain. Aspirin is available as compressed, soluble, pediatric, or buffered tablets. The soluble tablets contain calcium carbonate and citric acid. In the presence of water these additives react with effervescence and disperse the drug in a fine suspension. The buffered tablets are widely used, but there is no undisputed evidence that they are less irritating, more analgesic, or more readily absorbed. Aspirin tablets should be kept dry, as the drug gradually hydrolyzes in the presence of moisture to salicylic acid, which is a strong irritant.

Aspirin is an analgesic and antipyretic. It does not, as a rule, affect the heart, although some patients report tachycardia. The drug is not habit forming nor is it contraindicated in hypertension. It is absorbed readily from the gastrointestinal tract. Aspirin circulates in the blood until the esterases there break it down to salicylic acid and acetic acid. This occurs in 30 to 120 minutes. The greatest relief from the symptoms is obtained when the ester is intact.

Allergy to Aspirin. Some persons are allergic to aspirin, and occasional toxic reactions such as urticaria, angioneurotic edema, and vasomotor rhinitis have been observed. In hypersensitive patients, edema of the trachea has resulted in death.

Therapeutic Uses

1. The principal use of aspirin is as an analgesic in headache, neuralgia and arthralgic pain. The oral dose is 600 mg. (10 grains).

2. Grippal conditions, to relieve pain and reduce fever and make the patient more comfortable.

3. Rheumatic fever, in daily doses of 5 to 10 Gm.

Preparations

Aspirin Tablets, U.S.P.; Acetylsalicylic Acid Tablets, B.P.	75 and 300 mg. (1¼ and 5 grains)
Soluble Acetylsalicylic Acid Tablets, B.P.	324 mg. (5 grains)
Aspirin Capsules, N.F.	300 mg. (5 grains)

Two other salicylates are available at this time: choline salicylate (Arthropan) and aluminum acetylsalicylate (Aspirin Aluminum Dulcet, "Baby Aspirin"). Aluminum acetylsalicylate is available as small cherry-flavored tablets containing 75 mg. for children under three years of age. Calcium acetylsalicylic acid complex (Calurin) and ethoheptazine with aspirin (Zactirin) are complexes or mixtures containing acetylsalicylic acid.

Sodium Salicylate, U.S.P., B.P., I.P.

The action and therapeutic uses of acetylsalicylic acid and sodium salicylate are the same, although acetylsalicylic acid seems more effective in relieving headache. The usual oral dose of sodium salicylate is 600 mg. (10 grains), with a range of 300 mg. to 1 Gm. (5 to 15 grains), every two to four hours.

Preparations

Sodium Salicylate Injection	1 Gm. (15 grains) in 5 ml.; 2 Gm. in 10 and 20 ml.
Sodium Salicylate Tablets, U.S.P. (I.P.)	300 and 600 mg.

Salicylamide, N.F.

Salicylamide is the amide of salicylic acid. Its action is similar to that of aspirin (acetylsalicylic acid), and it may be substituted for that drug in patients who do not tolerate it because of gastric irritation. It is used as an analgesic, antipyretic, and antirheumatic drug. The toxicity of salicylamide resembles that of other salicylates, with the exception that patients allergic to aspirin may not be sensitive to salicylamide. However, upon repeated use, sensitivity may develop in patients who are allergic to other salicylates.

Dosage and Method of Administration. Salicylamide is administered orally with fluids, preferably after meals. The usual analgesic dose is 300 mg. to 1 Gm. (5 to 15 grains) orally three times a day. The antirheumatic dose is 2 to 4 Gm. (30 to 60 grains) orally three times a day, or 1 to 2 Gm. (15 to 30 grains) every four hours over a period of three to six days. Smaller doses are given to children.

Preparations

Hexett Salicylamide Tablets	64 mg.
Salicylamide Tablets, N.F.	300 and 600 mg.

Trade names: Algiamida; Salamide

OTHER ANALGESIC DRUGS

A number of aniline derivatives such as acetanilid, acetophenetidin (phenacetin), and acetaminophen have in common the actions of reducing body temperature and relieving headache and muscular pains.

Acetanilid

Acetanilid was first used as an antipyretic but is principally used today for its analgesic action. It is believed to produce this effect by raising the threshold to pain stimuli relayed from the thalamus to the cortex. Acetanilid is readily absorbed from the gastrointestinal tract and is converted, to a large extent, in the body to N-acetyl-p-aminophenol (acetaminophen), which is excreted in the urine in a conjugated form. Brodie has evidence to show that the analgesic and antipyretic actions of acetanilid (and acetophenetidin) perhaps are elicited by the metabolic product, N-acetyl-p-aminophenol (acetaminophen).

Dosage and Method of Administration. Acetanilid is administered orally in doses of 200 mg. (3 grains) with a range of 200 to 500 mg. (3 to 7½ grains). It is also given in combination with other drugs. It is seldom used today.

Toxicity. Acetanilid seldom causes acute toxic symptoms. If taken continuously, or in large doses, for a long time, it produces methemoglobin. Acetanilid Tablets, N.F., of 200 and 300 mg. (3 and 5 grains) are available.

Phenacetin, U.S.P., B.P. (I.P.)

Phenacetin is a modification of acetanilid. Thus the absorption, fate, and excretion discussed under acetanilid are the same as for phenacetin. It is useful as an analgesic and is similar in action and potency to aspirin. It can cause methemoglobinemia, especially in infants. It has been reported that repetitive administration of large doses over long periods has produced hemolytic anemia and nephrotoxicity and in some cases anuria. The usual oral dose is 300 mg. (5 grains) every four hours as necessary with a range of 300 to 500 mg. (5 to 7½ grains).

Preparation

Phenacetin Tablets, U.S.P. (I.P.)   300 mg. (5 grains)
             Trade name: Phenacetin
             Synonyms: Femidine; Femina; Phenidin; Phenin

Acetaminophen, N.F. (Tempra, Tylenol)

Acetaminophen is an active analgesic which may be used for the relief of fever, muscular aches and pains, and headache. It is nonirritating to the gastric mucosa, is well tolerated, and may be administered for long periods of time. It is useful for persons sensitive to aspirin. It is more soluble than aspirin or acetophenetidin and hence is available in solutions intended for pediatric use. It is used for the relief of fever and the common respiratory infections of infants and children and following inoculations. It may be given with antibiotics. It is available as two liquid dosage forms, a red wild-cherry-flavored elixir or solution and a syrup colored green and flavored with mint. The oral dose for infants under one year is 0.6 ml. of the elixir or solution or ½ teaspoonful of the syrup; for children one to three, 0.6 to 1.2 ml. or ½ to 1 teaspoonful; three to six years, 1.2 ml. or 1 teaspoonful; 6 to 12 years, 2.4 ml. or 2 teaspoonsful; three to four times a day as needed. For adults and older children tablets are available. The oral adult dose is 600 mg. every four hours: for children 6 to 12 years the dose is 150 mg. every four hours.

Preparations

Acetaminophen Elixir or Solution	Calibrated dropping bottles containing 60 mg. in 0.6 ml.
Acetaminophen Syrup	120 mg. in 1 tsp. (5 ml.)
Acetaminophen Tablets, scored	300 mg.

Trade names: Apamide, Tempra, Tylenol

COMPOUND ANALGESICS

Aspirin, acetophenetidin, and caffeine with or without codeine are used in combination in many headache and other pain remedies. The APC capsules contain these drugs. The need for such mixtures is open to question. Aceto-phenetidin has been omitted from Anacin because of the unfavorable reports of its deleterious action on the kidney and the blood.

Preparations

Aspirin, Phenacetin and Caffeine Capsules, N.F. (APC Capsules)	Aspirin, 200, 230, and 250 mg.; phenacetin, 120 and 150 mg.; caffeine, 15 and 30 mg.
Aspirin, Phenacetin and Caffeine Tablets, N.F.	Aspirin, 230 mg. (3½ grains); phenacetin, 150 mg. (2½ grains); caffeine, 15 and 30 mg. (¼ and ½ grain)

Trade names: APC Capsules; A.S.A. Compound; Empirin Compound

Compound Codeine Tablets, B.P.	Acetylsalicylic acid and phenacetin, 259 mg. (4 grains) each, and codeine phosphate, 8 mg. (⅛ grain)

Aminopyrine, Amidopyrine, I.P. (Pyramidon)

Aminopyrine is rapidly absorbed from the gastrointestinal tract and is perhaps the most powerful analgesic of this group of drugs. The usual oral dose is 300 mg. (5 grains) with a range of 130 to 500 mg. (2 to 5 grains). The minor side actions are gastrointestinal distress, skin rashes, and tremors.

Aminopyrine Agranulocytosis.   There are a number of drugs, such as the organic arsenicals, gold salts, and sulfonamides, that may produce severe and sometimes fatal cases of agranulocytosis. Of the analgesic antipyretics, aminopyrine is the only drug known definitely to cause this condition.

In susceptible individuals, aminopyrine causes a reduction in the white blood cells but usually no changes in the red blood cells or platelets. With the reduction in the number of white blood cells and the consequent weakening of the body's defenses, bacterial invasion results. The symptoms are pharyngitis and ulcerated mucous membranes. If a diagnosis of agranulocytosis is made, antibiotics are usually used prophylactically to prevent infections.

Because of the serious nature of this syndrome, the drug is little used—and then with extreme caution. Its use in proprietary remedies is prohibited.

Preparation

Aminopyrine Tablets (I.P.)   300 mg. (5 grains)
               Trade names: Aneuxol; Dipyrin; Pyramidon

Phenylbutazone (Butazolidin)

Phenylbutazone, a derivative of aminopyrine, is used principally in the treatment of arthritis. It is discussed on page 692.

Dextro Propoxyphene Hydrochloride (Darvon)

Dextro propoxyphene, an agent unrelated to the opium alkaloids or the synthetic narcotics, has approximately the same potency as codeine in relieving pain. It is not listed as a narcotic by the World Health Organization or by the United States Commissioner of Narcotics. It has not been shown to produce addiction, but it does decrease the withdrawal symptoms of morphine addiction.

Dextro propoxyphene is available for oral use and is readily absorbed from the gastrointestinal tract. It may produce drowsiness, nausea, vomiting, and a skin rash. In therapeutic doses it does not cause euphoria or tolerance and does not depress the respiration. It is not constipative like codeine. The symptoms of overdosage are respiratory depression, sedation, mental confusion, unconsciousness, and possibly convulsions. Nalorphine should be used to combat the respiratory depression. Symptomatic and supportive treatment may include gastric lavage, administration of oxygen and intravenous fluids, and maintenance of body temperature.

Dextro propoxyphene is used to relieve pain associated with chronic or recurring diseases such as myalgias, neuralgias, bursitis, and arthritis. It is also available in combination with aspirin, acetophenetidin, and caffeine.

Dosage and Method of Administration.   Oral doses of 32 mg. every four hours or 65 mg. every six hours are recommended for adults.

Preparations

Dextro Propoxyphene Capsules	32 and 65 mg.
Dextro Propoxyphene, Aspirin,	Dextro propoxyphene, 32 mg.; phena-
Phenacetin and Caffeine Pulvules	cetin, 162 mg.; aspirin, 227 mg.; and
	caffeine, 32.4 mg.

Trade names: Darvon, Darvon Compound

Ethoheptazine (Zactane)

Ethoheptazine, which is related to meperidine, is reported to be a non-addictive analgesic which does not produce sedation, suppression of the cough reflex, or change in the size of the pupil. The side effects noted are nausea, vomiting, and dizziness. Ethoheptazine with aspirin (Zactirin) is more effective than ethoheptazine alone and is used for the relief of minor aches and pains. The oral dose is one to two tablets three or four times a day.

Preparation

Ethoheptazine with Aspirin Tablets	75 mg. of ethoheptazine with 325 mg. of aspirin

Trade name: Zactirin

Neocinchophen

Neocinchophen is discussed under the treatment of gout on page 694.

REVIEW QUESTIONS

1. Explain the mechanism of action of analgesic antipyretics in the relief of pain.
2. Explain the mechanism of action of the analgesic antipyretics in reducing body temperature.
3. Give the dose and several therapeutic uses for acetylsalicylic acid.
4. Explain the mechanism of action of the salicylates in rheumatic fever.
5. What points related to salicylates should be included in the teaching plan of a patient receiving anticoagulants?
6. What drug is useful for alleviating pain and reducing fever in infants and children? Describe two preparations of this drug.

REFERENCES

SALICYLATES

Alvarez, A. S., and Summerskill, W. H. J.: "Gastrointestinal Hemorrhage and Salicylates," Lancet, 2:920, 1958.
———: "Salicylate Anemia," Lancet, 2:925, 1958.
Annotation: "Aspirin Plain and Buffered," Brit. M. J., 1:349, 1959.
Ladd, R. J.: "Some Aspects of the Pharmacology of Aspirin," Australasian J. Pharm., 35:350, 1954.

Line, F. G.: "Aspirin Poisoning in Children," *J. Tennessee M. A.*, **49**:307, 1956.
Queries and Minor Notes: "Sensitivity to Aspirin," *J.A.M.A.*, **162**:84, 1956.
Rodman, M. J.: "Vascular Headache," *R.N.*, **19**:56, 1956.

RHEUMATIC FEVER

Gold, H. (ed.) : "Treatment of Rheumatic Fever," *Cornell Conferences on Therapy*,
   Vol. II. The Macmillan Company, New York, 1947, p. 95.
Hart, F. D.: "Analgesics in Rheumatic Disorders," *Brit. M. J.*, **1**:1265, 1960.
Rantz, L. A.: *Rheumatic Fever* (Disease-a-Month Series). Year Book Publishers,
   Inc., Chicago, 1954, pp. 26–29.

ACETANILID

Gross, M.: *Acetanilid*. Hillhouse Press, New Haven, Conn., 1946.

ACETAMINOPHEN

Cornely, D. A., and Ritter, J. A.: "N-Acetyl-p-Aminophenol (Tylenol Elixir) as a
   Pediatric Antipyretic-Analgesic," *J.A.M.A.*, **160**:1219, 1956.

PROPOXYPHENE HYDROCHLORIDE

Boyle, R. W.; Solomonson, C. E.; and Petersen, J. R.: "Analgesic Effect of
   Dextropropoxyphene Hydrochloride in Elderly Patients with Chronic Pain Syndromes," *Ann. Int. Med.*, **52**:195, 1960.

17

The General Anesthetics

General anesthetics produce a reversible loss of consciousness, analgesia, and muscular relaxation. Some of them produce analgesia before loss of consciousness and continue their analgesic effect after loss of consciousness, so that sudden painful stimuli do not break through to produce reflex physiological changes that may reduce the safety of the operative procedure. No substances in medicine have contributed more to human comfort than the anesthetics. They have made modern surgery possible and have transformed the operating room from a place of misery to one of tranquillity and peace.

History of the Discovery of Volatile Anesthetics.   The discovery and introduction of volatile anesthetics into surgery occurred a little over a century ago. Prior to that time, opium and alcohol had been used to obtund the pain of surgery; however, since the lethal and the "anesthetic" doses of these substances differ only slightly, they cannot be used with safety. In 1776, Joseph Priestly, who isolated oxygen from the air, prepared the gas nitrous oxide. In 1800, Sir Humphry Davy observed its analgesic effect and suggested its use in surgery. Because of the exhilarating effects produced by its inhalation, he called it "laughing gas." In 1844, Horace Wells, a dentist, used nitrous oxide for the painless extraction of teeth. He attempted a public demonstration in 1845, which was unsuccessful. This militated against the use of nitrous oxide as a general anesthetic for some time.

Crawford Long, a physician of Georgia, administered ethyl ether by inhalation in 1842 and performed a painless operation, but he neglected the immediate adequate publication of his discovery. In 1846, William Morton, a dentist, anesthetized a patient for Dr. John Warren of Boston, in the Massachusetts General Hospital, with ethyl ether, by means of a glass inhaler. The complete success of the operation achieved the introduction of ether as an anesthetic for surgery. Simpson and Keith in England, in 1847, introduced chloroform into medicine for the relief of labor pains.

In the past hundred years several additional inhalation agents have been introduced. Substances that are commonly used in this manner to produce anesthesia are ethyl ether, nitrous oxide, vinyl ether, chloroform, cyclopropane, halothane, fluroxene, and methoxyflurane.

Certain other depressants of the central nervous system have proved useful

288

in the field of general anesthesia. Although these drugs produce little analgesia and muscular relaxation, they are very useful in the production of unconsciousness. They are thiopental, thiamylal, thialbarbitone, hexobarbital, and amobarbital, which are barbituric acid derivatives, and tribromoethanol.

Modern Balanced Anesthesia.   Dr. J. S. Lundy introduced the term "balanced anesthesia" in 1926. Drs. D. M. J. Little and C. R. Stephens[1] have described modern balanced anesthesia as "the adequate accomplishment of the objectives for the job at hand." Balanced anesthesia may require the simultaneous use of several different anesthetic agents and other drugs and techniques so that (1) the patient may undergo surgery safely and pleasantly, (2) the surgeon's work may be expedited, and (3) the patient may return to his preoperative physiological status as promptly as is practical.

In this type of anesthesia, two or more general anesthetics or analgesics may be administered simultaneously or in sequence with oxygen. Intravenous, inhalation, or rectal anesthetics may be combined and may be used in combination with local anesthetics. For example, thiopental may be used for induction and an inhalation anesthetic for the maintenance of anesthesia.

In addition to the drugs classified as general and local anesthetics, the anesthesiologist makes increasing use of other drugs to control secretions, blood pressure, heart rate, and rhythm, to promote muscular relaxation, and for other purposes.

Hypothermia.   In cardiac and brain surgery, profound cooling of the whole body (hypothermia) is produced during anesthesia by various methods. A decrease in the metabolic rate in the cooled tissues, which consequently require less oxygen and anesthetic because cellular activity is reduced to minimum levels, allows the occlusion of the circulation to a specific area for about 15 minutes without injury at that site due to hypoxia. In addition, a bloodless area is available to the surgeon. Decreases in heart rate, cardiac output, and blood pressure occur. The problem of excessive hemorrhage and increased intracranial pressure is reduced.

Certain antihistaminics facilitate body cooling by causing vasodilatation, depressing the temperature-regulating mechanism, and inhibiting the shivering of muscles. Examples are chlorpromazine and promethazine (Phenergan). A combination of these drugs with meperidine (Demerol) (50 mg. of chlorpromazine, 50 mg. of promethazine, and 100 mg. of meperidine) is known as a *lytic cocktail.* The intramuscular or intravenous injection of this combination causes a fall in body temperature and blood pressure as well as marked sedation. As a rule, a lytic cocktail is used in conjunction with cooling of the body in an ice bath.

Dangers Involved.   Increased irritability of the heart due to excessive

---

[1] Stephens, C. R., and Little, D. M. J.: "Modern Balanced Anesthesia: a Concept," *Anesthesiology,* **5**:246, 1954.

cooling often causes cardiac arrhythmias. Atrial fibrillation and flutter may occur at 30° C. or below, but normal rhythm returns on rewarming. Below 30° C. there is danger of ventricular fibrillation, which may cause death. The problems of rewarming are circulatory collapse, reactive bleeding, and the rapidity with which warming should be accomplished.

Preanesthetic Medication. The barbiturates, narcotics, or both are given to produce serenity and amnesia for the events preceding the operation and to act as a base for the anesthetic to be given. These drugs may be given orally, parenterally, or rectally. In addition, atropine or scopolamine is used to lessen the secretion of saliva and to reduce to a minimum undesirable reflex action through the vagus nerve. Scopolamine has the additional effect of producing amnesia. The dosage of these drugs is based upon the patient's size, age, general condition, and the anesthetic procedure contemplated.

The night before the operation sedation of the patient is desirable. A barbiturate such as secobarbital (Seconal), pentobarbital (Nembutal), or amobarbital (Amytal) is usually given to quiet and relax the patient and to produce sleep. The drug should be given after all other preoperative procedures have been completed so that it will have its maximum effect. Approximately 30 to 45 minutes before the operation is scheduled, a combination of a barbiturate and/or a narcotic and atropine or scopolamine is generally administered. The nurse should be sure that all preoperative procedures have been completed before giving the drugs because the patient will become drowsy and should not be allowed out of bed. This should be explained to him as well as the fact that his mouth will become dry.

RESPONSE OF THE CENTRAL NERVOUS SYSTEM TO GENERAL ANESTHETICS

Anesthesia is produced by progressively increasing the amount of the anesthetic in the inspired air and thus in the blood and brain. Loss of consciousness is one of its primary prerequisites. It results from the reversible reduction of the activity in the reticular activating system (RAS); see page 246. This prevents the activation of the cortex and thus induces loss of consciousness. The general anesthetics block the transmission of impulses more readily across synapses than conduction along the nerve fibers. The RAS is therefore more susceptible to their action because of its multineural or multisynaptic organization wherein impulses pass over one synapse after another. Laterally conducting impulses are not impaired and reach the cortex.

The administration of an anesthetic results in selective depression of the central nervous system, which may be preceded by varying degrees of excitation. These drugs first depress (1) the RAS, (2) the cerebral cortex, and (3) the midbrain. This is followed by depression of the spinal centers, which causes first sensory and then motor paralysis of the functions of the spinal cord from below upward. If the administration of the anesthetic is continued, the medullary centers are involved, and death may result from paralysis of the respiratory and vasomotor centers. Subhypnotic doses of many anesthetics may be used to produce analgesia.

STAGES OF ANESTHESIA

The action of the general anesthetics may be divided into four stages. These stages vary considerably in character and duration, depending upon the nature of the anesthetic as well as the speed of induction and the manner in which it is administered. They are best seen with use of chloroform and ether. When induction is rapid, as with cyclopropane, the early stages are less clearly defined. When anesthesia is induced by intravenous administration, unconsciousness occurs so promptly that the preliminary stages (particularly stage II) of anesthesia are not observed. The classification of stages and levels of anesthesia was originally developed by Dr. A. E. Guedel. He has indicated that while it is applicable to classical agents such as chloroform and ether, it does not adequately apply to such agents as thiopental, nor does it apply well to "balanced anesthesia."

Stage I: Analgesia. This is the period from the beginning of induction to the loss of consciousness. The patient is conscious and experiences sensations of warmth, remoteness, drifting, falling, and giddiness. There is a marked reduction in the perception of painful stimuli.

Stage II: Subconscious Excitement. This stage begins with the loss of consciousness. The inhibitory control of the higher centers is removed and the subconscious emotions take over. The responses in this stage vary with different individuals. This is a potentially dangerous stage. Some patients pass through this stage peacefully and quietly. Others become very excited and may cry or laugh. There may be excessive and even violent struggling movements. The blood pressure increases, the pulse is rapid and strong and perhaps irregular. The respiration is rapid and irregular. Often the breath may be held and then a deep breath may be taken. The roving movements of the eyeballs are at a maximum in this stage. The reflex pupillary dilatation may be increased with emotional excitement. All reflexes are present. Excessive salivation, swallowing, coughing, and vomiting may occur. It is desirable to pass through this stage as quickly as possible.

Stage III. Surgical Anesthesia. This is the stage of unconsciousness and repression or paralysis of reflexes. It is divided into four planes:

Plane 1. The appearance of full, rhythmical breathing marks the beginning of stage III. However, the respiratory rate and volume may be modified throughout the operation by preoperative medication and the type of surgery.

The roving movements of the eyeballs gradually diminish until they are lost at the end of this plane. With the beginning of this plane, the reflex dilatation of the pupils decreases, and the pupils, which were dilated in stage II, return to the anesthetic normal. The coughing, swallowing, vomiting, and conjunctival reflexes disappear. Muscular relaxation of the extremities but not of the abdominal muscles is observed.

Plane 2.   The respiration is regular and relatively deep. The muscles of the eyeball are relaxed and the eyes are fixed. Muscular relaxation is improved so that cutting of the skin or muscles does not usually produce reflex contraction. Most surgical procedures may be carried out at this level. Patients may be maintained in this plane for long periods of time without experiencing harmful effects.

Plane 3.   The respiration is regular, but the inspirations are not so deep as in plane 2 and there is an increase in the respiratory rate. Relaxation of the abdominal muscles is increased. Paralysis of the intercostal muscles occurs. Chest movements are diminished and abdominal breathing becomes more pronounced. Constriction of the pupil in response to light is lost in the middle of this plane. Anesthesia is, as a rule, never carried beyond this depth.

Plane 4.   The respiration is rapid and shallow and may be irregular. The inspirations are short and gasping. The breathing is abdominal. Dilatation of the pupils occurs, which may be due to loss of tone or to hypoxia due to respiratory depression.

Stage IV: Respiratory Paralysis.   This stage begins with central respiratory paralysis and ends with cardiac failure and death unless restorative measures are instituted. In this stage all functions of the central nervous system are depressed.

Recovery.   If the anesthetic is removed and the respiration is reestablished and sustained before the heart stops, the symptoms may be reversed. As recovery proceeds, the signs of the various stages occur in the reverse order. The patient is subject to reflex stimuli and recovery excitement, which may be caused or increased by pain.

INHALATION ANESTHESIA

There are two types of inhalation anesthetics:

1. Gases. These are gases under ordinary temperatures and are supplied in steel cylinders under high pressure. There is a color code indicating the contents of the cylinders.

2. Liquids. These are volatile liquids which are vaporized before use. They are supplied in suitable sealed containers.

Preparation for Inhalation Anesthesia. There should be a patent air-way so that adequate oxygen can reach the patient at all times and so that the anesthesia may be lightened or deepened as required. This may be provided by the insertion of an endotracheal tube through either the nose or the mouth. A local anesthetic such as lidocaine (Xylocaine) (see p. 248) may be used to obtund the laryngeal reflexes. Artificial or assisted respiration must be instituted if natural respiration is depressed or stops.

Methods of Administering Volatile Anesthetics. The methods of administering volatile anesthetics are as follows:

1. *Open Method.* The liquid anesthetic is dropped on a cotton or gauze mask held over the patient's nose or mouth. Air is the diluent and no anesthetic machine is required.

2. *Semiopen Method.* The mask is so constructed that the patient rebreathes some of the anesthetic mixture. Air is usually used as the diluent; hence the anesthetic machine is not generally used.

3. *Semiclosed Method.* The mask has a valve that permits expiration outside the system so that the patient breathes only the new anesthetic and oxygen mixture. The anesthetic machine is required.

4. *Closed Method.* The gaseous or liquid anesthetic is contained in a special apparatus which, when attached to the patient's nose and mouth, constitutes a closed system. The patient is continually rebreathing the contents of the system. Provision is made for the removal of carbon dioxide with soda lime and the addition of oxygen as needed. The anesthetic machine is required.

Distribution and Excretion of the Volatile Anesthetics. The volatile anesthetics obey the same general physical laws of pressure, diffusion, and solubility in fluids as do the inert gases. The tension or partial pressure of these agents in the blood influences the anesthetic effects produced.

The amount of anesthetic and the volume of air or oxygen with which it is diluted determine the partial pressure of the inhaled mixture. As a rule, it is desirable to increase the partial pressure as rapidly as possible in the beginning to shorten the undesirable and even dangerous effects that may occur during induction. However, it may sometimes be necessary to decrease the tension of the anesthetic during induction, when the irritating effects of the drug produce coughing, salivation, or closure of the glottis.

The anesthetic mixture, which is carried to the lungs during inspiration, is diluted with the air present in the lungs. Pulmonary ventilation then moves the drug into the alveoli and from there it diffuses across the alveolar membranes. Diffusion takes place because of the pressure gradient between the alveoli, where the tension is higher, and the pulmonary capillaries, where the tension is less. The anesthetic dissolves in the plasma, which is essentially aqueous in character, and on the surfaces of the red blood cells and is carried to the tissues. As the anesthetic is more soluble in oil than in water, it passes from the blood to the tissue lipids. The lipids are present in abundance in the central nervous system, particularly the brain, where a high concentration occurs. In addition, the circulation to the brain is relatively high, and so more drug is made available there (at least at first) than to the other lipoidal tissues in the body. The rate of accumulation and release of the anesthetic from the general body lipids is slower than that characteristic for the brain because of the poorer blood supply to the former.

The drug passes from the arterial blood to the tissues faster than from the tissues to the venous blood as long as the anesthetic gradient in the arterial blood in relation to the tissues is maintained. When the gradient no longer exists, the anesthetic leaves the tissues by way of the venous blood at the same rate as it is supplied to the tissues by the arterial blood. Thus anesthetic equilibrium may be established. This is rarely seen clinically.

Progressively smaller amounts of the anesthetic are required to maintain the steady anesthetic state for surgical procedures. When the anesthetic is removed, its tension in the inspired air disappears but the alveolar tension continues to supply progressively decreasing amounts to the arterial blood. The anesthetic tension in the arterial blood to the brain decreases, and the gradient outward from the brain tissues to the lower tensions in the venous blood is established. Thus the anesthetic may be redistributed from the central nervous system to other tissues of the body from which it is more slowly released and excreted.

Anesthetics, in general, are not appreciably altered by the body, as are most drugs, but are absorbed, transported, and excreted essentially unchanged. They are excreted almost entirely in the expired air. A small amount may be lost through the skin, in the perspiration, and in the urine. During surgical operations they may also be excreted from the body cavity. The rate of excretion is different for each anesthetic. As a rule, about one half is eliminated in the first 30 or 40 minutes after cessation of administration. The remainder is excreted more slowly.

If the drug has been administered for only a short time, the patient may awaken rapidly. He awakes by two mechanisms: (1) the redistribution of the anesthetic in the body and (2) its excretion by the lungs. If the anesthesia has been prolonged, the body tissues may be saturated with the anesthetic, which can be redistributed to the brain, and so awakening is delayed.

Mechanism of Action of Volatile Anesthetics. The more potent anesthetics, which may be administered with an abundance of oxygen, are distributed in the lipids of the central nervous system because they are more soluble in oil than in water (Meyer-Overton theory). This is a physicochemical action and is concerned with the distribution of anesthetics to the site at which they exert their effects. The exact mechanisms of action are not known but there seems to be an interference with the production and utilization of energy by the cells of the central nervous system. It is believed that the presence of the anesthetics in the central nervous system interferes with enzyme systems in the cells or on the surface of cells and disturbs the normal metabolic activities of nervous tissue in a reversible manner. In vitro experiments show that anesthetics depress the rate of oxygen utilization by nervous tissue. Different anesthetics may interfere with different systems and thus may differ in the exact mode of action.

INDIVIDUAL VOLATILE ANESTHETICS

Ether, U.S.P.; Anaesthetic Ether, B.P. (I.P.) (Ethyl Ether)

Ether, a clear, colorless fluid with a characteristic odor, is very volatile and its vapors are highly flammable. It is the most generally used of all volatile anesthetics, and is administered by inhalation. Ether is not decomposed in the body, but its presence in the cells of the central nervous system produces analgesia, unconsciousness, and excellent muscular relaxation.

Effects Produced by Inhalation of Ether. Ether progressively depresses the central nervous system, as described on page 290. The vasomotor and respiratory centers are depressed before the cardiac centers.

The stages of anesthesia listed on pages 291–92 are observed when ether is administered. The effects appear relatively slowly. The induction period with ether is longer than with other anesthetics and the recovery is also slower.

Ether vapors may be irritating to the respiratory tract; if it is administered in too high concentration, irritation of the pharynx and larynx may cause reflex breath holding, which will prevent its continued administration. This is a protective reflex to prevent the too rapid intake of an irritating substance. Its irritating properties may also produce a flow of mucus, which may be counteracted by the administration of atropine or scopolamine. As anesthesia progresses, the flow of mucus stops as a result of the action of ether on the salivary centers.

Systemic Respiratory Actions. Ether, at first, produces increased respiratory movements owing to reflex stimulation resulting from irritation of the bronchial tree; then the respiration becomes depressed and may cease. The drug causes depression of the respiratory center directly.

Cardiovascular System. The blood pressure rises and the heart rate increases, owing to excitement in the induction stage. With more prolonged administration, tachycardia, which is due to the release of vagal control, resulting from depression of the vagal centers, may be observed. In the deeper planes of anesthesia the heart muscle may be depressed directly. Ether does not sensitize the heart to epinephrine, and dangerous arrhythmias are not often seen. Peripheral vasodilatation occurs and the blood pressure falls.

Skeletal Musculature. Skeletal muscle relaxation is due to the action of ether on the pyramidal and extrapyramidal pathways and especially to its action on the neuromuscular mechanism. Ether exerts a curare-like blocking effect at the neuromuscular junction and produces profound muscular relaxation.

Gastrointestinal Tract. Ether produces a mild stimulant action on the gastrointestinal tract at first. Occasionally, if it is given too rapidly, nausea and vomiting may ensue. Nausea and vomiting and distention may also occur following recovery from the anesthetic. In moderate to deep anesthesia, a reduction in tone and activity may occur which may result in postoperative atony.

Kidney. The small amounts of ether that are excreted in the urine may cause some irritation of the kidney tubules, and red blood cells, albumin, and casts may appear for a few days postoperatively.

Hyperglycemia. A rise in blood sugar is often noted. This is caused by the secretion of epinephrine from the adrenal medulla and the epinephrine-induced glycogenolysis following the stimulation of sympathetic nerves to the liver.

Absorption, Fate, and Excretion. Ether is absorbed through the pulmonary epithelium and is carried to the brain and other tissues as described on page 293. More than 90 per cent is excreted unchanged in the exhaled air. The rest diffuses through the open cavity during surgery or through the skin or is excreted in the urine and perspiration. When the administration of ether is discontinued, the concentration in the blood decreases rapidly, and after two hours relatively little is found in the body. The odor of ether may persist about the patient for several days.

Therapeutic Uses. The principal use is to produce general anesthesia for prolonged operations requiring dependable muscular relaxation.

Administration. Ether is administered by inhalation with air or oxygen. Ether anesthesia may be continued for many hours without harm to the patient. It is administered by open drop or from vaporizers in rebreathing semiclosed or closed systems.

Ether has been administered rectally and intravenously. It is sometimes administered orally as a carminative.

Acute Toxicity. Toxicity results from overdosage and is due to the depressant action of ether on the medullary respiratory center, which may produce respiratory arrest. If ether is removed, redistribution between the lipids of the central nervous system and the body tissues including fat occurs and reduces the depressant effect on the respiratory center. Respiration may be resumed as rhythmical discharges arise in the center spontaneously. Oxygen and artificial respiration may be instituted to hasten the elimination of the anesthetic. There may be a significant decrease in the blood pressure and cardiac output, but respiratory failure, as a rule, precedes circulatory failure.

Advantages in the Use of Ether.   The advantages in using ether far outweigh the disadvantages.

Ether is safe for long operations. Its principal action is on the central nervous system, and it is sufficiently potent to permit high concentrations of oxygen in the anesthetic mixture. Abdominal relaxation is excellent. Ether is inexpensive and comparatively safe when administered under proper conditions.

Disadvantages in the Use of Ether.   Ether boils at a low temperature; hence it is difficult to administer in warm climates. The vapors are inflammable, and the drug is irritating to the mucous membranes. Since the induction period is often stormy, other anesthetics are used to induce anesthesia. A switch to ether after consciousness is lost is then smooth. Postoperative distress, especially vomiting, is very frequent with ether.

Contraindications to the Use of Ether.   (1) Acute or chronic infections of the respiratory tract, (2) diabetes or acidosis from any cause, (3) nephritis, renal insufficiency, (4) decreased liver function, and (5) diseases or injury to the brain accompanied by increased intracranial pressure. Increased intracranial pressure accompanies anesthesia particularly in the presence of hypoxia or carbon dioxide excess.

Preparation

Ether, U.S.P.   ¼-, ½-, and 1-lb. copper-lined tins

Nitrous Oxide, U.S.P., B.P., I.P.

Nitrous oxide is a noninflammable gas that is supplied in steel cylinders. It is administered by inhalation by a special apparatus, the anesthetic machine.

Effects Produced by Inhalation of Nitrous Oxide.   After the inhalation of nitrous oxide, there is a sensation of fullness in the head, giddiness, and whirling in space. Hallucinations and dreams may occur and sounds may be imagined. When nitrous oxide mixed with air is inhaled, it produces a condition similar to alcoholic intoxication. The individual is merry and laughs but does not go to sleep. When the pure gas is inhaled, the patient becomes pale and unconscious. If the administration is continued more than two minutes, cyanosis and death may result due to severe hypoxia.

Anesthesia is produced with nitrous oxide by using a mixture of 90 per cent nitrous oxide and 10 per cent oxygen. The induction period is short (two to three minutes), and recovery from anesthetic depression is rapid. Upon withdrawal the excretion is rapid; within five minutes there is no detectable amount present in the body. The respiration is stimulated. It is safe for operations up to 30 minutes if the oxygen is increased to 25 per cent or more.

Therapeutic Uses.   The principal uses for nitrous oxide are: (1) to induce anesthesia, (2) in dentistry, (3) in obstetrics, and (4) as a supplement to other anesthetics.

The disadvantages of its use are: (1) rise in blood pressure and increase in the pulse rate, which are dangerous in hypertension and in elderly people; and (2) difficulty in obtaining muscular relaxation required for major surgical procedures, when sufficient oxygen (20 per cent) is used to prevent hypoxia.

Contraindications to Nitrous Oxide–Oxygen Anesthesia.   If there is no reduction in the normal alveolar oxygen tension, there are no contraindications to its use.

Vinyl Ether, N.F., B.P., I.P. (Divinyl Oxide, Vinethene)

Vinyl ether is a colorless, volatile fluid that resembles ether in its action. It is more inflammable and explosive than ether. The action is more rapid than with ethyl ether, and loss of consciousness may occur in one or two minutes. Recovery is rapid and usually occurs without excitement.

Effects Produced by Inhalation of Vinyl Ether.   The effects on the respiration and circulation are similar to those produced by ethyl ether. At first the respiration is stimulated reflexly; then the respiration is diminished as the respiratory center is depressed. Paralysis of the respiration precedes circulatory failure. There are no significant effects on the heart. The skeletal muscles are only moderately relaxed.

Toxic Effects.   With prolonged administration, liver and kidney damage may be observed.

Therapeutic Uses.   Vinyl ether is used to induce anesthesia and in operations of short duration. It should not be used for longer than 30 minutes. It is most often used in children.

Advantages and Disadvantages in the Use of Vinyl Ether.   The advantages are ease of induction and prompt recovery. The disadvantages are: (1) the deep planes are easily reached, and therefore the patient should be watched carefully; (2) the drug has a low safety margin and may produce kidney and liver damage, particularly if administered over a long period of time or if administration is accompanied by hypoxia, (3) it frequently causes copious salivation and secretion of mucus, (4) muscle relaxation is inadequate for major surgery, and (5) it is expensive in comparison to other volatile liquids.

Contraindications to the Use of Vinyl Ether.   (1) For long operations, (2) for surgery requiring muscle relaxation, (3) in the presence of hepatic or renal insufficiency, and (4) in the presence of acute infections of the respiratory tract.

Preparation

Vinyl Ether, N.F.   10-ml. ampuls and 25-, 50-, and 75-ml.
                                           bottles with plastic droppers

Trade names: Vinethene; Vinesthene

Ethylene, N.F.

Ethylene is a colorless gas. It is nonirritating, and it is not unpleasant to inhale. A mixture of 80 per cent ethylene and 20 per cent oxygen is used. Anesthesia is produced rapidly, and the return to normal is prompt. The induction is smooth, and postoperative sequelae are few. Ethylene is often used in the poor-risk patient. There are no changes in the principal systems or functions of the body. It does not depress the respiration in any concentration. Skeletal muscle relaxation is fair, and deep anesthesia is impossible with adequate oxygen.

Therapeutic Use. The principal use of ethylene is in producing obstetrical analgesia.

Disadvantages in the Use of Ethylene. The principal drawbacks to the use of ethylene are: (1) it does not produce sufficient muscular relaxation; and (2) mixtures of oxygen and ethylene are very explosive. Tragic accidents have been caused by the ignition of oxygen-ethylene mixtures by static electric sparks.

Contraindications to the Use of Ethylene. There are none, if the patient is maintained without hypoxia. However, it should not be used with cautery or high-frequency units because the gas is highly flammable.

Ethyl Chloride, U.S.P., B.P., I.P.

Ethyl chloride is a colorless, extremely volatile, flammable liquid. When inhaled it is a powerful, rapidly acting general anesthetic. Induction is prompt, and recovery is rapid with little or no excitement. It possesses a narrow margin of safety. Ethyl chloride depresses the heart muscle directly and sensitizes the automatic tissue of the heart; hence arrhythmias, which are sometimes fatal, may occur.

Therapeutic Uses. Ethyl chloride is sometimes used to induce anesthesia in children. Its use for this purpose has been supplanted to a great extent by vinyl ether. It is used as a local anesthetic (see p. 432).

Contraindications to the Use of Ethyl Chloride. (1) The presence of any circulatory disturbances or disease, (2) procedures requiring the use of cautery or apparatus which may be a source of ignition, and (3) procedures requiring more than several minutes for completion.

Preparation

Ethyl Chloride, U.S.P., B.P., I.P.   Spray tube, with special cap, containing
                                           100 Gm.

Trade name: Kelene

Chloroform, N.F., B.P. (I.P.)

Chloroform is a heavy volatile liquid that is neither flammable nor explosive when mixed with air or oxygen. It may be carried in sealed tubes, which are opened as needed. Chloroform is more potent than ether and is more pleasant to take. It is not irritating to the respiratory tract. There is less excitement in the induction stage.

Effects Produced by Inhalation of Chloroform. Chloroform produces depression of the central nervous system. With adequate oxygenation it may produce all stages of surgical anesthesia. In the induction stage, overactivity of the vagus may cause marked slowing of the heart.

Absorption, Fate, and Excretion. Chloroform vapor is inhaled, absorbed and transported in the blood, and excreted essentially unchanged in the lungs in the same manner as ether. A very small amount is broken down in the body.

Therapeutic Uses. Chloroform is used (1) as a general anesthetic, (2) as an emergency anesthetic, (3) in convulsive seizures, and (4) in obstetrics in the home.

Advantages in the Use of Chloroform. The induction period is rapid and does not necessitate the use of a preliminary agent. Chloroform produces excellent relaxation of skeletal muscle and of smooth muscle of the genitourinary tract. It is not explosive.

Disadvantages in the Use of Chloroform. Chloroform may produce cardiac slowing and arrest, which may be prevented by the administration of atropine. It may also produce ventricular arrhythmias of various types. Older reports of liver damage have reduced greatly its use in the United States.

Contraindications to the Use of Chloroform. (1) Diseases of the heart, (2) hypertension or hypotension, (3) diabetes mellitus or acidosis from any cause, (4) diseases of the liver, (5) diseases of the kidney, and (6) acute or chronic diseases of the respiratory tract.

Re-evaluation of Chloroform. Chloroform has been studied by Dr. R. M. Waters, using modern techniques in anesthesiology. When properly administered with oxygen, no organ damage was observed, and he believes that chloroform should not be abandoned as an anesthetic.

Cyclopropane, U.S.P., B.P., I.P.

Cyclopropane is a gas which is very inflammable, and its mixtures with oxygen or air are explosive. As an anesthetic, it is more potent than nitrous oxide. It is easily inhaled and quickly produces unconsciousness and surgical anesthesia. Relaxation of the abdominal musculature is fair but not nearly so good as with ether.

Cyclopropane is administered by inhalation with the closed-system technique.

The induction is rapid and pleasant. A plethora of oxygen can be given, since anesthesia can be induced with 30 per cent and maintained with 15 per cent cyclopropane.

Therapeutic Uses.   Cyclopropane is used as an anesthetic for all forms of surgery. It is especially useful in chest surgery, in which quiet respiration and absence of muscle spasm are important. In obstetrics, it does not interfere with the contractions of the uterus or with the respiratory system of the fetus.

Advantages and Disadvantages in the Use of Cyclopropane.   The advantages far exceed the disadvantages in the use of cyclopropane. (1) The vomiting and nausea are less than with some anesthetics, (2) there is no visceral damage, (3) the induction is smooth and the recovery is rapid, (4) it tends to maintain blood pressure at normal levels in shock by offsetting vasodilatation, and (5) it produces quiet respirations.

The disadvantages are (1) mixtures of cyclopropane and oxygen are explosive, (2) cyclopropane is expensive, (3) it increases cardiac irritability and causes arrhythmias, (4) inadequate respiratory exchange can cause post-anesthetic "cyclopropane shock," and (5) there is no analgesic effect post-anesthetically. The patient is often restless, noisy, and apprehensive before he is capable of controlling his reaction to pain.

Contraindications to the Use of Cyclopropane.   (1) In cardiac disease, (2) in operations requiring the use of cautery, high-frequency units, or other equipment which may cause sparks or produce flames, and (3) when epinephrine or norepinephrine is necessary.

Trichloroethylene, U.S.P., B.P., I.P. (Trilene)

Trichloroethylene is a clear, volatile liquid that produces prompt analgesia and anesthesia when inhaled. Its action resembles that of chloroform, but it is less potent. It is suitable only as an analgesic. Trichloroethylene is not flammable when mixed with air, but it may be explosive when mixed with oxygen. The untoward effects are tachypnea, bradycardia, and serious cardiac irregularities. It produces poor muscular relaxation, mainly because insufficient amounts can be given to reach the deeper plane. It is widely used as an analgesic. It is administered by means of an inhaler controlled by the patient or an anesthetic machine controlled by the anesthetist.

Advantages and Disadvantages of the Use of Trichloroethylene. The main advantage of this compound is that it is a potent analgesic agent which can be easily administered.

Disadvantages are (1) it causes cardiac depression manifested by arrhythmias, (2) it is decomposed in the presence of soda lime and cannot be used in the closed system, (3) it may cause hepatotoxicity, and (4) its margin of safety is similar to that of chloroform when used for surgical anesthesia.

Preparations

Trichloroethylene, U.S.P.   6-ml. ampuls and 30-ml. bottles
Trichloroethylene Inhaler

Trade names: Chlorylen; Gemalgene; Trethylene; Trichlorethylene; Trielin;
        Triline; Trimar; Westrosol

Halothane, U.S.P., B.P. (Fluothane)

Halothane is a nonexplosive and nonflammable liquid the vapor of which has been used extensively as a general anesthetic for all types of surgical procedures. Induction is smooth and rapid and early intubation is achieved. With concentrations of 2 per cent, surgical anesthesia is obtained in about ten minutes and may be maintained with 0.5 to 1 per cent concentrations. It is a safe and predictable anesthetic if concentrations do not exceed 2 per cent. Secretions are absent or minimal, and there is a moderate degree of muscular relaxation. Adequate muscle relaxation is not obtained consistently without relaxants in which case succinylcholine chloride may be used. After removal of the anesthetic there is a prompt recovery of consciousness in about 5 to 20 minutes. There are no significant postoperative complications; the incidence of nausea and vomiting is minimal. Respiratory arrest, hepatic damage, cardiovascular collapse, cardiac arrest, or severe hypotension may occur with overdosage. Halothane may be administered by the open-drop method for short procedures. A gas machine with semiclosed absorption or nonrebreathing technique is used for longer procedures. Because of its potency and low margin of safety, halothane should be used in vaporizers calibrated so that safe concentrations can be carefully maintained. It is delivered in a gas mixture of nitrous oxide and oxygen with flow rates of 8 to 10 liters per minute.

Advantages and Disadvantages of Halothane. The advantages are that it (1) is nonflammable, (2) is nonirritating to the upper respiratory tract, (3) is characterized by rapid induction and recovery, (4) is potent— more potent than chloroform in regard to rapidity of induction, and (5) produces less nausea and vomiting postoperatively.

The disadvantages are (1) it causes depression of the respiration and circulation, (2) over-concentration leads to circulatory collapse, (3) it may be hepatotoxic, and (4) it increases irritability of cardiac automatic tissue predisposing to arrhythmias.

Contraindications to the Use of Halothane. (1) In the presence of cardiac disease or irregularities of rhythm, (2) in hypotension (shock), and (3) in emaciated "toxic," anemic, or acutely ill patients.

Preparation

Halothane, U.S.P., B.P.   Bottles containing 125 ml.
            Trade name: Fluothane

Fluroxene (Fluoromar)

Fluroxene is a liquid whose vapor is flammable in anesthetic concentrations. It may be used as a general anesthetic for any type of surgical anesthesia not requiring profound muscle relaxation. The induction is smooth, rapid, and pleasant. Coughing, excessive salivation, excitement, and laryngospasm are minimal. Analgesia is profound. The return to consciousness is rapid, pleasant, and free from side effects. Analgesia is present for a considerable period of time after the return to consciousness. There appear to be no specific toxic effects on the liver or kidneys, and the evidence of cardiac arrhythmias is minimal. Fluroxene is administered with one of the various types of anesthetic machines. Concentrations of 1.5 to 2 per cent produce analgesia; 7 to 8 per cent concentrations are required when the anesthetic is administered alone. When it is administered with 75 per cent nitrous oxide as a supplement agent, surgical anesthesia is obtained with 1 to 2 per cent fluroxene.

Precautions. The blood pressure may fall slightly, and tachypnea and decreased tidal volume may occur during deep anesthesia, so that blood pressure and respiration should be observed carefully and assisted, when necessary.

The vasopressors, ephedrine, epinephrine, levarterenol, and vasopressin, as well as the intravenous muscle relaxants may be administered during fluroxene anesthesia. Intravenous muscle relaxants may be necessary to obtain adequate ventilation for laryngoscopy and abdominal operations.

Contraindications to the Use of Fluroxene. (1) Presence of the cautery or other source of ignition, (2) shock from trauma or hemorrhage.

Preparation

Fluroxene   Bottles of 125 ml.
                           Trade name: Fluoromar

Methoxyflurane (Penthrane)

Methoxyflurane is a volatile liquid the vapor of which is nonexplosive and nonflammable in any mixture with air or oxygen. It is safe for use with cautery and diathermy apparatus. It is an excellent anesthetic. Anesthesia is best induced by concentrations of 1.5 to 3 per cent vaporized by a high flow of oxygen. The open-drop method has been used in infants and children.

Therapeutic Uses. It is used for general anesthesia and as an analgesic for obstetrics, in conjunction with nitrous oxide when nonflammable anesthetics are required.

Advantages of Methoxyflurane. (1) It is nonflammable, (2) it produces excellent relaxation as the sole agent without the aid of relaxants, (3) analgesia extends to the period of emergence and lasts several hours postoperatively, (4) nausea and vomiting are minimal post anesthesia, and (5) salivation is not excessive.

Disadvantages of Methoxyflurane. (1) It is characterized by a prolonged induction and excitation period, (2) there is prolonged somnolence during the emergence and recovery period, (3) some patients have headaches during the postoperative period, (4) methoxyflurane produces hypotension, and (5) it depresses the respiration during maintenance.

Contraindications. (1) Liver disease or insufficiency, (2) hypotensive states, and (3) situations in which rapid recovery is mandatory.

Preparation

Methoxyflurane   Bottles containing 125 ml.
                        Trade name: Penthrane

Xenon

Recently a rare and supposedly inert gas of the atmosphere, xenon, was shown by Dr. S. C. Cullen to possess anesthetic properties.

NONVOLATILE ANESTHETICS (INTRAVENOUS ANESTHETICS)

Intravenous use of anesthetics is not new. Ether, in diluted solutions, was injected intravenously in 1909. The injections were painful. Its volatility and insolubility presented difficulties. Later, nonvolatile anesthetic substances were used. Amobarbital (Amytal sodium) was administered intravenously in 1928. It produced a long sleep after the operation and predisposed the patient to respiratory complications. As the sedative effect subsided, the patient was often delirious.. It was replaced in 1932 by hexobarbital (Evipal sodium). The action produced by hexobarbital was shorter in duration. It was widely used until 1943, when thiopental sodium (Pentothal) was introduced.

Effects of Intravenous Anesthetics. Upon intravenous administration, these drugs produce sedation of the central nervous system and recovery in somewhat the same manner as the volatile anesthetics. They produce little or no analgesia and little abdominal relaxation (in safe doses). They depress the respiration. The rate and depth of breathing are decreased and the rhythm may become irregular. When they are injected rapidly, there is a fall in blood pressure. Laryngospasm occurs frequently. Anesthesia is induced rapidly and easily and, of course, without causing pulmonary irritation. Apprehension, fear, and unpleasant memories are reduced to a minimum. Repeated injections are made to maintain the anesthesia. The recovery is rapid and there is usually no postoperative nausea or vomiting. Intravenous anesthetics are usually given with oxygen and nitrous oxide. There is no fire or explosion hazard.

The thiobarbiturates owe their rapidity of action to a high lipid solubility. For this reason they pass rapidly from the blood to the lipids of the brain and, in addition, to the body fat. Therefore, the blood concentration decreases as the fat concentration increases. With a small dose, recovery is rapid. With large doses or repeated small doses, the fat may become saturated and the drug is slowly released to the blood and again to the brain and anesthesia is prolonged. The drugs are all metabolized, but rather slowly, in the body, primarily by the liver and partly by the other tissues.

Mechanism of Action.   It is not known exactly how the barbiturates and thiobarbiturates produce their depressant effects on the brain. It is believed that they interfere with the enzyme reactions that take place in the cells or on the cell membranes. In vitro experiments have shown that they inhibit the oxidation of glucose and pyruvate. They may inhibit the activity of cytochrome reductase or interfere with the synthesis of acetylcholine by blocking the reduction of pyruvate. Dr. J. H. Quastel has suggested that the narcotics and thiobarbiturates may inhibit respiration in the enzyme reactions responsible for the synthesis of adenosine triphosphate (ATP).

Therapeutic Uses.   The ultrashort-acting barbiturates are used (1) to produce general anesthesia of short duration, (2) as preanesthetic or basal anesthetic agents, (3) to control convulsions, and (4) for "narcodiagnosis" and "narcosynthesis" in psychiatry.

Sodium Thiopental, U.S.P., Thiopentone Sodium, B.P. (Pentothal Sodium)

Thiopental is one of the most widely used intravenous anesthetics. It is sometimes administered rectally.

Action of Thiopental.   Thiopental markedly depresses the cerebral cortex, and its depressant action on the motor areas is so prompt and dependable that it is used to combat the convulsions that may rarely occur under the volatile anesthetics, ether and vinyl ether. When administered intravenously, it produces anesthesia very quickly and the recovery is usually prompt. When small doses of thiopental are administered, awakening occurs early. This appears to be due to its redistribution in the body, as in the case of the general anesthetics. Thiopental is metabolized partly in the liver and partly by the cells of the other tissues of the body. There is evidence to show that its hourly metabolism is only about 15 per cent. Therefore, after thiopental has been given for prolonged periods of time, cumulative effects occur and the emergence from the effect of the drug is usually very slow.

Dosage and Method of Administration.   Thiopental is unstable in solution. It is marketed as a dry powder in combination with anhydrous sodium carbonate in sealed ampuls. The powder is dissolved in sterile distilled water just prior to its use. The usual intravenous dose of 2 to 3 ml. of a

2.5 per cent solution is injected at the rate of 1 ml. every five seconds and is repeated in about 30 seconds as required. Sleep is produced in one-half to one minute and lasts from 15 to 30 minutes. The needle is usually allowed to remain in the vessel to supplement the initial dose, if necessary. It is not recommended alone for operations of long duration. Its unsupplemented use is confined to procedures lasting no longer than 20 minutes. The total dosage is 0.5 to 1 Gm. for 20 to 30 minutes.

Thiopental is also administered rectally in a 10 per cent solution. For basal anesthesia, the rectal dosage is calculated on the basis of 45 mg. per kilogram of body weight or 0.45 ml. of a 10 per cent solution per kilogram of body weight. The maximum dose should not exceed 3 Gm. It is often used rectally for children.

Signs of Thiopental Anesthesia.   There are no reliable signs of thiopental anesthesia. The stages and planes applicable to inhalation anesthesia cannot be used as guides. The anesthetist must attempt to maintain the patient between a state of decreased reflex activity and respiratory and circulatory failure.

Therapeutic Uses.   Thiopental sodium is used (1) for operations of short duration, (2) to induce anesthesia, (3) as a basal anesthetic, and (4) to combat convulsions that occur under volatile anesthetics. Thiopental is easily supplemented with ether, nitrous oxide and oxygen, or cyclopropane.

Untoward Effects.   (1) Respiratory depression or failure due to overdosage or use of large quantities of the drug over long periods of time, (2) hypotension, (3) prolonged somnolence as the drug is excreted slowly, (4) twitching of muscles, and (5) slough at the site of injection due to extravascular injection of the solution.

Advantages.   (1) There is pleasant induction of basal narcosis for the patient. The induction is simple and rapid. (2) Postanesthetic emesis is reduced. (3) The drug does not stimulate production of secretions or irritate mucous membranes in the respiratory tract. (4) Recovery is prompt if minimal doses are used.

Disadvantages.   (1) Basal narcosis is uncontrollable since, once the drug is in the vein and overdosage has occurred, it cannot be retrieved, (2) all reflexes are not abolished, particularly those of the larynx and pharynx, and laryngeal spasm may develop, (3) the drug cannot be used as a sole agent because it is not analgesic and causes anesthesia by inducing a severe depression, and (4) muscular relaxation is not satisfactory unless general anesthetics or muscle relaxants are also used.

Contraindications to the Use of Thiopental.   (1) Aged persons with degenerative changes, (2) diseases of the heart with decompensation, (3) hypotension, and (4) chronic diseases of the respiratory tract.

Preparations

Sodium Thiopental for Injection, U.S.P.; Thiopentone Injection, B.P. (I.P.)
Ampuls containing 500 mg., 1, 5, and 10 Gm.

Trade names: Pentothal Sodium; Farmotal; Intraval; Nesdonal; Pharmotal; Thionembutal

Thiamylal Sodium (Surital Sodium)

Thiamylal is provided in vials as a mixture with sodium bicarbonate. It is an ultrashort-acting intravenous barbiturate for anesthetic procedures of short duration. Its action is rapid (20 to 60 seconds), and the recovery is rapid. Thiamylal is detoxified in the liver; therefore, it is contraindicated in liver disease. There are less circulatory and respiratory changes and a lower incidence of laryngospasm than with thiopental.

Dosage and Administration. Thiamylal is administered intravenously in doses of 3 to 6 ml. of a freshly prepared 2.5 per cent solution at the rate of 1 ml. every five seconds. Additional injections may be made intermittently with the needle in the vein. The maximum dose should not exceed 1 Gm. or 40 ml. of a 2.5 per cent solution.

Preparation

Thiamylal Sodium for Injection, N.F.
Vials containing 500 mg., 1, 5, and 10 Gm.
Trade name: Surital Sodium

Sodium Hexobarbital, N.F., I.P. (Evipal Sodium)

Hexobarbital is similar in action to thiopental, but it is less potent and very short acting. It is administered intravenously in doses of 2 to 4 ml. of a 10 per cent solution. The maximum dose is 10 ml.

Preparation

Sterile Sodium Hexobarbital, N.F.
Ampuls containing 1 Gm.
Trade names: Cyclonal; Evipal Sodium; Evipan; Methexenyl

Thialbarbitone Sodium (Kemithal Sodium)

Thialbarbitone is similar in action to thiopental. It is almost one half as potent and is said to produce less respiratory depression and less laryngospasm. It is administered in 5 or 10 per cent solution. This anesthetic is widely used in England. Secobarbital, pentobarbital, and amobarbital are also used intravenously. They are discussed on pages 316–23.

Methohexital (Brevital) Sodium

Methohexital is a potent, ultrashort-acting anesthetic. Recovery is exceptionally rapid. Anesthesia may be maintained either with intermittent injections of a 1 per cent solution or by constant-drip infusion using a 0.2 per cent solution. The dose (5 to 10 ml.) of a 1 per cent solution is administered at the rate of 1 ml. (10 mg.) in five seconds. Intermittent injections should be individualized, and usually 2 to 4 ml. are injected every four to seven minutes.

Preparation

Sodium Methohexital for Injection, N.F.   Ampuls containing 500 mg. and 2.5 Gm.

Trade name: Brevital

BASAL ANESTHETICS

Basal anesthetics are used to produce partial narcosis or sometimes light anesthesia prior to the administration of a general anesthetic. They lessen worry and anxiety, promote relaxation and a smoother induction, and permit the use of smaller doses of the general anesthetic. They are usually used with a general anesthetic but are sometimes used with block or spinal anesthesia. The drugs most often used are thiopental and tribromoethanol. They are generally administered rectally. Ether in oil, paraldehyde, and barbiturates may also be used.

Tribromoethanol, N.F. (Avertin)

Tribromoethanol is a solid that is very insoluble in water. Tribromoethanol Solution, U.S.P., contains 100 Gm. of tribromoethanol in 100 ml. of amylene hydrate. This solution is prepared for rectal administration by dissolving 2.5 ml. in 100 ml. of water at 37° C. It should be tested with a dye, Congo red, enclosed in the package, to see if it has decomposed. It is administered at body temperature by high enema, one-half hour preoperatively.

Action of Tribromoethanol. Tribromoethanol depresses the central nervous system and produces general anesthesia. The onset of narcosis is smooth, and the depth and duration of action depend upon the dose administered. A concentration of 5 mg. per cent in the blood produces partial narcosis; one of 8 to 10 mg. per cent, deep narcosis. Drowsiness and depression may continue for six hours or more. In anesthetic doses, the respiratory center is depressed. Because of this depressant action on the respiration, tribromoethanol is used only as a basal anesthetic, not as a general anesthetic. The vasomotor centers are depressed, there is some peripheral vasodilatation, and the blood pressure is decreased. Because it depresses the functional activity of the liver, it is contraindicated in liver and kidney diseases and in diseased conditions of the rectum and colon.

Absorption, Fate, and Excretion. Tribromoethanol is rapidly absorbed, 50 per cent in ten minutes and 95 per cent in the first half hour. It is conjugated by the liver with glucuronic acid and is excreted in the urine.

Seventy to eighty per cent is eliminated in the first 48 hours and the rest over a period of days.

Therapeutic Use. Tribromoethanol is used as a basal anesthetic. It is supplemented with ether, nitrous oxide, or cyclopropane. Its use appears to be diminishing.

Dose and Method of Administration. The average dose is 0.06 to 0.08 ml. per kilogram of body weight (6 to 8 ml. for women, 9 to 10 ml. for men). It is administered rectally.

Preparation

Tribromoethanol Solution, N.F.   100 Gm. of tribromoethanol in 100 ml. of amylene hydrate

Trade names: Avertin with Amylene Hydrate; Avertin Fluid

Hydroxydione Sodium Succinate (Viadril)

This agent is a steroid compound. It is administered intravenously as a basal anesthetic prior to the administration of other anesthetics, especially nitrous oxide. The side effects noted are hypotension and thrombophlebitis. The intravenous dose in 0.5 to 1 per cent solution is 50 to 150 ml. It is available as a powder in ampuls containing 500 mg.

POSTANESTHESIA COMPLICATION AND NURSING RESPONSIBILITIES

Once anesthesia is discontinued, the patient does not experience an immediate recovery from its effects. The length of the recovery period depends upon the type and amount of anesthetic received. During this time the patient needs intelligent nursing assistance. Haphazard and improper postoperative care may negate completely the results of surgery which was carefully planned and executed. The incidence of postoperative complications is highest during this period, and many complications which manifest themselves later have their inception in the hours immediately following surgery. Some of these complications may be related to drugs used before and during surgery. They include:

Respiratory Obstruction. The use of drugs such as atropine and scopolamine to dry secretions preoperatively and the irritating effects of the inhalation anesthetics on the respiratory tract may cause thick, tenacious mucus to be produced. Blockage of one of the bronchi by a mucus plug will result in atelectasis. Measures used to prevent this include deep breathing, coughing, suctioning, frequent turning after the vital signs are stable, and adequate hydration.

Relaxation of the tongue with consequent closure of the glottis occurs with any general anesthesia. An oral airway, side-lying position of the patient, or hyperextension of the neck with the mandible extended up and out as if to pull it in front of the maxilla is used to maintain an open airway.

Respiratory inadequacy may exist at the end of the operation if muscle relaxants such as tubocurarine and succinylcholine have been used. Pulmonary ventilation must be assisted to prevent hypoxia and is frequently accomplished through the use of intermittent positive-pressure breathing apparatus or medicinal antidotes to the muscle relaxants.

Laryngeal spasm with an increased amount of secretions in the area of the larynx may occur as a result of the tracheal intubation for inhalation anesthesia. Removal of the secretions by suctioning and administration of oxygen by positive pressure may be required to prevent hypoxia.

Any patient who has undergone a surgical procedure under general anesthesia may vomit in the immediate postoperative period; particularly is this true of those who have received ether. Vomiting results from the suppressant action of general anesthetics upon the normal peristaltic movements of the gastrointestinal tract. This predisposes to distention of the stomach with fluid and air. Postoperatively, the contents of the stomach are forced out by contractions of the abdominal muscles. Since the patient's gag reflex may be diminished or absent, it is imperative that aggressive action be undertaken to prevent aspiration of the vomitus.

Cardiovascular Complications.   The depressant action of anesthetics on the cardiovascular system may cause various problems. Cardiac arrhythmias occur occasionally when cyclopropane is given. It can also cause a bradycardia by its action on the vagus. Atropine is sometimes given to correct this decreased cardiac rate. Agents which affect the nerve impulse conduction to the blood vessels may cause a prolonged circulation time. Hypotension is not unusual postoperatively. It occurs frequently with the use of agents which relax the muscles of the blood vessels and cyclopropane if the carbon dioxide level in the blood is decreased rapidly. It may also result from change of the position of the patient early in the recovery period, motion during transportation, and the use of narcotics. Increasing the blood volume by the use of intravenous fluids; maintenance of a flat, still position; or, in severe situations, using a vasopressor are usual methods of treatment.

Pain.   Many persons experience pain before they are completely free of the effects of the anesthetic agent. However, the administration of usual amounts of narcotics can lead to reanesthetization and circulatory or respiratory depression during this period. Therefore, reduced amounts (one fourth to one half the usual dose) are given to alleviate pain and allay anxiety. Cyclopropane has no analgesic effect postanesthetically. Thus patients receiving this agent are very likely to experience pain early in their recovery.

Restlessness and Excitement.   All patients pass through a stage of excitement in recovering from the effects of a general anesthetic. Pain, preoperative drugs such as scopolamine, and the anesthetic cyclopropane prolong this period. Since involuntary movements by the patient may be very harmful, the alert attention of the personnel is particularly important in this stage of recovery. A quiet, soothing voice rather than massive restraints tends to be most effective in calming the patient.

━━━━━━━━━━━━━━━ Table 17 ━━━━━━━━━━━━━━━

Some Aspects of Anesthetic Agents in Use Today

Agent	Flammability	Anesthetic Concentration, per cent	Advantages	Disadvantages
Nitrous oxide	Nonflammable	50–95	*Good analgesic,* short acting, no depression of circulation, respiration, kidney, or liver function. Useful in dental surgery.	Low potency, danger of hypoxia owing to high concentrations needed, poor relaxation.
Ethyl ether	Flammable with oxygen explosive	3.5–4.5	Safest agent, cheap, excellent relaxation, stimulates respiration rather than depresses it in the lighter planes of anesthesia. No adverse effects on blood pressure, respiration, circulation, kidney, or liver at levels of anesthesia usually used for surgery.	Long induction and recovery, increased secretions, flammable, nausea and vomiting.
Vinyl ether	Flammable	4	Similar to ethyl ether but recovery and induction shorter.	After 30 minutes of anesthesia, danger of *liver damage.* Good only in short cases.
Ethylene	Flammable with oxygen explosive	80	Similar to nitrous oxide but more potent, good in obstetrical analgesia.	Poor muscle relaxation, *explosive, unpleasant odor.*
Ethyl chloride	Flammable with oxygen explosive	3.0–4.5	Potent, rapid induction and recovery.	*Difficult to control,* many anesthetic fatalities, powerful circulatory and respiratory depressant.
Chloroform	Nonflammable	1.5	Potent, rapid induction and emergence, excellent relaxation.	Hypotension, respiratory depression, *cardiac arrhythmias, liver damage.* Directly toxic to myocardium.

———————————— **Table 17 (continued)** ————————————

Some Aspects of Anesthetic Agents in Use Today

Agent	Flammability	Anesthetic Concentration, per cent	Advantages	Disadvantages
Cyclopropane	Flammable	15–30	Rapid induction and recovery, *no depression of blood pressure.*	Depression of respirations and pulse rate. Sensitizes myocardium to epinephrine. If increased CO_2, danger of "cyclopropane shock."
Trichloroethylene	Nonflammable with air, explosive with oxygen	5.0–7.5	Good analgesic, rapid-acting agent. Used *mainly* as analgesic.	Sensitizes myocardium to epinephrine, tachypnea, no relaxation. May be hepatotoxic or cardiotoxic.
Halothane	Nonflammable	0.4–1.5	*Potent, rapid induction, recovery,* low incidence of nausea and vomiting. Most used agent at present.	Contraindicated in obstetrics due to depression of uterine contractions and therefore predisposition to postpartum hemorrhage, hypotension, adversely affects placental circulation. Also in patients with liver disease.
Fluroxene	Slightly flammable	3–5	Similar to ethyl ether but more rapid acting, no adverse effects on liver or kidney, minimal secretions.	Flammable, some nausea and vomiting, moderate muscle relaxation, in deeper planes some respiratory and blood pressure depression.
Methoxyflurane	Nonflammable	0.1–1	Potent, good muscle relaxation, analgesic.	Slow induction and recovery, hypotensive in anesthetic planes.

REVIEW QUESTIONS

1. *What are some of the usual requirements of balanced anesthesia?*
2. *What drugs may be given in combination to produce this type of anesthesia?*
3. *What effects do the general anesthetics produce?*
4. *List the stages of anesthesia and give a brief description of the symptoms observed in each stage. During which stage is surgery performed?*
5. *What kinds of substances are used to produce general anesthesia? Name several. How are they administered and how are they excreted?*
6. *What is the mechanism of action of the general anesthetics?*
7. *What are the advantages of the use of intravenous anesthetics? What are the disadvantages?*
8. *During the admission of the patient to the recovery room, the nurse is told that ether was the anesthetic agent administered during surgery. During the postoperative period, the nurse should observe the patient for what side effects?*
9. *During the anesthetic induction period, the patient enters the second stage of anesthesia. What characteristics of this stage will the nurse in the operating room observe?*
10. *What are the nursing responsibilities in the care of the postanesthetic patient?*

REFERENCES

Adriani, John: *Techniques and Procedures of Anesthesia*, 3rd ed. Charles C Thomas, Publisher, Springfield, Ill., 1964.

Breckenridge, F. J., and Bruno, P.: "Nursing Care of the Anesthetized Patient," *Am. J. Nursing*, **62**:74, 1962.

Dripps, R. D.; Eckenhoff, J. E.; and VanDam, L. D.: *Introduction to Anesthesia*, 2nd ed. W. B. Saunders Company, Philadelphia, London, 1961.

Schafer, K. N., *et al.*: *Medical-Surgical Nursing*, 2nd ed. C. V. Mosby Company, St. Louis, 1961.

HYPOTHERMIA

Cohen, D., and Hercus, V.: "Controlled Hypothermia in Infants and Children," *Brit. M. J.*, **1**:1435, 1959.

Hellings, P. M.: "Controlled Hypothermia; Recent Developments in Use of Hypothermia in Neurosurgery," *Brit. M. J.*, **2**:346, 1958.

Little, D. M., Jr.: "Hypothermia," *Anesthesiology*, **20**:842, 1959.

Schackman, R.; Wood-Smith, F. G.; Graber, I. G., *et al.*: "The 'Lytic Cocktail': Observations on Surgical Patients," *Lancet*, **2**:617, 1954.

Sellick, B. A.: "A New Method of Hypothermia for Open Heart Surgery," *Lancet*, **1**:443, 1957; *J.A.M.A.*, **164**:707, 1957.

VOLATILE ANESTHETICS

Feldberg, W.: "A Physiological Approach to the Problem of General Anesthesia and Loss of Consciousness," *Brit. M. J.*, **2**:771, 1959.

Guedel, A. E.: *Inhalation Anesthesia*, 2nd ed. The Macmillan Company, New York, 1951.

Lundy, J. S.: *Clinical Anesthesia: a Manual of Clinical Anesthesiology*. W. B. Saunders Company, Philadelphia, 1942.

Waters, R. M. (ed.) : *Chloroform: a Study after 100 Years*. University of Wisconsin Press, Madison, 1951.

HALOTHANE

Abajian, J.; Brazell, E. H.; Dente, G. A.; and Mills, E. L.: "Experience with Halothane (Fluothane) in More than Five Thousand Cases," *J.A.M.A.*, **171**: 535, 1959.

———: "Safety of Halothane Anesthesia," *Modern Med.*, Dec. 1, 1959, p. 213.

Council on Drugs, New and Nonofficial Drugs: "Halothane (Fluothane)," *J.A.M.A.*, **170**:123, 1959.

Dixon, G. H., and Matheson, D. I.: "Fluothane and Other Nonexplosive Halogenated Hydrocarbons in Clinical Anesthesia," *Canad. M.A.J.*, **79**:365, 1958.

Hewer, C. L. (ed.) : *Recent Advances in Anesthesia and Analgesia*, 9th ed. Little Brown and Company, Boston, 1963.

Raventos, J.: "The Action of Fluothane, A New Volatile Anesthetic," *Brit. J. Pharmacol.*, **11**:394, 1956.

FLUROXENE

Dundee, J. W.; Linde, H. W.; and Dripps, R. D.: "Observations on Trifluoroethylvinyl Ether," *Anesthesiology*, **18**:66, 1957.

Krantz, J. C., Jr.; Carr, C. J.; Lu, G.; and Bell, F. K.: "The Anesthetic Action of Trifluoroethyl Vinyl Ether," *J. Pharmacol. & Exper. Therap.*, **108**:488, 1953.

Musser, Ruth D.; Park, C. S.; and Krantz, J. C., Jr.: "Stability of Trifluoroethylvinyl and Ethylvinyl Ethers in the Animal Body," *Anesthesiology*, **18**:480, 1957.

New Drugs: "An Inhalation Anesthetic Fluroxene (Fluoromar)," *J.A.M.A.*, **186**: 325, 1963.

METHOXYFLURANE

Artusio, J. F., *et al.*: "Clinical Evaluation of Methoxyflurane in Man," *Anesthesiology*, **21**:512, 1960.

New Drugs and Developments in Therapeutics: "Methoxyflurane (Penthrane)," *J.A.M.A.*, **184**:709, 1963.

NONVOLATILE ANESTHETICS

Dundee, J. W., and Riding, J. E.: "A Clinical Trial of Thiamylal as an Intravenous Anesthetic in 1,750 Cases," *Brit. J. Anaesth.*, **27**:381, 1955.

Mushin, W. W.; Henderson, A. G.; and Mapleson, W. W.: "Comparative Potencies of Thiamylal (Surital) and Thiopentone," *Brit. J. Anaesth.*, **27**:374, 1955.

Tovell, R. M.; Anderson, C. C.; Sadove, M. S.; Artuso, J. F.; Papher, E. M.; Coakley, C. S.; Hudon, F.; Smith, S. M.; and Thomas, G. J.: "A Comparative Clinical and Statistical Study of Thiopental and Thiamylal in Human Anesthesia," *Anesthesiology*, **16**:910, 1955.

METHOHEXITAL

Bellville, J. W., *et al.*: "Relative Potencies of Methohexital and Thiopental," *J. Pharmacol. and Exper. Therap.*, **129**:108, 1960.

HYDROXYDIONE SODIUM SUCCINATE

Dent, S.; Stephen, C. R.; and Wilson, W. P.: "Clinical Experience with Viadril," *Anesthesiology*, **17**:672, 1956.
Galley, A. H., and Rooms, M.: "An Intravenous Steroid Anesthetic. Experiences with Viadril," *Lancet*, **270**:990, 1956.

18

The Barbiturates and Other Sedative and Hypnotic Drugs

Hypnotics are drugs used to produce sleep. Sedatives are drugs that quiet and relax a patient without producing sleep. Both hypnotics and sedatives are to the emotionally upset individual what morphine is to the badly injured person. Both are able to relieve suffering. Inasmuch as a large percentage of persons in the civilized countries have problems that introduce highly undesirable or intolerable currents in their lives, these two groups of drugs, sedatives and hypnotics, have, since 1903, come into wide and extensive use.

Wakefulness or the conscious state is a function of the reticular formation (RF) in alerting the cortex (see p. 246). The RF receives impulses from collateral fibers from all kinds of sensory nerves and relays them to the cortex to maintain consciousness. It is believed that drugs which produce sleep block these impulses in the RF and prevent this arousing action. They also depress the sensory and motor areas of the cortex. In this way sleep and unconsciousness occur.

THE BARBITURATES

The barbiturates are the drugs most frequently prescribed to produce sedation of the central nervous system. These are white crystalline compounds with a slightly bitter taste. They are prepared from barbituric acid, a synthetic derivative of malonic acid and urea, which is not a hypnotic in itself but the derivatives of which are hypnotic and sedative. About 500 derivatives of barbituric acid have been prepared, about 60 of which have been used in therapeutics. They behave qualitatively in the same manner, but there are some important quantitative differences in their actions. The sodium salts have been prepared for intravenous administration.

The Generally Used Barbiturates. The barbiturates most often prescribed are phenobarbital (Luminal), pentobarbital (Nembutal), secobarbital (Seconal), amobarbital (Amytal), butabarbital (Butisol), mephobarbital (Mebaral), metharbital (Gemonil), and thiopental sodium (Pentothal Sodium).

Pharmacology of the Barbiturates. The principal action of the bar-

316

biturates is on the central nervous system. They act mainly by blocking impulses in the ascending reticular formation and thus preventing them from being transmitted to the cerebral cortex. They also directly depress the cells in the sensory and motor cortex. The response to the barbiturates may be mild sedation, hypnosis, or general anesthesia, depending upon the dose and method of administration. In orally therapeutic doses there is little action on the respiration. Large doses, particularly when administered intravenously, depress the respiration and death may result.

Oral therapeutic doses sufficient to produce sedation and sleep do not appreciably affect the circulation. The blood pressure is normal and there is no change in the heart rate, rhythm, or electrocardiogram. Large doses cause peripheral vasodilatation and a fall in blood pressure. When the drug is metabolized or excreted, the blood pressure returns to normal.

The constituents of the blood are not significantly influenced in therapeutic doses. Large doses may elevate the blood sugar. Neither renal nor hepatic function is impaired by therapeutic doses.

Classification of Barbiturates. The barbiturates are classified into four groups according to their duration of action. They are the long-acting compounds, such as barbital and phenobarbital; the short-acting compounds, such as pentobarbital and secobarbital; the intermediate-acting compounds, such as amobarbital; and the ultrashort-acting compounds, such as thiopental sodium.

──────────── **Table 18** ────────────

Classification, Onset, and Duration of Action of Commonly Used Barbiturates

Classification	Drugs	Onset of Action	Duration of Action
Long acting	Phenobarbital	1 hr. or longer	10 to 12 hr.
Intermediate acting	Amobarbital Butabarbital	¾ to 1 hr.	6 to 8 hr.
Short acting	Pentobarbital Secobarbital	10 to 15 minutes	3 to 4 hr.
Ultrashort acting, i.v. anesthetic	Thiopental	Seconds	Minutes

Absorption, Fate, and Excretion. The barbiturates are readily absorbed on oral administration and are evenly distributed in the tissues of the body. They are not concentrated in the brain where they exert their action.

The long-acting barbiturates are metabolized slowly and excreted mainly by the kidney. Twenty-five per cent of the phenobarbital ingested may be recovered in the urine unchanged. The excretion is slow and takes place over several days. The short-acting and intermediate-acting barbiturates are destroyed principally in the liver and are therefore contraindicated in liver disease. Only small amounts of pentobarbital, secobarbital, and amobarbital are recovered from the urine when administered in therapeutic doses. The ultrashort-acting barbiturates are metabolized rapidly, but their brevity of response is also related to their distribution in the body tissues including fat.

Untoward Effects. Not all persons react alike to barbiturates; however, as a rule, the response is predictable. In some the hypnotic dose is ineffective; in others, it may produce restlessness, excitement, delirium, and even hallucinations. Barbiturates should be used with caution in the elderly and in very young children as they produce a paradoxical excitement instead of depression. The doses vary, but death from the therapeutic dose is probably unknown. Deaths may occur from overdosage, either accidental or intentional.

The prevalence of poisoning with barbiturates is of great concern to the doctor and the nurse. Many accidental deaths and suicides have been caused by overdosage with these drugs and the number is increasing.

Poisoning with Barbiturates. The barbiturates kill by central depression of the respiration. Severe poisoning results from ten times the therapeutic dose; 15 times the therapeutic dose may cause death despite restorative measures.

The symptoms of poisoning are mental confusion, headache, and a period of excitement (which simulates drunkenness), then sleep. The reflexes are sluggish, the skin cool, moist, and cyanotic. The patient becomes comatose and the temperature falls as the coma deepens. As respiratory depression continues, the pulse becomes weak and rapid and peripheral collapse may result.

Treatment of Poisoning. The treatment of the patient includes maintaining adequate blood pressure and respiratory exchange and decreasing the amount of central depression. The body heat of the patient should be conserved. A patent airway must be maintained, and frequent suctioning and the side-lying position are necessary to prevent aspiration due to the lack of the gag reflex. If the drug has been taken orally, gastric lavage is indicated at times to remove the drug remaining in the stomach. Some clinicians advise against routine gastric lavage because little, if any, of the drug is present in the stomach by the time coma ensues, and many deaths have occurred owing to inhalation of gastric washings by comatose patients. In mild to moderate poisoning, only supportive measures may be necessary. In severe poisoning, artificial respiration and the administration of oxygen by an intermittent positive-pressure breathing apparatus may be lifesaving. The usual nursing measures such as turning, positioning, skin care, and passive exercises should be instituted to prevent pulmonary, circulatory, and skin complications.

If the poisoning is due to an overdose of phenobarbital, it may be well to give a diuretic along with intravenous glucose or physiological salt solution to enable the kidney to function more rapidly in the elimination of the drug, which is excreted mainly by the kidney. Hemodialysis by artificial kidney or peritoneal dialysis (see p. 644) may be used to remove the barbiturate from the blood when anuria occurs in barbiturate coma. Penicillin, 1,000,000 units, is administered prophylactically to prevent pneumonia.

Analeptic drug therapy appears to be of less importance than the foregoing procedures. If the patient responds to pain stimuli, and deep tendon jerks are obtainable, it is doubtful that the analeptic drugs are indicated. Some analeptic drugs (see pp. 401–5) that have been employed are:

Nikethamide (Coramine)
Pentylenetetrazol (Metrazol)
Picrotoxin
Bemegride (Megimide)

The current trend is to avoid the administration of analeptics that may themselves produce toxic effects. Recently, excellent results have been obtained by direct physiological treatment of the depressed respiration and circulation and by the use of drugs to increase the blood pressure.

Habituation and Tolerance. The nervous, emotionally upset individual is the type most likely to be given barbiturates. Doses of 15 to 30 mg. ($\frac{1}{4}$ to $\frac{1}{2}$ grain) three or four times a day will provide much comfort to some patients, restoring them to more contentment and efficiency. As long as the need for sedation exists, the mentally disturbed patient is going to desire their aid. Small doses of barbiturates used to control nervousness during the waking hours are not habit forming to most patients. Many persons, however, do not wish to begin their use or to use them regularly, believing that they will develop a dependence on these drugs.

Larger doses during the day cause drowsiness and therefore are not desired by most patients. They want to be alert and able to accomplish their work. If an ordinary sleep-producing dose (100 mg.) is taken when an individual must continue working, he may appear and feel much like the alcohol-intoxicated person. He may finally go to sleep at his job or at the car wheel just as would an inebriated person.

Doses of 100 mg. at bedtime now and then enable many patients to secure their needed sleep without the development of tolerance and the need for larger doses. Such occasional use does not cause habituation. However, some persons require doses of barbiturates every night to produce sleep. If the dose remains the same, the sleeping response will decrease. Tolerance can be carried quite far, and soon many times the original dose becomes necessary. The patient desires to sleep and so becomes habituated to the drug.

Barbiturate Addiction. Recognition of the fact that continued use of very large doses of barbiturates can cause addiction has resulted from the clinical and experimental work of Dr. Harris Isbell and his associates. This addiction occurs after the habitual ingestion of 800 mg. or more daily of the potent, rapidly acting barbiturates such as amobarbital, secobarbital, and pentobarbital. There is no evidence to show that it occurs in persons taking the usual therapeutic doses of these drugs for long periods of time. A personality defect may be the main factor. This addiction may be preceded by alcoholic or narcotic addiction, and often alcohol and the amphetamines are indulged in at the same time as the barbiturates (mixed addiction). Addicts usually take the barbiturates by mouth, but at times they may inject solutions of the drugs.

The symptoms of barbiturate addiction are similar to those of chronic alcoholism. These are impairment of mental efficiency, mental sluggishness, confusion, loss of emotional control, belligerence, tremors, blurred speech, and ataxia.

Very serious and dangerous symptoms may follow the abrupt withdrawal of barbiturates from an addicted person. These may include increasing anxiety and nervousness, muscle tremors and twitchings, and weakness. Convulsions of the grand mal type may occur. Following the convulsions, the patient is confused and may go to sleep and recover without any other symptoms. Others may become delirious and disoriented and may experience hallucinations before sleep intervenes. In some cases death has resulted. In treating this addiction, the patient should be hospitalized and the drug withdrawn cautiously and gradually. Rehabilitation procedures are the same as those described for narcotic addiction (see p. 273).

Therapeutic Uses

1. To provide sedation. To quiet a patient and relieve hyperirritability, tension, and anxiety without producing sleep in hyperthyroidism, epilepsy, peptic ulcer, high blood pressure, menopause, dysmenorrhea, hysteria, allergic disorders, and Parkinson's disease. Phenobarbital is the drug of choice. The barbiturates are also used in persons undergoing treatment for drug addiction.

2. In insomnia. To produce sleep when sleeplessness is due to worry, anxiety, or hyperexcitability. The drugs of choice are the rapidly acting barbiturates secobarbital or pentobarbital. Sleep occurs in about 10 to 15 minutes and lasts for three to four hours. The patient generally sleeps all through the night and is not drowsy in the morning owing to the effects of the drug. Some patients have no difficulty going to sleep but awaken in four or five hours. They may be given secobarbital as an "Enseal" which dissolves very slowly so that its effects are delayed for four to five hours. A longer-acting barbiturate such as amobarbital is sometimes used. A mixture of secobarbital and amobarbital called Tuinal is useful for both rapid and more prolonged action.

3. To combat convulsions. As invaluable lifesaving agents in combating convulsions resulting from overdosage with certain drugs and convulsions

from tetanus, eclampsia, or cerebral pathology. For these conditions the short-acting or ultrashort-acting drugs are injected intramuscularly or intravenously.

4. Preanesthetic medication prior to a general anesthetic. With local anesthetics to reduce the incidence of toxic reactions.

5. Surgical anesthesia of short duration. Thiopental is given intravenously.

6. In pediatrics. To sedate children during times of stress and illness and occasionally for routine examinations of the ears, nose, and throat.

7. In neuropsychiatry. To produce blurred consciousness. The inhibitions are released and the patients talk more freely. Amobarbital is the drug of choice.

Preparations and Dosage

Amobarbital, U.S.P.; Amylobarbitone, B.P.	100 mg. (20 to 300 mg.) once or twice daily, orally
Amobarbital Tablets, U.S.P.	8, 15, 30, 50, and 100 mg.
Amylobarbitone Tablets, B.P.	100 and 200 mg.
Amobarbital Elixir, N.F.	17.6 mg. in 4 ml.
Sodium Amobarbital, U.S.P.; Amylobarbitone Sodium, B.P.	200 mg. (20 to 500 mg.) once or twice daily, orally, intramuscularly, or subcutaneously
Sodium Amobarbital Capsules, U.S.P.	60 and 200 mg.
Sodium Amobarbital, U.S.P.	Ampuls containing 60, 125, 250, and 500 mg. and 1 Gm.

Trade name: Amytal

Aprobarbital, N.F.	60 and 130 mg. orally, hypnotic dose
Elixir Aprobarbital	8 mg. in each ml.

Trade name: Alurate

Barbital, N.F.; Barbitone (I.P.)	300 mg. orally; hypnotic dose
Barbital Tablets, N.F.	300· mg.
Sodium Barbital, N.F.; Barbitone Sodium, B.P.	300 to 600 mg. orally
Sodium Barbital Tablets; Barbitone Sodium Tablets, B.P.	300 mg.

Trade names: Diemal; Medinal; Veronal

Sodium Butabarbital, N.F. Butobarbitone, B.P.	30 mg. orally, sedative dose: 100 mg. orally, hypnotic dose (100 to 200 mg., B.P.)
Sodium Butabarbital Capsules, N.F.	100 mg.
Sodium Butabarbital Elixir, N.F.	6.6 mg. in each milliliter
Sodium Butabarbital Tablets, N.F.	15, 30, 50, and 100 mg.
Butabarbitone Tablets, B.P.	100 to 200 mg.

Trade names: Butisol and Bubartal Sodium

Heptabarbital	50 to 100 mg. orally b.i.d. or t.i.d. sedative, 200 to 400 mg. orally, hypnotic dose
Heptabarbital Tablets	200 mg.

Trade name: Medomin

Hexobarbital — 260 to 520 mg. orally at bedtime

Hexobarbital Tablets — 260 mg.

Sodium Hexobarbital, N.F., I.P. — 2 to 4 ml. (2 to 10 ml.) of a 10 per cent solution intravenously

Sterile Sodium Hexobarbital, N.F. — Ampuls containing 1 Gm.

Trade names: Evipal Sodium; Cyclonal; Cyclural; Dorico; Evipan; Hexanastab; Methexenyl; Somnalert Tobinal

Mephobarbital, U.S.P. — 30 mg. t.i.d. (30 to 250 mg. daily), anticonvulsant; 100 mg. t.i.d. (100 to 800 mg. daily), hypnotic and sedative

Mephobarbital Tablets, U.S.P. — 30, 100, and 200 mg.

Trade names: Isonal; Mebaral; Phemitone; Prominal

Metharbital, N.F. — 100 mg one to three times daily, orally for adults; 50 mg. one to three times daily, orally for children

Metharbital Tablets, N.F. — 100 mg.

Trade name: Gemonil

Sodium Pentobarbital, U.S.P.; Pentobarbitone Sodium, B.P. — 100 mg. (50 to 300 mg.) once or twice daily orally; 100 mg. (100 to 300 mg.) intravenously

Sodium Pentobarbital Capsules, U.S.P. — 50 and 100 mg.

Sodium Pentobarbital, U.S.P. — Ampuls containing 250 and 500 mg.

Sodium Pentobarbital Elixir, U.S.P. — 3.4 to 3.9 mg. in 1 ml.

Sodium Pentobarbital Injection, U.S.P. — 250 mg. in 5 ml.; 1 Gm. in 20 ml.; 2.5 Gm. in 50 ml.

Sodium Pentobarbital Tablets, N.F.; Pentobarbitone Tablets, B.P. — 30, 50, and 100 mg.

Trade names: Nembutal Sodium; Embutal; Isobarb; Iturate

Phenobarbital, U.S.P.; Phenobarbitone, B.P. — 30 mg. (15 to 100 mg.) up to four times a day

Phenobarbital Elixir, U.S.P. — 4 mg. in 1 ml.

Phenobarbital Tablets, U.S.P.; Phenobarbitone Tablets, B.P., I.P. — 15, 30, 60, and 100 mg.

Sodium Phenobarbital, U.S.P., I.P.; Phenobarbitone, B.P. — Dose is the same as for phenobarbital

Sodium Phenobarbital, U.S.P. (I.P.) Sodium Phenobarbital Injection, N.F.; Phenobarbitone Injection, B.P. (I.P.) — Ampuls containing 120 and 300 mg. 150 mg. in 2 ml.; 300 mg. in 2 ml.

Sodium Phenobarbital Tablets, N.F. (I.P.); Phenobarbitone Sodium Tablets, B.P. — 30, 60, and 100 mg.

Sodium Phenobarbital Tablets (H.T.) — 50 and 60 mg.

Trade names: Luminal; Fenemal; Gardenal; Phenobarbyl; Somonal

Sodium Probarbital — 250 mg. (50 to 500 mg.) orally three times a day

Sodium Probarbital Elixir — 13 mg. in each milliliter

Sodium Probarbital Tablets — 250 mg.

Trade name: Ipral Sodium

Secobarbital, U.S.P.	100 mg. (50 to 200 mg.) up to three times a day
Secobarbital Elixir, U.S.P.	4.5 mg. in 1 ml.
Sodium Secobarbital, U.S.P., Quinalbarbitone Sodium, B.P.	100 mg. (50 to 200 mg.) orally up to three times a day
Sodium Secobarbital Capsules, U.S.P.; Quinalbarbitone Tablets, B.P.	50 and 100 mg.
Sodium Secobarbital, U.S.P.	Ampuls containing 250 mg.
Suppositories Secobarbital Sodium	Containing 32.5, 65, 130, or 200 mg.

Trade names: Seconal and Evronal Sodium

Talbutal Caplets	30, 50, and 120 mg.

Trade name: Lotusate

Sodium Thiamylal	3 to 6 ml. of a freshly prepared 2.5 per cent solution; maintenance, 0.5 to 1 ml. as required
Sodium Thiamylal for Injection, U.S.P.	Ampuls containing 500 mg., 1, 5, and 10 Gm.

Trade name: Surital Sodium

Thialbarbitone Sodium	

Trade names: Intranarcon; Kemithal

Sodium Thiopental, U.S.P.; Thiopentone Sodium, B.P.	2 to 3 ml. of a 2.5 per cent solution intravenously at a rate of 1 ml. every five seconds; maintenance dose, 0.5 to 1 ml. as required. Rectal dose, 45 mg. (25 to 45 mg.) per kilogram of body weight in 10 per cent solution
Sodium Thiopental for Injection, U.S.P.; Thiopentone Injection, B.P.	500 mg. and 1, 5, and 10 Gm.

Trade names: Pentothal Sodium; Intraval

Vinbarbital, N.F.	60 mg. orally
Vinbarbital Capsules, N.F.	30, 100, and 200 mg.
Sodium Vinbarbital	60 mg. intramuscularly or subcutaneously
Sodium Vinbarbital Injection, N.F.	5-ml. ampuls and 20-ml. vials containing 60 mg. in 1 ml.

Trade name: Delvinal Sodium

OTHER HYPNOTIC AND SEDATIVE DRUGS

In addition to the barbiturates, a number of other drugs are used to produce sedation and sleep. They are chloral hydrate, chlorobutanol, paraldehyde, sodium bromide, carbromal, methylparafynol, methyprylon, ethchlorvynol, ethinamate, and glutethimide. Chlorpromazine, reserpine, meprobamate, and other sedatives are discussed in Chapter 19. Scopolamine (hyoscine), very useful as a sedative, is described in Chapter 30. Among the *antihistamine* drugs, discussed in Chapter 47, there are several that are used as sedatives, e.g., methapyrilene, promethazine (see also pp. 760, 762), and chlorcyclizine. Methapyrilene is available without a prescription under several trade names. Several nonbarbiturate sedative-hypnotic agents are presented in Table 19, page 328.

Chloral Hydrate, U.S.P., B.P., I.P.

Chloral hydrate, the first synthetic hypnotic, was prepared in 1832. It was not used as a hypnotic until 1869. Chloral hydrate is a white crystalline substance with a disagreeable odor and taste.

Absorption, Fate, and Excretion. Chloral hydrate is readily absorbed from the gastrointestinal tract. It is irritating to the gastric mucosa and so is contraindicated in gastric and duodenal ulcer and chronic indigestion. It is reduced in the body to trichloroethanol, which is thought to be the sleep-producing metabolite. Trichloroethanol is conjugated with glycuronic acid and is excreted in the urine as urochloralic acid.

Pharmacological Actions. Chloral hydrate depresses the sensorimotor areas of the cerebral cortex. It is an excellent sedative and hypnotic; none is safer and more dependable. Drowsiness and sleep occur in 20 to 30 minutes and sleep lasts for about eight hours. The effects are confined to the cerebrum in therapeutic doses. There is no adequate theory to explain its action.

Tolerance and Habituation. Tolerance and habituation may occur. Tolerance is due to the increased capacity of the liver to conjugate chloral and its alcohol; consequently, repetitious doses may cause damage to the liver.

Toxicity. Large doses of chloral hydrate produce depression of the respiration. Paralysis of the respiration is the cause of death in toxic doses. The margin of safety is large. The fatal dose is from 3 to 30 Gm. Chloral hydrate should be given with care to persons with cardiac, kidney, or liver disease. Small therapeutic doses of 500 mg. orally, however, do not aggravate pre-existing pathological conditions.

A combination of chloral hydrate and alcohol is known in the vernacular as a "Mickey Finn" or "knockout drops." The depressant effect of the two drugs is additive. The preparation is not used in therapeutics.

Dosage and Method of Administration. Chloral hydrate is administered orally or rectally (oil-retention enema in children). The usual oral dose is 500 mg. (7½ grains) with a range of 250 mg. to 1 Gm. three times a day. It is often prescribed in sweetened flavored solution. Soft capsules comtaining the drug in solution form are now available.

Therapeutic Uses

1. To produce sedation in hysteria and hyperexcitability.
2. As a hypnotic in insomnia caused by anxiety and worry.

Preparations

Chloral Hydrate Syrup, U.S.P.   500 mg. of chloral hydrate in each
                                                                teaspoonful
Chloral Hydrate Capsules, U.S.P. (red,   250 and 500 mg.
blue, green)
Chloral Hydrate Suppositories   Containing 1.3 Gm.

Trade names: Felsules; Lorinal; Noctec; Somnos

Paraldehyde, U.S.P., B.P.

Paraldehyde is a clear, colorless, oily liquid with a strong, pungent odor and a very disagreeable taste. It is sparingly soluble in water.

Pharmacological Actions. Paraldehyde depresses mainly the sensory areas of the cerebral cortex. It produces drowsiness and sleep in 10 to 15 minutes without preliminary excitement. The sleep lasts four to eight hours. The medullary centers are not depressed in therapeutic doses, and there are no effects noted on other tissues or organs of the body. When the hypnotic dose is increased, profound sleep and analgesia result. Paraldehyde is less potent than chloral hydrate. The sleep is normal and there are few, if any, aftereffects.

Absorption, Fate, and Excretion. Paraldehyde is readily absorbed from the gastrointestinal tract. From 11 to 28 per cent is excreted by the lungs hence the penetrating characteristic odor which is quite detectable when the patient is receiving the drug. A small amount is excreted in the urine. The remainder is metabolized, probably in the liver, to carbon dioxide and water.

Dosage and Method of Administration. Paraldehyde is administered orally in doses of 8 ml. (1 to 30 ml.) up to three times a day. It is administered orally in ice water, cold aromatic elixir, or syrup. Paraldehyde is administered rectally, dissolved in water or oil. Oil minimizes its rectal irritation. The intramuscular dose is 5 ml. The B.P. intramuscular dose is 2 to 8 ml. By rectal injection as a basal anesthetic, the dose is 15 to 30 ml.

Therapeutic Uses

1. As a sedative in bromide psychoses, maniacal hallucinations, morphine disorientation, and delirium tremens. It lessens fear, anxiety, and hysteria.
2. To produce sleep.
3. In obstetrics, during labor.
4. As a basal anesthetic.

Toxicity. Overdosage with paraldehyde may produce coma with depression of the respiration and circulation and a fall in blood pressure. Death is rarely caused by excessive overdosage. The margin of safety is wide, one patient having recovered after a dose of 150 ml.

THE BROMIDES

The use of bromides in medicine began almost a century ago. These white crystalline salts with a salty, pungent taste have been largely replaced by phenobarbital and other anticonvulsant and sedative drugs.

Pharmacological Action. The bromides are depressant to the sensori-motor areas of the cortex. Their action is due to the bromide ion. The depression may vary from mild sedation to coma, according to the size of the dose. Large therapeutic doses depress many reflexes of the brain and spinal cord. By reducing the hyperexcitability of the cortex the bromides reduce the number and frequency of seizures in epilepsy. They have little or no effect on the pain centers. The irritability of the cough center is lessened.

After bromides are given for some time, mental alacrity is decreased and the patient is relaxed and indifferent. There is a feeling of unconcern and imperturbability. Concentration is impaired and mental confusion results. Sleep may result, but the bromides are weak hypnotics. Ordinary doses have little effect on the circulation. Large doses depress the heart and the vasoconstrictor center.

Absorption, Distribution, and Excretion. The bromides are absorbed rapidly from the gastrointestinal tract. High concentrations produce irritation of the gastric mucosa; therefore, the drugs should be well diluted or given with a large amount of fluid. They circulate in the body and are widely distributed in the body fluids; they are excreted very slowly in the urine and small amounts may be found there for two or three months.

Acute Poisoning. Acute poisoning with bromides is rare. Very large doses may produce marked disorientation, stupor, and collapse without other neurological signs.

Chronic Poisoning—Bromism. The symptoms of chronic bromide poisoning are gastrointestinal upset, fetid breath, lacrimation, coryza, excessive salivation, and a skin rash. Toxic psychoses such as hallucinations, delusions, and maniacal symptoms may be observed. Overdosage with bromides may produce a change in personality pattern. Diagnosis of bromide poisoning should be confirmed by blood bromide content.

When symptoms of overdosage are observed, the drug should be discontinued and appropriately large amounts of sodium chloride administered to hasten the elimination of the bromide. If the patient cannot take sodium chloride because of cardiac involvement, ammonium chloride may be substituted.

Therapeutic Uses

1. Mild sedation to relieve nervous tension.
2. Anticonvulsant in epilepsy.

Dosage and Method of Administration. The bromides are given by mouth in the form of effervescent tablets or salts or in elixirs to disguise the disagreeable taste. They are given after meals with plenty of fluids. The usual oral dose of sodium bromide, the bromide salt most frequently used, is 300 mg. (5 grains) three times a day.

Preparations

Sodium Bromide Elixir, N.F. 700 mg. in 4 ml.
Sodium Bromide Tablets 300 and 600 mg. (5 and 10 grains)

Methylparafynol (Dormison)

Methylparafynol, a nonbarbituric acid hypnotic that produces sedation and sleep, is an oily liquid with a disagreeable odor and taste. It is sealed in green gelatin capsules which contain 250 mg.

Pharmacological Action. Methylparafynol is much more potent in producing sleep than paraldehyde and about two fifths as potent as pentobarbital. Sleep, which occurs in 10 to 60 minutes, may last two hours, but the patient generally sleeps through the night. The drug is of little value as a sedative in ambulatory patients because it is difficult to control the dosage at the sedative level.

Absorption, Fate, and Excretion. Methylparafynol is readily absorbed on oral administration. It appears to be almost completely metabolized to carbon dioxide and water by the action of the liver and kidneys. A smaller amount seems to be metabolized by the brain.

Toxicity. The acute toxicity is low. The margin of safety is wide, and the side actions are few. The drug does not produce drowsiness on the following morning. Habituation seems to be minimal.

Dosage and Method of Administration. Methylparafynol is administered orally in doses of 250 to 500 mg. It is used in chronic insomnia. Capsules containing 250 mg. are available.

Methyprylon, N.F., B.P. (Noludar)

This new agent has sedative effects upon the central nervous system which can be produced in mild degree for daytime quieting effects in doses of 50 to 100 mg. three or four times daily, and in greater degree as a hypnotic and somnifacient (sleep-producing drug) at bedtime in doses of 200 to 400 mg. A 50-mg. dose is roughly equivalent to 15 mg. of phenobarbital. Blood counts, including differential white cell counts, should be made in prolonged use of this agent. The total daily dose should not exceed 400 mg.

Preparations

Methyprylon Elixir, N.F. 50 mg. in 5 ml.
Methyprylon Tablets, N.F., B.P., Scored 50 and 200 mg.
Trade name: Noludar

Ethchlorvynol, N.F. (Placidyl)

This new agent is used for the treatment of ordinary insomnia, usually with oral bedtime doses of 500 mg. It acts rather promptly in most individuals, with a duration of action of approximately five hours. Ethchlorvynol is readily absorbed from the intestinal tract and metabolized and inactivated to an appreciable extent by the liver. The hypnotic effects are not so great or so predictable as with the barbiturates, but the drug appears to be safe and to produce no "hangover" effects the following day. Wide usage may reveal disadvantages that are not known at this time. Capsules of 100, 200, and 500 mg. are marketed.

Glutethimide, N.F., B.P. (Doriden)

This sedative is also alleged to produce sedation and tranquillity without lessening the individual's dexterity or acuity. It causes some autonomic nervous system depression but does not affect the blood pressure or heart rate in ordinary doses.

A dose of 250 mg, of glutethimide is used at bedtime for producing sleep, and is approximately equivalent in potency to 50 mg. of the faster-acting barbiturates such as secobarbital. Doses of 125 mg. several times daily may be effective in quelling hyperactive behavior and mental disturbances. Effects

---

Table 19

Additional Nonbarbiturate Hypnotic and Sedative Agents

Approved and Trade Names	Dosage and Methods of Administration	Preparations
Acetylcarbromal (Abasin, Car- based)	Orally 260 to 600 mg. t.i.d. or q.i.d.	Tablets: 260 and 300 mg.
Bromisovalum (Bromural)	Orally. Sedative: 300 mg. t.i.d. Hypnotic: 600 to 900 mg. at h.s.	Tablets: 300 mg. Powder: 1-oz. bottles
Carbromal, B.P. (Adalin, Broma- dal, Nyctal, Plan- adalin, Uradal)	Orally. Sedative: 300 to 600 mg. t.i.d. or q.i.d. Hypnotic 600 to 900 mg. at h.s.	Capsules: 300 mg.
Petrichloral (Pentaerythritol Chloral, Peri- chlor)	Orally. Sedative: 300 mg. t.i.d. Hypnotic: 600 mg. to 1.2 Gm. at h.s.	Capsules: 300 mg.
Ethinamate, N.F. (Valmid)	Orally, 500 mg. to 1 Gm. 20 min- utes before retiring	Tablets: 500 mg.

are immediate, as with simple sedatives, beginning two or three hours after ingestion and lasting for four to six hours. Tablets of 250 and 500 mg. are available.

ANTIHISTAMINES

Most antihistamines produce sedative actions as a side effect. Methapyrilene (see p. 762) and the phenathiazine antihistamines are used primarily for this effect.

Propiomazine Hydrochloride (Largon)

This agent, a phenothiazine antihistamine, is used as a hypnotic prior to general anesthesia for surgery, during parturition, and in nighttime sedation. It enhances the sedative effects of the barbiturates and other central nervous system depressants including morphine, meperidine, etc. Dosage of the barbiturates should be decreased to one half when used with propiomazine, and that of the narcotics by one quarter to one half. Due care of the patient made drowsy by the drug should be taken.

Dosage and Administration. Propiomazine is given intramuscularly and intravenously in doses of 10 to 30 mg. Repeated medication is usually not required in surgery, labor, or nighttime sedation, but doses may be given as needed every three or more hours.

Preparation

Propiomazine Hydrochloride Solution 1- and 2-ml. ampuls containg 20 mg. in 1 ml.

Trade name: Largon

Magnesium Sulfate, U.S.P., B.P.

Magnesium sulfate is used in the treatment of eclampsia and other convulsive syndromes. Side effects are depression of the heart and central nervous system, particularly the respiration. The intramuscular dose is 1 to 2 Gm. in a 25 or 50 per cent solution. This may be followed by 1 Gm. every 30 minutes until relief is obtained. The intravenous dose is 3 ml. of a 5 per cent solution, cautiously, until relaxation occurs. It is available as an injection containing 100 mg. in 20 ml., 500 mg. in 2 ml., 2.5 Gm. in 10 ml., 1 Gm. in 2 ml., 2.5 Gm. in 5 ml., and 5 Gm. in 10 ml.

REVIEW QUESTIONS

1. *Outline the pharmacological responses to the barbiturates.*
2. *Name four groups into which the barbiturates are classified. Give one example of each.*
3. *Discuss the fate of phenobarbital in the body.*

4. Explain the mechanism of action of pentobarbital medication prior to local anesthesia.
5. Name five clinical conditions for which barbiturates are administered.
6. Give the adult dose, principal use, route of administration, and another name for the following drugs:

Phenobarbital   _____   _____   _____   _____
Pentobarbital   _____   _____   _____   _____
Mephobarbital   _____   _____   _____   _____
Secobarbital   _____   _____   _____   _____
Amobarbital   _____   _____   _____   _____

7. Discuss habituation and tolerance to barbiturates.
8. Describe acute barbiturate poisoning and outline the treatment.
9. Name three other sedative and hypnotic drugs. Give dose and method of administration of each.

REFERENCES

BARBITURATES

Batterman, R. C.: "The Evaluation of Sedatives," *J. Am. Geriat. Soc.*, **4**:172, 1956.
Committee on Advertising: "Current Concepts in Therapy of Sedative Hypnotic Drugs," *New England J. Med.*, **255**:520, 1956; **256**:77, 1957.
Isbell, H.: "Addiction to Barbiturates and the Barbiturate Abstinence Syndrome," *Ann. Int. Med.*, **33**:108, 1950.
Isbell, H., and Fraser, H. F.: "Addiction to Analgesics and Barbiturates," *Pharmacol. Rev.*, **2**:355, 1950.
Louw, A., and Sonne, L. M.: "Megimide in the Treatment of Barbituric-Acid Poisoning," *Lancet*, **271**:961, 1956.
Plum, F., and Swanson, A. G.: "Barbiturate Poisoning Treated by Physiological Methods," *J.A.M.A.*, **163**:827, 1957.
Shulman, A.; Shaw, F. H.; Cass, N. M.; and Whyte, H. M.: "A New Treatment of Barbiturate Poisoning," *Brit. M. J.*, **1**:1238, 1955.
"Treatment of Barbiturate Poisoning" (editorial), *Brit. M. J.*, **2**:1107, 1956.

GLUTETHIMIDE

Cohen, H.: "Primary Glutethimide Addiction," *New York J. Med.*, **60**:280, 1960.

19

Drugs Used in the Treatment of Mental Illness

The value of drugs in treating patients with psychiatric problems has received considerable attention in recent years. Many medications have been introduced, some of which seem to be very effective with selected patients. At the present time, however, drugs should not be viewed as a panacea for mental illness. Rather, drugs are utilized in conjunction with other appropriate therapeutic measures. For information concerning other valuable treatment methods, students are referred to the literature on psychiatry and psychiatric nursing.

The physician's decision to prescribe drugs, the drug selected, and how it is administered vary according to the individual needs of the patient and the subsequent treatment goals.

Varying reactions to a drug may be observed in different persons. Significant side effects must be promptly and accurately reported. A disturbed patient may not indicate symptoms, particularly if he is very sick and has difficulty communicating with other people. Therefore, it is especially important for the individual working with the mentally ill patient to be familiar with the drug being administered and to observe the patient for untoward reactions. Side effects must not be ignored on the basis of the assumption that they are due to psychological factors.

The feelings a patient may possess regarding medication depend on many factors, primarily his past experiences and the attitudes of the doctor and the nurse regarding his medications. The effect of a medication not only depends on the physiological action but is influenced by the patient's expectations. For example, some people may feel that drugs are the solution to their problems, and become impatient if rapid improvement is not noted. Others may hesitate to take medication because of fear of becoming too dependent on the drug. These examples illustrate feelings related to medication which may be significant to specific patients. The preparation and administration of drugs by the nurse have been discussed in Chapter 5. An additional precaution is to be absolutely certain that the patient has swallowed his medicine because he may dispose of it or save it and accumulate an overdose. This is particularly important with patients who may have suicidal thoughts.

331

THE TRANQUILIZING DRUGS

The term *tranquilizer* came into use with the introduction of two new classes of drugs having activities not earlier known or appreciated. These drugs are also called *ataractics* or ataraxic (peace of mind) agents. The first of these groups consisted of the *Rauwolfia sepentina* alkaloids, of which the best knows is reserpine. Since this group has now become second in importance in the treatment of mental disease, it will be discussed after the more extensively used phenothiazine derivatives.

Drugs of the phenothiazine and *Rauwolfia* groups relieve much of the mental anguish, anxiety, and hallucinations without producing appreciable sedation. These effects are obtained in both neurotic and psychotic patients. Noisy and hyperactive patients in mental institutions have been changed by these drugs into calm, cooperative persons, many of whom are able to be discharged in a short time as compared with prolonged or permanent residency without tranquilizer therapy. Some of the treated patients can return to their jobs; some are quite manageable at home or in an institution and are for the first time receptive to the psychiatrist's attempts to understand and work out some of their emotional problems. Some patients who are withdrawn, depressed, and quiet are usually not benefited by these drugs. Their depression may be deepened. Stimulant drugs may be useful in these cases. Older stimulants are discussed in Chapter 23, and newer ones later in this chapter (see pp. 348–53). The terms "psychic energizers" and "psychostimulants" are used to classify this new group.

THE PHENOTHIAZINES

Chlorpromazine Hydrochloride, U.S.P., B.P. (Thorazine)

Chlorpromazine was first used in Europe, under the trade name Largactil, as a hypothermic agent. The temperature of the mammalian body can be lowered by proper doses of this and similar drugs. Hypothermia is used in some surgical procedures (see pp. 289–90). The drug was also found to suppress nausea and vomiting in many conditions and was introduced in the United States (1954), Canada, and abroad mainly for this use. The tranquilizing effects of the drug were seen with increasing frequency, and its usefulness in hyperactive mental patients and in anxiety neuroses was soon established.

Pharmacological Properties of Chlorpromazine. *On the Brain.* Chlorpromazine depresses the reticular formation and the profuse thalamic projection system and diminishes alertness. Thus the patient becomes less sensitive to troublesome situations that would cause emotional responses. The psychotic is protected from hallucinations and terrifying flights of the imagination. The drug acts on the hypothalamus, depressing the sympathetic nervous system centrally, which is partially responsible for the vasodilatation of the blood vessels and the fall in blood pressure. Its action on the hypothalamus also causes a lowering of body temperature and the basal metabolic rate. Chlorpromazine depresses the chemoreceptor trigger zone (CTZ) in the medulla (see p. 380) and prevents the nausea and vomiting caused by certain drugs and that which occurs in various diseases (see Table 25, p. 381).

Other Actions. Chlorpromazine blocks the neurohormones in the autonomic nervous system and produces adrenolytic (vasodilatation) and anticholinergic (antispasmodic—dry mouth, etc.) effects. In addition, it has an antihistaminic action. It also potentiates the action of narcotics, anesthetics, and hypnotics.

Use of Chlorpromazine in Mental Disease. Chlorpromazine has shown great tranquilizing effects in emotional upsets such as anxiety and tension, in neuroses characterized by hyperactivity, agitation, and similar effects, and in certain types of schizophrenias, manias, and toxic and senile psychoses. Psychiatrists warn against the use of chlorpromazine and reserpine in some cases of obsessional neurosis and hysteria and in the depressive states.

A majority of the agitated hyperactive patients are greatly benefited by chlorpromazine, with cessation of hallucinations, fears, and antisocial behavior. Grossly disorderly conduct and thinking may become organized along normal or near-normal patterns. Patients who have required institutional confinement and close observation are often so much improved that they are discharged with fairly normal living and working capacities. The earlier in the course of the mental disease treatment is begun, the greater the success achieved. However, some patients are treated quite successfully after many years of confinement.

Treatment is prolonged, often up to 15 months. The conventional measures of psychotherapy, occupational therapy, rehabilitation, and occasionally electroconvulsive therapy, etc., are still employed with some patients under drug treatment. The important feature is the accessibility of the patient to psychiatric measures, made possible by the drug.

Use of Chlorpromazine in Other Conditions. Chlorpromazine is used (1) to control nausea and vomiting (see p. 381); (2) with other drugs to relieve intractable pain, as in cancer; (3) in anesthesiology to potentiate the action of general anesthetics; (4) to control hiccups; (5) in the treatment of status asthmaticus; and (6) in the treatment of alcoholism. Since chlorpromazine potentiates the action of depressants of the central nervous system, the dosage of narcotics or sedatives should be reduced to one fourth to one half of the prechlorpromazine level.

Side Effects. A number of untoward reactions have been encountered during the prolonged periods of treatment required with chlorpromazine in mental disease and at times in other conditions. Table 20 shows the types of side effects seen.

———————————————————————— Table 20 ————————————————————————

Side Effects in Chlorpromazine (Thorazine) Therapy

Excessive sedation, drowsiness	Nausea and vomiting
Tachycardia (rapid heart)	Convulsions
Hypothermia	Edema of face and ankles
Dryness of the mouth	Hypotension
Dermatitis, rashes	Parkinsonism (see p. 371)
Photosensitivity of skin	Jaundice, liver damage
Psychoses, euphoria, depression	Blood dyscrasias
Enlargement of the breasts	Menstrual changes

The frequency of occurrence of the more severe conditions listed in Table 20 is rather low. Reduction in the dosage usually abolishes the milder side effects. Some may be treated as indicated for the same reactions to reserpine (Table 21, p. 343). Jaundice has occurred in 1 to 2 per cent of cases. It has been investigated by means of needle biopsies and found to be associated with variable degrees of swelling and necrosis of the cells of the minute bile channels, which may be followed by destruction of liver cells in the central portions of the lobules. The tests give results similar to those produced by biliary tract disease, an *obstructive* type of jaundice. This complication represents an allergy-like reaction to chlorpromazine in sensitive individuals. Jaundice should be an indication for discontinuing the drug, at least until signs of liver damage have disappeared. Another suitable drug can then be employed, or chlorpromazine can be reinstituted with lower dosage and with regular laboratory tests performed to detect the return of jaundice. Jaundice usually appears within the first two weeks of therapy but may occur later.

Chlorpromazine and other phenothiazine derivatives sometimes cause extra-pyramidal symptoms which are usually transient and easily reversed. Symptoms of motor restlessness as tapping of the feet, an inability to sit still, and insomnia are experienced frequently with small doses. When higher dosage levels are used, dystonias or symptoms resembling parkinsonism may occur. Symptoms of dystonia may include spasm of the neck or limb muscles, extensor rigidity of back muscles, carpopedal spasm, and difficulty in swallowing. Pseudoparkinsonism presents symptoms such as masked facies, tremors, drooling, pillrolling motion, and shuffling gait. Treatment of these conditions includes dosage reduction, temporary discontinuance of the drug, or the administration of barbiturates or antiparkinsonism drugs.

Because of the tendency of chlorpromazine to reduce blood pressure, more markedly when the patient is standing, he should be kept in bed for an hour or longer after each dose if the intramuscular route is being used. He may be told to remain in a reclining or sitting position until any feelings of faintness or rapid pulse have subsided. Phenylephrine or levarterenol may be useful in controlling very low pressures.

Blood dyscrasias are rare, but those occurring may be fatal. Anemia has been seen but can be corrected, although this condition bears careful watching. Depression or disappearanace of the granulocytic white blood cells has occurred. The incidence is undoubtedly higher in cases treated for prolonged periods or with higher doses. Most cases reported have occurred between the fourth and tenth weeks of therapy.

Deaths have occurred from this agranulocytosis. Symptoms of the conditions include fever and sore throat. When these are present in patients receiving the drug, they should always be checked by blood counts because a reduction in the granulocytes is a positive indication for discontinuing the drug.

Dermatitis in patients and their nurses has been reported. Skin involvement has apparently been caused by handling of chlorpromazine. This danger is present where tablets are crushed or if the solution is allowed to be sprayed during the removal of air from syringes just prior to injection. For these reasons great care on the part of the nurses should be exercised while preparing and administering the drug. The crushing or dissolving of tablets and the contact with syrups and solutions of the drug should be avoided. Sterile cotton should be wrapped around the needle when air is removed from the syringe.

Dosage and Methods of Administration.   Chlorpromazine may be administered orally, intramuscularly, and intravenously. The onset of some of its actions is rapid, particularly with parenteral administration. Dosage usually varies, according to the severity of the patient's condition. The usual oral dose is 25 mg. four times a day (10 mg. to 1 Gm. daily). The intramuscular or intravenous dose is 25 mg. (25 mg. to 1 Gm.) daily.

Parenteral administration is reserved for special cases, such as patients who will not or cannot cooperate in oral medication, or who are in need of rapid effects. When intramuscular injections are given, they should be made in the upper outer quadrant of the buttock, deeply in the muscle, and very slowly. The site should be massaged, for these injections are irritating and may be quite painful. A local anesthetic or physiological saline solution may be used to dilute the drug when the regular strength is not tolerated. Hyaluronidase (p. 766) has been tried for lessening the irritation. The regular-strength solution should not be given intravenously or subcutaneously.

In surgery and in hiccups, when intravenous administration is ordered, it should be made with diluted material and either in divided doses or as a slow infusion from drop bottles. Nurses in repeated contact with solutions of chlorpromazine should use rubber gloves because of the danger of dermatitis.

The drug must be used with caution in conjunction with alcohol, narcotics (morphine, meperidine, etc.), or barbiturates because of potentiating effects on this group of drugs.

Preparations

Chlorpromazine Hydrochloride Tablets, U.S.P., B.P.	10, 25, 50, 100, and 200 mg.
Chlorpromazine Hydrochloride Injection, U.S.P., B.P.	25 mg. in 1 ml.; 50 mg. in 2 ml.; 250 mg. in 10 ml.
Chlorpromazine Hydrochloride Syrup, U.S.P.	10 mg. in 5 ml.

Trade names: Thorazine; Ampliactil; Amplictil; Hibernal; Largactil; Megaphen; Propaphenin

ADDITIONAL PHENOTHIAZINE TRANQUILIZERS

Since the exploitation of the unforeseen value of chlorpromazine in the treatment of mental disorders, many phenothiazine tranquilizers have been developed in the hope of obtaining other drugs with the same tranquilizing actions but with fewer and less severe side effects, such as liver damage, hypotension, drowsiness, Parkinson's symptoms, etc. (see p. 371). Some of these new derivatives are less potent but most of them are more potent than the original compound. The appearance of liver damage, drowsiness, and hypotension has been reduced in some cases. However, with greater care in the use of the phenothiazines, side effects are kept at a lower level than formerly for all drugs of this group. It should be considered that any of the side effects listed in Table 20 can occur with the new derivatives, especially with prolonged use or elevated dosage.

Prochlorperazine (Compazine)

This drug is available as two salts, **Prochlorperazine Maleate, U.S.P., B.P.,** for oral administration, and **Prochlorperazine Edisylate, U.S.P.,** for oral and parenteral administration. It is less potent than chlorpromazine and produces less drowsiness. Jaundice rarely occurs; however, Parkinson-like symptoms are seen more frequently than with chlorpromazine. The drug is widely used in milder emotional conditions; in higher doses, in psychoses. It is also used as a preoperative and obstetrical tranquilizer and has a very favorable action as an antiemetic. The oral or intramuscular dose as a tranquilizer or antiemetic ranges from 15 to 40 mg. daily in divided doses. For children weighing 20 to 30 lb., the maximum daily dose is 7.5 mg.; for those weighing 85 lb., 15 mg. The rectal and intravenous doses are in the same general range. Large doses up to 175 mg. daily may be used in institutional cases.

Preparations

Prochlorperazine Maleate Tablets, U.S.P., B.P.	5, 10, and 25 mg.
Prochlorperazine Capsules (sustained release)	10, 15, and 30 mg.
Prochlorperazine Edisylate Injection, U.S.P.	10 mg. in 2 ml:; 50 mg. in 10 ml.
Prochlorperazine Edisylate Syrup, U.S.P.	5 mg. in 5 ml.
Prochlorperazine Suppositories	2.5, 5, and 25 mg.

Trade name: Compazine

Trifluoperazine, B.P. (Stelazine)

This drug has a more potent and prolonged action (about 12 hours) than chlorpromazine. The same side effects noted for chlorpromazine may be observed. The most common one is drowsiness. Dizziness and Parkinson-like symptoms occur with high dosages or prolonged use. The oral dose is 1 mg. twice daily. The intramuscular dose is 1 to 2 mg. every four to six hours. Tablets of 1 mg. and an injection containing 10 mg. in 1 ml. are available.

Perphenazine, B.P. (Trilafon)

This drug has the same actions and uses and is about twice as potent as chlorpromazine. It produces less sedation but more Parkinson-like symptoms. It is administered orally, parenterally, or rectally. The intravenous use should be reserved for very severe vomiting or retching in surgery or persistent hiccups. The oral adult dose is 6 to 64 mg. daily in two to four divided doses. For children one to six years old, the dose is 2 mg. two or three times a day; 6 to 12 years of age, 2 to 4 mg. three or four times a day. The intramuscular dose is 5 mg., and the intravenous dose is 1 mg. or less per minute (diluted) by slow-drip infusion. No more than 5 mg. should be given at one time. It is available as an injection, 5 mg. in 1-ml. ampuls or 10-ml. vials; as a syrup, with 2 mg. in 5 ml.; as tablets of 2, 4, and 8 mg., "Repetabs" of 8 mg.; and as suppositories of 4 and 8 mg.

Triflupromazine Hydrochloride, B.P. (Vesprin)

The actions and side effects of this drug are similar to those observed for chlorpromazine. It is used for the management of psychotic patients, in the control of nausea and vomiting in a variety of conditions, and in the management of persons under treatment for excessive use of alcohol. The oral dose for adults and children over 12 years of age is 10 to 50 mg. three times a day, according to age, severity of symptoms, and whether or not the patient is in an institution. The intramuscular dose is 5 to 10 mg. The intravenous adult dose is 1 to 3 mg., repeated after four hours, if required. For children the dose is 2 mg. It is available as tablets of 10, 25, and 50 mg.; capsules of 100 mg.; an emulsion, 10 mg. in 1 ml., as an injection containing 10 or 20 mg. in 1 ml., a ¾-ml disposable unit (intramuscular), and suppositories (rectal), 35 and 70 mg.

Thiopropazate Hydrochloride (Dartal)

The actions, uses, and side effects are generally similar to those observed with chlorpromazine. The oral adult dose is 2 to 10 mg. three or four times a day. It is available as tablets of 2, 5, and 10 mg.

Promazine Hydrochloride, N.F., B.P. (Sparine)

The actions, uses, and side effects are similar to those of chlorpromazine. There is less hypotension and no jaundice has been reported. The oral, intramuscular, or intravenous dose is 25 to 300 mg. daily in divided doses. The maximum dose is 1 Gm. The drug is available as tablets of 10, 25, 50, 100, and 200 mg.; as a syrup, 10 mg. in 5 ml.; as an injection containing 25 and 50 mg. in 1 ml.; and as "Tubex" units containing 50 mg. in 1 ml. (for intramuscular use only).

Mepazine Acetate, Hydrochloride (Pacatal)

This drug calms patients with neuroses and psychoses but is less potent than chlorpromazine. The side effects are similar but less pronounced and less frequent. The ones sometimes noted are blurring of vision, dizziness, tremors, and urinary retention. No jaundice has been reported. The oral or intramuscular adult dose is 25 mg. three or four times a day, increasing by 25 mg. daily until optimal effects are attained. In more serious hospitalized cases, the daily dose is 100 to 400 mg. daily. The drug is available as tablets of 25, 50, and 100 mg. and an injection containing 25 mg. in 1 ml. The acetate is used for injection.

Methoxypromazine (Tentone)

The uses and side effects are the same as those given for mepazine. The oral dose is 30 mg. to 1.5 Gm. It is available as tablets of 10, 25, and 50 mg.

Fluphenazine (Permitil, Prolixin)

The action and side effects of this drug are similar to those of chlorpromazine, but it is more potent. It is used as a tranquilizer, in the treatment of psychoses, as an antiemetic, and to potentiate the actions of sedatives, narcotics, and anesthetics. The oral dose is 0.5 to 10 mg. daily, usually in divided doses. In severe cases of psychosis, 20 mg. may be given. It is available as tablets, 0.25 mg. (Permitil), and 1, 2.5, and 5 mg. (Prolixin).

Thioridazine, B.P. (Mellaril, Melleril)

This drug, a mercapto derivative, is a tranquilizer in anxiety and tension states. It may be used in psychoneurotic and personality disorders, including agitated depression and also the manic states. It is useful in the treatment of schizophrenia and in behavioral problems of children. It may be administered with other drugs in the treatment of rheumatoid disorders, cardiovascular diseases, in certain types of asthma, chronic gastrointestinal disturbances, alcoholism, and in gynecology and obstetrics. It is not an antiemetic. The side effects are fewer than with chlorpromazine. Extrapyramidal symptoms, hypotension, blood dyscrasias, and jaundice have not been experienced, although they may occur in hypersensitive patients or with overdosage. The drug is contraindicated in severely depressed or comatose conditions. The oral dose is 10 to 75 mg. three or four times a day, depending upon the severity of the symptoms. In hospitalized patients, 100 to 200 mg. may be administered. It is available as tablets containing 10, 25, and 100 mg.

Promethazine Hydrochloride, U.S.P., B.P. (Phenergan)

This is a very potent antihistamine (see Chap. 47) and was first used as such. It has all the general actions of chlorpromazine except that it has less adrenolytic activity. This drug is used for all purposes enumerated for the phenothiazine derivatives except that it is little used in psychoses. It is frequently used preoperatively, in obstetrics as a tranquilizer, and in the treatment of motion sickness (see p. 378). No cases of jaundice, hypotension, or blood dyscrasias have been reported. The adult oral or rectal dose is 25 mg. (6 to 50 mg.) four times a day or 50 mg. at bedtime on the night before surgery. Children receive one half the adult dose, with less for smaller children. The parenteral dose is 25 mg. up to 1 mg. per kilogram of body weight.

Preparations

Promethazine Hydrochloride Injection, U.S.P., B.P.	25 mg. in 1 ml.; 250 mg. in 10 ml.
Promethazine Hydrochloride Syrup, U.S.P.	20 mg. in 5 ml.
Promethazine Hydrochloride Tablets, U.S.P., B.P.	12.5 and 25 mg
Promethazine Suppositories	25 and 50 mg.

Trade name: Phenergan

Acetophenazine Dimaleate (Tindal)

This member of the phenothiazine group is used in the symptomatic relief of anxiety, excessive apprehension, hyperexcitability, etc. The possible side effects are those listed for chlorpromazine (p. 334).

Dosage.   Dosage should be individualized but usually is adequate when 20 mg. are given three times daily.

Preparation

Acetophenazine Dimaleate Tablets   20 mg.
Trade name: Tindal

Prothipendyl Hydrochloride (Timovan)

This agent is chemically similar to the phenothiazines and is used for the relief of tension in ambulatory patients, adolescents, geriatric cases, and others with anxieties. It should not be used in acute alcoholism.

Dosage.   Doses of 100 to 400 mg. daily in divided amounts may be given orally, depending upon age and the severity of the condition.

Preparation

Prothipendyl Hydrochloride Tablets   25 and 50 mg.
Trade name: Timovan

Chlorprothixine (Taractin) resembles the phenothiazines in its chemical structure, actions, and side effects but is not a member of this class. Its sedative action is greater than that of the average phenothiazine derivative, and it is believed to produce an improved sleep pattern. It is recommended for the treatment of mild to moderate neuroses and severe neurotic and psychotic states, and for the relief of vomiting. The average oral or intramuscular dose is 10 to 50 mg. three or four times a day.

Preparations

Chlorprothixine Injection   25 mg. in 2-ml. ampuls
Chlorprothixine Tablets   10, 25, and 50 mg.
Trade name: Taractin

RAUWOLFIA AND ITS ALKALOIDS

For generations, the roots of plants now bearing the generic name *Rauwolfia* have been used in India for quieting persons who were mentally disturbed and hyperactive. Hypertension, although not so prevalent in that country as in the United States, many years ago was benefited by extracts of this plant, commonly called *snakeroot*. These reports in Indian medical journals were eventually investigated in Europe, where the value of *Rauwolfia serpentina* in hypertension was confirmed. The powdered roots were introduced in the United States in 1953 for this purpose. The hypotensive and tranquilizing activities are found in some of the many alkaloids present in these roots. These alkaloids are extracted and constitute a preparation used today and known as alseroxylon. Both alseroxylon and the powdered whole root of *Rauwolfia* are used in the treatment of mental disease and hypertension. The important alkaloids are *reserpine* and *rescinnamine*. The purified alkaloid, deserpidine, is obtained from another species, *Rauwolfia canescens*.

Reserpine, U.S.P., B.P. (Serpasil)

Reserpine is the most widely used pure alkaloid of the *Rauwolfia* group. It is a tranquilizer with calming and mood-altering effects in mental disease.

Pharmacological Actions of Reserpine. *Action on the Hypothalamus.* Reserpine acts on the hypothalamus to produce sedation and relaxation. It does not depress the reticular formation, as do chlorpromazine and the barbiturates, so there is less sedative action. The untamed, fighting animal becomes docile, yet not necessarily sedated, upon treatment with reserpine. Reserpine also acts on the vasoconstrictor or vasomotor centers, or both, and on the vagal centers. These actions cause relaxation of the blood vessels, a lowering of blood pressure, and a bradycardia (slowing of the heart).

Other Actions. Dilatation of the blood vessels in the nasal membranes causes nasal congestion; increased secretion of gastric acid may account for the development of peptic ulcer in some patients receiving this drug. It is further suggested that continued reserpine therapy effects a degree of "functional sympathectomy," or paralysis or weakness, of the sympathetic nervous system through the depletion of epinephrine and of norepinephrine from the sympathetic postganglionic nerve endings.

Mechanism of Action. Reserpine causes the release of norepinephrine and serotonin from its binding sites in all sympathetic nerves everywhere, as in the arterioles, heart wall, brain, intestines, and salivary glands. Once released from its protected bound sites, it is quickly inactivated by enzymes. The drug also causes depletion of epinephrine and other related amines. Thus reserpine reduces sympathetic nervous activity. The tranquilizing effects and possibly the central hypotensive actions of reserpine are most likely caused by the depletion of all or some of such amines from the brain.

The Use of Reserpine in Mental Disease. The principal effects of *Rauwolfia* and reserpine in anxieties, hyperactivity, agitated psychoses, etc., are similar to those described for chlorpromazine (p. 333). The reader is also referred to the general discussion of the tranquilizers as a newer class of agents, page 332.

The improvement in moderately disturbed mental conditions is not usually achieved immediately upon institution of therapy. It is most often delayed for days or weeks and may be dependent upon the finding of the correct dosage. Improvement may begin within a week, with noticeable quieting to the patients. In some, this phase is followed by a period in which the behavior reverts somewhat to the agitation, tension, delusions, etc., which characterized their conditions before treatment was administered. This has been called the *turbulent* phase. With careful continuation or intensification of the treatment, many cases emerge from this type of recession into an *integrative* period with more lasting amelioration of the pattern. Basic psychotherapy can then be conducted with considerable degrees of success in rehabilitating the patients and, in such cases, the psychiatrist and the patient may make progress which was not otherwise possible. This opportunity to establish meaningful relationships is perhaps as important as the reversal of the psychopathology by a medicament. Properly utilized, it may be a determining factor in the permanence of the improvement.

Therapeutic Uses. Reserpine is used (1) as a tranquilizing drug in normal persons under temporary stress or strain; (2) in delirium tremens; (3) in various psychiatric disorders such as schizophrenia and paranoid and manic states; (4) in some cases of epilespy; (5) in premenstrual tension; (6) in the menopausal syndrome; (7) sometimes in headache (hypertensive and tension) ; (8) in some itching dermatoses; and (9) for increasing the appetite and weight. Its use in hypertension is a very important one and is discussed on pages 555–57.

Dosage and Method of Administration. Dosage varies according to the requirements of the patient. The oral and parenteral doses usually range from 0.25 mg. to 1 mg. daily, in two to three divided doses, decreasing to the minimum required as early as feasible. Absorption from the intestines is satisfactory, and the drug is usually given by mouth. The intramuscular or intravenous route is used for more rapid effect or when the patient is either uncooperative or incapable of swallowing and retaining tablets or a liquid form. Larger doses are required in more severe cases.

Preparations

Reserpine Tablets, U.S.P., B.P.	0.1, 0.25, 0.5, 1, 2, 4, and 5 mg.
Reserpine Elixir	0.2 mg. per 4 ml.
Reserpine Injection, U.S.P.	5 mg. in 2 ml.; 25 and 50 mg. in 10 ml.

Trade names: Crystoserpine, Rauloydin, Raurine, Rau-Sed, Reserpoid, Roxinoid, Sandril, Serfin, Serolfia, Serpanray, Serpasil, Serpiloid, Serpine

Side Effects. With the extensive and chronic use of reserpine, a large number of side reactions have been encountered. It is important to know these in order that they may be recognized when they appear, and thus be related to the drug. These undesirable effects as well as the types of treatment that may be used to counteract them are listed in Table 21. Occasionally it becomes necessary to decrease the dose of reserpine or to discontinue it altogether, temporarily or permanently.

Gastric hyperacidity may be caused by continued use of reserpine in doses of 0.3 mg. daily, and ulceration of the stomach and more severe depression may result from daily doses of 0.5 mg. or more.

Table 21

Side Effects Caused by Reserpine and Types
of Agents Useful in Treating Them

Side Effect	Treatment
Generalized tremulousness	Anticholinergics, antihistaminics, etc.
Hypotension, bradycardia	Phenylephrine, levarterenol, etc.
Drowsiness, fatigue	Stimulants, analeptics
Nasal stuffiness	Decongestants
Abdominal cramps, diarrhea, nausea, vomiting, ptyalism	Anticholinergics, antiemetics
Dizziness, diarrhea	Decrease in dosage or withdrawal
Muscle cramps, twitching, paresthesia, urinary frequency	Anticholinergics
Edema	Antihistaminics
Increase or decrease in appetite, thirst	Dietary control or anorexic agents
Parkinson-like symptoms (extrapyramidal syndrome)	Antiparkinsonism agents
Dermatitis	Antihistaminics
Blurring of vision	Change of glasses if warranted
Impotence, lactation, menstrual irregularities	None, or decrease in dosage
Convulsions, peptic ulcer	Conventional measures and withdrawal of reserpine
Signs of disturbances in the midbrain (fever, ocular palsy, incoordinate movements, anorexia, confusion)	Withdrawal or decrease in dosage
Psychological effects, variable from deep depression, with suicidal attempts, to turbulence	Variable among agents above. Withdrawal of reserpine usually mandatory when depression occurs.

Rescinnamine, N.F. (Moderil)

This alkaloid has been extracted from *Rauwolfia serpentina* and is available for treatment of those conditions for which reserpine is used, namely, mental disorders and hypertension. It appears to have the same order of potency as that of reserpine, which it closely resembles, but is not so widely used. The side effects produced by rescinnamine are the same as those of reserpine, although sedation and bradycardia are usually less frequent and of milder degree.

Dosage and Method of Administration. Oral dosage is individualized and kept minimal in order to keep side effects minimal. The usual dose is 0.25 mg. twice daily for up to two weeks, followed by decreases compatible with the therapeutic aims.

Preparation

Rescinnamine Tablets, N.F.   0.25, 0.5, and 1 mg.
Trade name: Moderil

Deserpidine (Canescine, Harmonyl)

Deserpidine is the generic name now applied to canescine, an alkaloid from *Rauwolfia canescens*. It is very similar to reserpine and rescinnamine and approximately equal to them in potency and side effects. It is administered orally in mental and hypertensive patients, in doses of 0.1 to 3 mg. daily, in divided amounts, according to the severity of the condition. Two to three milligrams are given to psychotic cases in institutions.

Preparation

Deserpidine Tablets   0.1, 0.25, and 1.0 mg.
Trade name: Harmonyl

Rauwolfia Serpentina, N.F. (Raudixin, Rauserpa, Rauval, Rauwistan)

Rauwolfia is the powdered whole root. It produces the same therapeutic responses in emotional, mental, and hypertensive diseases as do the pure alkaloids. Most of these activities are accounted for by its reserpine and rescinnamine content. It is administered orally, usually in doses of 100 to 150 mg. twice daily. The minimum dose should be determined for each patient.

Preparation

Rauwolfia Serpentina Tablets, N. F.   50, 100 mg.
Trade names: Raudixin, Rauserpa, Rauval, Rauwistan

Alseroxylon (Rau-Tab, Rautensin, Rauwiloid)

Alseroxylon is the fat-soluble alkaloidal fraction of the roots of *R. serpentina* and owes its therapeutic actions and its side effects to reserpine and rescinnamine, which comprise most of the preparation. Its average oral adult dose is 2 to 3 mg. daily. Orally, 1 mg. is approximately equivalent to 0.2 mg. of reserpine.

Preparation

Alseroxylon Tablets   2 mg.
Trade names: Rau-Tab, Rautensin, Rauwiloid

DIPHENYLMETHANE DERIVATIVES

These drugs resemble the antihistamines and antispasmodics in action. They are recommended for oral use to relieve tension and anxiety and for parenteral use in acutely disturbed or hysterical patients. Drowsiness may occur, and the action of the barbiturates is potentiated. These agents are comparatively weak in action and have not gained widespread use.

————————————— **Table 22** —————————————

Diphenylmethane Derivatives

Approved and Trade Names	Dosage and Methods of Administration	Preparations
Azacyclonal Hydrochloride (Frenquel)	Orally: 20 to 100 mg. t.i.d. I.v.: 100 mg. q. 4 to 8 h. for 1 to 7 days	Tablets: 20 mg. Injection: 5 mg. in 1 ml. in 20-ml. ampuls
Hydroxyzine Hydrochloride (Atarax, Vistaril)	Orally: 25 mg. t.i.d. I.m: 50 to 100 mg. q. 4 h.	Tablets: 10, 25, and 100 mg. Syrup: 2 mg. in 1 ml. Injection: 25 mg. in 1 ml.; 10-mg. vials. Atarax (oral), Vistaril parenteral)
Benactyzine Hydrochloride (Phobex, Suavital)	Orally: 1 mg. q.i.d. to 5 mg. t.i.d.	Tablets: 1 and 5 mg.
Captodiamine Hydrochloride (Suvren)	Orally: 100 mg. t.i.d. or q.i.d.	Tablets: 50 and 100 mg.
Buclizine Hydrochloride (Vibazine)	Orally: 50 to 100 mg. q.i.d. to t.i.d.	Tablets: 25 and 50 mg.

Chlordiazepoxide Hydrochloride, N.F. (Librium)

Chlordiazepoxide hydrochloride is a new type of drug that is useful for the relief of irrational fears, anxiety, and tension. It promotes muscular relaxation and has a "taming" action on wild animals (e.g., tigers and monkeys) in doses considerably lower than those required to produce sedation.

Dosage and Method of Administration.   In the treatment of moderate anxiety and tension the drug is given orally in doses of 10 mg. three or four times a day. For geriatric patients and children, 10 mg. are given once a day; however, some children may require 10 mg. two or three times daily.

Side Effects.   Minor side effects, such as nausea, constipation, and skin rashes, are infrequent and mild and may be controlled quickly by reduction of dosage. In elderly and debilitated patients, ataxia and drowsiness have been reported.

Therapeutic Uses.   Chlordiazepoxide hydrochloride is used in low dosage to lessen moderate anxiety, tension, tension headache, and behavior disorders in children. In higher doses it is useful in chronic alcoholism, agitated depression, acute and chronic anxiety states, and hysterical or panic states. Up to 500 mg. a day may be given until agitation is controlled, at which time the dose should be reduced.

Preparation

Chlordiazepoxide Hydrochloride Capsules, N.F.   10 mg.

Trade name: Librium

THE MUSCLE-RELAXING TRANQUILIZERS

There is a group of mildly to moderately potent tranquilizers which have a relaxant effect upon the skeletal muscles of the body. Some observers have raised the question regarding the probability that the latter action may alone cause a feeling of complacency. Others feel that the depressant action, known to occur in the spinal cord and to cause muscle relaxation, may also occur in areas of the brain where suppression of activity may produce tranquilization. There are spinal suppressant drugs with muscle-relaxant effects that do not have tranquilizing effects. These are discussed in Chapter 20, along with the pharmacological properties of the entire group, as they relate to the nature of the suppression of certain spinal reflex activity.

Meprobamate, N.F., B.P. (Equanil, Miltown)

This drug has a depressant effect inside the spinal cord and in certain areas of the brain. It has a relaxant effect upon skeletal muscles because of this depressant action (see pp. 367–68). In this regard it is similar to mephenesin (p. 368) but is much longer acting. Meprobamate is employed also for its tranquilizing action, in the same sense as reserpine and chlorpromazine. The drug is not very effective in the more severe cases, but it is used in moderately tense and anxious patients, including alcoholics. The muscular relaxation ascribed to meprobamate is thought to provide better sleeping.

Toxic Effects.   Side reactions to meprobamate consist mainly of skin eruptions, some of which have been widespread and severe. These have been purpuric (skin hemorrhage), petechial (minute hemorrhage), and erythematous lesions. Itching and swelling have accompanied many of these reactions. Fever, chills, weakness of extraocular muscles with diplopia (double vision), drowsiness, excessive peristalsis, and diarrhea have been reported. Cases of overdosage with 6 to 38 tablets have been reported in which the patients were comatose, presented marked flaccidity of skeletal muscles, and had dangerously low blood pressure. They were successfully treated, the methods including the use of phenylephrine and nikethamide. It has been established that two tablets (800 mg.) do not impair driving skill, visual reaction time, steadiness, or depth perception.

Emotional dependence, tolerance with a tendency to increase the dosage of meprobamate, and withdrawal symptoms may occur if care is not exercised during the use of this agent. Convulsions have followed abrupt cessation of medication when excessive, e.g., 6.4 Gm. daily.

Dosage and Method of Administration.   For sedative effects and for decreasing muscle spasm, an oral dose of 400 mg. three or four times daily is usually sufficient. Twice this amount may be necessary, and even this may fail to produce desired results. Reserpine or chlorpromazine may be needed for greater effects.

Preparation

Meprobamate Tablets, N.F., B.P.   200 mg. and 400 mg.
Meprobamate Capsules   400 mg., sustained release
      Trade names; Equanil; Meprosan (sustained-release form), Miltown

Chlormezanone (Trancopal)

Chlormezanone represents an entirely new chemical group in pharmacology, the metathiazanones. It suppresses nerve impulses in the brain as well as in the spinal cord, and is a potent agent in relaxing spastic skeletal muscles associated with backache, intervertebral disk syndrome, neck pain, bursitis, arthritis, sprains, etc.

Chlormezanone has a tranquilizing action which is useful in the treatment of anxiety and tension states. It is effective in primary dysmenorrhea and premenstrual tension, and of some value in asthma and angina pectoris. The compound is rapidly absorbed after oral administration, acts within 15 to 30 minutes (if the stomach is empty), and is effective for four to six hours.

Side Effects. Side effects are rare, occurring in only 2 to 3 per cent of patients, and thus far they have not been serious. They include nausea, drowsiness, dizziness, weakness, rash, flushing, depression or nervousness, and constipation or diarrhea. Treatment has been continued in most patients exhibiting side effects; however, the dosage is often decreased.

Dosage and Method of Administration. At present the drug is given orally, 100 to 200 mg. three or four times daily in adults and half this amount in children.

Preparation

Chlormezanone Tablets (elongated,   100 and 200 mg.
peach)
              Trade name: Trancopal

Phenaglycodol (Ultran)

This compound, a weak muscle relaxant, is described as a tranquilizer with the usual actions in agitated, anxious patients with no effect upon mental acuity. It has been studied in normal persons by means of psychological techniques and found not to decrease efficiency of thought, reactions, finger dexterity, etc., at doses of 400 mg. four times daily. Meprobamate was included at equal doses with similar results. Phenaglycodol is effective against epilepsy associated with focal (localized) brain damage. Therapeutic results are usually attained at doses of 300 mg. three or four times daily in appropriate cases.

Doses of 400 to 600 mg. may be taken before retiring to promote sleep. Side effects have not thus far been encountered at these levels.

Preparation

Phenaglycodol Tablets	200 mg.
Phenaglycodol Capsules (turquoise and white)	300 mg.

Trade name: Ultran

MISCELLANEOUS ADDITIONAL TRANQUILIZERS

Several additional agents (Table 23) are included in the group of muscle-relaxing tranquilizers. They produce mild to moderate tranquilizing effects in the less severe emotional illnesses and the same side effects as meprobamate.

——— Table 23 ———

Approved and Trade Names	*Miscellaneous Tranquilizers* Dosage and Methods of Administration	Preparations
Ectylurea (Nostyn)	Orally: 400 mg. t.i.d. or q.i.d.	Tablets: 400 mg.
Ethylcamate (Nuncital, Striatran)	Orally: 400 mg. t.i.d. or q.i.d. with meals	Tablets: 200 mg.
Hydroxyphenamate (Listica)	Orally: q.i.d.	Tablets: 200 mg.
Mephenoxalone (Trepidone)	Orally: 400 mg. q.i.d.	Tablets: 400 mg.
Metaxalone (Skelaxin)	Orally: 400 mg. q.i.d.	Tablets: 400 mg.
Oxanamide (Quiactin)	Orally: 400 mg. t.i.d. or q.i.d.	Tablets: 400 mg.

THE PSYCHOSTIMULANTS

A group of drugs unrelated chemically has been recently developed which has a stimulating and energy-producing action found to be quite useful in patients with depression of mood. This condition can be quite severe and disabling and is seen rather frequently in medical practice. Prior to the development of these newer drugs, called *psychostimulants* or *psychic energizers*, apathetic and depressed patients were treated with caffeine and the amphetamines, which are discussed in Chapter 23. The amphetamines have the disadvantage of causing a rise in blood pressure, an increase in the heart rate, and a decrease in the appetite. Caffeine has less potency than the newer drugs.

Of these recently developed stimulants, the group of monoamine oxidase inhibitors has attracted the most attention.

MONOAMINE OXIDASE INHIBITORS

There are many new drugs having as their chief characteristic the ability to inhibit oxidation in the body of normal chemical compounds that have one amino group in their structure. Such chemical compounds are usually rendered inactive when oxidized; hence their functions in the body are prolonged and perhaps increased by the "protective" action of the monoamine oxidase (MAO) inhibitors. These drugs are notable by virtue of their actions as (1) stimulants of the central nervous system, (2) depressants of blood pressure, and (3) prophylactics in angina pectoris (see p. 546). Among the important amines spared from normal destruction in the tissues are epinephrine, norepinephrine, and serotonin, all of which have actions within the brain and in the regulation of blood pressure.

The monoamine oxidase inhibitors include isocarboxazid, nialamid, phenylzine dihydrogen sulfate, tranylcypromine, and pargyline. They may stimulate the mood in depression, relieve pain in angina pectoris, and are used in the treatment of rheumatoid arthritis. The side effects are the same for all with a few exceptions, which will be noted. They produce lowering of blood pressure, dizziness, vertigo, constipation, overactivity, jitteriness, insomnia, weakness, fatigue, dryness of the mouth, blurred vision, skin rashes, and hepatitis. Many of these are rare or mild. Nialamid may cause headache, sweating, and insomnia; phenylzine causes stomach upsets. There have been reports recently of severe and even fatal hypertension associated with severe headache and intracranial bleeding, particularly with tranylcypromine. Other symptoms observed are palpitation, stiffness and soreness of the neck, nausea, vomiting and sweating (sometimes with fever and sometimes with cold clammy skin), dilated pupils, photophobia, constricting chest pain, and tachycardia, bradycardia, and other arrhythmias. Phentolamine mesylate (5 mg.) intravenously or pentolinium tartrate (3 mg.) subcutaneously may be used to reduce blood pressure.

Contraindications. The drugs should not be administered to patients with a confirmed or suspected cerebrovascular defect or cardiovascular disease, hypertension, or pheochromocytoma.

Precautions. Hypertensive crises have occurred in patients receiving the drugs in this group after the ingestion of strong or aged varieties of cheese. This is thought to be due to the tyramine content of this food. Patients should be warned not to eat cheese or take drugs containing pressor amines (epinephrine, ephedrine) or certain antihistaminic agents as occur in cold remedies, hay fever preparations, or anorexiants, or drink alcoholic beverages.

Since these drugs may cause hypotension, they should not be given with other drugs having hypotensive actvity such as meperidine and other narcotic analgesics, barbiturates, phenothiazine derivatives and the thiazide diuretics.

They should not be given with reserpine or guanethidine (which releases norepinephrine) (see p. 556) or antidepressants such as imipramine and amitriptylene.

Dosage and Methods of Administration and Preparations

Isocarboxazid (Marplan	Orally. 30 mg. daily in single or divided doses; reduce to 20, 10, or 5 mg. daily if benefits permit. Liver-function test should be performed. Use care when other drugs are administered, as it may potentiate their action.	Tablets, 10 mg. (yellow)
Nialamid (Niamid)	Orally. 75 mg. daily in single or divided doses. Revise gradually upward or downward after one week.	Tablets, 25 mg. (pink) and 100 mg. (orange)
Phenylzine Dihydro-Sulfate, Phenelzine Sulphate, B.P. (Nardil)	Orally. 15 mg. three or four times a day, reducing if possible.	Tablets, 15 mg. (orange)

Tranylcypromine Sulfate (Parnate)

This is a potent monoamine oxidase inhibitor which acts more promptly than other members of the group. Its actions, side effects, and precautions in its use are the same as those listed above. Hypertensive crises have been noted more often with this drug than with others of this group.

Therapeutic Use.   The use of tranylcypromine should be reserved for the symptomatic treatment of patients with severe, disabling, and potentially fatal mental depression for whom electroconvulsive therapy is undesirable or inappropriate and who do not respond satisfactorily to other antidepressant therapy. It should be limited to patients under close observation, preferably in a hospital, or very cautiously in nonhospitalized depressed patients. The possibility of suicide is always present.

Dosage and Method of Administration.   The recommended initial dose is 20 mg. daily. Subsequent doses are adjusted in accordance with the patient's response.

Preparation

Tranylcypromine Sulfate Tablets   10 mg.
Trade name: Parnate

Pargyline (Eutonyl) is discussed with the hypertensive drugs (see p. 564).

ADDITIONAL PSYCHOSTIMULANTS

Imipramine Hydrochloride, N.F., B.P. (Tofranil)

This drug stimulates the mood in various types of depression without euphoria or psychokinetic stimulation. Its mechanism of action is not known at this time. The side effects are dryness of the mouth, rapid pulse, constipation, visual disturbances, tremors, weight gain, and urinary frequency and retention. Parkinson-like symptoms, skin rash, and transient jaundice have also been reported. The drug should be used with caution in glaucoma and prostatic hypertrophy. It should not be used in combination with or immediately following monamine oxidase inhibitors as psychotic reactions have been reported in these situations. The initial oral or intramuscular dose is 100 mg. daily. This can be increased by 25 mg. every few days up to 200 mg. daily in divided doses depending upon the patient's reaction.

Preparations

Imipramine Injection, N.F.	25 mg. in 2 ml.
Imipramine Tablets, N.F.	25 mg.

Trade name: Tofranil

Methylphenidate (Ritalin) Hydrochloride, N.F.

This agent is intermediate between caffeine and amphetamine (Chap. 23) in its stimulant effects upon the brain. It does not usually, but may, decrease the appetite, as does amphetamine. It is useful in treating depressions of various types, including those produced by the tranquilizers. It may improve the mood and mental alacrity in dejected persons. It has been employed to hasten recovery following surgery with barbiturate anesthesia (Chap. 18).

Side Effects. Nervousness, palpitation, insomnia, dizziness, headache, and nausea may occur but are infrequent with usual doses. Increase in blood pressure and pulse rate may occur during intravenous use.

Dosage and Methods of Administration. Adults may be given orally 10 mg. two or three times daily for mood elevation. When greater or more rapid effects are needed, as in deep drug-induced depressions, 10 to 50 mg. may be given subcutaneously, intramuscularly, or intravenously, as often as every 30 minutes. Parenteral solutions prepared by the pharmacist or nurse should be used within two months. A special solvent is supplied with lyophilized powder in vials. Solutions must not be added to barbiturate infusions.

Preparations

Methylphenidate Hydrochloride Tablets, N.F.	5, 10, and 20 mg.
Methylphenidate Hydrochloride Injection, N.F.	100 mg. in vials

Trade name: Ritalin

Pipradrol (Meratran) Hydrochloride, N.F.

Pipradrol is a cortical and subcortical stimulant with apparent beneficial effects in depression states. It may produce mild overactivity, insomnia, and anorexia if dosage is not well controlled. It is administered orally to adults in doses of 1 to 2.5 mg. three times daily. No dose is recommended for children at the present time.

Preparation

Pipradrol Hydrochloride Tablets	1 and 2.5 mg.
	Trade name: Meratran

Deanol Acetamidobenzoate (Deaner)

Deanol is thought to be the precursor of choline in the brain, where it is available for the synthesis of acetylcholine. This hormone is described on pages 442–43, with regards to role in the functioning of the autonomic nervous system. Its role in the brain is little understood.

Pharmacological Action. In man, deanol produces a mild stimulation after seven to ten days with a daily oral dose of 10 to 50 mg. This stimulation is associated with decreased fatigability and shorter sleeping time. In doses above 25 mg. per day, increased muscle tone may occur, particularly in the neck, the masseter (a chewing muscle), and the anterior thigh muscles (quadriceps). This may be associated with an increased action of acetylcholine at the motor end-plates (see p. 415). An increased ability to concentrate has been noted in normal volunteers. It should not be used in epileptic patients, with the exception of those with petit mal, who may be benefited by the drug.

Side Effects. These are (in order of decreasing frequency): occipital headache, constipation, the muscle tenseness described above, insomnia, itching, postural hypotension, and weight loss. The latter two are rare and are usually associated with overdosage.

Dosage and Method of Administration. Deanol is given orally. The initial daily (morning) dose is 50 mg. The maintenance dose is usually 25 to 100 mg. daily. Children may be given an appropriate lower dosage.

Preparations

Deanol Tablets	25 mg.
	Trade name: Deaner

Amitriptyline Hydrochloride (Elavil)

Amitriptyline hydrochloride, an anticholinergic agent (see text Chap. 30) is reported to have a stimulatory, mood-elevating action in depressions of various types (see p. 398). It is also believed to reduce anxiety and tension in certain cases. Side effects are generally mild at usual doses and include drowsiness, dizziness, nausea, excitement, lowering of blood pressure, headache, perspiration, and a skin rash. This agent should not be given to patients with glaucoma (see pp. 472 and 473) or urinary retention.

Dosage and Administration. Amitriptyline may be given orally and intramuscularly. Initial oral doses of 150 mg. daily may be required, but 25 mg. two to four times daily usually suffice for the less severe depressions. Often dosage can be reduced to 10 mg. four times daily and maintained for several months.

Preparations

Amitriptyline Hydrochloride Tablets 10 and 25 mg.
Amitriptyline Hydrochloride Injection 10-ml. vials, 10 mg. per ml.
Trade name: Elavil

NEUROPHARMACOLOGY AND NEUROCHEMISTRY

The study of the chemistry of the brain and of chemical agents in elucidating or altering the function of nerves, nerve cell bodies, synapses, and pathways and structures in the nervous system is approximately as old as other branches of biochemistry and experimental pharmacology. However, both disciplines have evolved new techniques that include refined chemical methods, behavior studies of variously trained animals, new drugs, and accurate placement of tiny wires in various parts of the brains of living animals and human schizophrenics. Such investigations have been increasing in scope with an increase in the number of trained workers in this field.

It is not possible to summarize adequately in this book the important developments in these fields. They include the discovery of *hallucinogenic* chemicals, notably LSD (lysergic acid diethylamide), which produced for limited periods in human volunteers mental aberrations that greatly resemble schizophrenia. Azacyclonol hydrochloride is capable of preventing this LSD-induced psychosis. Important advances in the understanding and treatment of mental disease have been and undoubtedly will continue to be announced.

REVIEW QUESTIONS

1. *Describe the results that may be obtained with reserpine and chlorpromazine in the "disturbed wards" of psychiatric hospitals. How would you distinguish the term "sedation" from the term "tranquilization"?*
2. *List several side effects seen with continuous use of reserpine and chlorpromazine.*
3. *What is the nature of the effects of meprobamate in the body and at what dose is the drug prescribed?*
4. *What are the features of the extrapyramidal syndrome (Parkinson-like symptoms) that may be produced by the phenothiazines, Rauwolfia preparations, and reserpine? Find in Chapter 20 (see pp. 371–75) and become familiar with this condition, which, if drug-induced, is reversible by withdrawing the tranquilizer responsible for it.*
5. *List all the drugs, or the general drug types, presented in this chapter, which*

have been known to or may cause jaundice. What organ is involved in jaundice and what observations could detect damage before jaundice appears?

6. *What agents would you consider appropriate for treating a 71-year-old woman with atherosclerosis (hardening of the arteries) as her only outstanding medical condition, but who is so depressed, giving complaints about her loneliness, that she does not eat unless forced, talk unless urged, or take any interest in her environment? What side effects could be anticipated with the drugs selected?*

7. *Give another name, the type of therapeutic action for which used, a possible side effect, and an average daily oral dose (total) for each of the following:*

Largactil	*Compazine*
Fluphenazine	*Deanol*
Reserpoid	*Equanil*
Trifluoperazine	*Ritalin*
Rescinnamine	*Isocarboxazid*
Imipramine	*Phenylzine*

REFERENCES

MENTAL DISEASE

Featherstone, R. M., and Simon, A. (eds.) : *A Pharmacological Approach to the Study of the Mind.* Charles C Thomas, Publisher, Springfield, Ill., 1959.

Himwich, Harold E.: "Tranquilizers and the Brain," *Med. World News,* June 17, 1960, p. 26.

Lynn, F. H., and Friedhoff, A. J.: "The Patient on a Tranquilizing Regimen," *Am. J. Nursing,* **60**:234, 1960.

Stafford-Clark, David: "Foundations of Research in Psychiatry," *Brit. M. J.,* **2**: 1199, 1959.

CHLORPROMAZINE

Ayd, F. J., Jr.: "Thorazine and Serpasil Treatment of Private Neuropsychiatric Patients," *Am. J. Psychiat.,* **113**:16, 1956.

Bower, W. H.: "Chlorpromazine in Psychiatric Illness," *New England J. Med.,* **251**:689, 1954.

Cohen, I. M.: "Complications of Chlorpromazine Therapy," *Am. J. Psychiat.,* **113**: 115, 1956.

Koetschet, P.: "Chlorpromazine in Clinical Medicine," *Internat. Rec. Med.,* **168**: 295, 1955.

FLUPHENAZINE

Darling, H. F.: "Fluphenazine: A Preliminary Study," *Dis. Nerv. System,* **20**:167, 1959.

PROCHLORPERAZINE

Vischer, T. J.: "Clinical Study of Prochlorperazine, a New Tranquilizer for the Treatment of Nonhospitalized Psychoneurotic Patients," *New England J. Med.,* **256**:26, 1957.

METHOXYPROMAZINE

Council on Drugs: "Methoxypromazine Maleate," *J.A.M.A.*, **172**:1519, 1960.

PROMAZINE

Graffeo, A. J.: "Three Years of Treatment of Chronic Hospitalized Psychotic Individuals with Promazine (Sparine)," *Am. J. Psychiat.*, **116**:842, 1960.

THIOPROPAZATE DIHYDROCHLORIDE

Mathews, F. P.: "Dartal: A Clinical Appraisal," *Am. J. Psychiat.*, **114**:1034, 1958.

THIORIDAZINE

Azima, H.; Durost, H.; and Arthure, D.: "The Effect of Thioridazine (Mellaril) on Mental Syndromes," *Canad. M.A.J.*, **81**:549, 1959.

TRIFLUOPERAZINE

Goddard, E. S.: "Trifluoperazine in Psychoneurotic Outpatients," *Canad. M.A.J.*, **81**:467, 1959.

TRIFLUPROMAZINE HYDROCHLORIDE

Goldman, H. I.: "Treatment of Postalcoholic Syndrome with Triflupromazine Hydrochloride," *J.A.M.A.*, **171**:1502, 1959.

ACETOPHENAZINE DIMALEATE

Sines, L. K., and Hamlon, J. S.: "Clinical Evaluation of a New Phenothiazine in Chronic Psychiatric Patients," *Dis. Nerv. System*, **21**:86, 1960.

PROTHIPENDYL HYDROCHLORIDE

Cohen, S.; Ditman, K. S.; Mooney, H. B.; and Whittlesey, J. R. B.; "Prothipendyl (Timovan®) in the Treatment of Alcoholism, Preliminary Report," *J. New Drugs*, **1**:235, 1961.

CHLORPROTHIXINE

Ma, J. Y., and Crandell, A.: "Clinical and Laboratory Evaluation of Chlorprothixine in Institutional Patients," *J. New Drugs*, **2**:26, 1962.

RAUWOLFIA ALKALOIDS

Barsa, J. A., and Kline, N. S.: "Treatment of 200 Disturbed Psychotics with Reserpine," *J.A.M.A.*, **158**:110, 1955.
Braun, M.: "Reserpine as a Therapeutic Agent in Schizophrenia," *Am. J. Psychiat.*, **116**:744, 1960.
Clough, P. W.: "Reserpine in the Treatment of Neuropsychiatric Disorders," *Ann. Int. Med.*, **43**:632, 1955.
Kline, N. S.: "Use of *Rauwolfia serpentina* Benth. *in* Neuropsychiatric Conditions," *Ann. New York Acad. Sc.*, **59**:107, 1954.

Symposium (F. F. Yonkman, consult. ed.): "Reserpine (Serpasil) and Other Alkaloids of *Rauwolfia serpentina:* Chemistry, Pharmacology and Clinical Applications," *Ann. New York Acad. Sc.,* **59**:1, 1954.

BENACTYZINE

Hargraves, G. R.; Hamilton, M.; and Roberts, J. M.: "Benactyzine as an Aid in Treatment of Anxiety States," *Brit. M. J.,* **1**:306, 1957.

HYDROXYZINE DIHYDROCHLORIDE

Robinson, H. M., Jr.; Robinson, R. C.; and Strahan, J. F.: "Hydroxyzine (Atarax) Hydrochloride in Dermatological Therapy," *J.A.M.A.,* **161**:604, 1956.

AZACYCLONOL HYDROCHLORIDE

Rinaldi, F.; Rudy, L. H.; and Himwich, H. E.: "Clinical Evaluation of Azacyclonol, Chlorpromazine and Reserpine on a Group of Chronic Psychotic Patients," *Am. J. Psychiat.,* **112**:678, 1956.
————: "The Use of Frenquel in the Treatment of Disturbed Patients with Psychoses of Long Duration," *Am. J. Psychiat.,* **112**:343, 1955.

CAPTODIAMINE HYDROCHLORIDE

Low, N. L., and Myers, G. G.: "Suvren in Brain-injured Children," *J. Pediat.,* **52**:259, 1958.

CHLORDIAZEPOXIDE

Keith, E. I., and Ardoline, G. A.: "Anticonvulsant Action of Methaminodiazepoxide Hydrochloride," *Fed. Proc.,* **19**:263, 1960.
Symposium: Methaminodiazepoxide Hydrochloride," *Dis. Nerv. System,* **21**:3, 1960 (suppl.).

MEPROBAMATE

Barsa, J. A., and Kline, N. S.: "Use of Meprobamate in the Treatment of Psychotic Patients," *Am. J. Psychiat.,* **112**:1021, 1956.
Borrus, J. C.: "Miltown in Mental Illness," *J.A.M.A.,* **157**:1596, 1955.
Selling, L. S.: "Clinical Study of a New Tranquilizing Drug (Meprobamate)," *J.A.M.A.,* **157**:1594, 1955.
Shane, A. M., and Hirsch, S.: "Three Cases of Meprobamate Poisoning," *Canad. M.A.J.,* **74**:908, 1956.
Stough, A. R.: "Possible Habituating Properties of Meprobamate," *J.A.M.A.,* **166**: 882, 1958.

CHLORMEZANONE

DeNyse, D. L.: "Chlormethazanone as a Skeletal Muscle Relaxant," *M. Times,* **87**:1512, 1959.
Lichtman, A. L.: "New Developments in Muscle Relexant Therapy," *J. Kentucky Acad. Gen. Prac.,* **4**:28, 1958.

PHENAGLYCODOL

Reitan, R. M.: "The Comparative Effects of a Placebo, Ultran and Meprobamate on Psychologic Test Performances," *Antibiotic Med. & Clin. Therap.*, **4**:158, 1957.

EMYLCAMATE

Young, R.: "Striatran (1-Ethyl-1-Methly Propyl Carbamate), a New Internuncial Blocking Ataraxic," *Internat. Rec. Med.*, **174**:345, 1961.

HYDROXYPHENAMATE

Cahn, B.: "Effect of Hydroxyphenamate in the Treatment of Mild and Moderate Anxiety States," *Dis. Nerv. System*, **22**:30, 1961.

MEPHENOXALONE (FORMERLY METHOXYDONE)

Shatin, L.; and Gilmore, T. H.: "Methoxydone (AHR-233) in Hospitalized Non-psychotic Patients," *Amer. J. Psychiat.*, **117**:833, 1961.

OXANAMIDE

Feuss, C. D., Jr., and Ivanov, C. J.: "Quiactin as an Outpatient Drug," *Marquette M. Rev.*, **23**:78, 1958.

Kristofferson, A. B., and Cormack, R. H.: "Some Effects of Quiactin on Normal Behavior," *Clin. Res.*, **6**:416, 1958.

MONOAMINE OXIDASE INHIBITORS

Brodie, B. B.; Spector, S.; and Shore, P. A.: "Interaction of Monoamine Oxidase Inhibitors with Physiological and Biochemical Mechanisms in Brain," *Ann. New York Acad. Sc.*, **80**:609, 1959.

Cole, Jonathan O.: "Therapeutic Efficacy of Antidepressant Drugs," *J.A.M.A.*, **190**:448, 1964.

Council on Drugs: "Reevaluation of Trancylcypromine Sulfate," *J.A.M.A.*, **189**:161, 1963.

"Drugs for Depression," *Brit. M.J.*, **2**:522, 1964.

Editorial: "New Drugs for Depression," *Brit. M. J.*, **1**:178, 1960.

"Hypertensive Reactions to Monoamine Oxidase Inhibitors," *Brit. M.J.*, **1**:578, 1964.

Symposium: "Amine Oxidase Inhibitors," *Ann. New York Acad. Sci.*, **80**:553-1039, 1959.

ISOCARBOXAZID

Ford, R. B.; Branham, H. E.; and Cleckley, J. J.: "Isocarboxazid: A New Anti-depressant Drug," *Clin. Med.*, **6**:1559, 1959.

PHENELZINE

Evans, W. L.: "Clinical Experience with Phenelzine in Psychosomatic and Psychophysiologic Disorders," *New York J. Med.*, **60**:865, 1960.

NIALAMID

Ayd, F. J.; Bianco, E.; and Zullo, L.: "Treatment of Depressive States in Ambulatory Patients," *Dis. Nerv. System*, **20**:1, 1959.

TRANYLCYPROMINE

Freyhan, F. A.: "The Modern Treatment of Depressive Disorders," *Am. J. Psychiat.*, **116**:1057, 1960.
Lurie, M. L., and Salzer, H. M.: "Tranylcyromine (Parnate) in the Ambulatory Treatment of Depressed Patients," *Am. J. Psychiat.*, **118**:152, 1961.

IMIPRAMINE

Pollack, B.: "Clinical Findings in the Use of Tofranil in Depressive and Other Psychiatric States," *Am. J. Psychiat.*, **116**:312, 1959.
Sloman, L.: "Myocardial Infarction During Imipramine Treatment of Depression," *Canad. M.A.J.*, **82**:20, 1960.
Straker, M., and Roth, E. M.; "Use of Imipramine (Tofranil) in the Aged Chronically Ill," *Canad. M.A.J.*, **82**:362, 1960.

METHYLPHENIDATE

Ferguson, J. T.: "Treatment of Reserpine-induced Depression with a New Analeptic: Phenidylate," *Ann. New York Acad. Sc.*, **61**:101, 1955.
Madi, M. L., and Kovitz, B.: "Experiences with Methyl-Phenidylacetate Hydrochloride in Psychotic Patients," *Antibiotic Med & Clin. Therap.*, **3**:309, 1956.

PIPRADROL

Fabing, H. D.; Hawkins, J. R.; and Moulton, J. A. L.: "Clinical Studies on α-(2-Piperidy) Benzyhydrol Hydrochloride, a New Antidepressant Drug," *Am. J. Psychiat.*, **111**:832, 1955.

DEANOL

Barsa, J. A., and Saunders, J. C.: "Deanol (Deaner) in the Treatment of Schizophrenia," *Am. J. Psychiat.*, **116**:255, 1959.
Council on Drugs: "Deanol Acetamidobenzoate," *J.A.M.A.*, **172**:1518, 1960.

AMITRIPTYLINE HYDROCHLORIDE

Dorfman, W.: "Clinical Experiences with Amitriptyline (Elavil)," *Psychosomatics*, **1**:153, 1960.

20

Drugs Used in Hyperkinesia. Treatment of Epilepsy. Skeletal Muscle Spasm. Parkinson's Disease

TYPES AND TREATMENT OF EPILEPSY

Epilepsy is a chronic disorder of the central nervous system characterized by transient episodes of unconsciousness, a specific type of psychic dysfunction, or localized or widespread convulsive movements. At times the etiology is unknown. On the other hand, injury to the brain, either mechanical or that following an acute infection, or a brain tumor may produce a focus of excitable tissue which initiates excessive abnormal electrical discharges periodically. These may be relatively localized or widespread over motor and sensory areas of the brain. During the resulting seizures, dysrhythmias or abnormal brain waves occur which can be recorded by the electroencephalogram (EEG). There are several types of epilepsy. Each presents a characteristic clinical picture and EEG pattern and responds to certain types of anticonvulsant drugs. Mixed seizures are often seen and require the administration of several drugs in combination.

Petit Mal. Petit mal is a form of epilepsy characterized by very short lapses of consciousness. There may be a sudden pause in conversation or movement lasting not more than 30 seconds. It occurs frequently in children, and the brief lapses may occur many times a day. Petit mal rarely causes a person to fall or show muscular spasm.

Grand Mal. Grand mal is the most frequent form of epilepsy. The seizure is characterized by a sudden loss of consciousness, tonic and clonic convulsions of all muscles, cyanosis, and frothing at the mouth. This is often preceded by an *aura*, which may be a certain taste, odor, headache, or other sensation, and which is usually the same for each patient. The patient may cry out as he falls. The convulsion begins in any part and spreads over the body. After the convulsion subsides, the patient is confused and falls into a deep sleep. The brain wave during the grand mal attack shows outstanding variations from normal.

Status Epilepticus. This is a condition in which grand mal convulsions follow one another without a return of consciousness in the intervals between

359

seizures. Brain damage may occur and convalescence with helplessness may take weeks. The patient may be paralyzed in most muscle groups and may be unable to speak for days after consciousness is regained.

Psychomotor Epilepsy. Psychomotor, or "temporal lobe," epilepsy is characterized by transient mental disturbances with abnormal behavior for a few minutes but without convulsions.

Jacksonian Epilepsy. In this type, also known as "focal epilepsy," a finger or limb may twitch or show spasmodic movement without loss of consciousness and without mental aberration.

Treatment. Epilepsy responds well to treatment with drugs unless it is caused by specific organic disease. The EEG is very helpful in diagnosing and aiding treatment. In the administration of drugs to the epileptic, it may be necessary to try several, or two or more in combination, in order to attain the best therapy because individuals vary greatly in their response to antiepileptic drugs. There are more than one million epileptics in the United States. With modern treatment seizures may be controlled in 80 to 85 per cent of the cases and patients can lead a reasonably normal life.

Until 1938 the treatment of epilepsy was confined to the use of two groups of drugs: the bromides and the barbiturates, chiefly phenobarbital. Both these drug groups depressed the sensory as well as the motor cortex and thus produced drowsiness and a decrease in mental alacrity. It is desirable to control the convulsions and other manifestations without interference in alertness.

DRUGS USED IN GRAND MAL EPILEPSY

Drugs used in the treatment of epilepsy are called antiepileptics or anticonvulsants. Most of them are central nervous system depressants.

Sodium Diphenylhydantoin, U.S.P.; Phenytoin Sodium, B.P., I.P. (Dilantin Sodium)

Diphenylhydantoin sodium is a synthetic compound somewhat related to the barbiturates. It is an anticonvulsant drug that is available for oral, intravenous, and intramuscular administration.

Pharmacological Action. Diphenylhydantoin produces depression of the motor cortex and inhibits the spread of the abnormal impulse without an appreciable effect on the sensory cortex and therefore does not cause decreased mental acuity. Thus it has an anticonvulsant action with little or no hypnotic effect. It improves the EEG only slightly.

Absorption, Fate, and Excretion. Diphenylhydantoin is readily absorbed from the gastrointestinal tract. A small fraction is metabolized and the remainder is excreted in the urine, mostly in the conjugated form.

Untoward Effects. The side effects include hyperplasia (overgrowth) of the gums with soreness, tenderness, and bleeding, gastric upsets, skin rash, and itching. Various effects due to its action on the central nervous system are dizziness, vertigo, nervousness, blurred vision, nystagmus, and, in rare cases, psychotic symptoms. Hypoxia and respiratory and circulatory depression may follow parenteral administration.

Therapeutic Uses and Doses

1. *Treatment of Epilepsy.* Diphenylhydantoin is more effective in grand mal than in petit mal. For adults, the dose is 100 mg. up to four times a day (100 to 600 mg. daily). For children, the dose is 30 to 60 mg. It is often given with phenobarbital.

2. *Treatment of Status Epilepticus.* The intravenous dose is 150 to 250 mg. A subsequent dose of 100 to 150 mg. may be given in 30 minutes, if necessary. Dosage for children is calculated according to body weight. After the convulsions have ceased, the drug may be administered intramuscularly. Upon return of the patient to consciousness, the drug may be administered orally.

3. *Prophylactic Control of Seizures in Neurosurgery.* The intramuscular dose to protect the patient from convulsions during surgery and postoperatively is 100 to 200 mg. three or four times during a 24-hour period. Oral administration replaces intramuscular injection as soon as possible.

Preparations

Diphenylhydantoin Oral Suspension, N.F.	25 mg. in 1 ml.
Sodium Diphenylhydantoin Capsules, U.S.P.	30 and 100 mg.
Sodium Diphenylhydantoin Sterile, U.S.P.	Vials containing 250 mg.

Trade names: Dilantin Sodium; Alepsin; Epanutin; Eptoin
Synonyms: Cansoin; Di-hydan; Dintoin; Diphantoin; Epilan-D; Eptal; Solantoin; Zentropil

Other Hydantoin Derivatives

Two other drugs, ethotoin and phenantoin, are comparable in actions and side effects to diphenylhydantoin. They are used as anticonvulsants in grand mal epilepsy and at times in jacksonian (focal) epilepsy.

Ethotoin, B.P. (Peganone). The adult oral dose is 2 to 3 Gm. daily, with food, in four to six divided doses. The dose for children is 500 mg. to 1 Gm. Tablets of 250 and 500 mg. are available.

Side effects include dizziness, headache, fatigue, skin rash, diplopia, nystagmus, diarrhea, fever, numbness, and chest pain. Nausea and vomiting are rare.

Phenantoin (Mesantoin). The oral adult dose is 200 to 600 mg. daily in four to six divided doses. The dosage for children is 100 to 400 mg. daily. Tablets of 100 mg. are available.

Side Effects. These include skin rashes, anemia, and agranulocytosis. To detect possible changes in the blood, periodic blood counts are recommended. They should include white cell count, differential count, and calculation of neutrophils.

Phenacemide (Phenurone)

Phenacemide depresses the central nervous system, reducing the severity of or preventing grand mal and petit mal convulsions in epilepsy. It is absorbed from the small intestine and is almost completely metabolized in the liver. The oral adult dose is 250 to 500 mg. three times a day. The average total daily dose rarely exceeds 3 Gm. In some cases the drug has serious side effects, such as personality changes, psychosis, hepatic damage, rash, and depression of the red and white blood cell count. It should not be given if the disease can be controlled by other anticonvulsants. It may be given in combination with phenobarbital, diphenylhydantoin, or paramethadione.

Preparation

Tablets Phenacemide   500 mg.
                    Trade names: Phenurone; Fenostenyl

Primidone, U.S.P., B.P. (Mysoline)

Chemically, primidone is closely related to phenobarbital, but it is not a barbiturate. The usual effective oral dose in the treatment of epilepsy is 125 mg. once daily, preferably at bedtime. The dose may be increased at weekly intervals until the maximum therapeutic response is obtained. There are no serious toxic effects, but there is a high incidence of drowsiness, anorexia, dizziness, headache, and ataxia. Tablets of 250 mg. are available.

Acetazolamide, U.S.P., B.P. (Diamox)

Acetazolamide is a useful drug in the treatment of certain cases of grand and petit mal epilepsy. It suppresses both the frequency and severity of seizures. It appears to produce a relative acidosis, as did the ketogenic diet used long ago, and may have a direct action on nerve tissue by inhibiting the activity of carbonic anhydrase, the enzyme that facilitates the removal of carbon dioxide. No direct sedative action or serious toxic effects have been observed. The daily oral dose is 250 to 500 mg. Its use as a diuretic is discussed on page 638; its use in glaucoma, on page 473.

Preparation

Acetazolamide Tablets, U.S.P., B.P.   250 mg.
                    Trade names: Diamox; Diomox

ADDITIONAL DRUGS IN GRAND MAL EPILEPSY

The barbiturates are still widely and effectively used in controlling grand mal seizures. Those most commonly employed are phenobarbital, mephobarbital, and metharbital.

Phenobarbital, U.S.P. (Luminal)

Phenobarbital, a long-acting barbiturate, causes continuous suppression of epilepsy without producing excessive drowsiness. However, in the chronic management of the disease the accompanying sedation may be undesirable and may necessitate the administration of another anticonvulsant such as diphenylhydantoin simultaneously. The dose of each drug may then be reduced accordingly. Dextro amphetamine is sometimes administered to counteract the sedative effects. Therapy with phenobarbital should be continuous without interruption because abrupt withdrawal might precipitate a grand mal seizure.

Phenobarbital is especially effective in grand mal epilepsy. It is often given simultaneously with diphenylhydantoin. It is not very useful in petit mal but may be given along with trimethadione in patients with both types of epilepsy.

The usual oral dose of phenobarbital is 15 to 100 mg. three or four times a day. For preparations see page 322.

Mephobarbital, N.F. (Mebaral)

Mephobarbital, a barbiturate with pronounced sedative and antispasmodic properties but mild hypnotic effects, has been widely employed in the control of grand mal and petit mal seizures. Patients do not experience the degree of drowsiness or the decrease in mental alertness and efficiency caused by other barbiturates. The drug is useful also in reducing tension in anxiety states and various manifestations of psychosomatic and nervous disorders.

Therapeutic Use and Dose. In the treatment of petit mal and grand mal epilepsy, the oral adult dose is 30 mg. three times a day (30 to 250 mg. daily). Drowsiness is less marked with mephobarbital than with phenobarbital.

Preparation

Mephobarbital Tablets, N.F.　　　　　　　30, 50, 100, and 200 mg.
　　　　Trade names: Mebaral; Isonal; Phemitone; Prominal

Mebaroin

Mebaroin, a combination of mephobarbital and diphenylhydantoin, is a sedative and anticonvulsant that causes little or no drowsiness. It is used in all forms of epileptic attacks. The oral adult dose is one to two tablets three times a day; for children over six years of age, the dose is one to three tablets daily; for younger children, one-half tablet is given once or twice daily.

Preparation

Mebarion Tablets (Scored)   90 mg. of mephobarbital and 60 mg. of diphenylhydantoin

Metharbital, N.F. (Gemonil)

Metharbital is a barbiturate derivative that shares the anticonvulsant activity of phenobarbital. It is converted in the body to barbital. The drug is helpful in various forms of epilepsy and may be used with other anticonvulsants such as trimethadione, paramethadione, or diphenylhydantoin. The oral dose for infants and small children is 50 mg. one to three times daily. The adult oral dose is 100 mg. one to three times daily. These doses may be gradually increased, depending on tolerance and effectiveness.

The untoward effects are drowsiness, dizziness, and irritability.

Preparation

Metharbital Tablets, N. F.   100 mg.

Trade name: Gemonil

DRUGS USED IN PETIT MAL EPILEPSY

Trimethadione, U.S.P.; Troxidone, B.P. (Tridione, Trimetin)

Trimethadione is an anticonvulsant drug used in the treatment of petit mal epilepsy. Administered by mouth, it is readily absorbed from the gastrointestinal tract and is almost completely metabolized in the body. Some is excreted in the urine unchanged. The side effects are not very severe and include a skin rash, gastrointestinal distress, and headache. Upon long-continued use, overdosage, or individual sensitivity, a patient may experience photophobia or a glare effect and may see everything as if it were covered with frost or snow. This disappears with discontinuance of the drug. A few cases of agranulocytosis and rare instances of aplastic anemia have been reported; hence blood examinations should be made repeatedly. Trimethadione is contraindicated in liver or kidney disease. It may aggravate grand mal seizures in mixed types of epilepsy.

Therapeutic Use and Doses. In the treatment of petit mal epilepsy, better results are obtained with children than with adults. The adult oral dose is 300 mg. three to six times a day. The dose for children is 150 to 300 mg. The optimum dosage should be determined for each patient.

Preparations

Trimethadione Capsules, U.S.P.   300 mg.
Troxidone Capsules, B.P.
Trimethadione Tablets, N.F.   150 mg.

Trade names: Tridione; Trimetin; Absentol

Paramethadione, U.S.P., B.P. (Paradione)

Paradione, a drug used in petit mal epilepsy, acts in a manner similar to trimethadione, to which it is related. There is less glare effect, and some individuals are controlled better with this drug than with trimethadione. The initial oral dose for adults is 900 mg. daily in divided doses. The dose may then be increased or decreased to give the smallest dose that will control the symptoms. For children the usual oral dose is 300 to 500 mg.

Preparations

Paramethadione Capsules, U.S.P.	150 and 300 mg.
Paramethadione Solution, U.S.P.	30 per cent

Trade names: Paradione; Petidon

Phensuximide, N.F. (Milontin)

This drug is moderately useful in petit mal epilepsy. It is relatively nontoxic, but may cause nausea, vomiting, weakness, and blood cell or urinary changes. The occasional skin eruptions and drowsiness may be controlled by reducing the dosage or withdrawing the drug temporarily. The initial oral dose is 500 mg. to 1 Gm. two or three times a day.

Preparations

Phensuximide Capsules, N.F.	500 mg.
Phensuximide Oral Suspension, N.F.	62.5 mg. in 1 ml.

Trade name: Milontin

Methsuximide, N.F. (Celontin)

Methsuximide, chemically related to phensuximide, is used in petit mal and psychomotor seizures. It increases grand mal attacks, as does trimethadione in some cases. It can be used with other drugs when petit and grand mal seizures occur in the same patient.

Side Effects.   These are approximately the same as those of phensuximide but, in addition, include ataxia, anorexia, psychic disturbances including psychosis, headache, diplopia (double vision) or blurring of vision, fever, hiccups, sweating, leukopenia, and possibly kidney and liver damage. Blood cell studies should be done regularly.

Dosage and Method of Administration.   Oral doses must be adjusted individually. One 300-mg. capsule is given daily with weekly increases of one capsule daily until four are taken (300 mg. four times daily). Capsules of 300 mg. are available.

Ethosuximide (Zarontin)

Primarily useful in preventing petit mal seizures, ethosuximide reportedly controls more than three fourths of the cases treated. It may be given with the agents used to suppress grand mal epilepsy when both forms are present. The side effects most frequently encountered have been gastric distress, nausea, drowsiness, dizziness, and headache. Less frequent effects are skin rash and granulocytopenia.

Dosage. Ethosuximide is administered orally. The initial dose for patients under six years of age is 250 mg. once daily, and for all those older, this amount twice daily. Thereafter increases by 250 mg. daily can be made every four to seven days until maximal control is achieved as permissible by any accompanying side effects. One to one and one-half grams may be required.

Preparation

Ethosuximide Capsules   250 mg.
Trade name: Zarontin

Amino-Glutethimide (Elipten)

This is an anticonvulsant which may be used in most forms of epilepsy. It may be given in combination with other antiepileptic drugs. The side effects during the first week or two of administration are sedation, ataxia, mental confusion, abdominal discomfort, headache, anorexia, and flushing of the face. Leukopenia occurs rarely. The oral adult dose is 125 mg. to 1.5 Gm. daily in divided doses. The dose for children is 62.5 to 750 mg. daily. There should be a gradual increase from the low dose to that required for maintenance. Tablets of 125 and 250 mg. are available.

Additional Drugs in Petit Mal Epilepsy

Several of the drugs described in the section on grand mal seizures are reported also to have varying effects upon the petit mal type. These are the barbiturates (methobarbital, metharbital, and phenobarbital), primidone, and acetazolamide.

DRUGS IN FOCAL PSYCHOMOTOR EPILEPSY

Drugs reported to be effective in focal or jacksonian epilepsy are the barbiturates, diphenylhydantoin, amino-glutethimide, and possibly ethotoin, phenacemide, and acetazolamide. Compounds often or occasionally useful in psychomotor forms are primidone, phenacemide, amino-glutethimide, and ethotoin.

DRUGS IN STATUS EPILEPTICUS

The occurrence of *status elipticus* seizures must be treated in a hospital. Short- or ultrashort-acting barbiturates or diphenylhydantoin is usually given intravenously in just sufficient dosage, with repetition, to stop seizures but not to add unnecessarily to the cerebral depression that follows the convulsions. Death may follow uncontrolled *status epilepticus.*

MIXTURES OF THE ANTIEPILEPTIC DRUGS

The physician has a choice of several types of agents for use in the different forms of epilepsy. He can alternate drugs until the most satisfactory one is found. It is often necessary to use two or more drugs in order to reduce the number of attacks to the minimum. Combinations are indicated when two or more types of the disease are seen in the same individual. With optimal medication and dosage, approximately 50 per cent of epileptics are completely controlled and the frequency and severity of attacks greatly reduced in another 35 per cent.

THE SKELETAL MUSCLE RELAXANTS

Skeletal muscle spasm has no relationship to epilepsy except during seizures. There is, however, a group of drugs, often with anti-petit-mal-epilepsy activity, that has a depressant effect upon certain circuits in the spinal cord and subcortical areas of the brain. These may be used to relax spastic or hypertonic muscles. In animal studies these drugs show anticonvulsant activity resembling that of the petit mal drugs. Few are used in epilepsy. Some have, in addition, mild to moderate tranquilizing properties.

Skeletal Muscle Spasm.   At rest, skeletal muscle is normally in a state of mild tone. A few of the fibers of a given resting muscle are receiving occasional nerve impulses through the nerves supplying the muscle. Furthermore, some muscles, e.g., those that hold our head and spine erect, are held in a state of considerable tone or contraction at all times unless we are lying very relaxed. In certain situations these normal but varying degrees of muscle tone are increased to such an extent as to be termed *spasm.* In some of these situations the abnormality is primarily within the muscle itself, resulting from strain, injury, or inflammation. On the other hand, pathology involving a joint, bursa, tendon, bone, or other structure may reflexly produce spasm in surrounding muscle groups. This is usually a protective mechanism serving to immobilize a diseased structure. A pain-spasm reflex condition may thus be set up, actually resulting in more pain, then increased spasm, etc., in a reinforced cycle of events.

Table 24

Conditions Often Associated with Skeletal Muscle Spasm

A. Those of muscles
  1. Strains, excessive use
  2. Contusions (bruises), postoperative spasm
  3. Torticollis (wry neck)
  4. Myositis (inflammation)
B. Those of joints and bone
  1. Arthritis (of limb, back, neck, etc.)
  2. Trauma, sprains, compression, fractures
  3. Low-back abnormalities (lumbar disk syndrome, etc.)
C. Those of additional structures
  1. Bursitis
  2. Fibrositis
  3. Tenosynovitis
  4. Cellulitis
  5. Infection of a viscus, e.g., appendicitis
D. Those of the nervous system
  1. Cerebral palsy
  2. Upper motor neuron lesion (e.g., apoplexy)
  3. Parkinson's disease
  4. Athetosis
  5. Multiple sclerosis
  6. Other spinal or brain lesions

In some cases of spasm of skeletal muscles—for example, in arthritis, cerebral palsy, trauma, pyramidal tract interruption (stroke), extrapyramidal (Parkinson's) disease, and anxiety states—it is desirable to relax the involved muscles. Agents capable of decreasing spasm by depressing the neuronal or "polysynaptic" activity in the cord or higher centers are now being referred to as "lissive agents." In ordinary doses they do not paralyze muscles nor do they seriously interfere with their contraction when movement is attempted. Their inhibitory action is within the central nervous system rather than at the nerve-muscle, or *neuromyal,* junction (synapse).

LISSIVE AGENTS

Mephenesin, N.F. (Myanesin, Tolserol)

Mephenesin, the oldest of the lissive agents, was introduced in 1948. It is administered orally or intravenously. The drug is well absorbed from the gastrointestinal tract, is metabolized rapidly, and appears to be free from side actions by this route. It is advisable to give oral preparations after meals or with milk in order to minimize gastric irritation. Upon intravenous injection, lightheadedness, weakness, double vision, nystagmus, and hematuria may occur. Mephenesin carbamate produces a more prolonged effect.

Therapeutic Uses

1. As a relaxant for spastic and neurological disorders, delirium tremens, Parkinson's disease, arthritis, tetanus, alcoholism, cerebral palsy, and trauma of the back, neck, and extremities.

2. With secobarbital to produce sleep in patients when secobarbital alone is not effective. It synergizes barbiturate sedation.

3. In anxiety tension states.

4. For occasional aid in *status epilepticus* and electroconvulsive therapy in psychiatric practice.

Dosage and Method of Administration.   The usual oral dose is 2 to 3 Gm. three or five times a day. The intravenous dose is 30 to 150 ml. of a 2 per cent solution at the rate of 6 or 7 ml. per minute.

Preparations

Mephenesin Tablets, N.F.	250 and 500 mg.
Mephenesin Capsules, N.F.	250 and 500 mg.
Mephenesin Elixir	100 mg. in 1 ml.
Mephenesin Solution	50- and 100-ml. ampuls containing 20 mg. in 1 ml.

Trade names and synonyms: Tolserol; Myanesin; Atensin; Curythan; Lissephen; Memphenesin; Mephesin; Myodetensin; Myolysin; Relaxar; Relaxil; Avosyl; Daserol; Dioloxol; Kinavosyl; Mepherol; Mephson; Myoten; Myoxane; Oranixon; Prolax; Sinan; Spasmolyn; Tolansin; Tolosate; Toloxyn; Tolulexin, Tolulox

Mephenesin Carbamate Tablets	500 mg.

Trade name: Tolseram

Methocarbamol (Robaxin)

This agent is identical with mephenesin carbamate except for the addition of one oxygen atom. It suppresses multisynaptic reflexes in the spinal cord, as does the parent compound. It is effective in treating the types of spastic muscular contractions described for mephenesin. In severely acute conditions, and in minor surgical manipulations such as dislocated shoulder or a simple fracture where muscle spasm is present, the drug is administered intravenously.

Side Effects.   On oral administration, side reactions occur in about 10 per cent of the patients and include dizziness, drowsiness, headache, blurred vision, fever, skin rashes, and nausea. These effects are usually mild and may subside with lowering of the dosage. Persons on full dosage should be warned about driving automobiles or operating dangerous equipment. When the drug is administered intravenously, flushing, a metallic taste, and some decrease in blood pressure and pulse rate may occur. The agent should not be given intravenously in the presence of significant renal disease.

Dosage and Methods of Administration.   Adults may be given 1.5 to 2 Gm. orally four times daily for two or three days. This dosage is then lowered to 1 Gm. four times daily if control of muscle spasm can be continued at this level. Children should be given approximately 30 mg. per pound of body weight, in divided doses daily. Adults may be given intramuscularly 0.5 Gm. in each buttock every eight hours; they may be given intravenously a 10 per cent solution at a rate not greater than 3 ml. per minute but for not more than three days at a time. The total daily dose should not be greater than that described for oral administration. Extravasation should be avoided, for the solution is irritating to subcutaneous tissue.

Preparations

Methocarbamol Tablets (white)   500 mg.
Methocarbamol Solution   10-ml. ampuls containing 1 Gm. in
                                       50 per cent polyethylene glycol-300
                    Trade name: Robaxin

Chlorozoxazone (Paraflex)

This drug has the same mechanism of action described for mephenesin. The therapeutic uses, except for the treatment of Parkinson's disease, epilepsy, and cerebral palsy, are the same. There is a low incidence of side effects, which may include nausea, vomiting, gastric burning, dizziness, headache, and lethargy. The oral adult dose is 250 to 750 mg. three or four times a day. The drug is available as tablets containing 250 mg.

Styramate (Sinaxar)

This is another carbamate with the same actions and uses of the other skeletal muscle relaxants. The side effects are similar and include mild gastrointestinal upsets, drowsiness, and dizziness. The oral dose is 200 to 400 mg. three or four times a day. Tablets of 200 mg. are available.

Orphenadrine Citrate (Norflex) and Hydrochloride (Disipal)

These are skeletal muscle relaxants with actions and therapeutic uses similar to those of mephenesin. They have a prolonged action and are given only twice a day. The oral dose is 100 mg. twice daily of orphenadrine citrate and 50 mg. three times daily of the hydrochloride.

Phenyramidol Hydrochloride (Analexin)

This drug relieves musculoskeletal pain and relieves tension. It is used in premenstrual tension and headache, postpartum pain, dysmenorrhea, and in many types of pain caused by muscle spasm. The incidence of side effects is infrequent. There may be mild gastrointestinal irritation and pruritus with or without rash. The oral dose is 200 to 400 mg. every four hours. Tablets of 200 mg. are available.

Carisoprodol (Rela, Soma)

This drug is used in the treatment of stiffness in muscle sprains, bursitis, low-back pain, and traumatic strains and bruises. It produces drowsiness that tends to disappear with reduction in dosage. The oral dose is 250 to 350 mg. three times a day and at bedtime. Tablets of 250 and 350 mg. are available.

TRANQUILIZING DRUGS

Some of the tranquilizing drugs have a relaxant effect on skeletal muscle. These drugs are discussed in Chapter 19.

PARKINSON'S DISEASE

Parkinson's disease is a condition caused by or associated with degeneration of the brain in the region of the corpus striatum. It may be caused by arteriosclerosis, which causes a diminution in the blood supply to an area, with resultant degeneration; it may follow encephalitis; or it may occur in the absence of either of these causes. The disease may progress slowly or rapidly. Among the symptoms are tremors, rigidity of skeletal muscle, cramps in the extremities, a fixed facial expression, salivation, a "pillrolling" motion of the hand, and a characteristic gait with short, fast steps. Some of these symptoms are amenable to drug therapy, at least partially. Physiotherapy and other measures are often of equal importance.

This disease is not cured under any known therapy, but the symptoms are relieved. The Parkinson syndrome may also be caused by the two most useful groups of tranquilizers, the phenothiazines and reserpine and its congeners (Chap. 19). Symptoms produced by these drugs disappear following discontinuation of the drug or possibly upon decreasing the dosage. They will usually decrease in severity when an anti-Parkinson drug is administered with the tranquilizer.

Trihexyphenidyl Hydrochloride, U.S.P., Benzhexol, B.P. (Artane, Pipanol)

Trihexyphenidyl is a synthetic anticholinergic drug that appears to be very useful in all types of Parkinson's disease, including postencephalitic, arteriosclerotic, and idiopathic types. It is an antispasmodic drug owing to the fact that it is a cholinergic blocking agent and also that it has a direct relaxant action on smooth muscle. It is useful in controlling both rigidity and tremors of skeletal muscle, partly because of its action on the cerebral motor centers. Trihexyphenidyl diminishes mental sluggishness, salivation, and depression. The drug is administered orally. The usual initial oral dose is 1 mg. the first day. The dosage is increased to 2 mg. on the second day with further dosage increases of 2 mg. on subsequent days until a total daily dose of 6 to 15 mg. is given. The daily dose is divided into three or four parts, and is given before or after meals. Doses of 12 to 15 mg, may be required with some postencephalitic patients. The side effects are dry mouth, nausea, mydriasis, blurred vision, and restlessness.

Preparations

Trihexyphenidyl Hydrochloride Elixir, U.S.P.	0.4 and 0.5 mg. of trihexyphenidyl in 1 ml.
Trihexyphenidyl Hydrochloride Tablets, U.S.P.; Benzhexol Tablets, B.P.	2 and 5 mg.

Trade names: Artane; Pipanol; Paralest; Peragit

Cycrimine Hydrochloride, N.F. (Pagitane)

This synthetic drug is closely related to trihexyphenidyl. Side effects such as dryness of mouth, blurring of vision, epigastric distress, and transient nausea usually subside with continued therapy. More serious side effects such as vertigo or disorientation make it necessary to reduce dosage or discontinue therapy. The oral daily dose is 1.25 mg. three times a day, but this is subject to individualization. The maintenance dose is determined by the physician. The drug is available as tablets containing 1.25 and 2.5 mg.

Benztropine Methanesulfonate, N.F., B.P. (Cogentin)

This drug appears to be a valuable adjunct in the treatment of Parkinson's disease. It is useful in relieving symptoms in all forms of the disease. It may be given alone or in combination with other drugs. Benztropine has a cumulative action, and it may take several days for the effects to be noted. The initial dose is 0.75 mg. Maintenance daily dose is 0.5 to 2 mg. orally, The drug produces drowsiness, dryness of mouth, and blurring of vision which may be controlled by dosage. Tablets of 2 mg. are marketed.

Ethopropazine Hydrochloride, B.P. (Parsidol)

This drug is very effective in controlling muscular rigidity and in elevating the mood of patients, but its action is less marked in controlling tremors and spasms. It is therefore often administered in combination with other related drugs. The initial oral dose of ethopropazine is 10 to 50 mg. four times a day, best given with meals. This is increased by 50 to 100 mg. daily every few days until a total daily dose of 500 mg. is attained in about three weeks.

The untoward effects noted are ataxia, gastrointestinal irritation, blurred vision, headache, and confusion.

Preparation

Ethopropazine Tablets, B.P.   10 and 50 mg.
　　　　　Trade names: Parsidol; Dibutil; Lysivane; Pardisol
　　　　　Synonym: Profenamine

Procyclidine Hydrochloride (Kemadrin)

This is a muscle relaxant and antispasmodic drug. It reduces both rigidity and tremor. The secretion of saliva is diminished and reflex swallowing is facilitated. The usual initial oral dose is 2.5 to 10 mg. three times a day. Occasionally 15 mg. may be given four times a day. The toxicity of procyclidine is low, but it may cause dizziness and disorientation. It is contraindicated in glaucoma and tachycardia. Tablets of 5 mg. are available.

Caramiphen Hydrochloride, B.P. (Panparnit)

Caramiphen, a synthetic belladonna-like alkaloid, controls rigidity in some cases of Parkinson's disease. It produces mild atropine-like effects on salivation, gastrointestinal motility, and the pupil. The principal action of caramiphen is in reducing muscular rigidity. It is not very useful in controlling tremors; hence it is given with atropine.

The initial dose of caramiphen is 12.5 mg. three times the first day. The dose is gradually increased to 50 mg. every two or three hours if needed, up to 600 mg. daily.

Such untoward effects as drowsiness, vertigo, nausea, dry mouth, blurred vision, and constipation occur in about two thirds of the patients. The drug is marketed in tablets of 50 mg. (scored).

New Synthetic Drugs

Three new drugs, chlorphenoxamine, biperiden, and orphenadrine, all have the same actions, side effects, and therapeutic uses as trihexylphenidyl. They should be used cautiously in glaucoma.

Chlorphenoxamine (Phenoxene). The oral dose is 50 mg. three times a day to 100 mg. four times a day. Tablets of 50 mg. are available.

Biperiden Hydrochloride (Akineton). The oral dose is 2 mg. three times a day. This dose is gradually increased until a maximum daily dose of 24 mg. is reached. Tablets of 2 mg. are available.

BELLADONNA ALKALOIDS

The belladonna alkaloids were used for half a century prior to the introduction of the synthetic drugs to reduce rigidity, salivation, and tremors. The side actions are dry mouth and blurred vision. In susceptible or older people, confusion and delirium may result. The dose of belladonna tincture or hyoscyamus tincture is 0.3 to 0.6 ml. (5 to 10 minims) four times a day. The dose may be increased slowly. Tablets of atropine or scopolamine are given in doses of 0.3 mg. four times a day. The dose may be increased cautiously to 0.6 mg. four times a day.

ANTIHISTAMINES

Several antihistamines have been found useful in Parkinson's disease because they produce sedation and drowsiness. Among the useful compounds are phenindamine tartrate, diphenhydramine hydrochloride, and promethazine. The dose of phenindamine is 10 to 50 mg. three times a day. The dose for diphenhydramine and promethazine is 25 or 50 mg. two to four times daily.

PHENOTHIAZINES

Certain of the phenothiazines have the capacity of alleviating the severity of the symptoms of Parkinson's disease. These are mepazine and promazine, discussed on page 338, and two others, ethopropazine and promethazine, discussed in this chapter.

STIMULANTS

The lethargy frequently seen in Parkinson patients is often treated with one of the amphetamines, pentylenetetrazol, methylphenidate, or another psychostimulant or analeptic.

COMBINATIONS OF DRUGS IN PARKINSONISM

Only early and mild to moderately severe cases of Parkinson's disease can be controlled with a single drug. Most require two or three together, and the particular combination and the doses must be individualized. Trihexyphenidyl or one of the other compounds described may be administered with an antihistamine, with or without a phenothiazine and a stimulant. Belladonna preparations may be added to certain of the possible combinations, and mephenesin or another spinal cord depressant that reduces skeletal muscle spasm (see p. 368) may be used with any of the above. Dosage of individual drugs may be lower in combinations than when the individual drugs are prescribed alone.

Surgery, using liquid nitrogen, and physical methods (radioactivity or ultrasound rays) are now being employed in selected patients with this disease. Certain structures in the basal ganglia of the midbrain are destroyed in order to diminish or abolish tremor, spasticity, and other features of parkinsonism.

REVIEW QUESTIONS

1. Define epilepsy. Name three types. What are the symptoms noted in (a) grand mal and (b) petit mal?
2. In what way do the drugs used in the treatment of epilepsy produce their desired effects?
3. Compare the effects produced by phenobarbital and diphenylhydantoin. What are the advantages gained by the administration of diphenylhydantoin? What are the disadvantages in its use?
4. What advantages do mephobarbital and metharbital have over phenobarbital and what are their dosages?
5. Give the use, dosage, and side effects of primidone and phenacemide.
6. What drugs are useful in petit mal epilepsy? Give their doses and side effects.
7. Why is it often necessary to try several drugs before selecting the one to be used for the individual patient?
8. What drugs may be used in combination?
9. Make a list of the agents that are used in each of the four types of epilepsy and give one trade name for each.
10. Discuss the mechanism by which various conditions can cause spasm of skeletal muscle and that by which the lissive agents can relieve it.
11. Name the five central relaxants of skeletal muscle described in this and the preceding chapter, and give their doses.
12. What are the symptoms of Parkinson's disease?
13. What drugs are useful in controlling these symptoms? Name four. Give dose, method of administration, and one dosage form for each.
14. Explain the mechanism of action of trihexyphenidyl in relieving the symptoms of Parkinson's disease.

REFERENCES

ANTICONVULSANT AGENTS

Baird, H. W., III: "Convulsions in Infancy and Childhood," Connecticut Med., 23:149, 1959.
Carter, C. H.: "Evaluating a New Anticonvulsant in a 'Therapeutic Community,'" Dis. of Nerv. Syst., 21:50, 1960 (Aminoglutethimide).
Everett, G. M., and Richards, R. K.: "Comparative Anticonvulsive Action of 3, 5, 5-Trimethoxazolidine, 2,4-dione (Tridione), Dilantin and Phenobarbital," J. Pharcol. & Exper. Therap., 81:402, 1944.
Lennox, W. G.: "The Petit Mal Epilepsies; Their Treatment with Tridione," J.A.M.A., 129:1069, 1945.
————: "Tridione in the New Treatment of Epilepsy," J.A.M.A., 134:138, 1947.

Livingston, S., and Petersen, D.: "Primidone (Mysoline) in the Treatment of Epilepsy," *New England J. Med.*, **254**:327, 1956.
Noshay, W. C.: "The Treatment and Employability of the Epileptic," *Current M. Dig.*, **23**:67, 1956.
Robertson, E. G.: "A Perspective of Epilepsy," *Postgrad. Med.*, **23**:31, 1959.
Smith, B., and Forster, F. M.: "Mysoline and Milontin," *Neurology*, **4**:137, 1954.
Weaver, L. C.; Swinyard, E. A.; Woodbury, L. A.; and Goodman, L. S.: "Studies on Anticonvulsant Drug Combinations, Phenobarbital and Diphenylhydantoin," *J. Pharmacol. & Exper. Therap.*, **113**:359, 1955.

SKELETAL MUSCLE RELAXANTS

Council on Drugs: "Methocarbamol," *J.A.M.A.*, **172**:60, 1960.
Gruenberg, Friedrich: "Chlormezanone (Trancopal) in Musculoskeletal Disorders," *Current Therap. Res.*, **2**:1, 1960.
Park, H. W.: "Clinical Results with Methocarbamol, a New Interneuronal Blocking Agent," *J.A.M.A.*, **67**:168, 1958.
Ryan, R. E.: "A New Agent for the Symptomatic Relief of Myalgia of the Head," *Clinical Med.*, **7**:323, 1960 (Methocarbamol).
Vazuka, F. A.: "Comparative Effects of Relaxant Drugs on Human Skeletal Muscle Hyperactivity," *Neurology*, **8**:446, 1958.

PARKINSON'S DISEASE

Corbin, K. B.: "Trihexyphenidyl: Evaluation of the New Agent in the Treatment of Parkinsonism," *J.A.M.A.*, **141**:377, 1949.
———: "Treatment of Paralysis Agitans with Chlorphenoxamine Hydrochloride," *J.A.M.A.*, **170**:38, 1959.
Doshay, L. J., and Contable, K.: "Treatment of Paralysis Agitans with Orphenadrine (Dispal) Hydrochloride," *J.A.M.A.*, **163**:1352, 1957.
Doshay, L. J.; Constable, K.; and Agate, F. J., Fr.: "Ethopropazine (Parsidol) Hydrochloride in the Treatment of Paralysis Agitans: Posology, Method of Administration and Effects," *J.A.M.A.*, **160**:348, 1956.
England, A. C., and Schwab, R. S.: "The Management of Parkinson's Disease," *A.M.A. Arch. Int. Med.*, **104**:439, 1959.
Stevens, Harold: "The Management of Parkinsonism," *Maryland M.J.*, **12**:494. 1963.

21

Drugs Used in the Treatment of Motion Sickness. Antiemetics

MOTION SICKNESS

Motion sickness is an abnormal sensitivity to one or more types of motion. The individual may be susceptible to only one type but frequently is affected by any type of motion that is severe enough. Rhythmic movements in linear directions are primary causes, and most persons are more sensitive to vertical displacements than to changes in horizontal movement. Examples of motion sickness are seasickness, carsickness, trainsickness, and airsickness. The syndrome is divided into two stages: (1) early sensitivity, which includes pallor, cold sweating, mental depression, excessive salivation and swallowing, headache, and subnormal pulse and temperature; and (2) nausea and vomiting.

Stimulation of the receptor organs in the labyrinth of the ear, which registers changes in rate of acceleration and deceleration and in the direction of motion, is partly responsible for motion sickness. As a result of this stimulation, impulses are sent by way of the vestibular pathway to the cerebrum and cerebellum. Responses initiated by these impulses cause the symptoms noted in the first stage. Frequently motion sensitivity symptoms end here. The second stage is initiated by impulses transmitted to the vomiting center in the medulla. Other contributing causes are psychic (fear), olfactory (stale and other unpleasant odors), and visual factors.

During World War II, when it was necessary for large numbers of military personnel to travel by land, sea, and air, much research on this problem was carried out, and new drugs effective in preventing or relieving these symptoms were introduced into medicine. These drugs seem to prevent the spread of the impulses to the brain. The drugs used today in the treatment of motion sickness are the belladonna alkaloids, cyclizine hydrochloride, meclizine hydrochloride, promethazine hydrochloride, diphenhydramine hydrochloride, and dimenhydrinate.

BELLADONNA ALKALOIDS

Atropine and scopolamine (hyoscine) are used in the treatment of motion sickness. Scopolamine is more effective, probably owing to its depressant effect on the central nervous system. It is given in doses of 0.6 mg. every four hours. No drugs are superior to these, but their use is limited to 24 to 36 hours by side effects such as dry mouth, giddiness, and blurred vision, which occur with longer use.

Cyclizine Hydrochloride, U.S.P., B.P. (Marezine)

Cyclizine hydrochloride is an effective antinauseant and antiemetic. Its ability to prevent seasickness and airsickness was shown by Dr. H. I. Chinn and his associates. Cyclizine does not produce (except at high doses) drowsiness, dry mouth, or blurred vision. The usual oral dose to prevent motion sickness on long trips is 50 mg. three times a day after meals; for short trips 50 mg, are taken one-half hour before departure. The dose for children is 10 to 25 mg. For nausea and vomiting of pregnancy and vertigo, the oral dose is also 50 mg. three times a day. The lactate is available for intramuscular injection for the treatment of motion sickness or vertigo caused by other vestibular disturbances. The intramuscular dose is the same as the oral dose for the hydrochloride.The rectal dose for adults is 100 mg.

Preparations

Cyclizine Hydrochloride Tablets, U.S.P.   50 mg.
Cyclizine Hydrochloride Suppositories   50 and 100 mg.
Cyclizine Lactate Injection   50 mg. in 1 ml.
Trade name: Marezine Hydrochloride or Lactate

Meclizine Hydrochloride, U.S.P.; Meclozine, B.P. (Bonine)

Meclizine hydrochloride possesses a mild and prolonged antihistaminic action and is mainly used to prevent motion sickness. It is useful in airsickness, seasickness, and some cases of Ménière's syndrome—recurring episodes of tinnitus, vertigo, nausea, incoordination, headache, and reduced hearing. There is a low incidence of side effects. Drowsiness is produced in some persons taking 50 mg. but is seldom noted with doses of 25 mg. The usual oral dose is 25 mg. (25 to 50 mg.) once a day. One or two tablets are given one hour before departure. The effects last 24 hours.

Preparations

Meclizine Hydrochloride Tablets, U.S.P.   25 mg.
Meclizine Hydrochloride Chewing Gum   25 mg.
Trade names: Bonine; Ancolan; Postafene

Promethazine Hydrochloride, U.S.P., B.P., I.P. (Phenergan)

Promethazine is a potent, sedative antihistaminic drug. It is highly effective in airsickness as a prophylactic drug, and the effects produced last 8 to 12 hours. It is also used with narcotics to potentiate their action. The usual oral dose is 25 mg. a day (6 to 50 mg.) up to three times a day. The dose for children is 10 mg. The side effects are minimal, although it does produce drowsiness. The parenteral dose is 25 mg. (up to 1 mg. per kilogram body weight).

Preparations

Promethazine Hydrochloride Tablets, U.S.P. (Scored) ; Promethazine Tablets, B.P.	12 mg. (also 12.5 and 25 mg.)
Promethazine Hydrochloride Injection, U.S.P.	25 mg. in 1 ml.; 250 mg. in 10 ml.
Promethazine Hydrochloride Syrup	1.25 mg. in 1 ml.
Promethazine Hydrochloride Suppositories.	25 and 50 mg.

Trade names: Phenergan; Lergigan; Fargan

Diphenhydramine Hydrochloride, U.S.P., B.P., I.P. (Benadryl)

Diphenhydramine is a very useful drug in motion sickness. The usual oral dose is 25 mg. (25 to 50 mg.) up to four times a day. The dose for children is 10 to 25 mg. The intravenous dose is 50 mg. (10 to 50 mg.) It has an atropine-like and a sedative action. Better results are obtained with a combination of diphenhydramine (25 mg.) and scopolamine (0.35 mg.) than with either drug alone. Diphenhydramine is also discussed on pages 374 and 761.

Preparations

Diphenhydramine Hydrochloride Capsules, U.S.P., B.P.	25 and 50 mg.
Diphenhydramine Hydrochloride Tablets (Delayed Action)	50 mg.
Diphenhydramine Hydrochloride Elixir, U.S.P.	2.5 mg. in 1 ml.
Diphenhydramine Hydrochloride Injection, U.S.P.	50 mg. in 1 ml.; 100 mg. in 10 ml.; 300 mg. in 30 ml.

Trade names: Benadryl Hydrochloride; Allergan; Allerginia; Amidryl; Benapon; Benodine; Dabylen; Dimedrol; Restamin

Dimenhydrinate, U.S.P., B.P., I.P. (Dramamine)

Dimenhydrinate, a theophylline derivative of diphenhydramine, is useful in the treatment and prophylaxis of motion sickness. It relieves nausea, vomiting, and dizziness in a large percentage of patients. The usual oral dose is 50 mg. (50 to 100 mg.) four times a day. The intramuscular dose is 50 mg. Prophylactically, it is administered one-half hour before departure on a trip. Results of extensive trials have not proved that this drug is more effective than diphenhydramine. It has been used in radiation sickness, for combating

380 DRUGS ACTING ON THE CENTRAL NERVOUS SYSTEM

drug-induced vomiting, with electroshock therapy, and in other procedures associated with vertigo and nausea.

The successful use of dimenhydrinate in motion sickness prompted its parenteral use for postoperative nausea and vomiting. It is injected in 50-mg. doses prior to surgery and 50-mg. amounts at the conclusion of the operation and every four hours thereafter for three doses.

Preparations

Dimenhydrinate Tablets, U.S.P., B.P.   50 mg.
Dimenhydrinate Injection, B.P.   5-ml. vials containing 50 mg. in 1 ml.
Dimenhydrinate Syrup, U.S.P.   3 mg. in 1 ml.
    Trade names: Dramamine; Amosyt; Bontourist; Chloranautine;
    Dramarin; Nautamine; Neptusan; Permital; Suprimal

SUMMARY

The anti-motion-sickness drugs usually are given three times a day for seasickness and airsickness, with the exception of promethazine, which is given twice a day, and meclizine, which is given once a day. All these drugs prevent airsickness when a single dose is given prior to flying. Since these drugs all produce drowsiness, 5 mg. of dextroamphetamine sulfate may be administered with them to lessen drowsiness. Persons receiving these drugs should be told of this possible drowsiness as it may affect their activities; for example, they should not drive an automobile.

A newer agent, trimethobenzamide, effective in motion sickness is described in the following section, since it is useful as well in other types of nausea and vomiting.

ANTIEMETICS

The nausea-vomiting complex is one of the most frequent symptoms of disease. It is often induced by certain drugs and occurs after operations, during pregnancy, and as the result of certain types of motion in hypersensitive persons. Often it is mild and self-limiting, but at times it is very disturbing and should be brought under control when possible.

The Vomiting Centers and Chemoreceptor Zones. Vomiting is a natural protective mechanism for expelling irritating and toxic materials from the stomach. It is brought about by a series of movements controlled by two closely related centers in the medulla: the vomiting center, which is located in the lateral reticular formation, and a specialized area, the chemoreceptor trigger zone (CTZ), found on the surface close to the vagal nuclei. Vomiting may be initiated from almost every part of the body. Impulses reach the vomiting center from the viscera by way of the vagus and sympathetic nerves and also from various parts of the brain. Apomorphine, a

---
Table 25

Recommendations for Antiemetic Therapy*

Source of Emesis	Recommended Agent	Dose, mg.†	Frequency
Drug-induced			
Digitalis	Chlorpromazine	10–25	q.i.d.‡
Antibiotics	Chlorpromazine	10–25	q.i.d.
Nitrogen mustard	Chlorpromazine	10–25	q.i.d.
Alcoholic states	Chlorpromazine	50–150	q.i.d.
Opiates	Meclizine	25–50	q.i.d.
	Cyclizine	50	t.i.d.
	Dimenhydrinate	100	q.i.d.
Infections	Chlorpromazine	10–25	q.i.d.
Toxicoses			q.i.d.
Diabetic acidosis	Chlorpromazine	10–25	q.i.d.
Uremia	Chlorpromazine	10–25	q.i.d.
Carcinomatosis	Chlorpromazine	10–25	q.i.d.
Radiation sickness	Chlorpromazine	10–25	q.i.d.
Other	Chlorpromazine	10–25	
Postoperative vomiting			
Prophylactic	Dimenhydrinate	50	t.i.d.–q.i.d.
	Diphenhydramine	50–100	t.i.d.–q.i.d.
	Cyclizine	50	t.i.d.
Therapeutic	Chlorpromazine	25–50§	t.i.d.
Pregnancy	Meclizine (with or without pyridoxine)	25–50	h.s.
Motion sickness			
Airsickness	Scopolamine	0.65–1.0	
	Meclizine	25	b.i.d.
Seasickness	Meclizine	50	q.d.

* Modified from Conner, P. K., Jr., and Moyer, J. M.: "A Therapeutic Appraisal of Antiemetic Agents," *GP*, **14**:138, 1956. Prochlorperazine (p. 336) and triflupromazine (p. 337) can also be used for those conditions for which chlorpromazine is listed. Trimethobenzamide, a new agent, is reportedly effective in all conditions listed.
† Refers to oral dose; parenteral doses are usually slightly less.
‡ q.d. = once per day; b.i.d. = twice daily; t.i.d. = 3 times a day; q.i.d. = 4 times a day; h.s. = bedtime
§ First dose usually administered parenterally.

powerful emetic, and other drugs such as morphine, digitoxin, and the salicylates, which cause nausea and vomiting as one of their side effects, and toxins from bacterial and other diseases activate the CTZ, which in turn stimulates the vomiting center. Chlorpromazine, the original phenothiazine (Chap. 19), depresses the CTZ and is widely used as an antiemetic.

Many other phenothiazines such as prochlorperazine, triflupromazine, and pipamazine are also effective. **Pipamazine (Mornidine)** is also a weak

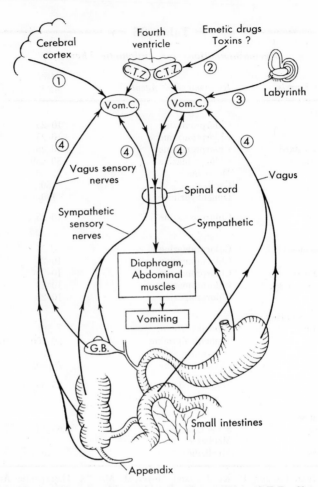

Fig. 11. Mechanisms in the initiation of vomiting. *C.T.Z.* Chemoreceptor trigger zones. *Vom. C.* vomiting center. *G.B.* gallbladder. *(1)* Cerebral stimulation of vomiting center; *(2)* drug stimulation of chemoreceptor trigger zone; *(3)* labyrinthine (motion, etc.) stimulation of vomiting center; *(4)* visceral afferent stimulation of vomiting center. The text describes the sites of action of the anti-emetics.

tranquilizer. It should be used with all the precautions recommended for chlorpromazine (see p. 333). The oral adult dose is 5 mg. The intramuscular or intravenous dose is 5 mg. injected over a five-minute period. It is available in 5-mg. tablets and as an injection containing 5 mg. in 1 ml.

Comparisons of the clinical effectiveness of various antiemetic drugs in vomiting associated with drug therapy, infections, toxicoses, surgical anesthesia, pregnancy, and motion sickness are summarized in Table 25.

Thiethylperazine Maleate (Torecan)

This compound is believed to suppress the chemoreceptor trigger zone (CTZ). It has been found useful in the control of vomiting in various infections, psychologically caused disturbances, pregnancy, surgery, radiation sickness, vertigo, and drug-induced emesis. It should not be used in severely depressed or comatose states or when a warning may be masked as in the vomiting of acute appendicitis. Side effects are occasionally seen at doses of 30 mg. or more daily, including disturbed gait, dryness of the mouth and nose, and lightheadedness. Higher doses may lead to extrapyramidal-type symptoms resembling parkinsonism in part (see p. 371). Dosage must be lowered or discontinued in the presence of troublesome degrees of these reactions.

Dosage and Administration. Thiethylperazine may be administered orally to adults in a dose of 10 mg. three times daily or intramuscularly in a dose of 10 to 20 mg. daily.

Preparations

Thiethylperazine Maleate Tablets   10 mg.
Thiethylperazine Maleate Solution   2-ml. ampuls containing 5 mg. in 1 ml.
                    Trade name: Torecan

Trimethobenzamide (Tigan) Hydrochloride

This is an entirely new compound in antiemetic therapy. It reduces or controls nausea and vomiting in pregnancy, motion sickness, gastrointestinal infections, radiation therapy, carcinomatosis, and specific toxicoses and those resulting from the administration of certain drugs.

Side Effects. These are minimal. Pain, burning, and erythema may occur at the site of injection.

Dosage and Methods of Administration. This drug may be given intramuscularly, if the patient is vomiting. The dose is 200 mg. to patients weighing 90 lb. or more. Children over 30 lb. may receive 50 mg. These doses may be repeated in two or three hours, or up to four times daily. Orally, 50 to 100 mg. may be given four times daily, depending upon the weight of the child or adult. The drug is available in capsules containing 100 mg. and as an injection containing 100 mg. in 1 ml.

REVIEW QUESTIONS

1. *What are some of the factors that cause motion sickness (airsickness, seasickness)?*
2. *Describe the symptoms experienced in motion sickness.*

3. *What drugs are useful in preventing these symptoms? Name four. Give dose, method of administration, and duration of action.*

REFERENCES

MOTION SICKNESS AND ANTIEMETICS

Abrams, W. B.; Roseff, I.; Kaufman, J.; Goldman, L. M.; and Bernstein, A.: "Clinical Evaluation of Trimethobenzamide, New Antiemetic Drug," *New York J. Med.*, **59**:4217, 1959.

Borison, H. L., and Wang, S. C.: "Physiology and Pharmacology of Vomiting," *Pharmacol. Rev.*, **5**:193, 1953.

Browne, D. C., and Sparks, R.: "Vomiting Mechanisms: A Clinical Study of Thiethylperazine," *South. M. J.*, **54**:953, 1961.

Chinn, H. I.: "Travel and Motion Sickness," *Internat. Rec. Med.*, **168**:523, 1955.

Commentary: "The Concept of Motion Sensitivity," *Internat. Rec. Med.*, **168**:371, 1955.

Doyle, O. W.: "Evaluation of Trimethobenzamide as an Antiemetic in Nausea and Vomiting Associated with Neoplasms," *Clin. Med.*, **7**:43, 1960.

Moyer, J. H.: "Effective Antiemetic Agents," *Med. Clin. North Amer.*, March, 1957, p. 1.

Wilson, W. L.; Shane, L. L.; and Moyer, J. H.: "The Use of Thioperazine as an Antiemetic," *Antibiotic Med. and Clin Therapy*, **6**:421, 1959.

22

The Alcohols

ETHYL ALCOHOL

Alcoholic beverages have been prepared and used by man as both beverages and medicinal agents since ancient times. At one time alcohol was thought to be a remedy for practically all diseases. During the past century its therapeutic use has diminished greatly, but its abuse as a beverage has become both a medical and a sociological problem.

Ethyl alcohol, or grain alcohol, is obtained by fermentation. It is formed by the growth of yeast in fruit and vegetable juices containing sugar or starch. The starch may be converted to sugar, which is oxidized to alcohol and carbon dioxide. Fermented, undistilled beverages such as wines and beers contain less than 14 per cent alcohol, unless alcohol is added; concentrations over 14 per cent inactivate the yeast and stop further production of alcohol. Port and sherry wines are "fortified wines" and contain about 22 per cent alcohol. Distilled liquors such as whisky, brandy, rum, and gin are made by distilling fermented grains, vegetables, or grapes and contain about 50 to 56 per cent alcohol.

Absorption, Fate, and Excretion. When alcoholic beverages are ingested, alcohol is rapidly absorbed, partially through the stomach wall and partially from the duodenal portion of the small intestine. Absorption is more rapid when the stomach is empty. The alcohol is carried to all parts of the body by the blood. Ninety to ninety-eight per cent of that absorbed is oxidized rapidly in the tissues of the body to carbon dioxide and water. Approximately 10 ml. an hour can be oxidized without symptoms. From 1 to 5 per cent of the ingested alcohol is excreted unchanged in the expired air and urine.

When there is no food in the stomach, ingested alcohol can be detected in the blood five minutes after its ingestion. The maximum concentration is reached in 30 minutes to one hour, depending upon the amount consumed. The concentration decreases as the alcohol is metabolized. Symptoms of intoxication are more noticeable when the concentration of alcohol in the blood is increasing.

A minute amount of alcohol is present in the blood and brain at all times. There is about 0.4 mg. per cent in the blood and 0.04 mg. per cent

385

in the brain. The substance is formed in an intermediate step in the oxidation of glucose.

The metabolism of alcohol in the body furnishes calories and energy. In this way it serves as a type of food and thus spares proteins, fats, and carbohydrates, which may be stored in the body.

Pharmacological Actions. *On the Central Nervous System.* In the amounts usually consumed, alcohol depresses the cells of the cerebral cortex. In larger quantities, its depressant action extends to the cerebellum, the spinal cord, and the respiratory center of the medulla. Alcohol kills by paralysis of the respiratory center, which controls normal breathing.

One effect of alcohol on the cerebral cortex is depression of inhibitory behavior. Small amounts often produce a feeling of well-being, talkativeness, greater vivacity, and increased confidence in one's ability. The powers of discrimination, judgment, self-criticism, and memory are reduced. There may be a disregard for certain moral and ethical concepts. Larger quantities of the drug may cause excitement and impulsive speech and behavior. The special senses become dulled and the person cannot hear normally and thus talks louder. The inebriated person may become boisterous, sentimental, or pugnacious. This sense of freedom from inhibitions has given alcohol the false reputation of being a stimulant.

Tests requiring conditioned reflexes are not performed well under the influence of alcohol. Judgment is impaired. After ingestion of 1 oz. of whisky, speed in typing is reduced and the number of errors is increased. Alcohol tends to make a person conform to his environment. It will produce sleep under favorable conditions.

The effect on the sensory areas extends to the motor areas and to the cerebellum. Irregularity in gait and lack of coordination occur. Still larger amounts in the blood cause a depressed respiration and stupor or coma.

The kidneys excrete alcohol, and attempts have been made to correlate its concentration in the urine with the degree of incoordination, impaired judgment, and depressed activity.

On the Heart and Circulation. Moderate amounts of alcohol produce little effect on the circulation. There may be a slight increase in the heart rate and blood pressure. The peripheral blood vessels are dilated and the blood passes from the viscera to the periphery. This produces a feeling of warmth and a flushing of the face in a warm room. Alcoholic beverages are sometimes used in peripheral vascular diseases to relieve constriction of the peripheral vessels. Some physicians recommend the use of alcoholic beverages for the relief of anginal pain.

On Body Temperature. Moderate amounts of alcohol produce no effect on body temperature, despite the feeling of warmth. Larger quantities cause a fall in body temperature due to the action on the heat center in the hypothalamus and peripheral vasodilatation.

On the Digestive Tract. Alcoholic beverages such as brandy and wine contain bitter substances that stimulate reflexly the flow of gastric juice and produce a sensation of warmth in the stomach owing to mild irritation. Small amounts of alcoholic beverages before meals depress the inhibitory centers, dispel worry and fatigue, and relieve tension. They stimulate the appetite and the secretion of hydrochloric acid. Thus patients with peptic ulcer are advised not to drink alcoholic beverages.

Alcohol, U.S.P., B.P. (I.P.) (Ethyl Alcohol)

Unless otherwise specified, the word "alcohol" in medical usage refers to 92 to 95 per cent ethyl alcohol and 5 to 8 per cent water by volume. It is an excellent solvent and mixes in all proportions with water.

Pharmacological Actions. *On the Nerve Trunks.* Degeneration of a nerve trunk is produced when 80 per cent alcohol is injected into or near the nerve, and insensibility to pain results. Pain stimuli passing over the nerve are blocked. The nerve trunk regenerates and pain may return. In facial neuralgia, relief from pain is afforded which may last for several months.

On the Skin. Alcohol has an astringent action on the skin. Ninety-five per cent alcohol absorbs water out of the skin and makes it dry. Seventy per cent alcohol is more antiseptic than other dilutions because it penetrates bacteria more readily. This concentration is the one most generally used for cleansing the body surface. It does not kill spores. It may be used as a lubricant for skin massage; however, its drying effect limits its use in this area. Frequently it is combined with a lanolin base. Since alcohol evaporates readily and produces a sensation of coolness, it is used in sponge baths to relieve an elevated temperature.

Therapeutic Uses

Uses of Alcoholic Beverages

1. In peripheral vascular diseases to dilate the blood vessels.
2. To improve the appetite and aid digestion.
3. To produce sleep in some people.
4. As reflex stimulants for the respiration and circulation in case of collapse.

Local Uses of Alcohol

1. As an astringent.
2. As a lubricant for skin massage.
3. As an antiseptic for cleansing the skin.
4. For the relief of pain. It is injected in or around the sensory nerve truck.
5. As an antifoam agent in pulmonary edema. When inhaled it changes a profuse frothy fluid to a small amount of liquid by lowering its surface tension.

Preparations

Alcohol, U.S.P., B.P.	Contains 94.9 per cent ethyl alcohol by volume
Diluted Alcohol, U.S.P., B.P.	Contains not less than 48.4 per cent and not more than 49.5 per cent ethyl alcohol by volume
Dehydrated Alcohol, B.P. (Absolute Alcohol)	Contains not less than 99 per cent ethyl alcohol
Whisky	Contains not less than 47 per cent and not more than 53 per cent ethyl alcohol by volume
Brandy	Contains not less than 48 per cent and not more thon 54 per cent ethyl alcohol by volume
Sherry Wine	Contains approximately 20 per cent ethyl alcohol

ACUTE POISONING AND CHRONIC ALCOHOLISM

Acute Poisoning (Drunkenness). Acute alcohol poisoning results from drinking excessive amounts of alcoholic beverages. The symptoms may be divided into two stages: (1) early excitement and (2) depression that may progress to coma. The individual may fall into a deep sleep or stupor. Sensations are lessened; hence pain may not be experienced. All muscles are relaxed. The face becomes cyanotic and the extremities are cold. The breathing is slow and snoring, and the pulse is rapid, strong, and bounding. Coma, with a rapid, weak, thready pulse, may follow. Death frequently results from respiratory failure due to the depressant action of alcohol on the respiratory center.

Treatment of Acute Intoxication. The liquor is removed from the stomach by gastric lavage. The patient is kept warm. Five to ten per cent glucose in 1 or 2 L. of saline may be administered. Twenty units of insulin and the contents of an ampul of vitamin B complex may be added to the saline solution to hasten the elimination of the alcohol and combat dehydration, which often occurs. Triiodothyronine (Cytomel) has also been used with limited success. It has been shown to hasten the removal of alcohol from the blood. Artificial respiration or oxygen may be administered to diminish the respiratory depression. Anticonvulsant therapy is recommended to prevent seizures that frequently occur when the patient is recovering from acute alcoholism.

The tranquilizing drugs are used to control anxiety, restlessness, and hyperirritability. They are particularly useful in the acute stage and in the period following withdrawal of the drug. The barbiturates are the sedatives of choice to combat insomnia. The smallest effective dose should be prescribed. Paraldehyde is given orally and rectally as a sedative. Chloral hydrate is also given orally as a sedative. The adrenocorticosteroids and ACTH are effective (1) in controlling the symptoms and reducing the period of disability in acute alcoholism, (2) in controlling the postwithdrawal symptoms, and (3) in delirium tremens. It is believed that improvement occurs because of the effect of the corticosteroids on the phenomena resulting from the severe stress that alcohol induces in man. The use of steroids and paraldehyde in alcoholism has decreased with the introduction of the tranquilizers.

The state of alcoholic depression that follows the withdrawal of alcohol may be treated with stimulants such as caffeine sodium benzoate, dextro amphetamine (Dexedrine), methylphenidate (Ritalin), and chlordiazepoxide (Librium).

Chronic Alcoholism.   Chronic alcoholism results from the constant use of the more potent alcoholic beverages. The habit is more prevalent in psychoneurotics and emotionally immature individuals who wish to escape from the realities, frustrations, and responsibilities of life. It may result from heavy social drinking over a period of years. There are about 60 million social drinkers in the United States. They drink because the presence of alcohol in the circulation reduces self-criticism and shyness and allows an escape from the unpleasant realities of life. With moderate drinkers, life becomes more pleasant because the alcohol produces relaxation and contentment, and minor irritations are minimized. Yet even social drinking may present a problem. It often causes a lowering of moral standards and a disregard for the rights of others. It is extremely dangerous to drive a motor vehicle after drinking. Twenty-seven persons are killed daily in the United States as the result of drinking by either drivers or pedestrians.

A chronic alcoholic is an unsuccessful social drinker. There are about four million chronic alcoholics in the United States. They drink alcoholic beverages excessively even though they know that this will injure their health and jeopardize their jobs, their family relationships, and their place in society. Alcoholic addicts are sick people and should be treated with sympathy and understanding. The main symptom is an intense craving for alcohol. Some persons show no signs of intoxication, while others appear to be drunk all the time.

Symptoms of Chronic Alcoholism.   Symptoms of chronic alcoholism are due to the direct effect of alcohol on the central nervous system, degenerative changes in the tissues, and inadequate diet. The most common manifestation is a redness of the nose, face, and conjunctiva. Nutritional deficiencies result from gastroenteritis, improper digestion of food, malnutrition, and inadequate absorption of thiamine (vitamin B_1), which may cause polyneuritis. Muscular tremors, peripheral and optic neuritis, various psychoses, and dulling of mental facilities result from nerve degeneration. About 15 per cent of the chronic alcoholics develop various psychoses, including delirium tremens.

Treatment of Chronic Alcoholism.   The treatment may be divided into three categories: (1) nutritional therapy, (2) psychotherapy, and (3) drug therapy.

NUTRITIONAL THERAPY.   A high-calorie diet supplemented with vitamins, especially thiamine chloride (B₁), is prescribed. Vitamin C (ascorbic acid) is also administered. The vitamins are given orally or intravenously, according to the needs of the patient.

PSYCHOTHERAPY.   This is the most difficult form of treatment. The physician is dealing with a person who has a problem or problems he wishes to avoid or forget. It is necessary to discover and remove the cause. A change in environment may be indicated.

In a great many cases, an organization called Alcoholics Anonymous (A.A.) meets a definite need in the treatment and prevention of relapse in alcoholism. Rehabilitated former alcoholics work with chronic alcoholics and offer the physical, mental, and spiritual aid necessary for their recovery. The national headquarters of A.A. is in New York City, and there are local clubs in most cities in the United States.

Approximately one half of the chronic alcoholics have a sincere desire to stop drinking and are able to do so immediately. About 40 per cent finally stop drinking after repeated trials and failures. About 10 per cent never stop.

Delirium Tremens.   Delirium tremens is an acute mania induced in the chronic alcoholic by the superimposing of unusual conditions of stress, such as exposure, overexertion, injury, an operation, or infection. The symptoms are restlessness, tremors, insomnia, delirium, and hallucinations of sight, touch, and hearing. The incidence of delirium tremens has diminished as a result of the use of tranquilizing drugs and corticosteroids in the treatment of chronic alcoholism.

Treatment of Delirium Tremens.   Alcohol is withdrawn and the patient is put on a light, nourishing diet. Fluids are administered intraveneously to assist in the restoration of water balance: 100 ml. of 5 per cent glucose in isotonic salt solution, to which 500 mg. of ascorbic acid, 200 mg. of thiamine chloride, and 100 mg. of nicotinic acid have been added. Sedatives such as phenobarbital in doses of 60 to 120 mg., paraldehyde in doses of 10 to 16 ml., or chloral hydrate in doses of 1 to 2 Gm. may be administered. Diphenylhydantoin sodium is administered in doses of 180 mg. as an anticonvulsant. The administration of corticosteroid preparations or chlorpromazine orally or parenterally has been very effective in controlling the symptoms.

ABSTINENCE-PRODUCING DRUGS

Disulfiram (Antabuse)

Disulfiram produces no apparent pharmacological effects when given alone, even after prolonged administration. In the recommended doses, it is slowly absorbed and slowly destroyed. After its administration for several days or weeks, ingestion of small amounts of alcohol produces very unpleasant, disconcerting, and even dangerous symptoms. These are flushing of the face;

gastrointestinal distress such as nausea, vomiting, and diarrhea; palpitation; dyspnea; fall in blood pressure; and, occasionally, collapse. The severity of the symptoms varies with the person and the amount of disulfiram and alcohol ingested. Disulfiram apparently interferes with the normal metabolism of alcohol in the body by retarding the metabolism of acetaldehyde. The increased concentration of acetaldehyde in the blood causes the symptoms.

Therapeutic Use. Disulfiram is used as an aid in the treatment of chronic alcoholism. The patient must consent to its administration and be informed of the symptoms to be expected if alcohol is ingested. The family must be advised of the danger of secret administration. The patient is premedicated with disulfiram for two or three weeks, whereupon a "test dose" of alcohol is administered, preferably in the hospital, to acquaint the patient with the symptoms that result from the ingestion of alcohol. A 15-ml. dose of 100-proof whisky is followed every 15 minutes by administration of the alcoholic beverages the patient is accustomed to taking, until symptoms occur.

Dose and Method of Administration. Disulfiram is given orally. No alcohol is taken 12 hours prior to its administration. A 500-mg. dose is given daily for two or three weeks. The usual maintenance dose is 250 mg. (125 to 500 mg.) daily. It may be necessary to continue the administration uninterrupted for several months or years.

Toxic Effects. Although disulfiram is usually nontoxic, severe symptoms have occurred in some patients from drinking alcoholic beverages after its administration. A few deaths have resulted due to circulatory and respiratory failure. Personality changes have also been noted. The drug is contraindicated in heart, liver, or kidney disease, epilepsy, diabetes, and various psychoses.

Preparation

Disulfiram Tablets   500 mg.
                 Trade name: Antabuse

Citrated Calcium Carbimide (Temposil)

This drug also interferes with the metabolism of alcohol and causes an accumulation of acetaldehyde in the body. It is less potent and produces fewer side effects than does disulfiram. The oral dose is 50 mg. twice daily. Tablets of 50 mg. are available.

OTHER SUBSTANCES PRODUCING ANTIALCOHOL EFFECTS

Recent reports on the antialcohol effects of the hypoglycemic sulfonylureas such as tolbutamide (Orinase), chlorpropamide (Diabinese), and also phenformin (DBI) re-emphasize the serious reactions that can occur when alcohol is taken with certain drugs. The widespread use of intoxicating beverages concomitant with the prevalent use of drugs in our present-day society necessitates the knowledge of drugs or other substances which will cause the so-called antialcohol reaction. The following substances may produce these reactions.

1. Tetraethyl lead (gasoline station attendants).
2. *Coprinus atramentarius* (edible mushroom).
3. Phenylbutazone (Butazolidin).
4. Isoniazid (INH).
5. Glyceryl trinitrate and certain organic nitrites.
6. Furazolidone (Furoxone).
7. Dimercaprol (BAL).
8. Chloramphenicol.

Although it is believed that most of these reactions are due to the inhibition of alcohol metabolism at the acetaldehyde level, it is possible that the antialcohol effect may not be due to the accumulation of acetaldehyde alone but may be related in part to the accumulation of other aldehydes arising endogenously such as certain catecholamine metabolites.

Methyl Alcohol (Wood Alcohol, Methanol)

Methyl alcohol was made years ago by the destructive distillation of wood. Now it is made synthetically from water and carbon monoxide under pressure. Although methyl alcohol has no value in medicine, it is used in various industries; this industrial use has led to accidental or industrial poisoning, since the substance is highly toxic.

Uses of Methyl Alcohol

1. To denature ethyl alcohol and make it unfit to drink.
2. As a solvent for shellac, varnishes, and paints, and as an antifreeze. Since it is dangerous to inhale vapors of methyl alcohol, adequate ventilation is necessary when products dissolved in it are used.

Poisoning with Methyl Alcohol. Toxic effects may be produced from drinking denatured alcohol or by inhaling the vapors. Methyl alcohol is not completely oxidized in the body as is ethyl alcohol. It is slowly metabolized to formaldehyde and formic acid. Formaldehyde is a tissue fixative and formic acid is toxic to the liver and kidney. Methyl alcohol has a specific action on the retina and may produce retinitis. Rapid degeneration of the optic nerve may cause blindness.

OTHER ALCOHOLS

There are many different alcohols, and their uses are many and varied. Our interest focuses on the few useful in the field of medicine.

Isopropyl and Butyl Alcohols

These are used as rubbing alcohols. They are also useful as solvents or diluents in the manufacture of lacquers, perfumes, cosmetics, and varnish removers. When they are taken internally, the symptoms of intoxication resemble those of ethyl alcohol. However, they are much more toxic.

Glycerin, U.S.P., B.P.

Glycerin is contained chemically in fat. It is a clear, viscid liquid that mixes with water in all proportions. It has a sweet, burning taste. Glycerin is used as a cathartic in the form of suppositories and in the treatment of dry hands (glycerin and rose water) and dry, coated mouth (glycerin and lemon). Since glycerin absorbs fluid, it softens and moistens the mouth. However, the end result may be a dry, irritated mouth as fluid is drawn from the mucous membrane. It is incorporated in salves, ointments, and lotions and is also used as a vehicle for other agents.

SUGAR ALCOHOLS

Sugar alcohols are white crystalline substances. *Mannitol,* which is obtained from manna, is a precursor of glycerin and may serve as a food. It has a cathartic action. *Sorbitol,* an isomer of mannitol, is present in the leaves of many plants, such as the mountain ash and the mulberry tree.

Sorbitol, U.S.P.

Sorbitol may be used in the diabetic diet, since some diabetics can tolerate sorbitol better than sugar, or glucose. Sorbitol is oxidized to fructose, which is polymerized in the liver and remains there a longer period of time. This allows more time for the mobilization of insulin to metabolize the sugar when it is present in the blood. The advantage of the use of sorbitol in the diabetic is that it delays postprandial hyperglycemia because the sugar is released more slowly. It is a matter not of "no calories" but of "slow calories."

Other Uses of Sorbitol. Sorbitol is used to prevent the curling of postage stamps, to disperse vitamins in cereals, to keep peppermint candy soft, and to keep tobacco from drying out.

Polysorbate 80, U.S.P. (Polyoxyethylene, 20 Sorbitan Mono-oleate, "Tween 80")

Polysorbate 80 is a complex mixture of polyoxyethylene ethers of mixed partial oleic acid esters of sorbitol anhydride. It is used as a dispersing agent for many oil-soluble foods and drugs. It promotes the absorption of fat and vitamin A from the gastrointestinal tract in patients with steatorrhea. Polysorbate 80 is comparatively nontoxic. The oral dose is 2 to 5 Gm. three times daily with meals. It may be administered in capsules or mixed with orange juice or water.

Therapeutic Uses

1. Nontropical sprue, where fat is not metabolized but passes in the feces.
2. Steatorrhea, 5 to 20 Gm., three or four times a day.
3. For infants who cannot utilize fat.
4. Subtotal gastrectomy in persons with gastric ulcer.

Preparation

Polysorbate 80 Capsules	500 mg.
Polysorbate Solution	1.5 Gm. in 5 ml.

Trade names: Monitan; Olothorb; Sorlate; Tween 80

REVIEW QUESTIONS

1. *What is "alcohol"?*
2. *Discuss the absorption of alcohol from the gastrointestinal tract and its fate in the body.*
3. *How does alcohol affect the circulation?*
4. *Discuss chronic alcoholism and its treatment.*
5. *Compare the fate of ethyl and methyl alcohols in the body.*
6. *What is the value of sorbitol in the diet?*
7. *Name several therapeutic uses for polysorbate 80.*
8. *A diabetic whose medication has been changed from insulin to Orinase asks the nurse why the doctor told him that he can no longer take an occasional social drink. How would you explain this to him?*

REFERENCES

Emerson, E. B.: *Alcohol and Man.* The Macmillan Company, New York, 1955.
Feldman, D. J.: "Drug Therapy of Chronic Alcoholism," *M. Clin. North America,* **41**:381, 1957.
Himwich, H. E.: "The Management of Alcoholism," *Modern Med.,* Nov. 1, 1959, p. 23.
Jellinek, E. M.: "Phases of Alcohol Addiction," *Quart. J. Stud. Alcohol,* **13**:673, 1952.
Lemkau, P. V.: "Alcoholism, a Medical and Social Problem," *Maryland State M. J.,* **1**:467, 1952.

23

Stimulants of the Central Nervous System: Caffeine, the Amphetamines, Anorexigenics, Respiratory Stimulants, and Therapeutic Gases

Central nervous system stimulants are drugs that increase the activity of some portion of the cerebrum, medulla, or spinal cord. When the frontal cortical areas of the brain are stimulated, there is an increase in mental alertness, the spirits are brightened, and mental fatigue is reduced. Examples of cerebral stimulants are caffeine and the amphetamines. The psychostimulants discussed in Chapter 19 are pharmacologically classified as central nervous system stimulants but are placed in the chapter concerning mental disease because of the orientation of general clinical thought toward their usage in that area.

The medullary centers may be stimulated directly or reflexly to cause an increase in the respiration or circulation. Some of the drugs used in threatened collapse are nikethamide (Coramine), pentylenetetrazol (Metrazol), and aromatic ammonia spirit.

The spinal cord may be stimulated and cause an increase in reflex activity. Strychnine produces this action primarily and was long used, but it is no longer recommended in therapeutics because of its toxicity.

CEREBRAL STIMULANTS

XANTHINE BASES

Caffeine, an alkaloid obtained from tea leaves, coffee beans, and other plants, is a xanthine derivative. Theophylline is also obtained from tea leaves. Theobromine comes from the chocolate plant. These drugs, which are closely related chemically, produce similar pharmacological responses. They are all cerebral stimulants, coronary artery dilators, diuretics, and cardiac and respiratory stimulants, but they are selective in producing varying degrees of response in different tissues. Theophylline acts mainly to relax smooth muscle such as the coronaries and bronchioles and is used in the treatment of bronchial asthma; theobromine, mainly as a diuretic; and caffeine, mainly as a psychic and respiratory stimulant.

395

Caffeine is a white crystalline substance with a bitter taste and has been made synthetically. It is a weak base and does not produce defined salts, but it is made more soluble by the addition of citric acid or sodium benzoate. A 50–50 mixture of citric acid and caffeine, called *citrated caffeine,* is administered orally; caffeine and sodium benzoate is administered parenterally.

Pharmacological Actions.   When caffeine is administered orally in doses of 200 mg. (100 to 500 mg.), its principal action is on the cerebral cortex. It is a mild cerebral stimulant. Caffeine increases mental alacrity, and drowsiness disappears without subsequent depression. Judgment is keener and more discriminating, and the ability to memorize is increased temporarily.

In oral therapeutic doses, caffeine produces no effect on the medullary centers. If caffeine and sodium benzoate in a dose of 500 mg. is injected subcutaneously, the respiration is stimulated, especially if it has been depressed by drugs. Caffeine also stimulates the vagus center. The cardiac slowing, which would be expected by this action, is antagonized by the stimulant action of caffeine on the heart muscle. The vasoconstrictor center is stimulated, but at the same time the peripheral blood vessels dilate owing to the direct relaxant action of caffeine on the smooth muscle of the blood vessels. The over-all effect is a transient fall in blood pressure. Caffeine produces diuresis mainly through its depressant action on the kidney tubules.

Caffeine does not produce analgesia directly; however, it will reduce cerebral blood flow, which is followed secondarily by a reduction in the cerebrospinal fluid pressure. Hence, caffeine is useful in the treatment of hypertensive headaches.

Absorption, Fate, and Excretion.   Caffeine increases acid secretion in the stomach and is readily absorbed from the gastrointestinal tract. It is widely distributed in the tissues of the body and is almost completely metabolized. About I per cent is excreted in the urine.

Toxicity.   Caffeine has a very large margin of safety. There is no record of poisoning resulting in death from therapeutic use.

A strong cup of coffee contains 100 to 180 mg. of caffeine, whereas a cup of tea contains about 30 mg. More caffeine is present in tea leaves, but the extraction is less efficient. Overdulgence in caffeine-containing beverages, particularly coffee, gives rise in susceptible individuals to palpitation and tachycardia. Repetitious stimulation of the central nervous system produces irritability, which may be accompanied by insomnia. Removal of caffeine from such individuals is desirable.

Therapeutic Uses

1. The principal use is to produce mild cerebral stimulation.

2. Caffeine and sodium benzoate is injected intramuscularly to combat toxic depressions of sedative drugs.

3. Caffeine is used in combination with other analgesics in various headache remedies (see p. 284).

Preparations

Citrated Caffeine Tablets, N.F.	300 mg.
Caffeine and Sodium Benzoate Injection, U.S.P.	2-ml. ampuls containing 500 mg.

THE AMPHETAMINES

A group of drugs more powerful than caffeine in stimulating the cerebral cortex and causing increased alertness or even excitation is one somewhat related chemically to epinephrine but exceeding it in cortical stimulation. The first of these drugs to be introduced was ephedrine, the main application of which is the raising of blood pressure and the relief of asthma, urticaria (hives), and other allergic conditions. Amphetamine followed. It has some stimulating action on the heart, as does epinephrine, and some pressor effect on the blood pressure. However, its cortex-stimulating features are far more pronounced than those of epinephrine or ephedrine. Amphetamine sulfate is used as a central nervous system stimulant.

Amphetamine Sulfate, N.F., B.P., I.P. (Benzedrine Sulfate)
Amphetamine Phosphate, N.F. (Raphetamine)

Small oral doses of amphetamine have little effect on the circulation and respiration. They definitely stimulate the sensory cortex and produce brighter spirits and may produce restiveness, volubility, and insomnia. Psychic stimulation may later be followed by depression or fatigue. Amphetamine may superimpose an excitability over fatigue, but it does not obliterate the need for rest. In normal individuals, amphetamine does not facilitate better mental performance, and the nervousness produced may be quite uncomfortable. Amphetamine stimulates the respiration and elevates the blood pressure. The actions of the drug on the autonomic nervous system are discussed on pages 459–60.

Untoward Effects. Amphetamine is contraindicated in patients with high blood pressure or cardiovascular disease. In nervous and hyperexcitable states, the drug should be avoided. Repetitious administration of amphetamine sulfate may cause hypertension, restiveness, irritability, and gastrointestinal distress, and collapse may result. Overdosage may produce dry mouth, pain in the chest, rapid heart, chills, and collapse.

Therapeutic Uses

1. As a cerebral cortical stimulant in mild psychogenic or depressive states such as are found in convalescence, old age, grief, and melancholia.

2. In narcolepsy, to combat drowsiness. The usual dose of the sulfate is 10 mg. (2.5 to 10 mg.) twice a day. The usual oral dose of the phosphate is 5 mg.

3. To depress the appetite in obesity.

Preparation

Amphetamine Sulfate Tablets, N.F., B.P.   10 mg.
> Trade names: Benzedrine Sulfate; Phenedrine; Aktedron; Elastonon; Orthedrine; Phenamine; Sympamine

Amphetamine Phosphate Tablets, N.F.   5 mg.
Dibasic Amphetamine Phosphate Tab-   5 mg.
lets, N.F.
Elixir Amphetamine Phosphate   1.25 mg. in each mililiter
> Trade names: Raphetamine Phosphate; Profetamine

Dextroamphetamine Sulfate, U.S.P.; Dexamphetamine Sulfate, B.P. (Dexedrine Sulfate)

The main action of dextroamphetamine is stimulation of the cerebral cortex. It has no action on the peripheral nervous system and thus does not affect blood pressure. When used in obesity, it may curb the appetite, which is a conditioned reflex originating in the higher cerebral centers. It depresses the sense of smell and sweet taste. Dextroamphetamine gives rise to brighter spirits and a determination to stick to a diet with fewer calories. Less food is eaten, and the patient loses weight. The physical activity of the patient is also increased.

Mechanism of Action. Dextroamphetamine sulfate inhibits aminoxidase, an enzyme that tends to oxidize certain amines to aldehydes. By lessening the production of the aldehydes, which apparently depress tissue respiration, the drug may allow the brain to function at a higher degree of activity.

Dangers Involved with Use of Dextroamphetamine. The patient who is tired and should rest may take the drug and no longer feel tired. The drug superimposes hyperexcitability over fatigue, which may, if overdone, result in collapse.

Therapeutic Uses

1. To depress the appetite in obesity.

2. As a psychic stimulant in depressed states, such as observed in convalescence, old age, grief, and melancholia, including withdrawal of alcohol from the alcoholic.

3. In Parkinson's disease along with anticholinergic drugs to elevate the mood and lift the spirits.

4. With antihistamines to combat drowsiness which often occurs as a side effect.

5. To increase the skill, judgment, and performance of athletes.

Dose and Method of Administration

The usual oral dose is 5 mg. (2.5 to 5 mg.) twice a day or 15 mg. in timed-release capsules (Spansules) may be administered once a day.

Preparations

Dextroamphetamine Sulfate Tablets, U.S.P.; Dexamphetamine Tablets, B.P.	5 and 10 mg.
Dextroamphetamine Phosphate Tablets, N.F.	5 mg.
Dibasic Dextroamphetamine Phosphate Tablets	5 mg.
Spansule Sustained Release Capsules Dexedrine Sulfate	15 mg.

Trade names: Dexedrine Sulfate; d-Amfetasul; Tridex; Timed Tridex

Methamphetamine Hydrochloride, U.S.P.; Methylamphetamine Hydrochloride, B.P. (Desoxyn)

This compound may be classified as a derivative of either amphetamine or ephedrine. Its action as a cerebral stimulant is similar to that of amphetamine, and it is more potent than ephedrine in raising blood pressure. The usual oral dose is 5 mg. (2.5 to 5 mg.) once or twice daily.

Therapeutic Uses

1. As a cerebral stimulant the uses are the same as those for dextroamphetamine.

2. To depress the appetite in obesity.

Preparations

Methamphetamine Hydrochloride Tablets, U.S.P.; Methylamphetamine Tablets, B.P.	2.5, 5, and 10 mg.
Methamphetamine Hydrochloride Sustained Release Tablets	5, 10, and 15 mg.

Trade names: Amphedroxyn; Desamine; Desoxyphedrine; Desoxyn; Desyphed; Dexoval; Dexstim; Drohese; Doxyfed, Dunalpha; Efroxine; Methedrine; Norodin; Pervitin; Semoxydrine; Syndrox

ANOREXIGENIC DRUGS

Obesity is generally caused by eating more food than is required. It may be psychic due to lack of affection or recognition, it may be due to family habits, or it may be hereditary. Lack of adequate exercise is also a factor. Although these drugs have been said to depress the appetite by acting on the control centers in the hypothalamus, this has not been adequately proved and many authorities believe that this effect is limited and that the main action is to stimulate the higher centers and distract the patient from overeating and encourage him to adhere to his diet. In addition, there is a tendency to increased activity, which tends to decrease the appetite. Some clinicians have suggested that these drugs are of no value. Others have recommended that they should be given for limited periods of time as adjuvants to a restricted diet. Tolerance has been noted and some drugs such as the amphetamines may be addictive. The side effects are insomnia, nervousness, dry mouth, blurring of vision, and, in some cases, constipation.

Contraindications. These drugs are not recommended for patients with coronary disease or hypertension and should be used with caution in highly nervous and agitated patients.

The use of amphetamine, dextro amphetamine, and methamphetamine in obesity has been discussed. Other synthetic drugs belonging to this group are listed in Table 26.

Table 26

Additional Anorexigenic Drugs

Approved and Trade Names	Dosage and Method of Administration	Preparations
l-Amphetamine Alginate (Levonor)	Orally: 5 to 10 mg. b.i.d.	Tablets: 5 mg.
l-Amphetamine Succinate (Cydril)	Orally: 21 mg. once a day in the morning	Capsules, timed release: 21 mg.
Benzphetamine HCl (Didrex)	Orally: 25 to 50 mg. t.i.d. before meals	Tablets: 25 and 50 mg.
Diethylpropion HCl (Tenuate, Tepanil)	Orally: 25 mg. t.i.d. or q.i.d. before meals and in midevening	Tablets: 25 mg.
(Tenuate Dospan, Ten-Tab)	75 mg. in the morning	Tablets, timed release: 75 mg.
Phendimetrazine HCl (Plegine)	Orally: 35 mg. t.i.d. before meals	Tablets: 35 mg.
Phenmetrazine HCl (Preludin)	Orally: 25 mg. b.i.d. or t.i.d. before meals or 75 mg. once a day	Tablets: 25 mg.; timed release, 75 mg.
Phentermine HCl (Wilpo)	Orally: 8 mg. t.i.d. before meals	Tablets: 8 mg.
As a complex resin (Ionamin)	15 to 30 mg. in the morning	Capsules: 15 and 30 mg.

DRUGS ACTING ON THE RESPIRATION

Respiration is the action of breathing, which includes taking atmospheric air into the lungs during inspiration and expelling modified air during expiration. The average respiratory rate in adults is 14 to 18 per minute. In health, the rate is increased by muscular exercise, the emotions, age, and the rate of the heart beat. In various diseased conditions and by the untoward actions of many drugs rate and depth are decreased; in other cases the rate may be rapid and shallow.

The main function of the respiration is to supply the cells of the body with oxygen and to remove an excess of carbon dioxide which results from oxidation in the cells. Air, which contains approximately 20 per cent oxygen, passes over moist membranes through the nose or mouth to the larynx, trachea, and lungs. External respiration involves the passage of oxygen from the alveoli of the lungs to the blood and that of carbon dioxide from the blood to the lungs and its elimination during exhalation. Internal respiration involves the exchange of gases between the systemic blood and the tissues, which includes passage of oxygen from the blood to the tissue cells and that of carbon dioxide from the tissue cells to the blood.

The respiratory center, located in the medulla, controls the depth and rate of respiration. It is sensitive to changes in the hydrogen ion concentration and the carbon dioxide and oxygen levels in the blood. Carbon dioxide is the main respiratory stimulant, and even slight increases in concentration produce an increase in the rate and depth of respiration. Lowering of the pH of the blood also stimulates the respiration. Nerve impulses reach the respiratory center from the sense organs as well as from the cerebral cortex and hypothalamus. The respiratory center sends impulses by way of the spinal cord and nerves to the intercostal muscles, those of the diaphragm, and the abdominal muscles to adjust the respiratory depth and rhythm to the body needs. Inspiratory movements initiate nerve impulses to the respiratory center which inhibit inspiration and thus bring about expiration. Other vagal impulses inhibit expiration, when necessary.

Chemoreceptors in the carotid and aortic bodies are sensitive to an excess of carbon dioxide or oxygen lack and, when stimulated, increase the frequency and depth of respiration. The carotid sinus and aortic arch receptors respond to changes in arterial pressure; as the pressure rises the pressor receptors are stimulated and the respiration is inhibited.

EMERGENCY RESPIRATORY STIMULANTS

Drugs which stimulate the respiration by their action on the respiratory center are carbon dioxide, pentylenetetrazol (Metrazol), nikethamide (Coramine), picrotoxin, bemegride (Megimide), and ethamivan (Emivan). Caffeine (see p. 396), amphetamine (see p. 397), ephedrine (see p. 458), and atropine (see p. 485) are also used for this purpose.

Carbon Dioxide

Carbon dioxide is an odorless, colorless gas present in the air which is produced as the waste product of metabolism. It is of great importance in the regulation of respiration and circulation. At low temperatures the gas becomes solidified and is known as carbon dioxide snow, or "dry ice," a caustic material. Supersaturated solutions of carbon dioxide (carbonated water) were used as medicinal preparations formerly. With the addition of flavoring and sweetening agents, these solutions have become the basis of the modern carbonated beverage industry.

Therapeutic Uses

1. In carbon monoxide poisoning to increase the tidal air and hasten the excretion of the poisonous gas.

2. In pneumonia to prevent atelectasis by causing the lungs to expand to their maximum.

3. As a respiratory stimulant during or after anesthesia; also in resuscitation of the newborn, threatened drowning, and certain cases of drug poisoning.

4. To control hiccups.

Dosage and Method of Administration. Carbon dioxide is administered by inhalation of concentrations of 5 to $7\frac{1}{2}$ per cent in oxygen, using the type of masks employed in anesthesia or simply an inverted funnel and rubber tubing. It is administered only for a fraction of a minute in higher concentrations, for the breathing will become quite rapid and labored if the gas is applied for a longer period. This procedure can be repeated at intervals as needed to stimulate deep breathing.

Untoward Effects. Inhalation of carbon dioxide may produce undesirable side actions such as dizziness, headache, dyspnea, irritation of the nasal passages, palpitation, diminution in vision, muscle twitching, and mental depression.

Preparation

Carbon Dioxide, U.S.P., B.P., I.P.	In the compressed state in steel cylinders; cylinders containing carbon dioxide and oxygen in varying proportions are available

Nikethamide, N.F., B.P. (I.P.) (Coramine)

Nikethamide is a clear, colorless, or pale-yellow liquid that is very soluble in water. It is a simple substance related chemically to a vitamin belonging to the B complex.

Action of Nikethamide. Nikethamide acts mainly on the central nervous system, principally on the medullary centers. It stimulates the vagal and vasoconstrictor centers, but its most important action is on the respiratory center. These centers are stimulated directly and reflexly through their action on the carotid body. Large doses of nikethamide stimulate the cerebrum and spinal cord, and convulsions may result. The drug produces an increase in blood pressure preceded by a transient fall. The effect on the circulation appears to be secondary to the improvement in the respiration.

Therapeutic Use. Nikethamide is used as a respiratory stimulant in emergencies such as barbiturate poisoning, threatened drowning, anesthetic accidents, and alcoholic intoxication. The dose is 1 to 5 ml. of a 25 per cent W/V solution, intravenously and intramuscularly.

Preparation

Nikethamide Injection, N.F., B.P.   375 mg. in 1.5 ml.; 1.25 Gm. in 5 ml.
Trade name: Coramine

Pentylenetetrazol, N.F. (I.P.) (Metrazol)

Pentylenetetrazol is a white crystalline compound that is made synthetically.

Pharmacological Action. The principal action of pentylenetetrazol is on the central nervous system. In therapeutic doses it has a prompt and powerful stimulating action on the medulla and midbrain. In excessive doses its action extends to the cerebrum and spinal cord, and convulsions are produced.

The principal use of pentylenetetrazol is to stimulate a failing respiration; it seems to stimulate the medullary respiratory center directly. Its action on the circulatory system apparently depends on the improvement of respiration.

Therapeutic Uses

1. As a respiratory stimulant in emergencies such as barbiturate poisoning, threatened drowning, anesthetic accidents, and alcoholic intoxication. The dose is 100 mg. (100 to 500 mg.) intravenously and subcutaneously.

2. In mental disorders (shock therapy). The drugs now available for mental disease have greatly decreased the use of shock therapy.

Preparation

Pentylenetetrazol Injection, N.F.;   100 mg. in 1 ml.; 300 mg. in 3 ml.;
Trade names: Metrazol; Cardiazol

Picrotoxin, N.F., B.P., I.P.

Picrotoxin is the active principle from the seeds of the *Anamirta cocculus*. The seeds have been used for the poisoning of fish; consequently the drug is sometimes called *fish berries*.

Pharmacological Action. The main action of picrotoxin is to stimulate the medullary centers. This action has been used to combat the depressed respiratory states resulting from an overdose of narcotics or hypnotic drugs. Its special use has been as an antidote in barbiturate poisoning. It is a convulsant drug that markedly stimulates the central nervous system and produces an "awakening effect." After this effect passes, the patient again lapses into a depressive state. The dose of picrotoxin may be repeated until the patient is out of danger. The action is potentially dangerous and "heroic"; therefore, the drug is used with constant medical supervision and, by some, only as a last resort.

The recommended dose of picrotoxin is 6 mg. (2 ml.) intravenously for the first dose, followed in 20 minutes by 6 mg. The third dose of 12 mg. is given 30 minutes later.

Preparation

Picrotoxin Injection, N.F., B.P.   3 mg. in 1 ml.

Bemegride, U.S.P., B.P. (Megimide)

In 1954, Dr. F. H. Shaw and co-workers at the University of Melbourne introduced bemegride (Megimide, mikedimide, methetharimide) as an antidote in barbiturate poisoning. This drug stimulates the respiration and reflex activity and reverses the electroencephalographic pattern of deep depression caused by overdosage with the barbiturates. It does not increase the rate of barbiturate elimination, nor does it lessen the duration of coma. Bemegride has had an extensive clinical trial, particularly in Australia, and some investigators believe that its stimulant effects on respiration and reflex activity combat deep coma and bring the patient to the "safe state"—a state of light anesthesia undisturbed by signs of shock.

Bemegride is administered intravenously. Normal salt solution containing 500 mg. in 100 ml. is infused at the rate of one drop per second. The maximum dose at a given time is 1.5 Gm. Subsequent doses may be administered according to the needs of the patient. Mental disturbances, mainly visual hallucinations and convulsive seizures, have been observed with overdosage.

Preparation

Bemegride Injection, U.S.P., B.P.   5 mg. in 1 ml. in 10-ml. vials and ampuls
                                           and 30-ml. vials
                   Trade names: Megimide, Mikedimide

Amiphenazole (Daptazole)

Amiphenazole (Daptazole) is a weak barbiturate antagonist and respiratory stimulant. It has been used by Drs. F. H. Shaw and A. Shulman in combination with bemegride. Daptazole and bemegride are injected intravenously at the rate of 1 ml. of Daptazole and 10 ml. of bemegride every three minutes until the level of light anesthesia is attained.

Ethamivan (Emivan)

Ethamivan (Emivan), the diethylamide of vanillic acid, is administered intravenously and orally as a central nervous system stimulant. Intravenously the effects are evanescent and last only up to 15 minutes, unless continuously administered. Orally the drug may be effective up to three or four hours. It is used in acute barbiturate poisoning and in overdosage with other central nervous system depressant drugs, in recovery from general anesthesia, in respiratory depression, and in hypoventilatory states associated with the accumulation of carbon dioxide. One gram dissolved in 250 ml. of saline or 5 per cent dextrose solution is administered by intravenous infusion at the rate of approximately 10 mg. per minute to restore consciousness or for complete arousal, or 2 mg. per kilogram may be administered intravenously at five-minute intervals until the desired level of consciousness or arousal is obtained. Ethamivan is administered orally in doses of 20 to 60 mg. two or three times a day for one to eight weeks in patients with chronic respiratory insufficiency.

Side Effects.   Coughing, sneezing, itching, flushing, and lightheadedness can be prevented by decreasing the speed of injection.

Preparations

Ethamivan Injection	2-ml. ampuls and 10-ml. vials containing 50 mg. in 1 ml.
Ethamivan Tablets	20 mg.

Trade name: Emivan

Toxic Effects of Respiratory Stimulants

The respiratory stimulants produce transient stimulation of the respiration, which lasts from 10 to 30 minutes. The most serious limiting factor for the use of these drugs is that on repeated administration, convulsions may result from overdosage. Clonic and tetanic convulsions, which are initiated by a direct stimulation of the medulla and spinal centers, occur. The periods of convulsions are alternated with periods of coma and exhaustion.

Reflex Respiratory Stimulants

Aromatic Ammonia Spirit, N.F.   Aromatic ammonia spirit is a hydroalcoholic solution of ammonia gas, ammonium carbonate, and oil of lemon. It is a volatile, irritant preparation that reflexly stimulates the circulation and respiration. The preferred method of administration is by inhalation. It is also administered orally in doses up to 2 ml. well diluted with water.

Camphor. Camphor is a gum that is obtained naturally as well as synthetically. A 20 per cent solution in oil is available for injection. A dose of 0.2 ml. is injected subcutaneously to stimulate the respiration and circulation reflexly.

Alcohol. Whisky and brandy produce reflex stimulation of the respiration and circulation by irritating the mucous membrane of the mouth, throat, and upper respiratory tract. These beverages are useful in milder cases of shock and collapse.

CONVULSANTS

ELECTROSHOCK THERAPY

Electroshock therapy is considered the treatment of choice by many physicians for most cases of depressive reactions. It reduces the time period required to tranquilize overactive, agitated patients.

Flurothyl Ether (Indoklon)

Flurothyl ether is a volatile liquid anesthetic which on inhalation causes convulsions that resemble the seizure produced by electroshock therapy. Since the clinical results are also similar, it is often used as a substitute for electroshock treatment of mentally ill patients. Convulsant therapy is thus simplified by having an anesthetic and convulsant effect in the same drug. Flurothyl ether is administered by inhalation.

Preparation

Flurothyl Ether   Vials containing 10 ml.

                Trade name: Indoklon

THERAPEUTIC GASES

Oxygen, carbon dioxide, and helium are gases administered by inhalation to improve the breathing and supply additional oxygen to the tissues when needed.

Oxygen

The fundamental importance of oxygen to animal life needs no explanation here. However, its clinical uses and indications should be noted. Normally it is continually supplied to the cells of the body by the circulation of the blood, which carries it both in physical solution and in chemical combination with the hemoglobin of the red blood cells. If the oxygen tension in the blood is reduced owing to a decreased concentration in the inspired air or if its transport to the cells is interfered with by disease or by poisoning with drugs, hypoxia (oxygen lack) or hypoxemia (lessened oxygen tension in the blood) results, and serious symptoms or even death may occur very quickly. If these conditions are acute, the prompt administration of oxygen may be lifesaving, or it may prevent the development of crippling conditions which could occur. If the cells of the body are deprived of oxygen for too long, the action is irreversible and the cells do not regain their function after oxygen is restored to them. The cells of the central nervous system are the most vulnerable, especially those in the brain. It is possible that they may not recover their activity after they have been deprived of oxygen for as little as five minutes.

Disease Conditions Causing Hypoxia.   The various disease conditions that cause deprivation of oxygen to the cells involve (1) the circulation, (2) the number of red blood cells and the amount of hemoglobin in the blood, (3) the lungs, and (4) both the central and peripheral nervous systems.

1. Inadequate circulation of the blood due to trauma or diseases of the heart and blood vessels is exemplified by hemorrhage shock, heart failure, coronary occlusion, cerebral thrombosis, and reflex spastic constriction of the peripheral blood vessels.

2. Reduction in the number of red blood cells and the amount of hemoglobin in the blood occurs in various types of anemia.

3. Inadequate oxygenation in the lungs may be due to (a) a reduction in the number of functioning lung units (alveoli). This may be caused by (i) compression of the alveoli by the distended pulmonary vessels, (ii) atelectasis (collapse of the lung), (iii) pneumonia, (iv) pulmonary cysts, (v) pulmonary infarcts, and (vi) consolidation of the lung. Or the inadequate oxygenation may rise from (b) improper mixing of the gases throughout the alveoli, as in emphysema; and (c) poor diffusion of gases across the alveolar-capillary membrane, as in pulmonary edema.

4. Diseases involving the nervous system cause injury to the brain, spinal cord, or some part of the peripheral nervous system. For example, poliomyelitic injury to the nerve cells of the spinal cord or medulla may cause destruction of the motor pathways to the respiratory muscles and thus interfere with breathing. Or a blockage of nerve impulses that normally cause contraction of skeletal muscles may result in respiratory depression or paralysis if the muscles involved are those concerned with breathing. Artificial respiration is indicated in these conditions.

Drugs and Poisonous Gases That Produce Hypoxia.   The central nervous system depressants (such as the narcotics) and the poisonous gases (such as carbon monoxide and hydrogen cyanide) produce hypoxia. Carbon monoxide combines with the hemoglobin of the blood to form carboxyhemoglobin, which prevents the combination of oxygen with hemoglobin to form oxyhemoglobin and so reduces the amount of oxygen carried to the tissues. Hydrogen cyanide interferes with the cellular uptake of oxygen.

Decreased Oxygen Tension.   A person who moves to the mountains usually adjusts gradually to the marked decrease in oxygen tension present in the atmosphere at high altitudes. The number of red blood cells increases and other necessary bodily adjustments also take place. However, the high altitudes reached in mountain climbing and aviation present too rapid an entrance into an atmosphere where the total barometic pressure is less; consequently, there is a reduction in the partial pressure of oxygen in the alveoli and eventually a decrease in the oxygen saturation of the blood. In these circumstances artificial measures must be used to supply oxygen to maintain normal body function.

Symptoms of Hypoxia.   The symptoms are increased pulse rate, rapid and shallow breathing, a decreased ability to concentrate, unstable emotions, fainting, analgesia, muscular incoordination, and cyanosis. Unconsciousness occurs as a result of the reduced function of the cerebral cortex, and finally the medullary centers are depressed and breathing becomes extremely difficult. These acute symptoms may be relieved almost immediately by the administration of oxygen, but until the fundamental cause of oxygen want is corrected, the symptoms will reappear upon discontinuing the oxygen.

Therapeutic Uses

1. At high altitudes (oxygen tanks are available to aviators and mountain climbers).

2. In lobar and bronchopneumonia, pulmonary edema.

3. For asthma resulting from bronchial constriction.

4. For carbon monoxide poisoning.

5. In circulatory disorders such as cardiac decompensation, coronary occlusion, and shock.

Methods of Administration.   Oxygen is supplied in a compressed state in steel cylinders fitted with reducing valves to deliver the gas. In the medical field the gas is administered in oxygen tents, by nasal catheters, or by face masks. It may be given under atmospheric pressure or under higher pressure with the use of an intermittent positive-pressure breathing apparatus. Compressed oxygen is very dry, and it must be humidified before being used by the patient. If this is not done, the patient's throat will become very dry and ulceration of the mucous membrane may occur. In generalized conditions, 40 to 60 per cent concentrations are administered. In ischemia, such as in coronary occlusion, higher concentrations up to 100 per cent may be necessary. The oxygen flow rate should be ordered by the physician.

Dangers in the Administration of Oxygen.   Sometimes high concentrations of oxygen over prolonged periods of time may cause substernal distress, tracheobronchitis, decreased vital capacity, hyperemia, and edema of the lungs. Other signs and symptoms of oxygen poisoning are fatigue, paresthesia in the hands and feet, joint pains, anorexia, nausea, and vomiting, Apnea or cessation of breathing may occur in patients whose respiratory centers are depressed or damaged so that respiration is being maintained reflexly by the

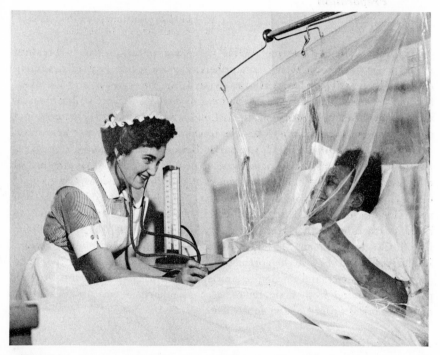

Fig. 12.   Oxygen tent. *(Courtesy of University Hospital, Art Department and School of Nursing, University of Maryland.)*

response of the chemoreceptor mechanism to hypoxia. The elimination of hypoxia by the administration of oxygen removes this last stimulus to the respiration, and artificial respiration is indicated. This may occur in patients with severe chronic pulmonary emphysema; hence they should not receive concentrations of oyxgen above 40 per cent. Administration of high concentrations of oxygen in incubators to premature infants many cause a type of blindness known as retrolental fibroplasia. Generally normal oxygen concentrations should be maintained in incubators. If a condition arises making additional oxygen necessary, the minimum amount for the shortest period of time should be used. Oxygen supports combustion; hence patients and visitors should be warned of the danger of smoking. Inflammable materials such as oil and grease should not come in contact with the apparatus used for the administration of oxygen.

Equipment and other appliances using electricity, such as call bells, electric heating pads, radios, and electric razors, should not be used in the presence of high concentrations of oxygen as they may produce sparks.

Preparation

Oxygen, U.S.P., B.P., I.P.	In cylinders containing not less than 99 per cent oxygen by volume

Oxygen Under Pressure (OHP). When pure oxygen is breathed under pressures greater than 1 atmosphere, a more severe type of poisoning occurs. The severity of the symptoms depends on the pressure and the duration of the time of exposure. The symptoms observed are facial pallor, nausea, vertigo, malaise, apprehension, a choking sensation, mood changes, and convulsions of the grand mal type. The mechanism of action is not known.

Controlled Studies in Hyperbaric Research.[1] Hyperbaric oxygenation, or the administration of oxygen at two to four times the pressure of atmospheric oxygen, is being investigated at certain universities and medical centers. Some of the potential indications for its use are (1) in carbon monoxide poisoning, (2) in barbiturate poisoning, (3) as an adjunct to radiation therapy in the treatment of malignant tumors, (4) in anaerobic infections (gas gangrene), (5) in cardiac surgery, (6) in peripheral vascular insufficiency, and (7) in hemorrhagic shock. The side effects encountered are oxygen toxicity and decompression sickness. Other hazards are fire, explosion, poisoning from toxic fumes, gaseous embolism, gaseous distention, and mechanical failure of the equipment.

Helium

Helium, an extremely light gas with a high rate of diffusion, is present in the atmosphere and in natural gases. It is an inert gas and owes its therapeutic usefulness entirely to its physical properties. A mixture of 80 per cent helium and 20 per cent oxygen is only about one third as heavy as air.

Therapeutic Uses

1. In *status asthmaticus* where a limited amount of air reaches the bronchioles.

2. In inflammatory obstructions to the air passages due to infection or mechanical irritation.

---

[1] "Controlled, Limited Studies Urged in Hyperbaric Research," *Medical News*, **184**:55, 1964.

3. In respiratory depression or unexpected obstruction to the air passages during anesthesia.

Dosage and Method of Administration. Helium is administered by inhalation in 80 per cent concentration with 20 per cent oxygen. The usual types of masks or an oxygen tent is used.

Preparation

Helium, U.S.P., B.P.
                    Cylinders containing helium and oxygen in the desired proportions

REVIEW QUESTIONS

1. *What effects are produced by stimulants of the central nervous system?*
2. *Explain the action of dextro amphetamine in obesity.*
3. *What are the advantages and dangers involved in the use of amphetamine?*
4. *What are emergency respiratory stimulants? Name two types and give two examples of each.*
5. *What is hypoxia? What are some of the disease conditions that cause hypoxia? What are the symptoms of hypoxia?*
6. *List some of the uses of oxygen. How is it administered?*
7. *For what purposes is carbon dioxide used and how is it administered?*

REFERENCES

Flemming, A. S.: "Amphetamine Drugs," *Public Health Rep.*, **75**:49, 1960.

Ivy, A. C., and Krasno, L. R.: "Amphetamine (Benzedrine Sulfate), a Review of its Pharmacology," *War Med.*, **1**:15, 1941.

Lands, A. M.: "The Pharmacological Activity of Epinephrine and Related Dihydroxyphenylalkyamines," *Pharmacol. Rev.*, **1**:279, 1949. ·

Leake, C. D.: "Newer Stimulant Drugs," *Am. J. Nursing*, **58**:966, 1958.

Maloney, A. H., and Tatum, A. L.: "Cardiazol (Metrazol) and Coramine as Cardiorespiratory Stimulants," *Arch. internat. de pharmacodyn, et de thérap.*, **42**:200, 1932.

Marshall, E. K., Jr.; Walzl, E. M.; and LeMessevier, D. H.: "Picrotoxin as a Respiratory Stimulant," *J. Pharmacol. & Exper. Therap.*, **60**:472, 1937.

Prinzmetal, M., and Alles, G. A.: "The Central Nervous Stimulating Effects of Dextro-amphetamine Sulfate," *Am. J. M. Sc.*, **200**:665, 1940.

Richards, R. K.: "Analeptics: Pharmacologic Background and Clinical Use in Barbiturate Poisoning," *Neurology*, **9**:228, 1959.

NARCOLEPSY

Prinzmetal, M., and Bloomberg, W.: "The Use of Benzedrine for the Treatment of Narcolepsy," *J.A.M.A.*, **105**:2051, 1935.

OBESITY

Kroger, W. S.: "Psychologic Factors in Obesity and Anorexic Drugs," *Am. Pract. & Digest Treat.*, **10**:2169, 1959.

Patterson, M.: "A Comparative Study of Phenmetrazine and Dextro-amphetamine in a Short Term Reducing Program in Medical Students," *Antibiotic Med.*, **6**:207, 1959.

Rendle-Short, J.: "Obesity in Childhood; a Clinical Trial of Phenmetrazine," *Brit. M. J.*, **5174**:703, 1960.

Rosenberg, P.: "The Further Use of Amphetamine (Benzedrine) Sulfate and Dextro-amphetamine in the Treatment of Obesity," *M. World*, **60**:210, 1942.

Rosenthal, G., and Solomon, H. A.: "Benzedrine Sulfate in Obesity," *Endocrinology*, **26**:807, 1940.

Rynearson, E. H., and Gastineau, C.F.: *Obesity*. Charles C Thomas, Publisher, Springfield, Ill., 1949, p. 22 ("Etiology").

IV DRUGS ACTING ON THE PERIPHERAL NERVOUS SYSTEM

In the foregoing section we have given consideration to the central nervous system, composed of the brain and the spinal cord. The peripheral portion of the nervous system is the aggregate of all the nerves that enter or leave the brain and cord. These are the peripheral nerves, carrying impulses from specialized receptors in the skin and the mucous membranes (e.g., those for touch, temperature, and pain) into the central nervous system, or from the central nervous system to the smooth and skeletal muscles and the glands. These nerves may be divided into two divisions: the somatic *nerves and the* autonomic *nerves. The somatic or "body" nerves are the group subserving the muscles and skin, while the autonomic nervous ·system concerns more closely the internal organs, glands, and the size of the blood vessels. We are able to use at will the somatic motor or muscle-moving nerves, while the autonomic system operates usually outside the influence of our will or planning. The autonomic system has many functions to perform for our benefit, such as assistance in digestion, movement of food along the intestine, regulation of blood pressure and heart rate, flow of saliva, and other work with which we are not usually consciously concerned. Of this important division we shall subsequently speak in further detail (see Section V, pp. 439–93).*

In the following two chapters we shall consider the means now at our disposal for altering the function of the somatic nerves. Chapter 24 deals with agents that can block the nerve impulses passing from the spinal cord or brain out along skeletal or somatic nerves to voluntary or skeletal muscles. These are the muscles of locomotion and of movement at our will. Agents that can paralyze these muscles (the neuromuscular blocking agents) have proved useful in surgical operations and in electric shock treatment of psychiatric patients. Less than paralyzing doses are employed, however, Drugs that can increase the number of nerve impulses arriving at the muscles in conditions in which the normal situation has been depressed by drug or disease are presented in Chapter 29.

In Chapter 25 are described pharmacological agents used for one purpose

413

only: to stop the passage of nerve impulses along the nerves. The object is to stop pain in a number of situations. If a tooth is to be drilled or removed, or a cyst removed from the skin, a local anesthetic is desired. In lower-abdominal operations, spinal anesthesia may be used; and in childbirth, a more limited form, caudal anesthesia, may be employed.

24

Neuromuscular Blocking Agents

The muscles of locomotion and other movements that are under voluntary control are innervated by somatic motor nerves from the brain and the spinal cord. The motor cranial nerves supply the external eye muscles, the facial muscles, and the muscles for chewing and swallowing. The spinal nerves from the first cervical to the last sacral nerve provide the control over most of the remaining skeletal muscles, with some overlapping.

Whereas the centrally acting relaxants discussed in Chapter 20 are often disappointing in cases in which a marked degree of relaxation of voluntary muscle is required, the drugs of the peripherally acting group readily paralyze muscles. One of these drugs to be discussed is present in curare, a material obtained from a South American plant and long used by natives there as an arrow poison. The rapidly produced nerve impulses from the brain, which normally activate the muscles, are blocked by the drug at the muscles. Drugs that can depress or inactivate the neuromusclar junction or synapse (motor end-plate) have considerable use in medicine and surgery. They may be divided into two groups on the basis of the two mechanisms by which they block transmission at the synapse. One group consists of *competitive inhibitor agents,* and because the forerunner of the blocking drugs, curare, is of this type, they are called *curariform agents.* These drugs compete with acetylcholine for the receptor sites at the end-plate and prevent acetylcholine from depolarizing them. Examples are tubocurarine, dimethyl-tubocurarine, and synthetic derivatives. A second group is composed of the *depolarizing agents.* They have an acetylcholine-like action and cause an initial depolarization which is prolonged and renders the end-plate region inexcitable.

In the resting state there is an increased concentration of Na ions on the outside and increased K ions on the inside of the cell membrane which causes a difference in the electrical charge on either side of the membrane. This is referred to as *polarization.* This condition is maintained by the normal metabolic processes in the cell (see p. 92). At this time the cell is ready to respond to the nerve impulse.

When acetylcholine, which is released from the nerve, reaches the motor end-plate, the cells become permeable to Na which then flows into the cell and neutralizes the electric charge. This is accompanied by an outflow of K ions.

415

The membrane thus becomes depolarized and the condition is referred to as *depolarization.* When one area becomes depolarized, currents flow into the surrounding polarized area and a wave of depolarization spreads over the surface of the muscle. This wave of depolarization causes the muscle to contract.

Acetylcholine is readily hydrolyzed by cholinesterase and the contraction is followed by a gradual return of Na ions to the outside by active transport "pumps" (see p. 93) and an inflow of K ions until *repolarization* occurs. The membrane is again polarized and ready to respond to the next nerve impulse.

Therapeutic Uses of Neuromuscular Blocking Agents

1. To widen the scope of less potent anesthetics and lessen the overall amount of anesthetic needed. These agents produce muscle relaxation on a lighter and safer plane of anesthesia.

2. To obtain relaxation for laryngoscopy and intubations.

3. To increase muscular relaxation during surgery. They are often used in orthopedic, eye, rectal, and general abdominal surgery.

4. For protection against trauma in convulsant therapy for psychiatric treatment.

5. To control convulsions or muscle spasms during anesthesia.

6. To produce relaxation of muscles following trauma from operative procedures and other pathological states, such as back strain, anterior poliomyelitis, and various spastic states. They are of limited value in spastic paralysis of apoplexy.

Danger of Overdosage with Neuromuscular Blocking Agents

Both the curariform drugs and the deporarizing ones, at sufficiently high dosage, cause paralysis of the respiratory muscles. Facilities for satisfactory artificial respiration must always be available before employing any of the muscle-paralyzing agents. The drugs should be administered only by persons thoroughly familiar with their dosage, effects, and dangers involved. No antidotes are available for the depolarizing agents.

CURARIFORM AGENTS

Curare alkaloids block neuromuscular transmission of nerve impulses at the motor end-plate by combining with the receptor sites normally occupied by acetylcholine. They thus compete with acetylcholine for the same receptors. Therefore, the normal amount of acetylcholine, liberated at the synapse by each nerve impulse, cannot exert its usual effect, the depolarization of the muscle portion of the end-plate and muscle contraction.

Curare

Curare, as previously mentioned, is the name applied to many South American arrowhead poisons, found in several plants indigenous to that continent. Curarized animals may be eaten without producing poisonous effects because the drug is destroyed in the stomach. Dr. Claude Bernard described the physiological action of the drug and, using frogs, located its site of action in 1840. Curare produces paralysis of skeletal muscle by its action at the neuromuscular junction. It was first available as a dark-brown extract. The composition of this crude extract was variable and its dosage was not dependable; consequently it was not used in clinical medicine until recently, when a standardized extract was made available. In 1935, Dr. H. King isolated the pure crystalline material, d-tubocurarine.

Prior to its introduction, abdominal muscular relaxation for surgical operations and relaxation of the jaw and larynx for tracheal intubation were achieved by means of deep anesthesia, which often was accompanied by many side effects. With the use of muscle relaxants less general anesthetic is required. However, they must be used in combination with anesthetic or analgesic agents because muscle relaxants are nonanesthetic.

Tubocurarine Chloride, U.S.P., B.P. (d-Tubocurarine)

The alkaloid tubocurarine is one of the active principles of curare plants. It has recently been synthesized. Its action is mainly on the neuromuscular receptor. To a lesser degree it interrupts transmission in the autonomic ganglia and partially blocks transmission between the parasympathetic postganglionic fibers and the effector cells in smooth muscle. Tubocurarine also often elicits as an untoward side effect a histamine-like response, bronchospasm. It produces muscular paralysis, slightly increased peristalsis, and some blocking of the afferent impulses to the brain so that shock may be considerably reduced in the curarized patient. Its action appears first on the muscles innervated by the cranial nerves, next on the muscles of the trunk and extremities, and lastly on the muscles having to do with respiration, especially the diaphragm. Recovery occurs in the reverse order and may require 20 to 30 minutes following the usual intravenous dose. The onset of action is rapid and its extent and duration is dependent upon the dose given. Relaxation is maintained by giving small doses as required. A cumulative effect may result from doses repeated at too short intervals. For therapeutic uses, see page 416.

Dosage and Methods of Administration. The intravenous administration of 6 to 9 mg. in solution produces complete abdominal relaxation. It is given in divided doses. After the effects wear off, 3 to 5 mg. additional may be given in three to five minutes. With ether anesthesia, only one third of the recommended dose should be used because the muscle-relaxant action of ether itself is so profound.

In electrically produced convulsions, as used in psychiatric cases, the usual dose is 3 mg. for each 40 lb. of body weight. This is given intravenously, over a period of not less than 90 seconds, to reduce the hazard of the breaking of bones during the convulsions. For spastic muscles in various conditions the same dose may be administered intramuscularly.

Side Effects. The side effects are occasional bronchospasm (caused by histamine release), a fall in blood pressure owing to capillary dilatation (muscle relaxation), and a rapid heart. Overdosage may produce paralysis of the muscles of respiration.

Preparation

Tubocurarine Chloride Injection, U.S.P.,   15 mg. in 1 ml.; 30 mg. in 10 ml.;
(B.P., I.P.)   60 mg. in 20 ml.
Trade names: Delacurarine; Tubadil; Tubarine

Depot Preparation of Tubocurarine Chloride.   In order to provide an injectable form of this agent, which would be more slowly absorbed from a muscle depot and thereby obviate the more frequent injections of the U.S.P. solution, the drug has been placed in an oil-beeswax menstruum. Each milliliter contains 25 mg. of the drug. Five-milliliter vials are available under the trade name Tubadil Injection.

Additional Product of Tubocurarine.   Intocostrin is a trade name for preparations containing specified amounts of tubocurarine or specified activity by bio-assay methods, expressed in units.

Dimethyl Tubocurarine Iodide, N.F. (Metubine)

This compound, representing a minor modification of tubocurarine, is three times more potent than the parent alkaloid and has a wider safety margin. Its actions are not appreciably different. The intravenous dose is usually one third that of tubocurarine, or 1.5 to 3 mg. with ether and 3 to 4 mg. with thiopental sodium and nitrous oxide.

Preparation

Dimethyl Tubocurarine Iodide Injection,   10-ml. ampuls containing 1 mg. in 1 ml.
N.F.   20-ml. ampuls containing 2 mg. in 1 ml.
Trade name: Metubine

Dimethyl Tubocurarine Chloride (Mecostrin)

This is the chloride of the previous compound and has the same action and uses as the iodide.

Preparation

Dimethyl Tubocurarine Chloride Solu-   10-ml. vials containing 1 mg. in 1 ml.
tion (Injection)

Trade name: Mecostrin

Gallamine Triethiodide, B.P., I.P. (Flaxedil)

Gallamine is one fourth to one third as active as tubocurarine, but its toxicity is less by an even greater ratio; hence its margin of safety is wider. It does not affect the autonomic ganglia or cause release of histamine and consequent bronchospasm. The average initial dose is 100 mg. intravenously. The dose may be augmented by additional amounts if required.

Preparation

Gallamine Triethiodide Injection   20-ml. vials containing 20 mg. in 1 ml.

Trade name: Flaxedil

Hexafluorenium Bromide (Mylaxen)

Hexafluorenium bromide resembles curare in its pattern of activity. It also inhibits the enzyme cholinesterase in the blood plasma but apparently not at the neuromuscular junction in skeletal muscle. In man, hexafluorenium potentiates the muscle-relaxant effects of succinylcholine and is used during anesthesia in surgery for this purpose. Smaller doses of succinylcholine are required and fewer side effects, such as muscular fasciculation, twitching, and postoperative muscle pain, are seen. Facilities for artificial respiration should always be on hand during the use of these agents.

Dosage and Administration. Hexafluorenium is given intravenously and intermittently following the induction of anesthesia. Approximately 0.4 mg. per kilogram (1 to 2 ml.) may be given at once and repeated if necessary in order to employ the minimum dosage of succinylcholine (see pp. 420–21).

Preparation

Hexafluorenium Bromide Solution   10-ml. vials sontaining 20 mg. in 1 ml.

Trade name: Mylaxen

Antidotes for Curariform Drugs

Antidotes for tubocurarine, gallamine, and the other curariform agents consist of compounds that inactivate the enzyme acetylcholinesterase, which breaks down the acetylcholine into inactive parts, acetic acid and choline. While the curare-like drug is at the end-plate, acetylcholine cannot act, although it is released each time a nerve impulse arrives. By inactivating the enzyme, acetylcholine is permitted to linger and build up its local concentration to the point of being capable of depolarizing the end-plate and thereby causing the muscle to contract. It thus breaks through the paralysis unless large over-doses of the curare agent have been given.

The *anticholinesterases,* or *cholinesterase inhibitors,* useful in combating the effects of curare compounds are neostigmine methylsulfate (1 or 2 ml., 1:2000 solution, p. 477), edrophonium (10 mg. in 1 ml. intravenously, p. 479), ambenonium (p. 480), and pyridostigmin (p. 479). Even these antidotes have dangers if given in doses higher than needed, and therefore, they must be used with caution. Their action is shorter than that of curariform agents and repetition of doses may be required. *Artificial respiration,* preferably with oxygen under positive pressure, should be carried out until it is safe to discontinue it.

DEPOLARIZING BLOCKING AGENTS

These compounds have the same effect as the natural mediator, acetylcholine, but of longer duration. The natural substance quickly depolarizes the muscle side of the end-plate causing muscular contraction and is then rapidly inactivated by the enzyme cholinesterase present at the neuromuscular junction. On the other hand, these drugs cause a persistent depolarization of the same membrane until they are washed away and excreted or are hydrolyzed and inactivated by pseudocholinesterase, an enzyme present in the blood.

Decamethonium Bromide; Decamethonium Iodide (Syncurine)

Decamethonium, also called C10, is four times more potent as a muscular relaxant than tubocurarine. The relaxation is more prompt and of shorter duration. It shows *stimulation* of muscle prior to depression. Fibrillary muscular twitchings are seen before relaxation. The agent produces less respiratory depression than tubocurarine, and no histamine response except at high doses. There is, accordingly, no bronchospasm and very little fall in blood pressure. Decamethonium is administered intravenously in doses of 2 to 2.5 ml. at the rate of 2 ml. (1 mg.) per minute until relaxation is obtained. Its earlier popularity has waned considerably.

Preparation

Decamethonium Bromide or Iodide, B.P.   10-ml. vials containing 1 mg. in 1 ml.
Trade names: Syncurine; Decontrax; Eulissin; Procuran; Synacur

Succinylcholine Chloride, U.S.P.; Suxamethonium Bromide and Chloride, B.P. (Anectine Chloride, Quelicin Chloride)

Succinylcholine chloride (diacetylcholine) is an ultrashort-acting relaxant of skeletal muscle. It is rapidly hydrolyzed and inactivated by the enzyme pseudocholinesterase, which is present in the blood. The duration of action of a single injection is two to five minutes. The first evanescent action is one of stimulation of certain muscle fibers or muscle fasciculations which may cause considerable soreness of the muscles. This is followed immediately by a flaccid paralysis. Succinylcholine does not cause the liberation of histamine. In rare cases, it may cause prolonged periods of muscular paralysis and apnea in patients who have a deficiency of the enzyme pseudocholinesterase in their blood. An occasional patient with liver disease may also exhibit a prolonged effect. There is no antidote available. Edrophonium (Tensilon) and neostigmine (Prostigmin) may actually intensify its effects. Artificial respiration must be given until the patient resumes breathing.

For therapeutic uses see page 416.

Dosage and Method of Administration. Succinylcholine chloride may be administered intravenously as a single dose of 10 to 40 mg. of a 2 per cent solution. This dose produces relaxation in less than one minute and lasts two minutes or slightly more, followed by rapid recovery. For prolonged procedures, a continuous intravenous drip infusion of a 0.1 per cent solution in 5 per cent glucose or sterile isotonic sodium chloride is used. The desired stage of muscular relaxation is obtained by allowing the solution to flow at the rate of 2 to 4 ml. per minute. The degree of relaxation can be changed in about 30 seconds by regulating the rate of infusion. The quantity varies with different patients and with the duration of relaxation required.

Advantages of the Use of Succinylcholine. These are: (1) it is short acting, and (2) it does not liberate histamine and cause bronchial spasm.

Disadvantages of the Use of Succinylcholine. (1) In some individuals apnea may occur, (2) no antidote is available, and (3) it must be given by intravenous infusion for a sustained effect.

Preparation

Succinylcholine Chloride Injection, 200 and 500 mg. in 10 ml. (1 Gm. in U.S.P.; Suxamethonium Chloride and 10 ml. also available) Bromide Injections, B.P.

Trade names: Anectine Chloride; Lysthenon; Quelicin Chloride; Scoline; Sucrostrin; Brevidil M (the bromide); Suxinyl

REVIEW QUESTIONS

1. *What is the pathway of the volleys of nerve impulses that result in the willful contraction of a skeletal muscle? At what point on this pathway do ether, cyclopropane, and other general anesthetics exert their effects, causing skeletal muscles to relax?*

2. *Between the site of action of the above anesthetics and the termination of the motor nerves, we can partially block the flow of nerve impulses to skeletal muscles (see Chap. 20). Review these agents and their mode of action. Discuss the differences between their fields of usefulness and those of the present compounds.*

3. *What effect should be produced if we could completely prevent the appearance of any acetylcholine at the synapse of the motor end-plate? What function does the enzyme cholinesterase (specially acetylcholinesterase) normally have?*
4. *Name the drugs that are termed "competitive blocking" or "curariform" agents?*
5. *What is meant by competitive inhibition and by noncompetitive (depolarizing) block of the neuromyal junction?*
6. *How is succinylcholine used?*
7. *Of what clinical usefulness are neuromuscular blocking agents? What dangers exist in their use? What lifesaving measures can be used when a patient has been given an overdose?*
8. *For which types of blocking agents are antidotes available? Why would there be little, if any, use for an antidote for succinylcholine overdosage?*

REFERENCES

Adriani, John: *Techniques and Procedures of Anesthesia,* 3 rd ed. Charles C Thomas, Publisher, Springfield, Ill., 1964.

Bourne, J. G.; Collier, H. O. J.; and Somers, G. F.: "Succinylcholine, Muscle Relaxant of Short Action," *Lancet,* **1**:1225, 1952.

Cleckley, J. J.; Orvin, G. H.; and Miller, W. C.: "Report on Five Thousand Consecutive Electro-shock Treatments Without Complications," *J. South Carolina M. A.,* **56**:1, 1960.

Council on Pharmacy and Chemistry: "Decamethonium Bromide, N.N.R.," *J.A.M.A.,* **162**:731, 1956.

Dripps, Robert D.; Eckenhoff, James E.; and Vandam, L. D.: *Introduction to Anesthesia,* 2nd ed. W. B. Saunders Company, Philadelphia, London, 1961.

Enderly, G. E. H.: "Muscle Relaxation with Decamethonium (C10)," *Anesthesia,* **14**:138, 1959.

Foldes, F. F.; Hillmer, N. R.; Molloy, R. E.; and Monte, A. P.: "Potentiation of the Neuromuscular Effect of Succinylcholine by Hexafluorenium," *Anesthesiology,* **21**:50, 1960.

Foldes, F. F.; Molloy, R. E.; Zsigmond, E. K.; and Zwartz, J. A.: "Hexafluorenium: Its Anticholinesterase and Neuromuscular Activity," *J. Pharmacol. & Exper. Therap.,* **129**:400, 1960.

Spencer, C. H., and Coakley, C. S.: "Clinical Evaluation of Syncurine® (Decamethonium Bromide): A Two Year Study," *Anesthesiology,* **16**:125, 1955.

Symposium: "Curare and Anticurare Agents," *Ann. New York Acad. Sc.,* **54**:297, 1951.

25

The Local Anesthetics

The nerve fiber is enclosed in a semipermeable membrane which is surrounded by tissue fluid. In the normal resting state which is maintained by the expenditure of energy (see p. 415). Na ions are concentrated on the outside and K ions are concentrated in the nerve fiber. Therefore, positive charges cover the external surface and negative ones the internal surface. The difference in potential between the inside and the outside of the membrane is referred to as *polarization* (see p. 415). In this condition the nerve is ready to respond to a stimulus entering the nerve fiber.

During the passage of the impulse which is initiated by acetylcholine the difference in permeability to Na^+ and K^+ is reversed; Na^+ are concentrated on the inside and K^+ are concentrated in the extracellular fluid and the difference in potential is reversed. This condition is referred to as *depolarization* (see p. 416). The impulse passes as a wave along with successive depolarizations in front of the impulse. Behind the impulse the original resting potential is restored. The nerve then becomes repolarized and is ready for the transmission of the next impulse.

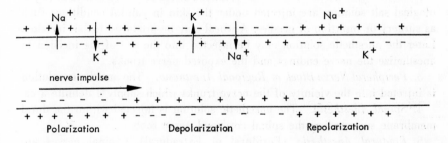

Impulses following one another are known as *volleys*. Their rate is usually of the order of 60 per second, ranging as high as 200 per second in the case of nerves to eye muscles, which are thus capable of very fast action. A nerve impulse is the same whether it is a sensory nerve carrying messages to the brain or a motor nerve taking impulses from the brain to the muscles, heart, etc. Under normal conditions these may continue almost indefinitely where fatigue is not a problem.

423

It has been postulated that local anesthetics act by stabilizing the membrane potential by combining with the lipoprotein membrane.

Local anesthetics are substances that reversibly block sensory impulses, especially pain, in a restricted area of the body. They block conduction along the sensory and motor fibers. If the concentration of the anesthetic is controlled, there is loss of sensation without motor paralysis, since the sensory fibers are affected before the motor fibers.

Local anesthetics may be divided into two groups according to their actions. Drugs such as cocaine and numerous synthetic derivatives act specifically on the sensory nerves or their endings. Other drugs such as ethyl chloride (Kelene), fluro-ethyl, and carbon dioxide snow cause local anesthesia by the production of cold. Ethyl chloride and fluro-ethyl, both liquids, are sprayed on the skin and evaporate so rapidly that they chill or even freeze the area.

Pharmacological Action. Local anesthetics manifest a selective action on nerve structures and interfere with nerve conductivity. They produce their effects wherever applied, as at sensory nerve endings, ganglionic synapses, myoneural junctions, or nerve trunks. The action is reversible. The mechanism of action is not clearly understood.

Methods of Administration. There are several methods for the administration of local anesthetics.

1. *Topical (Surface) Anesthesia.* The drug is applied directly to the mucous membrane of the eye, nose, or throat and occasionally to the urethra, rectum, or vagina. A solution may be painted or sprayed on a surface or instilled, as in the eye. Powders, ointments, creams, and lotions may be applied topically to the skin.

2. *Infiltration Anesthesia.* Weak solutions of the local anesthetics in physiological salt solution are injected under the skin in painful conditions such as surgery or insertion of needles. A wheal may be produced for an incision. Later the anesthetic solution may be injected into the site of the incision to anesthetize the nerve endings and the exposed nerve trunks.

3. *Peripheral Nerve Block or Regional Anesthesia.* The anesthetic solution is injected into the vicinity of the nerve trunks which supply a definite area.

4. *Spinal Anesthesia.* The anesthetic solution is injected within the dural membrane surrounding the spinal cord and nerve roots.

5. *Epidural Anesthesia* (Peridural or Extradural). Spinal nerves are blocked in the epidural space as they emerge from the dura and pass into the intervertebral foramina. The anesthetic solution is deposited outside the dura and within the bony spinal or caudal canal. The deposition of the anesthetic solution may be accomplished at the thoracic, lumbar, or caudal (sacral) area.

6. *Intravenous Procaine Analgesia.* A solution of procaine is injected intravenously. The purpose is mainly to alleviate the sensation of pain.

Toxicity of Local Anesthetics. Local anesthetics produce acute toxic effects if they are absorbed in sufficient quantities in the circulating blood. The type of anesthetic, the rate of injection, the concentration, the volume of the solution, and the site of injection are factors in poisoning. There are two types of toxic reactions: (1) on the central nervous system, producing cortical stimulation resulting in convulsions and medullary depression; and (2) on the heart, depressing the myocardium and interfering with the conducting mechanism, which causes slowing of the heart. Many of the drugs are destroyed by the esterases in the plasma and by the liver. Serious liver damage may be caused by overdosage. Some individuals are more sensitive to these drugs. In susceptible persons even small amounts produce acute poisoning.

Symptoms of Poisoning. The symptoms are mental confusion, laughter, and dizziness. Muscular movements are increased. Palpitation of the heart, rapid pulse, slowing of the heart, and irregular respiration are observed. The patient is pale and perspires freely. The pupils are dilated.

The more severe symptoms are delirium, difficulty in breathing, convulsions, and unconsciousness. Death may follow because of respiratory failure and may take place very quickly, or the patient may recover with treatment.

Treatment of Poisoning

1. To combat central nervous system stimulation, a quick-acting barbiturate is administered. As a prophylactic measure it is advisable to administer pentobarbital sodium orally, 100 mg., one-half hour before the administration of a local anesthetic. Convulsions may be checked with the intravenous administration of pentobarbital or thiopental. The minimum doses of these drugs should be given because they may increase the cardiovascular and respiratory depression.

2. Respiratory stimulants are used to counteract the depressant effect on the respiration.

3. Sympathomimetic amines are used to combat peripheral cardiovascular collapse.

SOLUBLE LOCAL ANESTHETIC SALTS

Cocaine, N.F., B.P., I.P. Cocaine HCl, B.P.

Cocaine is an alkaloid obtained from the leaves of *Erythroxylon coca.* The aboriginal Indians in Peru mixed the leaves with lime and chewed them to lessen hunger and fatigue. In 1860, Dr. A. Niemann isolated the alkaloid cocaine from the leaves.

Pharmacological Action. Cocaine blocks nerve conduction locally when it is applied to an abraded area of the skin or to the mucous membrane or when it is injected under the skin. The sensory paralysis is reversible and the nerves recover their normal function gradually. Ischemia is produced. Cocaine constricts the blood vessels and delays its own absorption and destruction. It is the only local anesthetic that possesses this property.

Therapeutic Uses. Cocaine is used to produce surface anesthesia. Owing to its high systemic toxicity and low penetrating power, cocaine hydrochloride is used only for instillation in the eye in a 2 or 4 per cent solution and for application to the mucous membranes of the nose and throat in 5 to 10 per cent solutions. It is used in those cases where vasoconstriction is important.

Toxicity. Acute toxicity results clinically from overdosage, too rapid absorption, and improper administration of cocaine solutions. The symptoms of poisoning are the same as those discussed under the toxicity of local anesthetics. Corneal opacities have recently been reported arising from cocaine instillation in the eye. Thus, the drug is no longer recommended for this use. Chronic poisoning or *addiction* to cocaine is serious. Therefore, all derivatives of coca leaves, including salts of cocaine, are included in the Harrison Narcotic Act. When cocaine is administered hypodermically or snuffed up the nose as "snow," there is a feeling of euphoria followed by depression. Psychic dependence on cocaine (habituation) is marked, but physiological dependence is not clearly demonstrable (as in the case of morphine addiction). However, the cocaine habit produces moral degeneration and is difficult to cure. Treatment should be carried out in a hospital or sanitarium.

Preparation

Cocaine Hydrochloride Tablets, N.F.   8 and 15 mg.

Procaine Hydrochloride, U.S.P., B.P., I.P. (Novocain)

Procaine is a synthetic local anesthetic that has approximately one eighth the activity of cocaine. It is poorly absorbed from the mucous membranes and is not used for surface anesthesia. However, upon injection, local anesthesia lasting about one hour is produced in two to five minutes. Procaine is less toxic than cocaine and is widely used for infiltration, spinal, and various types of nerve block anesthesia. Its low toxicity is due to its rapid destruction by the esterases of the tissues and the blood.

Procaine hydrochloride is administered subcutaneously in a 0.25 to 1 per cent solution in doses up to 1 Gm. It is administered intrathecally in a 1 to 5 per cent solution in doses up to 150 mg.

Intravenous Procaine. Procaine hydrochloride may be injected intravenously as an analgesic. Because procaine reduces cardiac irritability, it may be administered to prevent cardiac arrhythmias under cyclopropane anesthesia and during chest operations. The intravenous administration of this drug allows a reduction in the amount of a spinal anesthetic or thiopental sodium injected.

The intravenous dose for procaine hydrochloride is 4 mg. per kilogram of body weight, administered slowly over a period of 20 minutes as a solution of 0.1 per cent in isotonic salt. There is a sensation of warmth throughout the body, flushing of the head and neck, laughter, hilarity, and a feeling of light-headedness. This method of administration may be dangerous, and the solution should be injected with extreme caution.

Preparations

Procaine Hydrochloride Injection, U.S.P.	1 or 2 per cent in 30 and 100 ml.
Procaine Hydrochloride and Epinephrine Injection, U.S.P. (I.P.); Procaine and Adrenalin Injection, B.P.	30-ml. vials containing 1 per cent procaine hydrochloride solution with 1:100,000 epinephrine hydrochloride
Procaine Hydrochloride, U.S.P.	Ampuls or vials containing 50, 100, 150, 200, 300, and 500 mg. and 1 Gm.
Procaine Hydrochloride Tablets, N.F.	20, 50, 75, and 150 mg.

Trade names: Novocain; Ethocaine; Kerocaine; Neocaine; Novocaine; Planocaine; Syncaine

Tetracaine Hydrochloride, U.S.P., I.P.; Amethocaine Hydrochloride, B.P. (Pontocaine)

Tetracaine hydrochloride is a local anesthetic with actions similar to those of procaine hydrochloride, but it is much more potent and more toxic and produces a prolonged, intense local anesthetic action when applied to the mucous membranes. It is used for surface anesthesia in the eye, nose, and throat and for prolonged spinal and continuous caudal anesthesia.

A 2 per cent solution is sprayed in the nose and throat and a 0.5 per cent solution is instilled in the eye. The 2 per cent solution is tinted blue to prevent accidental parenteral use because serious reactions have resulted from the subcutaneous injection of the drug. A 0.5 per cent solution is injected to produce spinal anesthesia. The dose is 2 to 20 mg. For continuous caudal anesthesia a 0.15 per cent solution is used.

Preparation

Tetracaine Hydrochloride for Injection, U.S.P.	2-ml. ampuls containing 1 per cent tetracaine hydrochloride; 100-ml. bottles containing 0.15 per cent tetracaine hydrochloride
Tetracaine Hydrochloride	Ampuls containing 10, 15, or 20 mg.
Tetracaine Hydrochloride Solution	2 per cent solution tinted blue
Tetracaine Hydrochloride Tablets	100 mg. for making solutions
Tetracaine Hydrochloride Ophthalmic Ointment	0.5 per cent

Trade names: Pontocaine; Pantocaine; Anethaine

Lidocaine, U.S.P.; Lignocaine Hydrochloride, B.P. (Xylocaine)

Lidocaine is more potent than procaine and slightly more toxic. It is stable in solution for long periods of time and may be autoclaved. It is the only local anesthetic that does not cause vasoconstriction or vasodilatation, and it may be used by all methods of administration without the addition of epinephrine. Lidocaine is useful for surface, infiltration, nerve block, and spinal and low caudal anesthesia. Clinically, it produces a more prompt, intensive, and extensive anesthesia than procaine. The side effects, which are rare, are nausea, muscular twitching, and chilling. Untoward effects may occur due to unusual sensitivity, too rapid or accidental intravenous injection, or overdosage. Reactions resulting from systemic absorption are due to stimulation and/or depression of the cerebral cortex and medulla. Excitatory symptoms such as dizziness, tremors, and convulsions may occur with slow onset, while severe depression leading to respiratory arrest, cardiovascular collapse, and cardiac arrest may occur rapidly without warning. Concentrations of 0.5 per cent are used for infiltration anesthesia; 1 per cent, for topical anesthesia; and 1 to 2 per cent, for block anesthesia. A 5 per cent ointment is available for burns, abrasions, skin lesions, and anorectal and otological conditions. A 2 per cent jelly produces profound anesthesia of the mucous membranes and is especially useful for administration to the urethra. An aqueous viscous solution, available for oral administration, quickly induces surface anesthesia of the upper gastrointestinal tract. It is used to control hiccups and reflex vomiting including severe vomiting of pregnancy and to relieve the discomfort of laryngoscopy, esophagoscopy, and gastroscopy. The usual oral dose is 1 tablespoonful of a 2 per cent solution.

Preparations

Lidocaine Hydrochloride Injection, Lignocaine Hydrochloride Injection, B.P.	0.5, 1, and 2 per cent in 20 ml.; 0.8 and 1.2 per cent in 30 ml. (with and without epinephrine)
Lignocaine and Adrenalin Injection, B.P.	2 per cent with 1:125,000 adrenalin
Lidocaine Jelly	2 per cent in tubes containing 30 ml.
Lidocaine Ointment	2.5 and 5 per cent in tubes containing 35 Gm.
Lidocaine Viscous	2 per cent solution in 100- and 450-ml. plastic bottles.

Trade names: Xylocaine, Duncaine, Lignostab, Xylotox

Dibucaine Hydrochloride, U.S.P.; Cinchocaine Hydrochloride, B.P. (Nupercaine)

Dibucaine produces a prolonged action upon application to the mucous membranes or upon injection. It is more potent and more toxic than cocaine and should be used in high dilutions. For infiltration anesthesia, 1 to 50 ml. of a 1:1000 solution is used; for topical anesthesia, a 0.5 to 2 per cent solution or a 0.5 per cent ointment is applied to the conjunctiva. For intraspinal injection, 10 ml. (6 to 15 ml.) of a 1:1500 solution or 1.5 ml. (1 to 2 ml.) of a 1:200 solution is used.

Preparations

Dibucaine Hydrochloride Injection, U.S.P. 1:200 in 2 ml.; 1:1500 in 20 ml.

Dibucaine Ophthalmic Ointment, U.S.P.   0.5 per cent

Trade name: Nupercaine

Piperocaine Hydrochloride, B.P. (Metycaine)

Piperocaine produces prompt local anesthesia upon injection or topical application. It is instilled in the eye in 2 to 4 per cent solutions, applied to the throat in 2 to 10 per cent solutions, and to the urethra in 1 to 4 per cent solutions. For infiltration anesthesia, 0.5 to 1 per cent solutions are used; for nerve block, 1 to 2 per cent solutions; and for spinal anesthesia, 1.5 to 2 per cent solutions.

Preparations

Piperocaine Hydrochloride Injection   1.5 per cent in 200 ml.; 2 per cent in 30 ml.

Piperocaine Hydrochloride Ophthalmic Ointment   4 per cent

Trade name. Metycaine

OTHER SOLUBLE LOCAL ANESTHETIC SALTS

Butethamine Formate (Monocaine Formate). Butethamine formate is similar in action to procaine, but it is more potent and therefore more toxic. It is used as a spinal anesthetic. The drug is available as a 5 per cent solution in 2-ml. ampuls and in ampuls containing 50, 100, 200, 300, and 500 mg. of the crystals. Butethamine Hydrochloride, N.F. (Monocaine Hydrochloride), is used for nerve block anesthesia in dentistry and other minor surgery. Butethamine Hydrochloride and Epinephine Injection, N.F. (Monocaine Hydrochloride), is available in 1 and 1.5 per cent solutions with epinephrine in 2-, 3-, and 5-ml. ampuls and in 60- and 125-ml. bottles.

Chloroprocaine Hydrochloride (Nesacaine). This local anesthetic is about twice as potent as procaine and its effects occur more rapidly. It is used to produce analgesia or surgical anesthesia and is administered by infiltration, field block, and regional nerve block including caudal and epidural block. It may be used with or without pressor drugs such as epinephrine or phenylephrine. One, two, and three per cent solutions are used. The volume of the solution injected varies with the concentration of the solution, the purpose for which the anesthetic is administered, and the area to be anesthetized. The drug is suitable for topical application to the skin and mucous membranes.

Hexylcaine Hydrochloride, N.F. (Cyclaine). Hexylcaine hydrochloride is suitable for surface anesthesia in 5 per cent solution, for infiltration and nerve block anesthesia in 1 per cent solution, and for spinal anesthesia in 2.5 per cent solution. Solutions of the drug are available in the following concentrations: 1 per cent in 30-ml. vials, 2.5 per cent with 10 per cent dextrose in 2-ml. ampuls, and 5 per cent for topical administration in 60-ml. bottles.

Mepivacaine (Carbocaine). Mepivacaine is two to four times more potent than procaine and is less toxic. It is used for prolonged local anesthesia. It is administered for nerve block (epidural, dental, sciatic, etc.). It is available as cartridges (carpules which contain 3 per cent in 1.8 ml.) and vials (30 and 50 ml. containing 1 and 1.5 per cent solution and 20 ml. containing 2 per cent solution).

Ravocaine Hydrochloride (2-Propoxy Procaine). This drug is much more active and also more toxic than procaine or lidocaine. It is generally used as a 0.1 per cent solution for infiltration and 0.5 per cent for nerve block as in dentistry.

VASOCONSTRICTOR DRUGS

Vasoconstrictor drugs are often added to the preparations of synthetic local anesthetic drugs that produce vasodilatation. Their function is to prevent the rapid absorption of the local anesthetic and thus prolong its action at the site of injection. This precaution also reduces the risk of toxic reactions due to too rapid absorption. Epinephrine is the drug most often used.

SOLUBLE LOCAL ANESTHETICS FOR TOPICAL ADMINISTRATION ONLY

Benoxinate Hydrochloride, U.S.P. (Dorsacaine). Benoxinate hydrochloride is a surface anesthetic used in ophthalmology. It is less irritating to the conjunctiva than tetracaine. One or two drops of a 0.4 per cent isotonic solution are instilled in the eye for the measurement of intraocular tension (tonometry) and for the insertion of contact lenses. The drug is available as a 0.4 per cent ophthalmic solution.

Butacaine Sulfate (Butyn) and Nitromersol. This is a nonirritating, antiseptic ointment which produces local anesthesia of long duration when applied to the mucous membranes, especially the cornea. It is used for painful ocular conditions and postoperatively to prevent infection and relieve pain.

Preparation

Butacaine Sulfate Ointment 2 per cent with nitromersol, 1:3000 in lanolin and mineral oil in ⅛-oz. tubes.

Trade name. Butyn

Cyclomethycaine Hydrochloride (Surfacaine). Cyclomethycaine hydrochloride is a local anesthetic that is effective on damaged or diseased skin, burns, and the rectal and vaginal mucosa. It is used as an aerosol cream or ointment in the relief of pain of thermal and chemical burns, various skin lesions, and itching conditions of the skin. It is used in gynecology and obstetrics for its local anesthetic and analgesic action on the mucous membranes. The drug is available as a 1 per cent ointment, 0.5 per cent cream, 0.75 per cent jelly, suppositories containing 10 mg., and 0.25 per cent solution. **Cyclomethycaine Sulphate, B.P. (Surfathesin).**

Dimethisoquin Hydrochloride, N.F. (Quotane). Dimethisoquin hydrochloride is used topically to allay itching, irritation, burning, or pain in certain skin diseases and mild sunburn. It is applied topically to the skin as a 0.5 per cent lotion or ointment. One application usually affords relief for two to four hours. It is available as a 0.5 per cent ointment and lotion.

Diperodon Hydrochloride (Diothane). Diperodon produces effects similar to those of cocaine, but its action is more prolonged. It is used to relieve pain and irritation in abrasions of the skin and mucous membranes and in nonoperative cases of hemorrhoids and following hemorrhoidectomy. It is available as 0.5 and 1 per cent solutions in sodium chloride and as a cream for topical application as a surface anesthetic and analgesic.

Dyclonine Hydrochloride (Dyclone). This agent is applied locally to the skin and mucous membranes. It is used to relieve pain and itching in various skin diseases, minor burns, and trauma, and in itching of the anus or vulva. It may also be employed to anesthetize the mucous membrane prior to the insertion of instruments. It does not produce miosis or mydriasis and may be instilled in the eye to produce anesthesia. Dyclonine hydrochloride is administered topically in a 1 per cent concentration in vanishing cream and in 0.5 per cent aqueous solutions.

Naepaine Hydrochloride, N.F. (Amylsine). Naepaine solutions instilled in the eye produce prompt anesthesia with little smarting. They do not produce mydriasis nor do they increase intraocular tension. A 2 or 4 per cent solution is used in ophthalmology when mydriasis is not desired. Naepaine hydrochloride is available as a powder in vials containing 5 Gm. or as a 4 per cent solution.

Phenacaine Hydrochloride, N.F. (Holocaine Hydrochloride). Phenacaine solutions, which are self-sterilizing, produce a prompt and prolonged anesthetic action when instilled in the eye. They are slightly irritating and cause hyperemia and lacrimation. A 1 per cent solution is used to anesthetize the eye while foreign objects are removed or after corneal lacerations.

Pramoxine Hydrochloride (Tronothane). This agent is applied topically to the skin and mucous membranes to relieve pain and itching which occur with certain skin diseases, minor burns, wounds, and anal lesions. It is used to anesthetize the mucous membranes prior to rectal examination or the insertion of instruments. Concentrations of 1 per cent are administered as solutions, creams, or jellies. The solutions are applied by spraying or by gauze pads soaked in the solution. The creams and jellies are used for digital dilatation and for the lubrication of instruments before insertion into body canals or tubes (e.g., the uretha, ureters, and anus).

Proparacaine Hydrochlorde (Ophthaine). This is instilled in the eye in 0.5 per cent solution for tonometry, for removal of sutures, or in cataract extraction.

SLIGHTLY SOLUBLE LOCAL ANESTHETICS

These slightly soluble local anesthetics are applied to wounds, ulcers, the mucous membranes, and the skin in the form of dusting powders, solutions in oils, or ointments.

Ethyl Aminobenzoate, N.F., I.P.; Benzocaine, B.P. Ethyl aminobenzoate is nonirritating and nontoxic and produces effective anesthesia of the skin, mucous membranes, and abraded areas. It absorbs ultraviolet rays; therefore, ointments or solutions of the drug in oil are used to prevent sunburn. It is also used as a dusting powder or ointment on abraded and denuded areas of the skin and mucous membranes, in hemorrhoids, and to relieve itching in various skin diseases. **Ethyl Aminobenzoate Ointment, N.F.,** is 5 per cent in strength. The drug is also available as a 10 to 20 per cent dusting powder and as vaginal and rectal suppositories containing 180 and 300 mg.

Butyl Aminobenzoate, N.F., B.P., I.P. Butyl aminobenzoate is diluted with talc and used as an anesthetic dusting powder. It is also available in the form of troches, suppositories, and ointments.

Butamben Picrate (Butesin Picrate). Butamben picrate is used almost exclusively in the treatment of minor burns. It is available as a 1 per cent ointment with nitromersol 1:5000, which stains yellow.

Ethyl Chloride, U.S.P., B.P., I.P. (Kelene); Fluro-Ethyl

Ethyl chloride (see p. 299) and fluro-ethyl are gases at ordinary temperatures, although they are volatile liquids when under pressure in special glass containers. Under pressure of their own vapors they are sprayed on the skin and produce surface anesthesia in 30 to 60 seconds by freezing the tissues due to their rapid evaporation from the skin.

Either drug may be sprayed on "trigger zones" to relieve muscle spasm in certain acute regional muscular disorders such as sprains or strains and in the treatment of painful back syndromes particularly of the paravertebral muscles in the region of the cervical and lumbar areas of the spine. Fluro-ethyl appears to be replacing ethyl chloride.

Preparations

Ethyl Chloride, U.S.P., B.P., I.P.	Spray bottle, with special cap, containing 100 Gm.
	Trade name: Kelene
Fluro-Ethyl	Spray bottle, with special cap, containing 100 Gm.

SPINAL ANESTHESIA

Cocaine hydrochloride was first injected into the spinal fluid in 1899, at which time it was the only local anesthetic available. Owing to its toxicity, there were many accidents. Since many patients were killed and some were permanently maimed, the method was abandoned.

With the introduction of new synthetic local anesthetics, which proved to be much safer and less toxic, there was a renewal of interest in spinal anesthesia. Today it is one of the most generally used procedures to produce anesthesia and muscular relaxation.

Spinal anesthesia is produced by the injection of a solution of a local anesthetic into the subarachnoid space. A temporary paralysis of the sensory, autonomic, and motor fibers in the anterior and posterior roots emanating from the area bathed by the drug results. These nerves are blocked in the order mentioned. The activity returns in the reverse order; the patient can move his extremity while it is still numb.

Spinal anesthesia may be produced by a single injection or intermittently over longer periods of time through a spinal catheter.

Therapeutic Uses of Spinal Anesthesia.   It is used (1) most often for operations performed on the lower portions of the body, such as the perineal area, lower extremities, and groin. (2) in intra-abdominal operations because of excellent muscle relaxation, contracted bowel, and quiet breathing, (3) in patients with a full stomach in whom general anesthesia would be dangerous because of the possibility of aspiration, and (4) in muscular patients or alcoholics who require excessive quantities of general anesthetics.

Administration of a Spinal Anesthetic.   The local anesthetic is injected into the subarachnoid space between two vertebral spinous processes, in the lower thoracic or lumbar areas of the spine. First the skin is cleansed and made sterile; then a 2 per cent solution of procaine or a 0.5 per cent lidocaine solution is injected intradermally to anesthetize the area so that there will be no pain with the insertion of the needle. Spinal fluid equal to the volume of the drug to be injected is withdrawn. This prevents increased pressure in the spinal canal and danger of undesirable effects on the vital centers in the medulla. The drug, which may be dissolved in the spinal fluid which is withdrawn, is injected slowly and produces nerve block. Procaine hydrochloride, in doses of 120 to 150 mg., produces anesthesia that lasts for about one hour. Tetracaine hydrochloride, in 2- to 20-mg. doses, prolongs the anesthetic action up to three hours. For other drugs used see Table 27, p. 437.

A vasopressor drug as part of the solution injected into the subarachnoid space will increase the duration of spinal anesthesia. Epinephrine, 0.3 to 0.5 mg., may be used for this purpose.

Symptoms Produced.   After the injection of a spinal anesthetic, there is a loss of sensation with a feeling of numbness below the site of injection. The skeletal muscles become flaccid and relaxed. There are profound relaxation and absence of pain in about ten minutes. Any anxiety or fear in the patient should be relieved with enough thiopental sodium, cyclopropane, or nitrous oxide and oxygen to blur consciousness.

Owing to the blocking action on the sympathetic nerves which control arteriole constriction, the blood vessels dilate and the blood pressure falls slowly. This fall in blood pressure may be controlled by the injection of sympathetic stimulants such as ephedrine sulfate, 50 to 100 mg. intravenously, or phenylephrine hydrochloride, 5 to 10 mg. subcutaneously. The vagal tone is increased and bradycardia (slowing of the heart) occurs. Tachycardia (rapid heart) indicates hemorrhage, in which case the blood volume should be augmented by the administration of whole blood or plasma.

Respiratory failure is usually the cause of death occurring during spinal anesthesia.

Control of the Level and Intensity of Anesthesia.   Six extrinsic factors may be varied to affect the level and intensity of anesthesia.

1. Volume of solution injected. The greater the volume of solution used with a given weight of drug, the higher the level of anesthesia.

2. Rate of injection. Rapid injection causes the drug to ascend to higher levels of the spinal canal.

3. Specific gravity of the solution. The specific gravity of the spinal fluid averages 1.006 but ranges from 1.003 to 1.009. If the specific gravity of the solution injected is greater than that of the spinal fluid, it is termed hyperbaric; if it approximates that of the spinal fluid, isobaric; if it is less, hypobaric.

4. Position of the patient after injection. This factor depends upon the specific gravity of the solution employed. The object is to prevent the solution from diffusing cephalad into the cervical region.

a. Hyperbaric solutions. For low-spinal anesthesia the patient is placed in a flat or Fowler's position so that the solution gravitates caudad. For high-spinal anesthesia the Trendelenburg position with head sharply flexed is employed.

b. Isobaric solutions. Flat position is employed. The level of anesthesia is difficult to control by varying the position.

c. Hypobaric solutions. The Trendelenburg position is employed to ensure a caudad diffusion of the drug.

5. Dosage of drugs. The greater the amount of drug, the higher the level and the greater the intensity of the paralysis.

6. The period immediately following injection is a crucial time. Straining or movement on the part of the patient may raise the level of anesthesia.

Advantages of Spinal Anesthesia

1. It provides excellent muscular relaxation.
2. It is accompanied by little disturbance of metabolic processes.
3. It dispenses with the inhalation of irritating drugs.
4. The patient is conscious.
5. Excessive secretions, excitement, and postanesthetic nausea are absent.
6. It allows the use of cautery and electrical equipment.
7. It may be administered by the surgeon if the anesthesiologist is not available.

Disadvantages of Spinal Anesthesia

1. It is uncontrollable. Once anesthesia has been instituted, it cannot be terminated.
2. Its duration is always somewhat uncertain; thus the patient may be submitted to supplemental anesthesia.
3. The possibility of failure due to technical errors exists.
4. Motor paralysis at high levels is a possibility, causing respiratory depression or failure.
5. There may be circulatory changes such as peripheral circulatory failure due to paralysis of the muscles and of the autonomic nervous system.
6. It is occasionally followed by postoperative neurological complications, due to the effect of the drug on the spinal cord, trauma from needles, or infection.
7. The vagal pathways from the viscera are not blocked during abdominal surgery. Retching, nausea, and vomiting may follow traction on the viscera.

Contraindications to Spinal Anesthesia

1. Cardiovascular diseases, since circulatory depression is a common disturbance in spinal anesthesia.

2. Neurological diseases, since severe damage may be caused.

3. Diseases of the respiratory system accompanied by a decrease in vital capacity. Intercostal paralysis may decrease the tidal exchange and further decrease vital capacity.

4. In anemia, as the oxygen-carrying power of the blood is reduced. Hypoxia may occur in a high spinal if intercostal paralysis is present.

5. Reduction in blood pressure as in hemorrhage or shock. Severe hypotension may ensue as the compensatory mechanisms which attempt to readjust the vascular system to normal are disturbed by spinal anesthesia.

6. Psychically disturbed patients. They are disturbed during the operation and may become restless.

7. In children, as their circulatory system is more labile and the level of anesthesia is difficult to control.

8. Infections about the vertebral column or when anatomical abnormalities are present.

Types of Spinal Anesthesia. *Continuous Lumbar (Epidural) Anesthesia.* The drug is not injected into the subarachnoid space but in the vicinity of the nerves at some point along the spinal canal, paralyzing the nerve trunks and their branches at or beyond their point of exit from the spinal cord. Although this type of anesthesia is slower in onset, it appears to reduce the hazard of nerve damage and make less likely a fall in blood pressure.

Caudal Anesthesia. This is referred to as caudal, epidural, or sacral block. The anesthetic solution is injected in the epidural space in the sacral canal and blocks the lumbosacral and coccygeal plexus. This type of anesthesia is used for operations on the bladder, rectum, and genitalia and in lessening labor pains in obstetrics. The local anesthetics most often administered are piperocaine (1 per cent), procaine (2 per cent), chloroprocaine (3 per cent), lidocaine (1.5 per cent), and mepivacaine (1 per cent).

Continuous Caudal Anesthesia. Anesthetics are injected into the caudal canal by means of a urethral-type catheter or needle which is allowed to remain in place so that repeated injections may be made. Used principally in obstetrics, this type of anesthesia permits greater flexibility of dosage. Smaller amounts of the drug are administered at first, which may be augmented as required. Almost any soluble local anesthetic may be used for this type of anesthesia. See Table 27, page 437.

Saddle Block Anesthesia. In saddle block anesthesia, the perineal and buttock areas are anesthetized. The patient is given the injection in the upright sitting position and must not be put in lithotomy, Sims's, or other position for ten minutes after the injection. This type of anesthesia is used in rectal, urological, and gynecological procedures, in obstetrics and surgery involving the perineum, rectum, and scrotum. The drugs administered are procaine, piperocaine, or butethamine for short procedures; tetracaine or dibucaine for long procedures.

Postoperative Sequelae. Deaths from spinal anesthetics are few, but there are many postoperative sequelae, rarely serious. These sequelae include: (1) headache, which occurs in about 30 per cent of the patients and may last for days or weeks; (2) nausea and vomiting; (3) fever; (4) urinary retention, which is usually transient; (5) meningitis due to infection; (6) neuritis due to irritation of the nerves, paresthesia of the extremities, paralysis of the speech center, and double vision; and (7) permanent paralysis.

Table 27

Injectable Local Anesthetics

Drug	Spinal Block	Nerve Block Including Extradural and Paravertebral Block	Infiltration Anesthesia
PERCENTAGE STRENGTHS OF SOLUTIONS USED			
Butethamine Formate (Monocaine)	2% (100 to 150 mg.)		
Butethamine HCl, N.F. (Monocaine)		1 to 1.5%*	0.5 to 1%*
Dibucaine HCl, U.S.P.; Cinchocaine HCl, B.P. (Nupercaine)	1:1500 and 1:200 0.1 and 0.5	0.1%*	0.03 to 0.1%*
Hexylcaine HCl, N.F. (Cyclaine)	2.5% (15 to 50 mg.)	1%	1%
Lidocaine HCl, U.S.P.; Lignocaine HCl, B.P. (Xylocaine)	2 to 5%	1 to 2%* 0.5 to 2%*	0.5%* 0.5 to 2%*
Parethoxycaine HCl (Intracaine)	2.5%	0.5 to 1.5%	0.5%
Piperocaine HCl, U.S.P. (Metycaine)	1.5 to 5% (50 to 100 mg.)	1 to 2%	1%
Procaine HCl, U.S.P.; B.P. (Novocaine)	1 to 5% (50 to 200 mg.)	0.5 to 2%	0.25% to 1%
Tetracaine HCl, U.S.P.; Amethocaine HCl, B.P.	0.5 (4 to 20 mg.) 0.5 to 0.1%	0.1%	0.03 to 0.1%

* With epinephrine.

REVIEW QUESTIONS

1. *(a) Give two general methods of rendering a section of the skin insensitive to pain. (b) Explain: topical or surface anesthesia; infiltration of an anesthetic, as at the base of a finger; regional or larger anesthesia; epidural anesthesia.*
2. *What is meant by idiosyncrasy? What symptoms may be expected if a person idiosyncratic to local anesthetics of the procaine class has a reaction to such a drug? How can this reaction be treated?*
3. *Name a local anesthetic (a) with low toxicity, (b) of considerable potency when instilled into the conjunctival sac for corneal anesthesia. Name all agents useful for anesthetizing mucous membranes by surface (topical) application.*
4. *A sympathomimetic amine such as levarterenol or epinephrine is used with some local anesthetics for constricting the arterioles in the subcutaneous area being infiltrated. Explain the value of this vasoconstriction.*
5. *Explain the main features in administering spinal anesthesia. Why should the blood pressure fall and how may the fall be combated?*
6. *Name the postoperative complications or sequelae of spinal anesthesia.*

REFERENCES

Adriani, J.; "Local Anesthetics," *Am. J. Nursing*, **59**:86, 1959.

————: *The Pharmacology of Anesthetic Drugs: a Syllabus for Students and Clinicians*. Charles C Thomas, Publisher, Springfield, Ill., 1952.

————: *Techniques and Procedures of Anesthesia*, 3rd ed. Charles C Thomas, Publisher, Springfield, Ill., 1964.

Artusio, Joseph F.: "Anesthetics," in Modell, W. (ed.): *Drugs of Choice 1964–1965*, C. V. Mosby Company, St. Louis, 1964.

Breckinridge, F. J., and Bruno, P.: "Nursing Care of the Anesthetized Patient," *Am. J. Nursing*, **62**:74, 1962.

Bryce-Smith, R.: "Local Anesthetic Drugs," *Brit. M. J.*, **1**:1039, 1960.

Burstein, C. L.: *Fundamental Considerations in Anesthesia*, 2nd ed. The Macmillan Company, New York, 1955.

Greene, N. M.: "The Pharmacology of Local Anesthetic Agents, with Special Reference to Therapeutic Use in Spinal Anesthesia," *Anesthesiology*, **16**:573, 1955.

Lundy, J. S.: *Clinical Anesthesia*. W. B. Saunders Company, Philadelphia, 1942.

Schafer, K. N., *et al.*: *Medical and Surgical Nursing*, 2nd ed. C. V. Mosby Company, St. Louis, 1961.

Vandam, L. D., and Dripps, R. D.: "Long-Term Follow Up of Patients Which Received 10,098 Spinal Anesthetics," *J.A.M.A.*, **161**:586, 1956.

V DRUGS ACTING ON THE AUTONOMIC NERVOUS SYSTEM

There is still another division of the nervous system, the autonomic, which is partly within the central system and partly peripheral to it. It may be termed the involuntary, visceral, vegetative, or "automatic" nervous system. It is widespread throughout the body, and, in general, performs functions that are below the level of consciousness. The autonomic nervous system controls many of the functions of the thoracic and abdominal organs, as well as the size of the blood vessels, and the secretions of glands. It serves more to regulate the inner functioning of the body and the automatic adjustment of the organism to its environment. Each type of autonomic nerve has a specific function which may be altered.

The autonomic nervous system is an integral part of the central nervous system. Impulses to the brain from the various senses, such as hearing, sight, and touch, initiate visceral impulses that may alter the rate of the heart or respiration, dilate the arterioles and capillary networks, constrict the bronchioles, or produce abdominal cramping. Emotional responses caused by unhappy surroundings and experiences may produce stress that may change the functions and physiological responses of organs and tissues and thus produce cardiovascular changes, high blood pressure, or asthma. This autonomic imbalance can be corrected or modified by the administration of the drugs discussed in Chapters 27 to 30.

26

The Function and Innervation of the Autonomic Nervous System. The Eye

FUNCTION

The autonomic nervous system consists of two parts: the *sympathetic* and the *parasympathetic* divisions. This classification is based upon the anatomical origins of the nerves and their physiological functions. The sympathetic nerves originate in the thoracolumber regions of the spinal cord; therefore, the sympathetic division may also be called the *thoracolumbar* division. The parasympathetic nerves originate in the area of the midbrain, medulla, and sacral portion of the spinal cord; consequently the parasympathetic division may be called the *craniosacral* division.

The autonomic nervous system controls many fundamental processes by regulating the function of important organs and other structures in the body. The sympathetic and parasympathetic divisions have different roles. The parasympathetic division has many unrelated functions: it controls the ciliary muscle, which changes the shape of the lens of the eye; it causes constriction of the pupil to protect the retina from excessive light; it is called into action in emptying the urinary bladder; it slows the heart when the appropriate nerves are stimulated from within the medulla of the brain; it can increase blood flow in various areas by dilating blood vessels; and it increases the amount of salivary and lacrimal secretions under appropriate conditions. One of its major functions which concerns us in medicine is its role in the digestive process. The secretion of acid and the enzyme pepsin by the stomach, the rhythmic waves of contraction of the stomach during its phase of digestion, the tone and opening of the pyloric sphincter, and the movements of the intestines are vital functions over which the vagus, a cranial parasympathetic nerve, exerts control. We can both increase and decrease all these and other effects by pharmacological agents. Figure 13 shows the innervation of the various organs and tissues by the two divisions of the autonomic nervous system.

The sympathetic division functions mainly as an entire unit, often exerting its effects simultaneously in all areas it supplies. This is in contradistinction to the many discrete functions of the parasympathetic division.

The sympathetic division controls the mechanism for responding to in-

440

creased energy requirements of the body and to emergencies. In times of stress, in fear and anger, sympathetic nerves are stimulated. As a result, certain body functions are accelerated, thus facilitating a response such as quick movement or fighting. Epinephrine is secreted, which accelerates the circulation. The skeletal muscles are supplied with more blood. Glycogen is converted in the liver to supply the muscles with glucose for oxidation and liberation of energy. The pupils are dilated to increase the field of vision. In a less dramatic way, these functions prevail in ordinary activity.

INNERVATION

The autonomic nerves are composed of two types of fibers: the preganglionic and the postganglionic. In the sympathetic division the synapses between the pre- and postganglionic fibers are located outside the central nervous system either as two ganglionic cords lying on either side or in front of the vertebrae or as ganglia in the abdomen (see Fig. 14). In the parasympathetic division, the synapses of the motor fibers are found in ganglia close to or within the organ they innervate.

Transmission of Nerve Impulses by Chemical Mediators.   Under the influence of nerve impulses chemical substances which are synthesized and stored in the nerve fibers are released at the nerve endings. These substances, called mediators or neurohormones, transmit the impulses at the autonomic ganglia (synapses between the pre- and postganglionic fibers) and from the ends of postganglionic fibers to the effector cells (smooth and cardiac muscles and exocrine glands). Acetylcholine (AC) is the transmitter in the ganglia of both sympathetic and parasympathetic systems.

Cholinergic and Adrenergic Fibers.   Nerve fibers are classified on the basis of the mediator released from them. Those which release AC are called cholinergic; those which release norepinephrine and epinephrine are named adrenergic.

Cholinergic Fibers.   The cholinergic fibers are the postganglionic fibers of the parasympathetic division. They initiate their response at the effector cells of the organ by the liberation of acetylcholine at the "target" cells. These cells (e.g., smooth muscle, heart, glandular cells, etc.) are stimulated to act by this substance, which is the hormone of the parasympathetic nervous system. There are cholinergic fibers in the sympathetic system that dilate the arterioles in skeletal muscle which they innervate and those innervating the sweat glands and the uterus.

Acetylcholine is inactivated in the tissues by an enzyme, cholinesterase, which hydrolyzes it to choline and acetic acid. This action is prompt; hence the action of acetylcholine when it is released by the nerve impulse is brief. When cholinesterase is inactivated, the action of acetylcholine is intense and prolonged.

Adrenergic Fibers.   The adrenergic fibers are the postganglionic fibers of the sympathetic division which produce their response in the effector cells of the innervated organ by liberating predominantly norepinephrine and, to a lesser extent, epinephrine. These two substances are the hormones of the *sympathetic nervous system*. They are inactivated by enzymes, as is acetylcholine, but not so rapidly. They must, like acetylcholine, be formed repeatedly during the activity of the sympathetic nervous system.

The sympathetic division supplies nerves to nearly all areas supplied by the parasympathetic division. In many of these areas the two divisions exert opposite effects. Proper functioning of the structures thus doubly innervated is attained by an appropriate but variable degree of influence by these two opposing systems.

There is a close relationship between the autonomic nervous system and hormonal secretion. Some endocrine glands are influenced by autonomic innervation, and, in turn, the secreted hormones influence the degree of responsiveness of the autonomic nervous system.

The Hormones.   Acetylcholine plays a very important role in the autonomic nervous system and also in other parts of the body. It is synthesized and stored in the bound form in nerve tissues. Upon activation of nerve impulses it performs the following functions:

1. It provides synaptic transmission of nerve impulses in all ganglia of the parasympathetic and sympathetic systems.

2. It provides transmission from postganglionic fibers of the parasympathetic fibers and a few sympathetic fibers to cell receptors of organs.

3. It provides transmission from motor fibers to cell receptors in skeletal muscles.

4. It provides central synaptic transmission.

5. It is associated with the initiation and maintenance of cardiac rhythm.

It has been postulated that there are three types of receptors based on their reactions with cholinergic blocking agents. The alkaloid, muscarine, obtained from the mushroom *Amanita muscarinia* upon injection produces effects similar to those of acetylcholine on smooth muscles, heart muscle, and exocrine glands. These responses are called muscarinic, and the receptors on which muscarine produces its effect are blocked by atropine and are called *atropine sensitive*. Nicotine first stimulates and then blocks transmission in the autonomic ganglia and also at the neuromuscular junction of skeletal muscle as does acetylcholine. These effects are called *nicotinic*. The ganglionic receptors are blocked by hexamethonium, while the receptors at the neuromuscular junction are blocked by d-tubocurarine.

Norepinephrine and epinephrine, the hormones and natural stimulators of the sympathetic system, are catecholamines. They are formed and stored

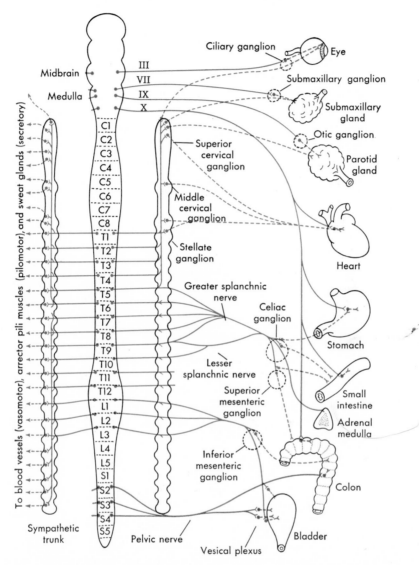

Fig. 13. Diagrammatic representation of some of the chief conduction pathways of the autonomic nervous system. For clarity, the nerves to blood vessels, arrector pili muscles, and sweat glands are shown on the left side of the figure, and the pathways to other visceral structures only on the right side. The sympathetic division is shown in red, the parasympathetic in blue. Solid lines represent preganglionic fibers; broken lines represent postganglionic fibers. (Kimber, D. C.; Gray, C. E.; Stackpole, C. E.; and Leavell, L. C.: *Anatomy and Physiology*, 14th ed. The Macmillan Company, New York, 1961. Modified from *Bailey's Textbook of Histology*, 13th ed., revised by P. E. Smith and W. M. Copenhaver. Courtesy of The Williams & Wilkins Company.)

as granules in the sympathetic nerve fibers (primarily norepinephrine), in the cells of the adrenal medulla and other chromaffin cells (primarily epinephrine), and in the nerve cells in the brain (primarily norepinephrine). Splanchnic nerve impulses mediated through the central nervous system cause a release of acetylcholine, which stimulates the adrenal glands to release the catecholamines. Epinephrine is the predominant hormone liberated from the

Table 28

Site and Response of Cholinergic Receptors

Cholinergic Receptors	Location of Receptors	Responses
Atropine sensitive	Smooth muscles, heart muscle	Muscarinic
Hexamethonium sensitive	Autonomic ganglia	Nicotinic
d-Tubocurarine sensitive	Neuromuscular junction of skeletal muscle	Skeletal muscle (nicotinic)

adrenal glands while norepinephrine is the principal mediator released at the postganglionic effector cells. Since some of the tissues innervated by sympathetic nerves are stimulated while others are inhibited upon stimulation, it has been suggested that there may be two types of receptors of the effector organs: (1) *alpha receptors,* which are primarily concerned with vasoconstriction and respond to norepinephrine and epinephrine and are blocked by alpha adrenergic blocking agents, and (2) *beta receptors,* which relax smooth muscle, especially the bronchi, which respond to isoproterenol (Isuprel) and epinephrine but do not respond to the alpha adrenergic blocking agents. There are two exceptions: the receptors in the heart are beta but do not respond to the beta adrenergic blocking agents, while those in the intestines are alpha receptors.

Table 29

Responses of the Effector Organs to Nerve Impulses*

Effector System	Adrenergic Nerve Impulses	Cholinergic Nerve Impulses
Eye		
Iris	Mydriasis	Miosis
Ciliary muscle	Lessens tone, eye relaxed for far vision(?)	Increases tone, eye accommodated for near vision
Intraocular tension		Decreased
Heart		
Rate	Accelerated	Slowed
Stroke volume	Increased	Decreased
Rhythm	Ventricular extrasystoles, tachycardia, fibrillation	Bradycardia, AV block, vagal arrest

Responses of the Effector Organs to Nerve Impulses*

Effector System	Adrenergic Nerve Impulses	Cholinergic Nerve Impulses
Blood vessels		
Coronary	Dilated	Dilated
Skin and mucosa	Constricted	Dilated
Skeletal muscle	Dilated, constricted	Dilated (?)
Cerebral	Constricted	Dilated (?)
Pulmonary	Constricted	Dilated
Abdominal viscera	Constricted	Dilated (not by vagal impulses)
Lungs		
Bronchial muscle	Relaxed	Constricted
Bronchial glands	Inhibited (?)	Stimulated
Stomach		
Motility and tone	Decreased	Increased
Sphincters	Contracted as a rule	Relaxed as a rule
Secretion	Inhibited	Increased, particularly enzymes
Intestine		
Motility and tone	Decreased	Increased
Sphincters	Contracted as a rule	Relaxed as a rule
Secretion	Inhibited (?)	Increased
Gallbladder and ducts	Relaxed (?)	Contracted
Urinary bladder		
Detrusor	Relaxed	Contracted
Trigone and sphincter	Contracted	Relaxed
Uterus (human), pregnant	Stimulated	Stimulated
Skin		
Pilomotor muscles	Contracted	—
Sweat glands	Stimulated	Stimulated
Adrenal medulla	—	Secretion of epinephrine and norepinephrine
Skeletal muscle	—	Stimulated
Liver	Glycogenolysis	—
Spleen capsule	Constricted	—
Salivary glands	Stimulated (sparse, thick, mucinous secretion)	Stimulated (profuse, watery secretion)
Lacrimal glands	—	Stimulated
Nasopharyngeal glands	—	Stimulated

* Modified from Goodman, L. S., and Gilman, A.: *The Pharmacological Basis of Therapeutics*, 2nd ed. The Macmillan Company, New York, 1958.

Table 30

Principal Autonomic Drugs

Autonomic Ganglia	Sympathetics	Parasympathetics
STIMULANTS	ADRENERGIC AGENTS	CHOLINERGIC AGENTS
Nicotine, prototype (small doses) Acetylcholine	A. *Catecholamines*, direct action Epinephrine, prototype Levarterenol (Levophed) Isoproterenol (Isuprel) B. *Phenylalkylamines*, indirect action Ephedrine, prototype Phenylephrine (Neo-Synephrine) Amphetamines Methoxamine (Vasoxyl) Mephentermine (Wyamine) Metaraminol (Aramine)	A. *Cholinergic agents* Acetylcholine, prototype Methacholine (Mecholyl) Carbachol (Doryl) Bethanechol (Urecholine) Pilocarpine *Pharmacological tool* Muscarine B. *Anticholinesterase agents* Physostigmine, prototype Neostigmine (Prostigmin) Pyridostigmine (Mestinon) Edrophonium (Tensilon) Ambenonium (Mytelase) Isofluorophate (DFP) Demecarium (Humorosol)
GANGLIONIC BLOCKING AGENTS	ADRENERGIC BLOCKING AGENTS	CHOLINERGIC BLOCKING AGENTS
Hexamethonium, prototype Mecamylamine (Inversine) Chlorisondamine (Ecolid) Pentolinium (Ansolysen) Trimethidinium (Ostensin) Tetraethylammonium (Etamon) *Pharmacological tools* Nicotine (large doses) Acetylcholine (large doses)	A. *Alpha receptors* Ergotamine (Gynergen), prototype Phentolamine (Regitine) Tolazoline (Priscoline) Phenoxybenzamine (Dibenzyline) Azapetine (Ilidar) B. *Beta receptors* *Pharmacological tools* Dichloroisoproterenol (DCI), prototype Pronethalol (Nethalide)	Atropine, prototype Scopolamine (hyoscine) Homatropine Propantheline (Pro-Banthine) and other synthetic atropine-like compounds

Response to Drugs. The principal responses produced by the action of drugs on the sympathetic and parasympathetic nervous systems are outlined in Table 29. Drugs are classified according to their action in simulating or opposing the action of the mediators of these systems and will be discussed in the following chapters under the following headings:

Adrenergic agents
Adrenergic blocking agents
Cholinergic agents
Cholinergic blocking agents

Since the responses of the two systems are antagonistic physiologically and pharmacologically, like effects are observed when the sympathetic nervous system is stimulated or the parasympathetic nervous system is depressed. For example, both epinephrine, which stimulates the sympathetic, and atropine, which depresses the parasympathetic system, dilate the pupil, accelerate the heart rate, dilate the bronchi, and decrease the motility and tone of the gastrointestinal tract.

The ganglionic blocking agents prevent the passage of all or some of the impulses across the synapses in both sympathetic and parasympathetic systems. Blockage of the sympathetic ganglia causes a relaxation of the tension of the smooth muscle of the blood vessels, a decrease in peripheral resistance, and a fall in blood pressure. This is the most pronounced effect produced by these drugs, which makes them valuable in the treatment of hypertension and peripheral vascular disease.

The side effects, which are mainly caused by blockade of the parasympathetic system, are blurring of vision, dry mouth, and constipation.

The two systems respond to drugs with a considerable amount of specificity. Table 30 lists the principal drugs that act on the autonomic nervous system, the type of response noted, and the division of the autonomic nervous system which responds to their action.

INNERVATION OF THE EYE

Autonomic Control of the Intraocular Muscles. The iris, a contractile circular diaphragm that forms the colored portion of the eye, controls the amount of light reaching the retina. It is composed of thin layers of smooth muscle which adjust the diameter of the central opening, or pupil. The iris is made up of two types of muscle:

1. The radial muscles, which are innervated by adrenergic fibers. Fibers from the upper dorsal nerves reach the sympathetic chain and pass through the inferior cervical ganglion to the middle and superior cervical ganglia to

the adrenergic fibers. When these fibers are stimulated, the pupil is dilated (mydriasis).

2. The circular muscles, which are innervated by cholinergic fibers. Fibers, which leave the brain by the oculomotor nerve, pass to the ciliary ganglia and thence to the circular muscle of the iris by way of the cholinergic fibers. When these fibers are stimulated, the pupil is constricted (miosis).

Pupillary Reflexes. Mydriasis (dilatation of the pupil) normally takes place as the eye adjusts its vision in a darkened room. It also occurs under stress, pain, and strong emotions and under the influence of certain drugs. Adrenergic drugs, e.g., epinephrine (when increased in the blood stream) and cocaine and ephedrine (when instilled in the eye), and cholinergic blocking agents, e.g., atropine and homatropine, produce mydriasis.

Miosis (constriction of the pupil) occurs in response to light and as part of the adjustment of the eye to near vision. It also occurs under the influence of cholinergic drugs, e.g., pilocarpine, physostigmine, and neostigmine.

Accommodation Reflex. The parasympathetic innervations to the ciliary muscle play an important part in the accommodation of the eye for far or near vision. The normal eye will bring the images of both near and distant objects to a focus on the retina. The necessary adjustment is made by altering the curvature of the lens. Thus images of objects are not blurred, regardless of distance.

The lens is a doubly convex, transparent body enclosed in an elastic capsule behind the iris. The fibers of the suspensory ligament attach this capsule to the ciliary body, which in turn is attached to a circular (ciliary) muscle. The ciliary muscle is composed of smooth muscle innnervated by branches of the oculomotor or third cranial nerve.

When the eye is at rest or accommodated for far vision, the lens is kept in a more flattened state by the pull of the elastic fibers in the suspensory ligament. Constant intraocular pressure in the eye keeps the coats of the eyeball distended so that the ciliary body is pulled forward and the fibers of the suspensory ligament remain taut.

Accommodation for near vision is brought about by the contraction of the ciliary muscle upon stimulation of its parasympathetic fibers. The inner edge of the ciliary muscle is drawn inward and toward the lens and slightly forward toward the cornea. This movement loosens the tension of the fibers of the suspensory ligament on the lens, which bulges forward and becomes more spherical, owing to its own elasticity. By increasing the curvature of the lens, the eye is accommodated for near vision. Cholinergic drugs such as pilocarpine, physostigmine, and neostigmine tend to adjust the eye for near vision. Cholinergic blocking agents such as atropine and related drugs paralyze accommodation and thus fix the eye for far vision. Cycloplegia is the term describing paralysis of accommodation.

Changes in Intraocular Pressure. The intraocular fluid (aqueous humor) is a limpid, watery substance that fills the space between the cornea and lens (anterior and posterior chambers). It is formed partly by filtration from the ciliary vessels and partly from some secretory activity of the ciliary body. The fluid passes through the posterior chamber and pupil into the anterior chamber. Some of the fluid is absorbed by the blood vessels and some passes through the spaces of Fontana and filters into the venous canal of Schlemm. One cause of increased intraocular tension and "hardening" of the eyeball (glaucoma) may be faulty drainage of the aqueous humor. Miotic drugs when instilled in the eye diminish this increased tension by drawing the smooth muscle of the iris away from the canal of Schlemm (in the angle formed by the iris and the cornea) and establishing better drainage of the aqueous humor through this channel.

Additional agents that decrease intraocular tension are described on pages 473–74.

REVIEW QUESTIONS

1. *List as many functions as you can for both the sympathetic and the para-sympathetic nervous systems.*
2. *What drugs mimic or reinforce each of these two divisions of the autonomic nervous system?*
3. *What drugs depress each division?*
4. *What is meant by the following terms?*

Adrenergic drug	*Cholinergic drug*
Adrenergic blocking agent	*Anticholinergic agent*
Cycloplegic agent	*Sympathomimetic*
Miotic agent	*Parasympathomimetic*
Mydriatic agent	

5. *What are the effects of blocking (a) the sympathetic ganglia? (b) The parasympathetic ganglia?*

REFERENCES

Ahlquist, R. P.: A Study of Adrenotropic Receptors," *Am. J. Physiol.*, **153**:586, 1948.

Brown, C. H.: "New Blocking Agents," *Am. J. Nursing*, **57**:877, 1957.

Jackson, D. E.: *Experimental Pharmacology and Materia Medica.* C. V. Mosby Company, St. Louis, 1939. See Fig. 690, "Schematic Representation of the Innervation of the Eye," p. 544; Fig. 691, "Diagrammatic Representation of the Structure and Innervation of the Eye," p. 546.

Moe, G. J., and Freyburger, W. A.: "Ganglionic Blocking Agents," *Pharmacol. Rev.*, **2**:61, 1950.

Paton, W. D. M.: "The Paralysis of the Autonomic Ganglia, with Special Reference to the Therapeutic Effects of Ganglion-Blocking Drugs," *Brit. M. J.*, **1**:773, 1951.

"Symposium on Neurohumoral Transmission," *Pharmacol. Rev.*, **6**:1, 1954.

Texter, E. C., Jr., and Ruffin, J. M.: "Drugs Affecting the Autonomic Nervous System: Part I. Clinical Application in Gastrointestinal Disorders," *South. M. J.*, **49**:910, 1956.

27

Stimulants of the Sympathetic Nervous System (Adrenergic Agents)

Adrenergic or sympathomimetic drugs stimulate one or several structures in the body innervated by the sympathetic nervous system. They produce effects that simulate the physiological responses to impulses transmitted by the adrenergic postganglionic nerves. For the various effects of such stimulation see Table 30, page 443. Epinephrine and norepinephrine, which are the hormones of this system, and some other naturally occurring substances are widely used clinically, in addition to numerous synthetic compounds related chemically to and resembling the catecholamines in their action.

PRESSOR AMINES

Epinephrine, U.S.P.; Adrenaline, B.P., I.P. (Adrenalin)

Epinephrine, the first hormone to be isolated, is the predominant hormone of the medullary portion of the adrenal gland. Smaller amounts of norepinephrine are present. Although the hormone has been synthesized, the natural form (levorotatory epinephrine), obtained from the adrenal glands of domestic animals, is more active than the synthetic (racemic) form and is the product used in medicine. This preparation contains about 0.1 per cent norepinephrine. It is unstable and is marketed in brown bottles which should be kept in the refrigerator.

Absorption, Fate, and Excretion. Epinephrine is destroyed in the gastrointestinal tract; hence it is not absorbed upon oral administration. However, the absorption is prompt upon subcutaneous or intramuscular administration. In the body, epinephrine is inactivated by o-methyl transferase enzymes and by amine oxidases. It is also conjugated with sulfuric or glucuronic acid, and the conjugated forms and some free epinephrine are excreted in the urine.

Pharmacological Actions. *On the Circulation.* The most prominent effects of epinephrine are those upon the heart and the vascular bed. Ordinary *subcutaneous* doses in man decrease the tone in most arterioles of the body, with a resultant fall in diastolic blood pressure (see p. 451). Arterioles in

450

most skeletal muscles and the heart are dilated by epinephrine. Those in the skin and mucous membranes as well as some in the viscera such as the lungs and kidneys are constricted. Thus blood is diverted from the skin and mucous membranes and viscera to the brain, liver, heart, and skeletal muscles which are most active in an emergency. With the fall in diastolic pressure, there is a rise in systolic blood pressure (see below), which is produced by the action of the drug on the heart. This action is twofold. Epinephrine increases the rate of the heart beat and, in addition, the force of contraction. The first is known as the *chronotropic* action and the second, the increased force, as its *inotropic* action. The inotropic action resembles the strengthening action of the digitalis alkaloids. These actions on the heart cause an increased cardiac output of blood into the aorta and systemic arteries, and thus an increase in systolic blood pressure. Epinephrine increases the irritability of the myocardium and in larger doses may cause disorders in cardiac rhythm. It may also sensitize the heart muscle to arrhythmias under cyclopropane or almost any other hydrocarbon anesthetic.

Epinephrine is not used in therapy for raising blood pressure because it is mainly by cardiac stimulation, or overstimulation, that this is accomplished. It is occasionally used as a cardiac stimulant and is sometimes effective in controlling Adams-Stokes attacks in which there is a defect in conduction of the motivating electric impulses to the ventricles (see Chap. 32).

Slow intravenous infusions of epinephrine may cause speeding of the heart (tachycardia) and peripheral dilatation of the majority of blood vessels, but only the systolic blood pressure is significantly altered. This is markedly increased, whereas diastolic pressure may remain unchanged or rise slightly. A more *rapid intravenous* injection of epinephrine, as when a subcutaneous dose is accidentally given into a vein, produces a *marked rise* in both systolic and diastolic pressure. Both may be more than doubled or even tripled. Most of the arterioles that are dilated by small quantities of the hormone are intensely constricted by larger amounts. Brain hemorrhage and small extravasations of blood elsewhere may occur. The cardiac rate is greatly accelerated after a brief slowing (bradycardia), temporarily caused by reflex action via the vagus fibers to the heart. Irregularities of the heart beat are frequently a consequence. Cardiac dilatation and ventricular fibrillation may result from the direct action on the myocardium. It is therefore extremely important to make certain not to inject subcutaneous doses of epinephrine into a vein. The plunger of the syringe should be pulled back much farther than usual in order to aspirate blood if a vein has been entered.

Epinephrine is sometimes used in the revival of patients in threatened drowning or collapse. In threatened collapse, 2 or 3 ml. of a 1:10,000 solution are injected into a large vein and washed in with saline. In cardiac arrest, 0.5 to 1 ml. of a 1:1000 solution of epinephrine injected into the right atrium, with cardiac massage, may cause the heart to start beating again. This must be done very quickly.

The capsule of the spleen, which contains sympathetically innervated smooth muscle fibers, is contracted by the catecholamines, expressing much of the blood pooled in that organ. This blood is thus a small reserve supply which can be made available in need.

The constriction of the arterioles, capillaries, and venules in and beneath the skin, which epinephrine produces, is useful in the treatment of urticaria, hives, and angioneurotic edema, which is thought to be caused by histamine or a histamine-like substance that dilates the capillaries and permits fluid to exude into the tissues. The rash, itching, and swelling are rapidly relieved by the injection of epinephrine.

Local Effect. The local application of epinephrine to the mucous membrane causes a prompt vasoconstriction. It is used as a hemostatic to check nasal hemorrhage. A small piece of cotton saturated with 1:1000 epinephrine is inserted in the nasal cavity. Spraying a 1:10,000 or a 1:1000 solution on the membranes of the nose or throat during surgical procedures will check bleeding. In the nasal catarrh, a 1:1000 solution will produce shrinking of the turbinates.

Epinephrine is often used with local anesthetics to produce ischemia (decreased blood supply). This allows the anesthetic to remain longer at the site of local surgery.

On Bronchial Muscle. The bronchioles are innervated by the adrenergic fibers, which are relaxant to these structures. When the effector cells are stimulated by the injection of epinephrine, the bronchioles, especially those which are constricted due to histamine, cholinergic drugs, or nervous reflexes, or by disease such as bronchial asthma, dilate. Epinephrine also constricts the blood vessels to the lungs and thus increases their vital capacity by decreasing vascular congestion of the bronchial mucosa.

Epinephrine is a prompt and dependable agent in the acute asthmatic attack. One-tenth milliliter or more of a 1:1000 solution is injected subcutaneously. Aerosols or fine mists of 1:1000 or 1:100 epinephrine may be sprayed or atomized in the mouth for rapid relief. However, epinephrine "fastness" is a limiting factor.

On the Gastrointestinal Tract and the Bladder. After an injection of epinephrine, the sphincters of the gastrointestinal tract and the bladder are contracted. The musculature of the intestines and the bladder is relaxed; thus, quieting of peristalsis results, and urinary flow retention is increased.

On the Uterus. Epinephrine generally causes contraction of the human uterus. If injected at the time of expected delivery, it causes relaxation and dilatation of the cervix. The action is transient. Two-tenths to three-tenths milliliter of a 1:1000 solution is injected subcutaneously.

On Metabolism.   Epinephrine stimulates fat, protein, and carbohydrate metabolism. It stimulates the glycogenolytic fibers to the liver; thus, sugar is set free in the blood and may be eliminated in the urine.

Minor Actions.   Epinephrine in physiological situations (e.g., cold, fear) causes erection of hair and secretion of tears. Dilatation of the pupil results from the stimulation of the sympathetic fibers to the radial muscle of the iris.

The saliva secreted under sympathetic nerve influence is thick and turbid and contains about 6 per cent organic solids. (That produced under parasympathetic stimulation is quite watery by contrast.)

Side Effects.   Epinephrine may cause fear, anxiety, nervousness, trembling, and pallor in therapeutic doses. An overdose will cause a rise in blood pressure in an elderly individual which may result in a cardiac or circulatory catastrophe. Tachycardia, dyspnea, and pulmonary edema may occur. Cardiac dilatation may follow. Paroxysmal ventricular tachycardia and multiple ectopic premature systoles may result in ventricular fibrillation and death.

Dosage and Methods of Administration.   Epinephrine hydrochloride (1:1000 aqueous solution) is usually administered subcutaneously or intramuscularly in doses of 0.5 mg. (0.2 to 1 mg.) up to every four hours. It may be administered intravenously in greatly reduced dosage in emergencies (0.05 to 0.1 ml. of a 1:1000 solution diluted with 5 ml. of normal salt solution). In cardiac arrest, 0.5 to 1 ml. of a 1:1000 solution may be injected into the right atrium. The intramuscular dose of an oil suspension is 2 mg. (0.4 to 3 mg.) every 8 to 16 hours. For its local action, 1:1000 to 1:10,000 aqueous solutions of epinephrine hydrochloride are applied to the mucous membranes to relieve congestion or to abraded areas to control capillary bleeding. Aerosols (1:100) are inhaled in bronchial asthma. Epinephrine bitartrate is applied locally as a 1 per cent ophthalmic ointment or as a 2 per cent ophthalmic solution. *Epinephrine preparations should never be used if they are brown in color or contain a precipitate.*

Therapeutic Uses

1. In bronchial asthma.
2. For urticaria, angioneurotic edema, hives, and serum sickness.
3. For acute cardiac arrest.
4. For hay fever, rhinitis, and sinusitis.
5. To check local hemorrhage.
6. To prolong the action of local anesthetics.

Preparations

Epinephrine Inhalation

Epinephrine Injection, U.S.P.; Adrenaline Injection, B.P., I.P.

Epinephrine Solution, U.S.P.; Adrenaline Solution, B.P.

1:100 solution

1-ml. and 30-ml. ampuls containing 1 mg. in 1 ml. (1:1000)

30-ml. bottles containing a 1:1000 solution

Sterile Epinephrine Suspension (in Oil)   1-ml. ampuls (1:500)
Epinephrine Bitartrate Ophthalmic Oint-   1 per cent
ment, N.F.

Trade names: Adrenalin Hydrochloride; Adrin; Epirenan; Hemisine; Renaglandin;
Vasoconstrictine

Synonyms: Adnephrine; Adrenine; Suprarenine; Suprarenaline

Levarterenol Bitartrate, U.S.P., I.P.; Noradrenaline Acid Tartrate, B.P. (Levophed Bitartrate)

Levarterenol is another name for norepinephrine, which was adopted when it was synthesized and became available as a drug in 1951. Prior to that time it had been isolated in the pure form from the medullary extracts of the adrenal glands of cattle.

Pharmacological Actions. Levarterenol causes constriction of arterioles and veins in most of the vascular beds of the body and thereby raises both systolic and diastolic blood pressure. In addition, it increases the contractile force of the heart, increasing its output. At the same time the rate of the heart is reflexly decreased by the increased blood pressure owing to the action on the vagus brought about by the inhibitor reflexes which arise in the carotid sinuses. As a result of the bradycardia, there may be no over-all increase in cardiac output. There is a concomitant increase in coronary blood flow, largely due to the increased diastolic blood pressure, and also to a direct dilating effect of levarterenol on the coronary arteries. The increase in coronary blood flow is of considerable importance in myocardial infarction and shock (see p. 496). The rise in blood pressure produced by levarterenol increases the blood flow to the brain, which is urgently needed in severe shock.

Side Effects. Excessive amounts of levarterenol may raise blood pressure, particularly in elderly persons, to dangerous levels at which circulatory accidents may occur. Like epinephrine, it may sensitize the heart muscle to arrhythmias and ventricular tachycardia under hydrocarbon anesthesia. Excessive extravasation of the drug, if untreated, may cause necrosis, tissue sloughing, and ulceration of the skin, and when this occurs, the area should be infiltrated with 5 to 10 mg. of phentolamine in 10 to 15 ml. of saline.

Therapeutic Use. Levarterenol bitartrate is used to control blood pressure in hypotensive states resulting from trauma, hemorrhage, myocardial infarction, and central vasomotor depression.

Dosage and Method of Administration. Levarterenol bitartrate is administered only by intravenous infusion. A 0.2 per cent solution (containing 0.1 per cent of the base) is diluted with 5 per cent dextrose solution in distilled water or 5 per cent dextrose in saline solution, so that 1 ml. contains 2 to 4 mcg. of the drug. This solution is then administered at the rate of 5 mcg. (1 to 10 mcg.) per minute, the rate depending on the pressor response. The blood pressure should be watched carefully, and must be taken frequently, with the rate of flow being adjusted so that a normotensive blood pressure is maintained. The site of infusion needs to be observed closely for signs of infiltration such as blanching and swelling. If they occur, the site of infusion should be changed.

Preparation

Levarterenol Bitartrate Injection, U.S.P., I.P.	4-ml. ampuls containing 8 mg. (to be diluted before infusion)

Trade names: Levophed Bitartrate; Hydroxyoctopamine

OTHER PRESSOR AMINES FOR THE TREATMENT OF SHOCK

In addition to epinephrine and levarterenol, a number of synthetic pressor amines are available for the treatment of shock. All are less potent and longer acting than levarterenol. The lower potency and prolonged activity are the bases for their use in some cases of shock, for they permit intramuscular and perhaps subcutaneous administration in addition to the intravenous route.

Metaraminol (Aramine) Bitartrate, U.S.P.

Metaraminol is a potent vasopressor drug with a prolonged action. It constricts the blood vessels and has a direct beneficial effect on the heart muscle (inotropic effect). Upon injection it increases both systolic and diastolic blood pressure. As a result, cerebral, renal, and coronary flows are improved. It does not appear to cause cardiac arrhythmias.

Side Effects. Overdosage may cause an excessive increase in blood pressure. Necrosis from leakage from the vein is rare.

Therapeutic Uses. Metaraminol is used in the treatment of shock associated with trauma, hemorrhage, and septicemia, and that accompanying myocardial infarction. It is also used to sustain blood pressure in patients during spinal and general anesthesia and other hypotensive states. It is applied topically as a nasal decongestant in rhinitis, sinusitis, hay fever, etc.

Dosage and Methods of Administration. Metaraminol is administered subcutaneously, intramuscularly, intravenously, and topically. The subcutaneous or intramuscular dose is 2 to 10 mg. The intravenous dose is 15 to 100 mg. diluted with 500 ml. of saline or 5 per cent dextrose (intravenous drip). In emergencies 0.5 to 5 mg. may be injected at once. Intranasally, two to three drops are applied in each nostril four times a day.

Preparations

Metaraminol Bitartrate Injection, U.S.P.	10 mg. in 1 ml. in 1-ml. ampuls and 10-ml. vials
Metaraminol Solution (nasal)	0.25 per cent

Trade name: Aramine

Methoxamine Hydrochloride, U.S.P. (Vasoxyl)

Methoxamine produces a prompt and prolonged pressor response due to increased peripheral resistance. The heart is slowed, perhaps reflexly. The drug is not a central nervous system stimulant. If it is used during cyclopropane anesthesia, it does not cause arrhythmias. The usual intramuscular dose is 15 mg. (5 to 20 mg.); the usual intravenous dose is 5 mg. (2.5 to 10 mg.). Methoxamine is used to sustain the blood pressure in shock and hypotension of spinal anesthesia. To relieve nasal congestion, one to three drops of a 0.25 per cent solution are applied to each nostril three or four times daily. It is available as an injection (20 mg. in 1 ml.) or as a 0.25 per cent solution (nasal).

Mephentermine Sulfate, N.F., B.P. (Wyamine)

Mephentermine has a positive ionotropic action on the heart and increases its force of contraction and cardiac output. The blood vessels are constricted, except for the coronaries, which are dilated. As a result of these actions the blood pressure is increased. Mephentermine has a unique antiarrhythmic action on the heart. It also stimulates the central nervous system and elevates the mood.

Therapeutic Uses

1. To raise the blood pressure in the treatment of cardiogenic shock accompanying myocardial infarction.
2. In the treatment of postural hypotension.
3. To elevate the mood in chronically ill geriatric patients.
4. As a nasal decongestant.

Dosage and Methods of Administration.   The usual intravenous or intramuscular dose is 20 mg. (20 to 80 mg.). As a decongestant the drug may be used in the form of a 0.5 per cent solution or the free base, which is volatile, in an inhaler.

Preparations

Mephentermine Sulfate Injection, N.F., B.P.	1- and 10-ml. ampuls containing 20 mg. in 1 ml.
Mephentermine Inhaler	250 mg.

Trade names: Wyamine; Mephine

Phenylephrine Hydrochloride, U.S.P., B.P. (Neo-Synephrine)

Phenylephrine is a synthetic substance closely related to epinephrine chemically and producting the same pharmacological responses. It raises the blood pressure by peripheral vasoconstriction. It may produce slowing of the heart. Its action on the central nervous system is minimal.

Dosage and Methods of Administration. Phenylephrine is administered intramuscularly, subcutaneously, orally, and topically. The usual subcutaneous or intramuscular dose is 5 mg. (1 to 10 mg.) three times a day. The usual oral dose is 10 to 25 mg. three times a day. Intranasal solutions, 0.25 to 0.5 per cent, are used every four hours. The ophthalmic solutions vary from 0.125 to 10 per cent.

Therapeutic Uses

1. To sustain blood pressure during spinal anesthesia (5 mg. subcutaneously).

2. To sustain blood pressure in other hypotensive states (20 to 50 mg. orally).

3. Topical administration to nasal mucosa in sinusitis, rhinitis, and hay fever (0.25 to 0.5 per cent solution).

4. In ophthalmology, as a decongestant (0.125 per cent), as a mydriatic (1 to 2.5 per cent), and as a vasoconstrictor (10 per cent) as a solution or as an emulsion.

5. With local anesthetics as a vasoconstrictor (1:2000) to localize and prolong their action.

Preparations

Phenylephrine Hydrochloride Injection, U.S.P.	4 mg. in 2 ml., 10 mg. in 1 ml., and 50 mg. in 5 ml.
Phenylephrine Hydrochloride Solution, U.S.P.	0.25 and 1 per cent
Phenylephrine Capsules	10 and 25 mg.

Trade names: Neo-Synephrine, Isophrin, Neophryn

Ephedrine Sulfate, U.S.P.; Ephedrine Hydrochloride, B.P.

Ephedrine is an alkaloid obtained long ago from a Chinese plant called *ma huang* (*Ephedra equisetina, Ephedra sinica*). It is now made synthetically. Ephedrine is a sympathomimetic drug which simulates the many actions of epinephrine on the organs stimulated by the sympathetic system. The drug stimulates the central nervous system and the skeletal muscles. It is a pressor amine but is not used in shock.

Pharmacological Actions. When injected, ephedrine causes a rise in blood pressure, which is prolonged for two to three hours. The heart rate and cardiac output are increased and the peripheral blood vessels are constricted. Upon repeated injection the vasopressor response to ephedrine diminishes with each dose (tachyphylaxis). It is thought that ephedrine acts by releasing norepinephrine at the receptor sites and that its prolonged action may cause exhaustion of this transmitter which may be responsible for this decreased effect. The activity of the drug is about one one-hundredth that of epinephrine; however, its oral activity expands its field of usefulness. Ephedrine stimulates the medullary respiratory center directly and is used to combat respiratory depression caused by hypnotic drugs. The drug also stimulates the sensory cortex, with excessive doses producing a condition similar to alcoholic inebriety. Ephedrine dilates the bronchioles, this response being more prolonged, although not so prompt, as that obtained with epinephrine; thus the drug is used in routine prophylactic therapy for the asthmatic, particularly the diabetic asthmatic, since it does not cause an increase in the blood sugar. Ephedrine produces pupillary dilatation by stimulating the effector cells in the radial muscle of the iris, which is innervated by the adrenergic fibers. Cycloplegia (paralysis of accommodation) is not produced. Ephedrine, 10 per cent solution, is instilled in the eye for ophthalmoscopic examination of the retina. Ephedrine increases the tone of the skeletal muscles and is used in the treatment of myasthenia gravis. Solutions of the drug are active nasal decongestants, as their local application constricts the capillaries and diminishes hyperemia.

Side Effects. The side effects noted are palpitation of the heart, nervousness, irritability, insomnia, and headache.

Therapeutic Uses

1. To elevate the blood pressure in hypotension during convalescence and in spinal anesthesia.
2. In asthma.
3. In coughs and colds.
4. To increase muscular tonus in myasthenia gravis.
5. Topically as a nasal decongestant.
6. To produce mydriasis for ophthalmoscopic examination.
7. To increase the pulse rate in Adams-Stokes disease.

Dosage and Methods of Administration. Ephedrine is administered orally, subcutaneously, and topically. The usual oral or subcutaneous dose is 25 mg. with a range of 25 to 50 mg. As a decongestant, 0.5 to 1 per cent aqueous or oily solutions are applied locally. Ophthalmic solutions are 10 per cent in strength.

Preparations

Ephedrine Sulfate Capsules, U.S.P.	25 and 50 mg.
Ephedrine Sulfate Injection, U.S.P.	1-ml. ampuls containing 25 or 50 mg.
Ephedrine Sulfate Tablets, N.F.	25 and 30 mg.
Ephedrine Sulfate Solution, N.F.	3 per cent solution
Ephedrine Sulfate Jelly, N.F.	1 per cent

Racephedrine Hydrochloride, N.F.

Racephedrine hydrochloride (*racemic* ephedrine hydrochloride) is applied topically to dilate the pupils of the eyes and to afford relief from nasal mucosal congestion. The drug is sometimes useful in preventing asthmatic attacks. It is administered in the treatment of hay fever and urticaria and is used to sustain blood pressure in certain types of hypotension. The usual adult oral dose is 25 mg. every three or four hours. For topical administration to the nasal mucosa, 0.5 to 2 per cent solutions are used. Four per cent solutions are instilled in the eye.

Preparations

Racephedrine Hydrochloride Capsules,   25 mg.
N.F.
Racephedrine Hydrochloride Solution,   1 per cent in Ringer's solution
N.F.

Pseudoephedrine (Sudafed)

Pseudoephedrine, related closely to ephedrine, is used orally as a nasal decongestant in colds, etc., and as a bronchodilator in asthma. Side effects are those of ephedrine. The dosage for adults is usually 30 to 60 mg. t.i.d.

Preparation

Pseudoephedrine Tablets   30 and 60 mg.
                    Trade name: Sudafed, Isoephedrine

ADDITIONAL PRESSOR AMINES

A number of sympathomimetic amines with vasoconstrictor activity are available for the oral treatment of chronic low blood pressure, for decongestant action on the nasal membranes, and to prolong the presence of local anesthetic agents in sites of surgical procedures. One group of related compounds, the amphetamines, produces these effects as well as central nervous system stimulation. A miscellaneous group of agents useful in decongesting turgescent nasal mucous membranes is presented on pages 463–64.

Amphetamines

The action and uses of amphetamine sulfate and amphetamine phosphate on the central nervous system have been discussed on pages 397–98. Amphetamine acts on the effector cells innervated by the sympathetic nerves and produces the same actions as epinephrine and ephedrine. It constricts the blood vessels, elevates the blood pressure, produces mydriasis, and inhibits the smooth musculature of the gastrointestinal tract. Its relaxant action on the bronchial musculature is less than that of epinephrine or ephedrine. In barbiturate poisoning, amphetamine sulfate is administered in doses of 10 mg. (10 to 50 mg.) by intramuscular injection. As an analeptic to overcome profound central depression due to barbiturates or other related drugs, the usual dose of amphetamine phosphate is 20 to 50 mg. intravenously or intramuscularly every 30 to 60 minutes until consciousness returns.

Preparations

Amphetamine Phosphate Injection, N.F.   100 mg. in 10 ml.
Amphetamine Sulfate Injection, U.S.P.   20 mg. in 1 ml.
For trade names see p. 398.

Methamphetamine Hydrochloride, U.S.P. (Desoxyn)

Methamphetamine stimulates the central nervous system (see p. 399). It is more potent in raising the blood pressure than ephedrine. The oral dose to sustain the blood pressure during spinal anesthesia is 2.5 to 5 mg. For preparations, see page 399. The B.P. intramuscular or intravenous dose is 10 to 30 mg. An injection is official in the B.P.

Hydroxyamphetamine Hydrobromide, U.S.P. (Paredrine)

This compound is used primarily for its action on the eye. It produces mydriasis without cycloplegia, which occurs in one-half hour and lasts from three to four hours. It is applied topically as a 0.25 to 1 per cent solution.

Therapeutic Uses

1. In ophthalmology as a mydriatic.
2. In combination with atropine to produce mydriasis and cycloplegia of short duration.

PRESSOR AGENT

Angiotensin Amide (Hypertensin)

This agent is a peptide consisting of eight amino acid molecules. It is a potent constrictor of the arterioles, especially those in the viscera and the skin. It increases the blood pressure without increasing the heart rate.

Side Effects and Precautions. This is a very potent drug and may cause dangerous hypertension. The blood pressure should be taken every two minutes after infusion is begun until the pressure is restored to normal and then every five minutes.

Therapeutic Use. Angiotensin amide is used in the treatment of shock and collapse in which low blood pressure must quickly be raised to normal or near normal levels. A rise in blood pressure generally occurs within 20 to 40 seconds. It is not recommended in shock associated with myocardial infarction.

Dosage and Method of Administration. The drug is infused intra-venously. To prepare the solution 5 ml. of sterile distilled water are added to the vial containing the lyophilized drug. The vial is gently rotated to assure complete solution, and the desired amount is withdrawn and added to the perfusion fluid. The average dosage is 3 to 10 mcg. per minute. The rate of flow is adjusted to maintain a desired blood pressure, and the drug is administered until the patient is able to maintain an adequate pressure, which may be a few hours and, in some cases, a day or more.

Preparation

Angiotensin Amide Lyophilized Powder   2.5 mg.

Trade name: Hypertensin

VASODILATOR SYMPATHOMIMETIC AMINES

Two drugs, nylidrin and isoxsuprine, which relax the arterioles and increase the blood flow to the tissues are used in peripheral vascular disease (see pp. 547–48.

Isometheptene Hydrochloride and Mucate (Octin)

This drug, by virtue of its stimulating action on the sympathetic nerves which are inhibitory to the hollow viscera and its direct action on their smooth muscle, produces a prompt relaxation of the smooth musculature of the genitourinary, gastrointestinal, and biliary tracts. It is used in vesical and ureteral spasm and may aid in the passage of ureteral stones. It is also used in irritable colon and migraine headache. Its action in migraine may be due to the dilatation of the blood vessels which are constricted in this condition. The side effects are a rise in blood pressure, palpitation, nervousness, light-headedness, and nausea. The dose of the oral solution of the hydrochloride is 15 to 20 drops every half-hour for a total of four doses. The intramuscular dose is 50 to 100 mg. The mucate is administered orally in doses of 120 mg. every half-hour for a total of four doses. The rectal dose is 250 mg.

Preparations

Isometheptene Hydrochloride Injection	100 mg. in 1 ml.
Isometheptene Hydrochloride Solution	10 per cent
Isometheptene Mucate Tablets	120 mg.
Isometheptene Mucate Suppositories	250 mg.

Trade name: Octin

THE BRONCHODILATOR SYMPATHOMIMETIC AMINES

A number of amines have been synthesized which relax the bronchioles but have little effect, if any, on the blood pressure. Isoproterenol is the one most widely used in the treatment of asthma.

Isoproterenol Hydrochloride, U.S.P.; Isoprenaline Hydrochloride, I.P. (Isuprel)

Isoproterenol is closely related to epinephrine but, unlike epinephrine, it does not cause constriction of the blood vessels. The drug does not cause a rise in blood pressure, but there is an increase in pulse pressure. Cardiac acceleration is produced and severe tachycardia may result. The principal use of isoproterenol is to dilate the bronchi in asthmatic spasm. The drug is useful in the treatment of heart block including Adams-Stokes syndrome. It causes a stimulating action, similar to that of epinephrine, upon the electrical conducting system of the heart. The ventricular rate is increased, and the circulation of blood is improved.

Side Effects. Tachycardia (rapid heart rate) may be produced, and in some individuals this may be extreme especially after injection. There may be precordial distress, palpitation, shock, dizziness, nausea, excitement, and tremors.

Dosage and Methods of Administration. Sublingually in asthma, 10 mg. to 20 mg. may be given three or four times daily. By inhalation, up to 0.5 ml., or up to 15 inhalations of a 1:200 solution (less of a 1:100 solution), may be aerosolized with oxygen over a 15- to 20-minute period. Doses of 0.2 mg. may be injected intramuscularly or subcutaneously in cardiac disorders. *Isoproterenol inhalant should never be used if it is brown in color or contains a precipitate.*

Preparations

Isoproterenol Hydrochloride Tablets (Sublingual), U.S.P.	10 and 15 mg.
Isoproterenol Hydrochloride Inhalation, U.S.P.	1:100 in 10-ml. bottles and 1:200 in 10- and 50-ml. bottles
Isoproterenol Sulfate Tablets (Sublingual); Isoprenaline Tablets, B.P.	10 and 15 mg.
Isoproterenol Hydrochloride Injection, U.S.P.	0.2 mg. in 1 ml.; 1 mg. in 5 ml.
Isoproterenol Hydrochloride Aerosol (Mistometer)	0.1 mg. of the base in each inhalation, 10-ml. vials
Isoproterenol Sulfate Aerosol (Medihaler-Iso)	0.06 mg. of the base in each inhalation, 10-ml. vials
Isoproterenol Sulfate Inhalation, N.F.	10, 25 per cent

Trade names: Isuprel; Iludrine; Isonorin; Isorenin; Isupren; Neodrenol; Neoepine; Norisodrine; Sanasma

Ethylnorepinephrine Hydrochloride (Bronkephrine)

Ethylnorepinephrine hydrochloride is useful as a bronchodilator in asthma. The drug does not cause a rise in blood pressure, nor does it produce central nervous stimulation. It is administered by subcutaneous, intramuscular, or slow intravenous injection (1 ml. in three or four minutes in *status asth-maticus* or persistent severe episodes). The usual adult dose is 1 ml., repeated as needed.

Preparation

Ethylnorepinephrine Hydrochloride Injection   10-ml. vials containing 2.0 mg. in 1 ml.

Trade name: Bronkephrine (formerly Butanephrine)

Methoxyphenamine (Orthoxine) Hydrochloride

Methoxyphenamine is a bronchorelaxant that is administered orally. It is not a cerebral stimulant and does not cause a rise in blood pressure in the usual doses. The side effects are palpitation, drowsiness, nervousness, dryness of the mouth, nausea, and faintness. The drug is used in the treatment of asthma, allergic rhinitis, and urticaria. The usual oral adult dose is 50 to 100 mg. every three or four hours. For children the dose is 25 to 50 mg. every three or four hours. Tablets of 100 mg. and a syrup containing 10 mg. in 1 ml. are available.

Protochylol (Caytine)

Protochylol is a new bronchodilator that is administered orally, by injection, and by inhalation. It is used in the treatment of bronchial asthma, chronic obstructive emphysema, and other bronchoconstrictor disorders. Occasionally a slight decrease in blood pressure, tachycardia, palpitation, and dizziness may occur as side effects. The oral dose is 2 to 4 mg. three times a day with meals. The intramuscular or subcutaneous dose of 0.25 to 1 mg. is followed by inhalation or the oral administration of tablets. For inhalation five to ten drops are placed in the open end of a nebulizer. Tablets of 2 mg., an injection containing 0.5 mg. in 1-ml. ampuls, and a 1:100 solution for inhalation are available.

VASOCONSTRICTOR DRUGS USED AS DECONGESTANTS

A miscellaneous group of drugs is used topically for decongesting the nasal mucous membranes in allergic and inflammatory conditions such as acute rhinitis and sinusitis. These drugs should be used cautiously even as nasal decongestants in patients with cardiac disease, hypertension, arteriosclerosis, or diabetes. They are instilled as drops in the nose or are administered by inhalation or nebulization. Some of these drugs produce a burning sensation. Side effects are rare with the usual dosage. However, with overdosage, they may cause a rise in blood pressure and stimulation of the heart. The decongestant preparations of epinephrine, mephentermine, metaraminol, methoxamine, phenylephrine, ephedrine, and racephedrine have been discussed earlier in this chapter.

Preparations

Cyclopentamine Hydrochloride, N.F. (Clopane)	Solution (nasal) 0.5 and 1 per cent
Methylhexaneamine (Forthane)	Inhaler: 250 mg.
Naphazoline Hydrochloride,* † N.F. (Privine)	Jelly (nasal) 0.05 per cent
	Nebulizer: 0.05 per cent
	Solution (nasal) 0.05, 0.1 per cent
Phenylpropanolamine (Propadrine)	Solution (nasal) 1 per cent
Phenylpropylmethylamine Hydrochloride (Vonedrine)	Solution (nasal) 2.8 per cent
Propyhexedrine, N.F. (Benzedrex)	Inhaler: 250 mg.
Tetrahydrozoline Hydrochloride†, N.F. (Tyzine)	Solution (nasal) 0.05, 0.1 per cent
Tuaminoheptane (Tuamine)	Inhaler: 325 mg.
Xylometrazoline Hydrochloride (Otrivin)	Solution (nasal) 0.05, 0.1 per cent

* This drug is also used in the eye for its vasoconstricting effect in 0.1 per cent ophthalmic solution.

† These drugs may produce rebound and refractory congestion after a few days' consecutive use.

NICOTINE

Nicotine, the principal alkaloid in the leaves of tobacco, concerns us in medicine chiefly as a stimulant of the sympathetic nervous system. This is because the amounts absorbed from the lungs and oropharyngeal membranes can produce vasoconstriction by stimulation of the autonomic ganglia. Smoking is often forbidden in vasospastic diseases (see Chap. 33).

REVIEW QUESTIONS

1. List the effects of epinephrine upon the following structures or functions: (a) smooth muscle cells of arterioles with adrenergic innervation, (b) blood pressure, (c) force of cardiac contraction, (d) heart rate, (e) bronchioles, (f) sphincters of the gastrointestinal tract and bladder, (g) uterus.
2. Discuss the dosage and routes of administration of epinephrine and list its major uses.
3. List the actions of levarterenol bitartrate (Levophed). Describe its administration and dosage.
4. What are the indication, advantages, disadvantages, dose, and methods of administration of isoproterenol (Isuprel)?
5. Discuss the actions and uses of ephedrine sulfate.
6. What are the actions of the amphetamines? Name several and give their dose and any special features.

REFERENCES

Brofman, B. L.; Hellerstein, H. D.; and Caskey, W. H.: "Mephenteramine, an Effective Pressor Amine," *Am. Heart J.*, **44**:396, 1952.

Ebert, R. V.: "The Mechanism and Treatment of Shock Associated with Infection," *South. M. J.*, **49**:485, 1956.

Foland, J. P.: "Bronkephrine in the Management of Bronchial Asthma," *Postgrad, M. Ed.*, **18**:397, 1955.

Gaddum, J. H., and Kwiatkowski, H.: "The Action of Ephedrine," *J. Physiol.*, **94**:87, 1938.

Haggerty, R. J.: "Levarterenol for Shock," *Am. J. Nursing*, **58**:1243, 1958.

Kurland, G. S., and Malach, M.: "The Clinical Use of Nor-epinephrine in the Treatment of Shock Accompanying Myocardial Infarction and Other Conditions," *New England J. Med.*, **247**:383, 1952.

Page, I. H., and Bumpus, F. M.: "Angiotensin," *Physiol. Rev.*, **41**:331, 1961.

Rosenberg, A. A.: "The Treatment of Shock in Acute Myocardial Infarction," *J. M. Soc. New Jersey*, **53**:138, 1956.

Simard, O. M.: "Nursing Care During Levarterenol Therapy," *Am. J. Nursing*, **58**:1244, 1958.

Talmers, F. N.; Regan, T. J.; and Hellems, H. K.: "Review of Pathophysiology and Treatment of Shock Accompanying Myocardial Infarction," *J. Michigan M. Soc.*, **55**:283, 1956.

28

Depressants of the Sympathetic Nervous System (Adrenergic Blocking Agents)

Drugs which block the postganglionic sympathetic nerve impulses at the receptor sites and also prevent the effects of circulating or injected epinephrine or norepinephrine are called *adrenergic blocking agents*. They do not destroy the catecholamines nor do they act on the autonomic ganglia. Some of these drugs antagonize the effects of the circulating catecholamines by producing vasodilatation of the peripheral vessels without exerting a significant effect on sympathetic tone. The more potent ones combine with the effector cells to prevent the transmission of sympathetic nerve impulses and thus produce extensive vasodilatation and a fall in blood pressure. Drugs that block the vasoconstricting action of the catecholamines are phentolamine (Regitine), tolazoline (Priscoline), phenoxybenzamine (Dibenzyline), azapetine (Ilidar), and the ergot alkaloids. They are useful in the diagnosis and treatment of peripheral vascular disease, causalgia, and some types of hypertension (those caused by excessive epinephrine or norepinephrine in the circulation due to adrenal tumors). Bretylium tosylate (Darenthin) and guanethidine (Ismelin), which are postganglionic depressants used in the treatment of hypertension, are described in Chapter 34.

Phentolamine Mesylate, U.S.P.; the Hydrochloride and Methanesulfonate, B.P. (Regitine)

Phentolamine is a moderately effective adrenergic blocking agent. It is readily absorbed upon oral administration and is useful in diagnosing tumors of the adrenomedullary tissue (pheochromocytoma) which secrete norepinephrine and variable amounts of epinephrine. The release of the catecholamines into the circulation causes a rare form of hypertension which may be either spasmodic or persistent. The symptoms are weakness, palpitation, substernal pain, sweating, and dizziness. If the increase in the blood pressure is caused by epinephrine or norepinephrine, the pressure will fall after the administration of phentolamine. A vasopressor such as levarterenol (Levophed) should be available for immediate use, if necessary, as peripheral

466

━━━━━━━━━━━━━━━━━━━━ **Table 31** ━━━━━━━━━━━━━━━━━━━━

Classification of Adrenergic Blocking Agents

I. Alpha receptor blocking agents
   1. Phentolamine (Regitine)
   2. Tolazoline (Priscoline)
   3. Phenoxybenzamine (Dibenzyline)
   4. Azapetine (Ilidar)

II. Beta receptor blocking agents
   1. Dichloroisoproterenol (DCI)
   2. Pronethalol (Nethalide)

III. Norepinephrine-releasing or -depleting agents
   1. Reserpine (Serpasil)
   2. Syrosingopine (Singoserp)
   3. Guanethidine (Ismelin)

IV. Norepinephrine release inhibitor
   1. Bretylium (Darenthin)

V. Norepinephrine synthesis inhibitor
   1. Methyldopa

vascular collapse can occur. If the hypertension is produced by other causes, there is no appreciable decrease in blood pressure following the administration of phentolamine. After diagnosis, the tumor is removed by surgery.

Side Effects.   The side actions are tachycardia, orthostatic hypotension, nasal stuffiness, nausea, vomiting, and diarrhea.

Therapeutic Uses

1. In peripheral vascular disease (see Chap. 33).

2. For diagnosis of epinephrine and norepinephrine-secreting tumors (pheochromocytomas) of the adrenal gland.

3. For treating ischemia caused by levarterenol.

Dosage and Methods of Administration.   Phentolamine is administered orally, intravenously, or intramuscularly. The usual oral dose is 50 mg. (50 to 100 mg.) four to six times a day. The usual intravenous or intramuscular dose is 5 mg. (5 to 30 mg.).

Preparations

Phentolamine Hydrochloride Tablets, N.F.   50 mg.

Phentolamine Mesylate for Injection, U.S.P.   Ampuls containing 5 mg. (to be dissolved in 1 ml. water for injection)

Trade names: Regitine, Rogitine

Tolazoline Hydrochloride, B.P. (Priscoline)

Tolazoline is a moderately active adrenergic blocking agent. It also produces some histamine-like and cholinergic effects which are responsible for the side effects. It blocks the action of epinephrine and norepinephrine and tends to restore the normal caliber of spastic blood vessels. Unlike other drugs of this class, it has a direct dilating effect upon the walls of small blood vessels. Its principal action is dilatation of the peripheral arterioles. Thus, it lessens pain by reducing angiospasm and promotes the return of function by increasing the blood supply to the extremities.

Side Effects. The untoward effects include palpitation, angina flushing of the skin, sweating, pain, a feeling of being chilly, even with "goose flesh," sensations of pins and needles in the fingers and toes, an increase in gastric acidity, possibly with nausea, and tachycardia. The symptoms are generally mild and usually disappear with continued therapy.

Therapeutic Uses

1. In peripheral vascular disease. The conditions in which it is useful are frostbite, acrocyanosis, ulcers of the extremities, Buerger's disease, Raynaud's syndrome, thrombophlebitis, and causalgic states (see Chap. 33).

2. In tinnitus aurium (ringing in the ears). This is sometimes relieved by increasing the blood supply to the areas involved.

3. As a diagnostic agent to determine the advisability of performing a sympathectomy in peripheral vascular disease.

Dosage and Methods of Administration. Tolazoline is administered orally and intravenously. The usual oral or intravenous dose is 25 mg. (25 to 50 mg.) one to four times a day. The dose should be individualized and adjusted to the response of the patient. Therapy should be initiated with cautious increase in dosage until the optimal effect is obtained as evidenced by the appearance of flushing. The patient should be kept warm to increase the effectiveness of the drug. In selected cases, the drug is given intra-arterially.

Preparations

Tolazoline Hydrochloride Tablets   25 mg.
Tolazoline Hydrochloride Longtabs   50 mg.
Tolazoline Hydrochloride Injection   25 mg. in 1 ml.; 10-ml. vials
Trade names: Priscoline; Priscol; Vasimid; Vasodil

Phenoxybenzamine Hydrochloride, B.P. (Dibenzyline)

Phenoxybenzamine is a long-acting adrenergic blocking agent that is very effective upon oral administration. It increases the peripheral blood flow, raises the skin temperature, lowers the blood pressure, and relieves causalgic pain. It may produce fatigue, tachycardia, pallor, miosis, nausea, nasal congestion, and sedation.

Dosage and Method of Administration.   The usual daily dose varies from 20 to 60 mg. orally.

Therapeutic Uses

1. For peripheral vascular disease (see Chap. 33).
2. For hypertension (rare use).
3. For chronic ulceration of the extremities.
4. For causalgia.

Preparation

Phenoxybenzamine Hydrochloride   10 mg.
Capsules, B.P.

Trade names: Dibenzyline, Dibenyline

Azapetine Phosphate (Ilidar Phosphate)

Azapetine phosphate, another adrenergic blocking agent and direct vasodilator, is useful in the same conditions as are the foregoing compounds. It may produce hypotension, vertigo, nasal stuffiness, drowsiness, and conjunctival congestion. Azapetine and other such agents should not be used in patients with severe coronary disease and only with caution in the presence of asthma and peptic ulcer.

Dosage and Method of Administration.   Twenty-five milligrams may be given orally three times daily, with gradual increase to 75 mg. three times daily.

Preparation

Azapetine Phosphate Tablets   25 mg.
Trade name: Ilidar Phosphate

ERGOT ALKALOIDS

The ergot alkaloids are adrenergic blocking agents but they are not used clinically for these effects. If epinephrine is injected following their administration, a fall in blood pressure is noted rather than the usual rise. This is known as the "epinephrine reversal." The blood vessels have both alpha (excitatory) and beta (inhibitory) receptors, and epinephrine affects both. When the alpha receptors are blocked by the ergot alkaloids, the beta receptors which cause vasodilatation respond to epinephrine and the blood pressure falls. Since norepinephrine acts mainly on the alpha receptors, adrenergic blocking agents inhibit some of its actions but do not cause a vasodepressor response. Ergotamine tartrate (Gynergen) is used for the treatment of migraine (see p. 548) and ergonovine maleate (Ergotrate) is used for its effect on the uterus (see p. 602).

Guanethidine, Bretylium, and Methyldopa

These drugs interfere with the synthesis and release of norepinephrine at the nerve ending and are sometimes used in hypertension (see pp. 563–65).

REVIEW QUESTIONS

1. *What is meant by adrenergic blockade?*
2. *What is a pheochromocytoma and what are its effects? How may it be diagnosed?*
3. *Describe the actions and uses of tolazoline, phentolamine, and phenoxy‑benzamine.*

REFERENCES

Black, D. A.: "Adrenergic Blockade," *Am. Heart J.*, **59**:153, 1960.
Boura, A. L.; Capp, F. C.; and Green, A. F.: "New Antiadrenergic Compounds," *Nature*, **184**:70, 1959.
Goodman, L. S., and Nickerson, M.: "Clinical Application of Adrenergic Blockade: A Critical Appraisal," *M. Clin. North America*, **34**:379, 1950.
Soffer, A.: "Regitine and Benodaine in the Diagnosis of Pheochromocytoma," *M. Clin. North America*, **38**:375, 1954.

29

Stimulants of the Parasympathetic Nervous System (Cholinergic Agents)

Drugs that stimulate the parasympathetic nervous system emulate the action of its hormone, acetylcholine, and are *parasympathomimetic* or *cholinergic* agents. Acetylcholine is not used in therapeutics because it is unstable, the dose is exceedingly small, and its actions (see p. 442) are very transient. However, many closely related compounds have been synthesized, and a few of them, such as methacholine, carbachol, and bethanechol, are useful therapeutic agents. Other cholinergic drugs produce their effects by inactivating cholinesterase and prolonging the activity of acetylcholine itself. These drugs —physostigmine, neostigmine, DFP, and TEPP, for example—are known as anticholinesterases.

CHOLINE ESTERS AND RELATED COMPOUNDS

Choline produces the same pharmacological responses as acetylcholine, but since its potency is one-thousandth to one one-millionth that of the hormone, it is not used in therapeutics as a cholinergic agent. However, it plays an important role in liver metabolism and, consequently, is used in chronic diseases of the liver. The more active esters of choline are used as cholinergic drugs.

Methacholine Bromide, N.F.; Methacholine Chloride, N.F. (Mecholyl)

Methacholine, a synthetic derivative of acetylcholine, is not so potent as that agent, although its action is more prolonged because of slower hydrolysis by cholinesterase. Methacholine causes slowing of the heart, owing to its action on the cardiac vagus. It also stimulates the receptor cells of the cholinergic fibers of the sympathetic nerves to the arterioles and causes vasodilatation. The slowing of the heart and the dilatation of the blood vessels are responsible for the fall in blood pressure.

Methacholine stimulates the smooth muscle of the (1) gastrointestinal tract, causing increased tonus and peristalsis; (2) the detrusor muscle of the bladder, causing it to contract and expel urine; and (3) the bronchi, pro-

471

ducing bronchial constriction. The secretions of the gastric and bronchial glands are increased. Methacholine does not stimulate the autonomic ganglia or skeletal muscle as does acetylcholine.

Toxic Effects. Large doses of methacholine may produce nausea and vomiting. The drug may cause dyspnea and precipitate an asthmatic attack because it constricts the bronchi and increases the secretions of the respiratory tract. Increased urination, abdominal pain, and diarrhea result from the increased activity of the bladder and urinary and gastrointestinal tracts.

Methacholine is not administered intramuscularly or intravenously because its rapid absorption may cause collapse, resulting from low blood pressure, or atrial fibrillation, heart block, or stoppage, owing to its potent action on the heart.

Therapeutic Uses

1. For paroxysmal tachycardia. This is the principal use.

2. In peripheral vascular disease. Its use in this disease is limited. The adrenergic blocking agents are used more often.

3. For postoperative urinary retention following spinal and general anesthesia and in patients with injury of the spinal cord. It has been replaced, to a large extent, by bethanechol.

Dosage and Methods of Administration. Methacholine is slowly absorbed from the gastrointestinal tract, where it may produce nausea and vomiting. The usual oral dose is 200 mg. two or three times a day, although 50 to 100 mg. three times a day may be adequate to relieve vascular spasm after moderate exposure to the cold. The larger doses are required in ulcers, scleroderma, and Raynaud's disease. For its action on the heart, the drug is given subcutaneously in doses of 20 mg. It is occasionally administered by iontophoresis.[1]

Contraindication and Treatment of Poisoning. Methacholine is contraindicated in asthma. Atropine, in doses of 0.5 to 1 mg., is administered intravenously to counteract symptoms of poisoning.

Preparations

Sterile Methacholine Chloride, N.F.   Ampuls containing 25 mg.
              Trade names: Mecholyl Chloride; Amechol
Methacholine Bromide Tablets, N.F.   200 mg.
              Trade names: Mecholyl Bromide, Amechol

Glaucoma. The intraocular pressure is maintained by the production of aqueous humor in the eye (see p. 448). Glaucoma is an eye disease in which faulty drainage of the fluid within the eye causes increased intraocular tension,

---

[1] In medicine, the method of introducing charged particles into the skin or other tissues by means of an electric current.

with the production of a harder eyeball. This condition may cause blindness. Cholinergic drugs such as carbachol, pilocarpine, physostigmine, neostigmine, isoflurophate, demecarium, and phospholine reduce intraocular pressure by producing miosis (constriction of the pupil) (see p. 447) and increasing the tone of the ciliary muscle. These effects improve drainage through the canal of Schlemm (see p. 448). Pilocarpine also increases the reabsorption of fluid through the trabecular membrane.

The carbonic anhydrase inhibitors, acetazolamide (Diamox), ethoxzolamide (Cardrase), methazolamide (Neptazane), and dichlorphenamide (Daramide), decrease aqueous humor by inhibiting carbonic anhydrase, one of the substances necessary for its production. These drugs are given orally. The effects from a single dose last from six to eight hours. The side reactions, which are not severe, are lethargy, anorexia, and numbing and tingling of the face and the extremities. The doses and preparations of these drugs are:

Acetazolamide (Diamox)	250 mg. b.i.d. to q.i.d.	Tablets: 250 mg.
Ethoxazolamide (Cardrase)	62.5 to 125 mg. b.i.d. to q.i.d.	Tablets: 62.5 and 125 mg.
Methazolamide, U.S.P. (Neptazane)	50 to 100 mg. b.i.d., t.i.d.	Tablets: 50 mg.
Dichlorphenamide, U.S.P., B.P. (Daramide)	25 to 100 mg. 1 to t.i.d.	Tablets: 50 mg.

Acetazolamide is also used in the treatment of epilepsy (see p. 362) and as a diuretic in cardiac edema (see p. 638).

Epinephrine may reduce the production of aqueous humor by causing vasoconstriction of the blood vessels. It may be used with the miotics for this purpose.

Carbachol, U.S.P., B.P., I.P. (Carbaminoylcholine Chloride, Doryl)

Carbachol, another synthetic choline derivative, simulates the action of acetylcholine but is more potent. It stimulates the autonomic ganglia and the innervation of skeletal muscle. Carbachol is seldom administered orally or parenterally because of its toxicity.

Therapeutic Use.   Carbachol is used as a miotic in glaucoma. It is applied topically in 0.75 to 3 per cent solutions.

Preparation

Carbachol Solution (Ophthalmic)   0.75 to 3 per cent
     Trade names: Carcholine; Doryl; Isopto Carbachol; Lentin; Moryl

Demecarium Bromide (Humorsol)

Demecarium is a potent and long-acting miotic used only locally in the eye for the reduction of intraocular pressure in glaucoma. One or two drops of a 0.25 per cent solution instilled in the conjunctival sac once every other day to twice daily may control the condition.

Preparation

Demecarium Bromide Solution   0.25 per cent, 5-ml. vials
Trade name: Humorsol

Echothiopate Iodide, U.S.P. (Phospholine)

Echothiopate is also a potent and long-acting miotic used locally in the eye for the reduction of intraocular pressure. It is instilled into the conjunctival sac in concentrations of 0.1 to 0.25 per cent. Aqueous solutions are stable and will keep for several weeks at room temperature. The drug is available as a powder for making solutions.

Other drugs used in glaucoma are discussed on page 445.

Bethanechol Chloride, U.S.P. (Urecholine Chloride)

Bethanechol is related to methacholine, and its effects are essentially the same. However, its main action, which is more prolonged because the drug is not hydrolyzed by cholinesterase, is on the smooth muscle of the gastrointestinal and urinary tracts. Bethanechol is recommended for counteracting some of the untoward effects of the ganglionic blocking drugs used in the treatment of hypertension. These effects include urinary retention and decreased movement of the intestines, leading to constipation or even paralysis of the gut (paralytic ileus). The drug should be employed quickly in the event of one of these complications, before the appearance of acute symptoms, and may be given orally, sublingually (beneath the tongue), or, if urgent, subcutaneously. *It must not be given intramuscularly or intravenously.* Small doses repeated with close observation every 15 to 30 minutes at the beginning of therapy can indicate the needs for each case and thus the size of subsequent doses.

Side Effects.   After subcutaneous injection these include headache, flushing, sweating, abdominal cramps, diarrhea, asthmatic breathing, and occasionally a fall in blood pressure. Atropine should be available for prompt parenteral administration.

Contraindications.   The drug is contraindicated in asthma, hyperthyroidism, obstruction of the vesical neck of the bladder, and mechanical obstruction in the gastrointestinal tract.

Dosage and Methods of Administration.   The usual oral dose is 10 mg. (5 to 30 mg.) three times a day; the maximum 24-hour dose is 120 mg. The usual subcutaneous dose is 2.5 mg. (2.5 to 5 mg.); the maximum 24-hour dose is 40 mg.

Therapeutic Uses

1. For postoperative urinary retention and that caused by ganglionic blocking drugs.

2. For gastric retention following vagotomy and gastric surgery.

3. For postoperative abdominal distention and intestinal atony associated with ganglionic blockade.

Preparations

Bethanechol Chloride Injection, U.S.P.   5 mg. in 1 ml.
Bethanechol Chloride Tablets, U.S.P.   5 and 10 mg.

       Trade names: Urecholine Chloride; Mecothane

Pilocarpine Nitrate, U.S.P., I.P., and Pilocarpine Hydrochloride, U.S.P.

Pilocarpine is the alkaloid obtained from the leaves of *Pilocarpus jaborandi,* a Brazilian plant. It is one of the oldest cholinergic drugs but is seldom used today. The nitrate is the most stable salt.

Pharmacological Actions. Pilocarpine stimulates the receptor cells of the organs innervated by the cholinergic fibers and thus mimics the action of acetylcholine in the periphery. It stimulates the smooth muscles of the bronchi and the intestinal tract, thus causing their contraction; stimulates the vagus; and increases all secretions (saliva, sweat, tears, mucus, gastric juice, and pancreatic juice), Pilocarpine constricts the pupil of the eye and produces spasm of accommodation.

Diaphoretic Action. Pilocarpine produces marked sweating by a direct action on the sweat glands. Several liters of sweat may be eliminated through the skin when a 5-mg. dose is injected subcutaneously. It was formerly used to relieve edema in hydremic nephritis. Slowing of the heart, bronchiolar constriction, pulmonary edema, and fluid and electrolyte imbalance are real hazards to its use.

Poisoning. *Symptoms.* The symptoms of overdosage with pilocarpine are salivation, sweating, nausea, vomiting, and a slow heart. The breathing becomes difficult because of bronchiolar spasm and mucus flow. The drug kills by paralyzing the cardiac muscle or causing pulmonary edema.

Treatment. The best antidote is atropine, 0.5 to 1 mg. intravenously. Glucose and saline fluids are administered intravenously or orally to restore electrolyte and water balance.

Therapeutic Uses

1. In glaucoma. Five-tenths per cent to 2 per cent solutions, generally 2 per cent, are instilled in the eye every two or three hours to maintain proper drainage.

2. After refraction of the eye, to combat cycloplegia and mydriasis caused by atropine or homatropine.

Preparation

Pilocarpine Solution, U.S.P. (Ophthal-   0.5 to 2 per cent
mic)

Arecoline

Arecoline is one of the alkaloids of the betal nut (*Areca catechu*). It emulates the action of pilocarpine. The drug is not used in human medicine but is employed as a laxative and vermifuge in veterinary medicine.

ANTICHOLINESTERASES

Anticholinesterase drugs inhibit the enzyme cholinesterase, thus preventing the inactivation of acetylcholine and prolonging its effect. There are many drugs and poisons that do this, including "nerve gases" of chemical-warfare importance, certain insecticides, and some therapeutic agents. Some of these substances, such as physostigmine and neostigmine, combine temporarily with the enzymes and produce reversible inhibition. Others, such as DFP and TEPP, form a lasting chemical combination; consequently, their effect is irreversible. New enzymes must be synthesized by the body to replace those inactivated.

Physostigmine Salicylate, U.S.P., B.P., I.P. (Eserine Salicylate)

Physostigmine is an alkaloid obtained from the dried, ripe seed or bean of *Physostigma venenosum*, a plant that grows in West Africa along the banks of the Calabar River. Physostigmine salicylate is the most stable salt. The solutions that turn pink on standing are irritating and should be discarded.

Pharmacological Actions. Physostigmine is readily absorbed and widely distributed in the body. As stated above, the drug inactivates cholinesterase and allows acetylcholine to accumulate in the tissues and produce its effects on the organs and tissues innervated by cholinergic fibers. The effects noted are slowing of the heart, vasodilatation, increased intestinal activity, increased glandular secretion, pupillary constriction, and paralysis of accommodation of the eye. Small doses sensitize the effector cells at the myoneural junction to the action of acetylcholine; hence, skeletal muscle contracts. Owing to this action on skeletal muscle, physostigmine counteracts the effects produced by curare and may be used as an antidote in curare poisoning. It was formerly used in the treatment of myasthenia gravis, but it has been replaced by neostigmine.

Poisonous Effects of Overdosage.   In poisonous doses, physostigmine causes marked muscular weakness. Nausea, vomiting, and a slow pulse are noted. The blood pressure is lowered, the breathing is labored, and convulsions may occur. Death is generally caused by paralysis of the respiration. Atropine is the best antidote. Intravenous glucose and isotonic salt solution may also be administered.

Dosage and Methods of Administration.   The usual oral or subcutaneous dose is 2 mg. (1 to 3 mg.) up to three times a day. In ophthalmology, 0.02 to 1 per cent solutions are used to produce miosis.

Therapeutic Uses

1. As a miotic in glaucoma. It reduces intraocular pressure rapidly, and the effects last for 12 to 36 hours. Solutions of 0.1 to 1 per cent are instilled in the eye.

2. To combat mydriasis and cycloplegia caused by atropine and homatropine, when these drugs are used to refract the eyes.

3. To increase the motility of the intestine and relieve distention in paralytic ileus following anesthesia and operations.

Preparations

Injection of Physostigmine Salicylate, 10-ml. vials containing 2 mg. in 1 ml.
I.P.
Physostigmine Salicylate (H.T.)   0.65 and 1.3 mg.
Physostigmine Salicylate Powder   Tubes containing 324 and 650 mg.
                  Trade name: Eserine Salicylate

Neostigmine Bromide, U.S.P., B.P., I.P. (Prostigmin Bromide), and Neostigmine Methylsulfate, U.S.P., B.P. (Prostigmin Methylsulfate)

These are synthetic drugs that are soluble in water. Neostigmine bromide is administered orally; neostigmine methylsulfate is administered subcutaneously or intramuscularly.

Pharmacological Actions.   Neostigmine inactivates cholinesterase reversibly, as does physostigmine, and therefore produces the same effects as that drug. The response is very rapid. Neostigmine is effective in the treatment of myasthenia gravis and as an antidote in curare poisoning.

Poisoning.   The toxic symptoms and their treatment are the same as for physostigmine. Atropine is the best antidote. Severe muscular fasciculations are not affected by atropine. Artificial or controlled respiration may be necessary.

Dosage and Methods of Administration.   Neostigmine is administered orally, subcutaneously, intramuscularly, and by instillation in the eye. The usual oral dose of neostigmine bromide is 15 mg. three times a day; the usual subcutaneous or intramuscular dose of neostigmine methylsulfate is 0.5 mg. (0.25 to 1 mg.) every four to six hours; 5 per cent solutions are instilled in the eye.

Therapeutic Uses

1. In *myasthenia gravis*. It is used in the diagnosis and treatment of the disease.
2. As an antidote for curare poisoning.
3. In postoperative urinary retention.
4. For peripheral vascular disease.
5. For paroxysmal atrial tachycardia.
6. As a diagnostic agent in suspected pregnancy, organic disease, or endocrine disorders.
7. To stimulate the contraction of skeletal muscle in poliomyelitis.
8. As a miotic, chiefly in glaucoma (a 5 per cent solution).

Myasthenia Gravis. Myasthenia gravis is a relatively rare chronic disease. It bears this name because it is a severe or "grave" weakness ("asthenia") of muscles. The condition is characterized by a progressive, abnormal fatigability, and flaccidity of skeletal muscles. The defect responsible for the condition is located at the endings of the involved motor nerves in their respective muscle groups and resembles in many respects the effects of curariform agents. The transfer of impulses from nerve to muscle across the motor end-plate is greatly reduced, if not, at times, nonexistent. If only a small number of the continuous volleys of impulses sent out from the motor nuclei of the spinal cord and cranial nerves are conducted across the synapse, then the muscle is not caused to inaugurate or maintain contraction for some useful purpose. Therefore, facial contours may change as the numerous muscles of the face become weak. The muscles that move the eyes, elevate the lids, effect swallowing and speaking movements, and produce respiration, locomotion, and arm-hand activities are usually all involved in moderate and severe cases. The disease may progress to motor paralysis, or there may be remissions which are sometimes prolonged. Drugs now in use in this condition are neostigmine, pyridostigmin (Mestinon), and ambenonium (Mytelase). The latter two have the advantage of activity longer than that of neostigmine. Ephedrine was used before the effectiveness of neostigmine was discovered and is occasionally combined with it now.

Neostigmine in Myasthenia Gravis. This anticholinesterase has, by virtue of the mechanism of action described above, prolonged the lives for years and decades and dramatically strengthened the deprived muscles of all patients in whom it has been properly used. The disease varies markedly in severity in each case. There are exacerbations, with increased severity of the lesion, followed in time by remissions in which marked spontaneous improvement occurs. Thus the dose of neostigmine needed varies from patient to patient and from month to month or year to year (hour to hour in rapidly changing cases in crises).

Preparations

Neostigmine Bromide Tablets, U.S.P.	15 mg.
Neostigmine Tablets, B.P.	
Neostigmine Bromide, Ophthalmic Solution	5 per cent bottles with dropper
Neostigmine Methylsulfate Injection, U.S.P., B.P., I.P.	0.5 mg. in 1 ml.; 5 and 10 mg. in 10 ml.

Trade names: Prostigmin; Proserine; Vasostigmine

Edrophonium Chloride, U.S.P., B.P. (Tensilon)

Edrophonium resembles neostigmine in its pharmacological actions. It is used as an antidote in overdosage with curariform drugs but not with succinylcholine chloride or decamethonium. In therapeutic doses, edrophonium produces a stimulant action on skeletal muscle and may be used as a diagnostic agent in *myasthenia gravis*. As an emergency measure, it is used in myasthenic crisis; however, its action is too transient for use in the treatment of the disease. In toxic doses, edrophonium produces paralysis of the skeletal musculature and death by respiratory paralysis. However, the margin of safety between the stimulant and depressant action is 40- to 80-fold. Since the drug is short acting, there is less incidence of side effects than with neostigmine.

As an antidote for curariform drugs and as a diagnostic agent in suspected *myasthenia gravis*, the intravenous dose is 10 mg. In myasthenic crises, the drug should be administered by intravenous drip for the duration of the emergency.

Edrophonium should be used very cautiously in bronchial asthma or cardiac disease because it may cause increased salivation and bronchial constriction, bradycardia, and cardiac dysrhythmias.

Preparation

Edrophonium Chloride Injection, U.S.P.   10 mg. in 1 ml.
Trade name: Tensilon

Pyridostigmin Bromide, U.S.P., B.P. (Mestinon Bromide)

The duration of activity of this drug is slightly longer than that of neostigmine. The latter must often be given to myasthenic patients at intervals during the night for their safety against too weak respiratory movements. While the cholinergic stimulation of the intestines is less with pyridostigmin than with neostigmine, untoward effects (cramps) may still be produced, and often warn of overdosage. These effects and increased salivation produced by the drug may be abolished by atropine and other anticholinergic agents. The anticholinesterases cause fasiculations (twitching) of skeletal muscles, often at the muscle-strengthening doses.

Dosage and Method of Administration. Tablets are administered orally and the dose very carefully adjusted for each patient. Thus, 60 mg. once to three times daily may help the very mild case. The usual dose range is 180 to 600 mg. daily, in four or five divided amounts. The drug is about one fourth as potent as neostigmine.

Preparation

Pyridostigmin Bromide Tablets, U.S.P.,   60 mg.
B.P.

Trade name: Mestinon Bromide

Ambenonium Chloride (Mytelase Chloride)

This anticholinesterase, introduced in 1956 after two years of clinical study, has shown advantages over the foregoing compounds in the treatment of *myasthenia gravis*. Dr. Robert Schwab, director of the Myasthenia Gravis Clinic at the Massachusetts General Hospital, Boston, has found this agent to be more potent than neostigmine and about twice as long in duration. Some patients require one fifth to two thirds as much ambenonium as neostigmine. There are more nausea and vomiting than with neostigmine but less cramping and diarrhea. The significant advantages of ambenonium are the effectiveness in cases unsatisfactorily treated with other agents, the longer duration of action which requires fewer doses and makes unnecessary the awakening of patients at night for medication, and the lower incidence of griping and diarrhea.

The treatment of myasthenic patients requires accurate knowledge of the disease and of the actions and dangers of the drugs discussed. Both underdosage and overdosage are associated with muscular weakness, which may be fatal in either case. Optimal neuromuscular transmission is the goal; side effects in many cases seem unavoidable at doses giving best results at the motor end-plates. *Crises* of the disease itself occur, with increased demand for an anticholinesterase, tracheal suction, and even "iron lungs." *Cholinergic crises* are produced by excessive doses of the drugs, whereupon the doses must be withheld and lowered when reinstituted. Atropine, 0.5 to 1.0 mg. ($\frac{1}{120}$ to $\frac{1}{60}$ grain), should be used in cholinergic crises.

Dosage and Method of Administration. Ambenonium is given by mouth at three- to six-hour intervals. The mild case may require only 5 or 10 mg. at each dose, while severe cases may need up to 75 mg. per dose.

Preparation

Ambenonium Chloride Tablets (Scored)   10 and 25 mg.
Trade name: Mytelase Chloride

Benzpyrinium Bromide, N.F. (Stigmonene Bromide)

Benzpyrinium bromide is chemically related to neostigmine, and its pharmacological actions are the same.

Dosage and Method of Administration. Benzpyrinium bromide is administered intramuscularly in doses of 2 mg. every three or four hours.

Therapeutic Uses

1. For postoperative abdominal distention.
2. For postoperative urinary retention.
3. For simple delayed menstruation.

Preparation

Benzpyrinium Bromide Injection, N.F.   2 mg. in 1 ml.
Trade name: Stigmonene Bromide

IRREVERSIBLE PHOSPHATE ANTICHOLINESTERASES

A number of organic phosphates are potent inhibitors of cholinesterase. Two of these salts are used clinically.

Isoflurophate (Diisopropyl Fluorophosphate, DFP)

DFP permanently inactivates cholinesterase and thereby produces stimulation of the cholinergic fibers by allowing a more intensified and prolonged action of acetylcholine. The drug is too toxic for systemic use. Its miotic action is more potent and prolonged than that of pilocarpine or physostigmine.

Method of Administration. A 0.01 to 0.1 per cent solution in oil is instilled in the eye.

Therapeutic Uses

1. As a miotic to combat mydriasis of homatropine and atropine.
2. In glaucoma to decrease intraocular pressure. The effects may last two or three weeks.
3. To aid in the correction of convergent strabismus (internal squint of the eyes) caused by excessive accommodation effort.

Preparation

Isoflurophate Ophthalmic Solution, N.F.   0.15 per cent in suitable oil
Isoflurophate   Ophthalmic   Ointment,   0.025 per cent
N.F.
Trade names: Dyflos; Floropryl

Tetraethylpyrophosphate (TEPP)

TEPP is a more potent anticholinesterase than DFP. It is unstable on exposure to the air, but solutions in peanut oil or propylene glycol are stable for months. The drug is readily absorbed on oral administration and is metabolized by the liver. It has been investigated for the treatment of *myasthenia gravis* but is rarely, if ever, used clinically. It may be used as an insecticide.

The toxic effects are the same as those of the other anticholinesterases.

Dosage and Methods of Administration. The usual oral dose is 10 mg. in propylene glycol; the usual intramuscular dose in 2.5 mg. in peanut oil or water. The dose may be repeated in 6 to 24 hours, after which a third dose may be given one hour later.

REVIEW QUESTIONS

1. *What is methacholine and what are its actions? Why is it a parasympathomimetic or cholinergic drug?*
2. *What is the mechanism by which cholinergic drugs reduce the fluid pressure in the eye in glaucoma? Should atropine and other anticholinergic drugs ever be used in glaucoma?*
3. *Give the uses of bethanechol and pilocarpine.*
4. *Discuss the fundamental action of anticholinesterases. List the reversible and irreversible drugs in this category.*
5. *What is the action of physostigmine, neostigmine, and DFP locally in the conjunctival sac?*
6. *Discuss the treatment of* myasthenia gravis.
7. *What are the uses of edrophonium?*

REFERENCES

Bilbao, C.; Cano, M.; Monteavaro, L. F.; *et al.*: "Postoperative (Adynamic Ileus; Its Prevention by Ambenoniumchloride." *Surgery*, **46**:1043, 1959.

Burger, A. S. V.: "The Mechanism of Action of Anticholinesterase Drugs," *Brit. J. Pharmacol.*, **4**:219, 1949.

Douglas, W. W., and Paton, W. D. M.: "The Mechanism of Motor End-Plate Depolarization Due to a Cholinesterase Inhibiting Drug," *J. Physiol.*, **124**:325, 1954.

Holmstedt, B.: "Pharmacology of Organophosphorus Cholinesterase Inhibitors," *Pharmacol. Rev.*, **11**:567, 1959.

Hunt, C. C., and Kuffler, S. W.: "Pharmacology of the Neuromuscular Junction," *Pharmacol. Rev.*, **2**:96, 1950.

Koelle, G. B., and Gilman, A.: "Anticholinesterase Drugs," *Pharmacol. Rev.*, **1**:166, 1949.

Rodin, F. H.: "Eserine: Its History in the Practice of Ophthalmology (Physostigmine)," *Am. J. Ophth.*, **30**:19, 1947.

Schwab, R. S., and Chapman, W. P.: "Clinical Uses of Neostigmine," *M. Clin. North America*, **31**:1238, 1947.

Starr, I., Jr., and Ferguson, L. K.: "Beta-Methylcholine Urethane: Its Action in Various Normal and Abnormal Conditions, Especially Postoperative Urinary Retention," *Am. J. M. Sc.*, **200**:372, 1940.

Wescoe, W. C., and Riker, W. F., Jr.: "The Pharmacology of Anti-Curate Agents," *Ann. New York Acad. Sc.*, **54**:438, 1955.

GLAUCOMA

Chandler, P. A.: "Long-Term Results in Glaucoma Therapy," *Am, J. Ophthal.*, **49**:221, 1960.

Leopold, L. H., and Comroe, J. H., Jr.: "Use of Diisopropyl Fluorophosphate ('DFP') in the Treatment of Glaucoma," *Arch. Ophth.*, **36**:1, 1946.

McDonald, P. R.: "Treatment of Glaucoma with Di-Isopropyl Fluorophosphate (D.F.P.)," *Am. J. Ophth.*, **29**:1071, 1946.

Stone, W. C.: "Use of Di-Isopropyl Fluorophosphate (DFP) in the Treatment of Glaucoma," *A.M.A. Arch. Ophth.*, **43**:36, 1950.

MYASTHENIA GRAVIS

Churchill-Davidson, H. C.: "Motor End Plate Changes in Myasthenia Gravis," *Am. J. Phys. Med.*, **38**:159, 1959.

Osserman, K. E.: "Studies in Myasthenia Gravis. I. Physiology, Pathology, Diagnosis and Treatment," *New York J. Med.*, **56**:2512, 1956.

Pinckney, C.: "Myasthenia Gravis," *Proc. Roy. Soc. Med.*, **52**:639, 1959.

Schwab, R. S.; Marshall, C. K.; and Timberlake, W.: "WIN 8077 (Mytelase) in the Treatment of Myasthenia Gravis," *J.A.M.A.*, **158**:625, 1955.

"Symposium on Myasthenia Gravis," *Am. J. Med.*, **19**:655, 1955.

30

Depressants of the Parasympathetic Nervous System (Cholinergic Blocking Agents)

The drugs in this group block the action of acetylcholine at the effector cells or the neuromuscular junction of tissues and organs (smooth and cardiac muscles and glands) innervated by the postganglionic cholinergic nerves. As a result, all functions controlled by these nerves are depressed. The heart rate is more rapid, the involuntary (smooth) muscles are relaxed, the secretions of the exocrine glands are checked, and the pupils of the eyes are dilated. These drugs do not prevent the formation of acetylcholine, nor do they destroy it. Rather, they compete for the sites on the receptor cells which acetylcholine normally excites in the propagation of impulses.

The cholinergic blocking agents are atropine, scopolamine, other belladonna alkaloids, and synthetic drugs that have been prepared as substitutes for atropine.

THE BELLADONNA GROUP

A number of plants of the potato or *Solanaceae* family contain alkaloids of similar chemical constitution which dilate the pupil of the eye. These are called *mydriatic* alkaloids. The plants of this group which are used in medicine are *Atropa belladonna* (deadly nightshade), *Datura stramonium* (Jimson weed), *Hyoscyamus niger* (henbane), and various species of *Scopola* The principal alkaloids in these plants are atropine, scopolamine (hyoscine), and hyoscyamine.

Belladonna Leaf, U.S.P. (B.P., I.P.)

Belladonna leaves are obtained from *Atropa belladonna*, a bushy perennial. The word "belladonna" means "beautiful lady" and reportedly comes from the ancient custom of instilling belladonna preparations in the eyes of ladies to dilate the pupils and thus make them more attractive. Preparations of belladonna, such as belladonna tincture, belladonna ointment and belladonna extract, have been used for many years.

484

Atropine Sulfate, U.S.P., B.P., I.P.

The most important alkaloid of belladonna is atropine. It is made synthetically.

Pharmacological Actions.   Atropine is one of the most effective antagonists to the action of acetylcholine. The effects produced by its administration are numerous and similar to those obtained when the sympathetic nervous system is overactive or when epinephrine is injected. Responses are elicited in the central nervous system, cardiovascular system, smooth muscle (bronchi, gastrointestinal tract, gallbladder, bile duct, and urinary tract), glands, eyes, and sensory nerve endings.

On the Central Nervous System.   Atropine stimulates the cerebral cortex and the medulla. In therapeutic doses (0.5 to 1 mg.), there is seldom any action on the psychic functions. In larger doses, atropine stimulates the cells of the cerebral cortex. With toxic doses, the patient becomes talkative and restless and has hallucinations; delirium and even mania may occur. This excitant stage is followed by depression, stupor, and coma due to exhaustion.

Therapeutic doses of atropine stimulate the medullary respiratory center; hence the breathing is faster and deeper. Large or repeated doses depress the respiration, and death may result from respiratory paralysis. The vagus center is stimulated and produces slowing of the heart. The vasoconstrictor center is stimulated briefly and then is depressed.

In very large doses, the stimulation of the central nervous system extends to the spinal cord. Reflex activity is increased, and muscular twitchings result.

The efficacy of atropine in controlling tremors and rigidity in Parkinson's disease suggests that the drug may depress the areas in the central nervous system that control muscle tone and movement.

On the Cardiovascular System.   The primary action of atropine on the heart is to change its rate. Therapeutic doses depress the vagus peripherally, whereupon the pulse is quickened. After an initial stimulation of the vagus centrally, atropine paralyzes the vagus peripherally and removes the heart from vagus control. It is used in bradycardia (slow heart) owing to vagus hypertonicity or vagotonia.

Atropine will antagonize the action of drugs that slow the heart through direct or indirect vagal stimulation. Some of these drugs are ammonia, physostigmine, pilocarpine, and neostigmine.

In therapeutic doses, atropine has little effect on the blood vessels or blood pressure. It will, however, antagonize the peripheral vasodilatation and fall in blood pressure caused by the choline esters. Large doses and sometimes therapeutic doses will cause dilatation of the cutaneous blood vessels of the face and neck. With toxic doses, the blood pressure falls because of depression of the vasomotor center.

On the Bronchi. The cholinergic nerves cause contraction of the muscle fibers surrounding the bronchi and bronchioles and effect secretion of the mucous cells in the membrane lining these same structures. Atropine, which blocks cholinergic activity, dilates the bronchioles and diminishes the secretion of mucus, thus allowing free passage of air. Drugs belonging to the belladonna group have been used for many years in the treatment of asthma; however, there are more effective ways of dilating these narrowed tubes (see discussion of sympathomimetic agents, pp. 452, 458, 461).

On the Gastrointestinal Tract. Cholinergic nerves are motor and secretory to the stomach and motor to the intestines. By this is meant that these nerves cause normal contractions of the stomach wall (via its smooth muscle layer), closure of the pyloric canal, peristaltic movement of the intestines, and secretion of gastric acid and pepsin. Since atropine blocks the action of cholinergic nerves, it lessens motor activity and diminishes gastric secretion. It tranquilizes the hypermotility of an excessively active gastrointestinal tract. Small doses may be administered for years, with or without acid neutralizers, to ulcer patients. Tolerance does not seem to develop, and untoward effects such as dry mouth are minor.

On the Gallbladder, Bile Duct, and Urinary Tract. Atropine produces relaxation of the gallbladder, bile duct, and ureters and may allow the passage of gallstones and kidney stones. The drug is indicated in incontinence of urine caused by excessive vagus tone, since it relaxes the bladder wall and increases the tone of the vesical sphincter.

On Secretions. Atropine combats perspiration and tends to lessen all secretions from glands innervated by cholinergic fibers (tears, mucus, saliva, gastric juice, and pancreatic secretions). It has no effect on urine flow, bile, or secretin.

On the Eye. When atropine is administered orally or subcutaneously in sufficient amount or when a diluted solution (0.5 to 1 per cent) is instilled in the eye, mydriasis and cycloplegia result. The mydriasis produced by atropine is caused by the relaxation of the sphincter muscle of the iris, which is innervated by cholinergic fibers. The radial muscle, which is innervated by adrenergic fibers, is then unopposed and the pupil widely dilates. The iris is pushed back against the cornea, blocking the cornea-iris angle where the canal of Schlemm lies and thus preventing the proper drainage of fluid from the anterior to the posterior chamber of the eye. This results in an increase in intraocular pressure; hence atropine is contraindicated in glaucoma.

When the ciliary (circular) muscle relaxes, the suspensory ligament of the lens is tightened. The lens becomes flatter and the eye is fixed for far vision. Cycloplegia (paralysis of the ciliary muscle) is produced by atropine.

When the eye is thus *refracted* with atropine, the ciliary muscle is relaxed. If there is an irregularity in the shape of the eyeball, the ciliary muscle can no longer struggle to overcome this irregularity and correct errors in vision. If the eye is not refracted, the strain under which the ciliary muscle is acting cannot be detected. After 45 or 50 years of age, the ciliary muscle loses tone and atropine is no longer needed for eye examinations. This is why one becomes more "farsighted" with age.

On the Sensory Nerve Endings.   Preparations containing belladonna extract or atropine, when applied locally to the skin or mucous membranes, relieve pain by paralyzing the sensory nerve endings. Belladonna ointment and suppositories are used in painful hemorrhoids. Belladonna plasters relieve low-back pain by producing a sensation of warmth or heat.

Absorption, Distribution, and Excretion.   Atropine is readily absorbed from the gastrointestinal tract upon oral administration. It is also absorbed when applied locally to the skin and mucous membranes and upon subcutaneous injection. It leaves the blood quickly and is widely distributed to the tissues throughout the body. About one third of the ingested drug is excreted unchanged in the urine, and the rest is metabolized in the body, probably by the enzymes in the liver.

Poisonous Effects from Overdosage.   Acute poisoning results from overdosage with atropine or drugs containing atropine. The symptoms occur promptly, as a rule, and continue for many hours. The earliest symptoms are excessive thirst, because of dryness of the mouth; difficulty in swallowing; and a flushed skin, especially of the face and neck. The respiration is rapid at first and later becomes slow and shallow. The pupils are dilated and there is dimness of vision.

With large doses, talkativeness and disorientation occur. Occasionally hallucinations and delirium appear. The excessive excitement is followed by unconsciousness, coma, and respiratory failure, which is the cause of death.

Treatment of Poisoning.   When the drug has been taken by mouth, the stomach should be washed out with 5 per cent tannic acid or strong tea, or the "universal antidote" for adsorption of the poison. An icecap may be applied to the head or sponging with alcohol may be used to aid in reducing fever. Respiratory stimulants may be used cautiously. Artificial respiration and the administration of oxygen may be necessary. Sedatives such as chloral hydrate, paraldehyde, or the short-acting barbiturates are given to lessen excitement. Neostigmine methylsulfate is given subcutaneously in doses of 0.5 to 1 mg., repeated every two or three hours if necessary. As the patient improves, 15 mg. of neostigmine bromide are administered orally.

Contraindications.   Atropine is usually contraindicated in patients with glaucoma, prostatic hypertrophy, or other obstructions at the neck of the bladder, and pyloric or duodenal obstructive lesions.

Dosage and Methods of Administration. Atropine sulfate is usually given orally, but solutions may be injected subcutaneously or intravenously. The usual dose is 0.5 mg. (0.3 to 1.2 mg.). For action in the eye, 1 to 2 per cent solutions are instilled in the conjunctival sac.

The oral dose of belladonna tincture is 0.6 ml. (0.3 to 2.4 ml.) and that of the extract is 15 mg. Belladonna extract is given in tablets or capsules, often in combination with other drugs in the treatment of colds.

Therapeutic Uses

1. For hypermotility of the gastrointestinal tract, pylorospasm, and reflex spasticity of the colon.

2. To relieve spasm of the bile ducts and ureters (biliary and renal colic).

3. For peptic ulcer, to diminish gastric secretion of acid.

4. For incontinence of urine resulting from hypertonicity of the bladder wall and sphincter.

5. In asthma, as a prophylactic measure, except status asthmaticus, which it aggravates.

6. As a preanesthetic medication to diminish salivary, nasal, and bronchial secretions.

7. To check nasal secretions and provide symptomatic relief in colds and hay fever.

8. In bradycardia and vagotonia (increased vagus influence).

9. In Parkinson's disease (see p. 374).

10. To effect refraction of the eyes for ophthalmoscopic examination for glasses. Homatropine is more widely used in adults for this purpose.

11. In infections of the cornea (keratitis) and iris (iritis), to prevent adhesions between the iris and the cornea. Homatropine or atropine may be used alternately with physostigmine.

12. As an antidote to cholinergic drugs.

Preparations

Atropine Sulfate Injection, U.S.P.	8 mg. in 20 ml.
Atropine Eye Ointment	1 per cent
Atropine Sulfate Tablets, U.S.P. (B.P., I.P.)	0.3, 0.4, 0.5, 0.6, and 1.2 mg. ($\frac{1}{200}$, $\frac{1}{150}$, $\frac{1}{120}$, $\frac{1}{100}$, and $\frac{1}{50}$ grain)
Belladonna Extract, N.F.	
Belladonna Tincture, U.S.P.	

Scopolamine Hydrobromide, U.S.P.; Hyoscine Hydrobromide, B.P., I.P.

Scopolamine, another of the alkaloids occurring in the plants of the belladonna group, acts like atropine on the parasympathetic nervous system. In therapeutic doses, it is a cerebral depressant, producing drowsiness, amnesia, or sleep which lasts several hours.

Dosage and Methods of Administration. The usual oral and sub-cutaneous dose is 0.5 mg. (0.5 to 0.6 mg.) repeated once very four hours, if necessary. The drug is instilled in the conjunctival sac in 0.2 per cent solution.

Therapeutic Uses

1. As preanesthetic medication for general and spinal anesthesia. Scopola-mine is given with morphine or one of the barbiturates. It lessens annoying secretions, thus decreasing the dangerous aspiration of saliva and bronchial mucus into the lungs.

2. For partial anesthesia or twilight sleep in obstetrics. It is given with meperidine.

3. For sedation of patients with delirium tremens.

4. In motion sickness (see p. 377).

Preparation

Scopolamine Hydrobromide Injection, U.S.P.; Hyoscine Injection, B.P., I.P.	0.3, 0.4, 0.6 mg. in 1 ml.
Scopolamine Hydrobromide Tablets, N.F.	0.6 mg.
Hyoscine Ointment, B.P.	0.25 per cent

SYNTHETIC SUBSTITUTES FOR ATROPINE

ANTISPASMODICS

Many synthetic drugs have been prepared to emulate the action of atropine on smooth muscle. (See Table 32, p. 490.) These drugs are called *anti-spasmodics* (spasmolytics). All are anticholinergics.

The antispasmodics relieve gastrointestinal hypertonicity, pylorospasm, and hyperirritable conditions of the urinary bladder. In certain patients, atropine produces undesirable side effects, such as rapid heart, dry mouth, and visual disturbances, which may be lessened or avoided in some cases by substituting these synthetic drugs.

Some of these drugs lessen gastric secretion and relieve pain produced by excessive acid in the stomach and hence are frequently used in the treatment of gastric and duodenal ulcer (see p. 570). The side effects that these various synthetic agents may produce are listed in Table 33. Excitement and euphoria are not caused by all compounds in the table because some do not pass from the blood into the brain. Side effects are frequent in systemic medication.

Contraindications. The anticholinergic drugs are usually contrain-dicated in patients with glaucoma, prostatic hypertrophy, or other obstructions at the neck of the bladder, and pyloric or duodenal obstructive lesions.

MYDRIATICS AND CYCLOPLEGICS

Some of these synthetic atropine substitutes are used locally in the eyes for cycloplegic action in refraction and for pupillary dilatation in ophthalmoscopic examinations (see atropine, p. 487). Side effects rarely occur with topical administration.

Table 32

Synthetic Anticholinergic Agents

(Antispasmodics)

Generic and Trade Names	Dosage and Methods of Administration	Preparations
Adiphenine hydrochloride (Trasentine)	Orally: 50 to 150 mg. t.i.d. a.c.	Tablets: 75 mg.
	I.m. or subcut.: 50 mg. q.2–4h.	Ampuls: 50 mg. in 1.5 ml.
Ambutonium bromide	Orally: 10 mg. (5 to 25 mg.) q.i.d.	Tablets: 10 mg.
Amprotropine phosphate (Syntropan)	Orally: 100 to 200 mg. (3 to 4 times daily)	Tablets: 50, 100 mg.
	I.m. or subcut.: 10 mg.	Powder: 5- and 25- Gm. bottles
Carbofluorine aminoester (Pavatrine)	Orally: 125 to 250 mg. (3 to 4 times daily)	Tablets: 125 mg.
Dybutoline sulfate (Dibuline)	I.m.: 25 mg., repeated if necessary after 20 minutes	Solution (injection): 25 mg. in 1 ml., 5-ml. vials
Dicyclomine hydrochloride (Bentyl)	Orally: Adults—20 mg. q.i.d. Infants—5 to 10 mg. q.i.d.	Capsules: 10 mg. Syrup: 10 mg. in 5 ml.
	I.m.: 20 mg. q.4–6h.	Solution (injection): 10 mg. in 1 ml., 2-ml. ampuls
Diphemanil Methylsulfate, N.F. (Prantal)	Orally: 100 mg. q.4–6h.	Tablets: 100 mg. (plain and prolonged action)
	I.m. or subcut.: 15 to 25 mg. q.i.d.	Solution (injection): 25 mg. in 1 ml., 1-ml. ampuls and 10-ml. vials
	Locally to skin: 1 to 3 times daily	Cream (topical): 2 per cent
Hexocyclium methylsulfate (Tral)	Orally: 100 mg. daily in divided doses	Tablets: 25 mg. plain; 50 mg. for sustained release
Homatropine methylbromide, N.F.	Orally: 5 mg. q.i.d. (10 to 80 mg. daily)	Tablets: 2.5 and 5 mg. Elixir: 0.5 mg. in 1 ml.
Isopropamide iodide (Darbid)	Orally: 5 mg. q.12h. or as required	Tablets: 5 mg.

━━━━━ **Table 32** *(Continued)* ━━━━━

Synthetic Anticholinergic Agents

(Antispasmodics)

Generic and Trade Names	Dosage and Methods of Administration	Preparations
Levohyoscyamine sulfate (Levsinex)	Orally: 0.375 mg. morning and night	Tablets: (extended action): 0.375 mg.
Mepenzolate methylbromide (Cantil)	Orally: 25 mg. q.i.d. or as required	Tablets: 25 mg.
Methantheline bromide, N.F. (Banthine)	Orally: 50 mg. (25 to 150 mg.) (3 to 4 times daily)	Tablets: 50 mg. Powder (for injection): 50 mg.
Methscopolamine bromide (Lescopine, Pamine)	Orally: 2.5 to 10 mg. t.i.d. ½ hour a.c. and h.s. I.m. or subcut.: 0.25 to 1 mg. q.6–8h.	Tablets: 2.5 mg. Solution (injection): 1 mg.
Methscopolamine nitrate (Skopolate)	Orally: 2 to 4 mg. t.i.d. ½ hour a.c. and h.s. (total, 12 mg. daily) I.m. or subcut.: 0.25 to 5 mg. (3 to 4 times daily)	Tablets: 2 mg. (plain and sustained action) Solution (injection): 5 mg. in 10 ml.
Oxyphencyclimine hydro-chloride (Daricon)	Orally: 10 mg. morning and h.s. or as required	Tablets: 10 mg.
Oxyphenonium bromide (Antrenyl)	Orally: Adults—10 mg. q.i.d., reducing after a few days	Tablets: 5 mg. Syrup: 1.25 mg. in 1 ml.
	Infants and children—1 to 5 drops t.i.d. according to age I.m. or subcut.: 1 to 2 mg. q.6h.	Pediatric drops: 1 mg. in 1 drop Solution (injection): 2 mg. in 1 ml., 10-ml. vials
Penthienate Bromide, N.F. (Monodral)	Orally: 5 to 10 mg. q.i.d.	Tablets: 5 mg. Elixir: 0.5 mg. in 1 ml.
Pipenzolate methylbromide (Piptal)	Orally: 5 mg. t.i.d. and 5–10 at h.s.	Tablets: 5 mg.
Piperidolate hydrochloride (Dactil)	Orally: 50 mg. t.i.d., a.c., and h.s.	Capsules: 50 mg.
Poldine methylsulfate (Nactisol, Nacton)	Orally: 4 mg. 3 or 4 times daily a.c. and h.s.	Tablets: 4 mg.
Propantheline bromide, U.S.P., B.P. (Pro-Banthine)	Orally: 15 mg. t.i.d. and 30 mg. at h.s. (up to 60 mg. q.i.d.) Parenteral: 30 mg. q.6h.	Tablets: 15 mg. Powder (for injection): 30 mg. (dissolve in 10 ml. of Water for Injection)

491

━━━━━━━━━━━━━━━━━━ **Table 32** (*Continued*) ━━━━━━━━━━

Synthetic Anticholinergic Agents

(Antispasmodics)

Generic and Trade Names	Dosage and Methods of Administration	Preparations
Tricyclamol chloride (Elorine, Tricoloid)	Orally: 50 mg. q.i.d., increasing to 250 mg. q.i.d. as required	Tablets: 50 mg. Capsules: 50, 100 mg.
Tridihexethyl chloride (Pathilon)	Orally: 25 to 100 mg. q.i.d. I.v., i.m., or subcut.: 10 to 20 mg. q.6h.	Tablets: 25 mg. Powder (injection): 10 mg. in 1 ml.
Valethamate bromide (Murel)	Orally: 10 to 20 mg. (3 to 4 times daily) I.v. or I.m. 10 to mg. q.4–6h.	Tablets: 10 mg. Solution (injection): 10 mg. in 1 ml., 5-ml. vials

Homatropine Hydrobromide, U.S.P., B.P., I.P.

Homatropine hydrobromide is a synthetic drug closely related to atropine. Its mydriatic and cycloplegic actions are prompt and not so prolonged. One drop of a 2 per cent solution is instilled in the eye every ten minutes for an hour prior to ophthalmoscopic examination.

━━━━━━━━━━━━━━━━━━━━ **Table 33** ━━━━━━━━━━━━━━━━

Side Effects of Anticholinergic Drugs

Dryness of the mouth and nose	Dilatation of the pupils
Flushing and dryness of the skin	Blurring of vision (cycloplegia)
Rapid heart (tachycardia)	Dizziness, nausea
Urinary retention	Excitement, euphoria
Difficulty in defecation	

Eucatropine Hydrochloride, U.S.P. (Euphthalmine)

Eucatropine is a synthetic mydriatic drug used for the routine ophthalmoscopic examination of the retina. It does not produce cycloplegia. It is applied locally as a 2 per cent solution.

Cyclopentolate Hydrochloride, U.S.P. (Cyclogyl)

Cyclopentolate hydrochloride produces rapid and intense cycloplegia and mydriasis of moderate duration. It does not cause undesirable local or systemic effects and appears to be nonirritating and nonsensitizing. Solutions of 0.5 to 1 per cent are instilled in the conjunctival sac for refraction of the eyes and in the treatment of keratitis, iritis, and other diseases of the eye.

Preparation

Cyclopentolate Hydrochloride Ophthal-   0.5 and 1 per cent
mic Solution, U.S.P.

Trade name: Cyclogyl

Tropicamide (Mydriacyl)

Tropicamide (Mydriacyl) produces rapid and short-acting dilatation of the pupil upon instillation in the eye. The cycloplegic effect lasts only two to four hours; so recovery of accommodation is relatively short. Several drops of a 0.5 to 1 per cent solution are instilled in the eye prior to ophthalmoscopic examination, which should be made within 20 to 30 minutes after the last drop has been instilled. It is available in 0.5 and 1 per cent solutions in 7.5-ml. dropping bottles.

OTHER CHOLINERGIC BLOCKING AGENTS

Trihexyphenidyl and caramiphen are discussed on pages 371 and 373.

REVIEW QUESTIONS

1. Discuss the actions of anticholinergic or cholinergic blocking agents in general. What are mydriatic alkaloids?
2. List the actions of atropine sulfate on various organs, systems, and structures. Discuss the associated clinical uses.
3. How have synthetic substitutes for atropine and other belladonna alkaloids improved the treatment of smooth-muscle spasm in various organs?
4. List as many antispasmodics as you can, giving their principal uses and usual doses.

REFERENCES

Bachrach, W. H.: "Anticholinergic Drugs," Am. J. Digest. Dis., 3:743, 1958.

Bargen, J. A.: "Psychosomatic Aspects of Digestive Disorders," Gastroenterology, 13:604, 1948.

Brown, C. H., and Collins, E. N.: "The Use of Banthine in the Treatment of Duodenal Ulcer: Preliminary Report on Its Use in 137 Patients," Gastroenterology, 18:26, 1951.

Council on Drugs: "Oxphencyclimine Hydrochloride (Daricon)," J.A.M.A., 172:564, 1960.

Cummins, A. J.: "Use and Abuse of Anticholinergic Drugs in the Management of Gastrointestinal Disease," *Am. Int. Med.*, **46**:356, 1957

Douthwaite, A. H., *et al.*: "Long Continued Inhibition of Gastric Secretion by Poldine Methyl Sulphate in Patients with Peptic Ulcer," *Brit. M.J.*, **1**:1575, 1961.

Gettes, B. O.: "Tropicamide; Comparative Cycloplegic Effects," *A.M.A. Arch. Ophth.*, **65**:632, 1961.

Goisser, V. W., *et al.*: "Management of Uncomplicated Peptic Ulcer," *M. Clin. North America*, **45**:1459, 1961.

Grossman, M. I.: "Inhibition of Gastric and Salivary Secretion by Darbid," *Gastroenterology*, **35**:312, 1958.

Hufford, A. R.: "Clinical Evaluation of Monodral in the Treatment of Gastrointestinal Diseases," *Am. J. Gastroenterol.*, **26**:199, 1956.

Kirsner, J. B, and Palmer. W. L.: "Certain Problems of the Medical Management of Peptic Ulcer," *South M. J.*, **49**:817, 1956.

Melrose, G., *et. al.*: "Clinical Evaluation of Poldine Methylsulphate," *Brit. M.J.*, **1**:1076.

Riese, J. A.: "The Treatment of Peptic Ulcer and Other Gastrointestinal Conditions with Tridal," *Am. J. Gastroenterol.*, **33**:62, 1960.

Texter, E. C., Jr.: "Psychosomatic Aspects of Peptic Ulcer," *Am. J. Digest Dis.*, **1**:126, 1956.

Texter, E. C., Jr., and Ruffin, J. M.: "Drugs Affecting the Autonomic Nervous System. Part I. Clinical Application in Gastrointestinal Disorders," *South M. J.*, **49**:910, 1956.

———: "Drugs Affecting the Autonomic Nervous System. Part II. Clinical Application in Gastrointestinal Disorders," *South M. J.*, **49**:1076, 1956.

Texter, E. C., Jr.; Smith, H. W.; and Barborka, C. J.: "Evaluation of Newer Anticholinergic Agents," *Gastroenterology*, **30**:772, 1956.

VI DRUGS ACTING ON THE CARDIOVASCULAR SYSTEM

The cardiovascular system consists of the heart and the vascular tree from aorta to capillaries to vena cava. With blood as the vehicle, the function of the cardiovascular system is to supply each cell of the body with the needed amounts of oxygen, food materials, and other vital substances and to remove waste products such as carbon dioxide and ammonia from these cells. The total functioning of the body is directly dependent upon this system—without its adequate, constant, automatic action man could not exist.

For adequate body functioning, blood must be maintained within a normal range in regard to volume and quantity and quality of the red cells, their oxygen-carrying pigment, hemoglobin, and other plasma factors. The clotting mechanism, necessary for the control of bleeding, must at times be altered by the physician. Chapter 31 presents the problems involved in these activities and their management with drugs.

In the remaining three chapters of this section, the treatment of various types of heart disease and peripheral vascular conditions will be discussed. Because of the dynamic principles, both mechanical and electrical, which are involved in heart and blood vessel physiology and pathology, attention will be given to background material in discussing the pharmacological actions of the cardiovascular drugs.

31

Drugs Acting on the Blood and the Blooding-Forming Organs

The blood supplies all the tissues and organs of the body with oxygen and nourishment. It also removes from the tissues waste products of cellular metabolism which are not needed and carries them to the lungs, kidneys, liver, bile, and skin for elimination.

Whole blood consists of a cellular fraction and a fluid portion, which is the plasma. The cellular consists of erythrocytes, leukocytes, and thrombocytes.

The chief constituent of the red blood cells is hemoglobin, an iron and protein compound which combines with oxygen at the alveolar-capillary level of the lungs transporting it to the cells where oxygen is exchanged for carbon dioxide. There are normally 4,500,000 to 5,000,000 red blood cells per cubic millimeter and about 15 Gm. of hemoglobin per 100 ml. of blood. A deficiency in the number of red blood cells or a reduction in the amount of hemoglobin is known as *anemia*.

Phagocytosis is the primary function of the leukocytes. Normally there are 5000 to 10,000 white cells in each cubic millimeter of blood. This number can be rapidly increased when there is an infectious process in the body.

The blood platelets, upon disintegration, set free a factor that is essential for the clotting of blood. This factor in the presence of a number of other substances in blood causes coagulation of shed blood normally in three to five minutes.

SHOCK

Shock is a common entity and can be described as a complex clinical picture having numerous sources of causation. Although studied over half a century, the basic mechanisms are but incompletely comprehended. Underlying all forms of shock is a disturbance in the normal ratio between the circulating blood volume and the capacity of the vascular bed which results in tissue hypoxia and circulatory failure; e.g., the blood volume may decrease, or the vascular bed capacity may increase. The cardinal symptom is a distinct decrease in an individual's normal blood pressure. This can be readily grasped if one understands that maintenance of adequate blood

496

pressure depends upon effective heart action, sufficient circulating blood volume, and appropriate peripheral resistance. A defect in any of these essential factors precipitates arterial hypotension or shock.

A reduction in blood volume as caused by hemorrhage, dehydration, or plasma loss from burned areas may be classified as *hematogenic shock*. Shock following spinal anesthesia, extreme pain, or a sympathectomy is characterized by vasodilatation as a result of diminished vascular tone and is considered *neurogenic shock*. *Cardiogenic shock* is due to failure of the heart to pump an adequate amount of blood through the vascular tree.

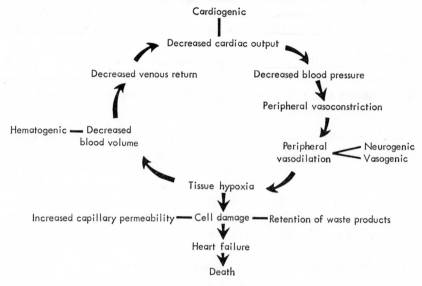

Fig. 14.   Shock cycle.

Examples of this type are seen in patients with myocardial infarction or acute cardiac decompensation. Shock resulting from the action of toxic substances, such as drugs and bacteria, or from the effect of a clot in a peripheral vessel causes vasodilatation and loss of vasomotion and can be considered *vasogenic* in nature.

Signs and symptoms common to all types of shock include decreased blood pressure; increased, weak, thready pulse; pallor; cyanosis; coldness of the extremities; restlessness and apprehension; decreased urinary output; and ringing in the ears.

Based on the underlying cause, treatment may include: restoration of adequate blood volume by using substances such as whole blood, plasma, and plasma expanders; vasoconstrictor drugs; cardiac stimulants, antibiotics; or anticoagulants.

If allowed to persist, shock becomes irreversible and no therapy will restore the blood pressure to normal levels. Figure 14 outlines the occurrences in the shock cycle.

USES OF BLOOD

Whole blood has three main uses:

1. As the treatment of choice in acute hemorrhage.
2. To restore the oxygen-carrying capacity of the blood when other measures are not adequate, as in bone marrow depression due to drugs or leukemia. Here packed cells are most commonly used to avoid increased blood volume.
3. In the correction of coagulation disturbances. Fresh normal or fresh frozen plasma may be used in this situation as it also contains the various clotting factors which may be lacking such as fibrinogen, prothrombin, and antihemophilic globulin.

Although much research has been done in the area of blood substitutes, there is, at the present time, no solution which can carry out the function of the red blood cells. The substitutes that are available should only be used in an emergency situation until whole blood can be obtained. The decision to give blood is not one lightly made. The benefits derived from blood transfusions must be weighed against the risks inherent in the transfusions for the individual patient. (Blood should never be given as a tonic.)

RESPONSIBILITIES OF THE NURSE

When the patient receives blood the nurse has certain responsibilities related to this therapy. She must be sure that the correct blood is given to the right person. Even with the precaution of typing and cross-matching many transfusion reactions occur because of human error. If the physician orders the transfusion rate in milliliters per hour, the nurse will want to convert this to number of drops per minute so that she can maintain a proper rate.

Because a possible hemolytic reaction usually occurs early, the first 50 to 100 ml. of a transfusion should be given at a slow rate, 2 to 4 ml. per minute, and the patient should be observed very closely during this period for adverse effects. If these are apparent, the infusion should be discontinued immediately as the severity of the reaction is dependent upon the amount of blood received.

The physical condition of the patient must also be considered in relation to the rate of flow. Children, older adults, and persons with cardiac conditions are not able to tolerate rapid infusions of large amounts of blood.

When too much blood is given too rapidly, circulatory overloading occurs. If the right side of the heart is not able to handle the greater volume of blood being returned to it, symptoms such as increased venous pressure, systemic edema, and engorged liver result. Pulmonary edema occurs when the right side of the heart is able to handle the increase but the left side is not. The observant nurse can prevent such an occurrence by regulating the rate of flow and reporting early signs and symptoms to the physician.

Before the transfusion is begun, the blood should be inspected for hemolysis, abnormal color, or cloudiness. It is best not to add any medication to the blood, for if a reaction should occur, it would be difficult to tell whether the blood or the drug was the precipitating factor. Blood should be refrigerated until just prior to its use as rapid warming destroys the red blood cells.

When caring for a patient receiving blood, the nurse should be alert to signs and symptoms of the various types of reactions (see Table 34) ranging from mild to very severe. She must also observe the site of the transfusion for a hematoma indicating infiltration of the blood into the subcutaneous tissue. This can occur if the movements of the patient cause the needle to become dislodged from the vein. It may also happen when the needle is withdrawn at the completion of the transfusion if adequate pressure is not applied. Such an occurrence prevents the use of the surrounding veins for intravenous therapy as well as causing discomfort to the patient.

BLOOD DERIVATIVES

Preserved whole blood and blood fractions are available for transfusions. Blood serum and plasma may be preserved as a lyophilized, sterile dry powder.

Normal Human Plasma, U.S.P.; Dried Human Plasma, B.P.

This is a cell-free plasma in dry form, which is restored to volume by the addition of sterile, pyrogen-free 0.1 per cent citric acid solution. It is used in the treatment of shock, with or without hemorrhage; extensive burns with loss of plasma; and hypoproteinemia. The usual intravenous dose is 500 ml. It may be dispensed as liquid, frozen, or dried plasma.

Preparations

Normal Human Plasma (Dried)	Equivalent of 50, 250, and 500 ml., respectively, of restored plasma packaged with 0.1 per cent citric acid
Normal Human Plasma (Citrated)	Equivalent of 50, 250, and 500 ml. of pooled plasma with 5 per cent dextrose
Lyovac Human Plasma (Irradiated)	Bottles of dried plasma packaged with 50, 250, and 500 ml. of 0.1 per cent citric acid

Table 34

Common Blood Transfusion Reactions

Cause	Type, Signs, and Symptoms	Treatment
	HEMOLYTIC	
Intravascular hemolysis of recipient's or donor's erythrocytes (usually donor's) due to incompatibility of blood	(Occurs early during transfusion) Severe pain in lumbar and substernal areas, flushing of the face, dyspnea, chills and fever, throbbing in the head, apprehension, abdominal pain, restlessness, nausea and vomiting, rapid pulse, decreased blood pressure (Later) Hemoglobinuria, hemoglobinemia, jaundice, oliguria-anuria	Stop transfusion, prevent or treat shock, correct electrolyte imbalances, hemodialysis if renal shutdown occurs
	ALLERGIC	
Hypersensitivity of recipient to unknown component in donor's blood	(May occur early in, during, or after transfusion) Urticaria, pruritus, edema of the face, laryngeal edema, bronchial spasm, difficulty in breathing, fall in blood pressure	Stop transfusion, antihistamines, epinephrine, antipruritics, maintain patent airway
	PYROGENIC (contaminated blood)	
Bacteria or their nitrogenous products from blood or contaminated equipment	(May occur late during, or after transfusion) Chills and fever, flushing of the skin, malaise, nausea and vomiting, apprehension, marked prostration.	Warmth, antipyretics, antihistamines, sedatives, antibiotics
	FEBRILE	
Causes unknown, most common type of reaction	(Occurs during or 1-2 hours after transfusion) Elevated temperature	Usually mild and self-limiting, application of cold, antipyretics
	TRANSMISSION OF DISEASE	
Disease-causing organisms in blood as: Serum hepatitis Syphilis Malaria	Signs and symptoms of individual disease occur after suitable incubation period	Usual treatment for disease, prevent by careful screening of donors, serological testing

500

Normal Human Serum Albumin, U.S.P.

This is serum albumin prepared from normal blood with serum globulin reduced to a minimum and most of the salt removed. The usual intravenous dose is equivalent to 25 to 50 Gm. of albumin. It is injected intravenously for the treatment of shock, nephrosis, cirrhosis of the liver, and hypoproteinemia.

Preparation

Normal Serum Albumin, U.S.P.

20 and 50 ml., equivalent to 100 and 250 ml. of plasma; 250 and 500 ml., equivalent to 250 and 500 ml. of plasma

PLASMA EXPANDERS OR SUBSTITUTES

Plasma expanders or substitutes are compounds of high molecular weight which exert sufficient osmotic pressure when they are present in blood to retain fluid in the circulation and thus maintain an adequate blood volume. The plasma expanders most often used are dextran and gelatin solutions.

Dextran, U.S.P. (Expandex, Gentran, Plavolex)

Dextran is a polymer of glucose which is soluble in water. It is used as emergency treatment in hemorrhage and traumatic shock. Fifty per cent of the dextran is excreted in the urine in 24 hours. The remainder is slowly oxidized over a period of a few weeks. Untoward reactions are not usually observed; however, occasionally symptoms such as pruritus, urticaria, and joint pain have been noted. With large doses hemorrhage due to decreased coagulation may occur. Solutions of dextran are easily stored and do not require refrigeration. They are readily available in emergencies until whole blood or plasma can be obtained.

Dosage and Method of Administration. Dextran is administered intravenously as a 6 per cent solution in isotonic sodium chloride. The usual dose is 500 ml. infused at the rate of 20 to 40 ml. a minute, as rapid expansion is needed. Repeated injections may be given, if necessary. The effects of a single injection usually last about 24 hours.

Preparation

Dextran Injection, U.S.P., B.P.

250- and 500-ml. bottles containing 60 mg. in 1 ml. of isotonic salt solution; 250-ml. bottles containing 120 mg. in 1 ml.

Trade names: Expandex; Gentran; Plavolex

Special Intravenous Gelatin Solution

This is a 6 per cent sterile, pyrogen-free, nonantigenic solution of gelatin in isotonic sodium chloride solution. It is used as an infusion colloid to restore blood volume in various types of shock, in emergencies, when whole blood or plasma is not available. Gelatin solutions are largely excreted in the urine. Two or three days after administration, gelatin is no longer found in the blood or urine. They are contraindicated in kidney disease as they may cause damage to the renal tubules and should be used with care in cardiac impairment. Tests for blood typing or cross-matching should be carried out before the administration of intravenous gelatin solutions because they may cause pseudoagglutination.

Dosage and Method of Administration. Special intravenous gelatin solution should be warmed to about 50° C (122° F.). Although it is fluid at body temperature, it gels at lower temperatures and, consequently, must be kept warm for prolonged intravenous drip. The usual dose of 500 ml. is given by intravenous infusion at the rate of 30 ml. a minute. About half of the gel remains in the circulation after 24 hours. A single infusion may be effective for 24 to 48 hours.

Preparation

Special Intravenous Gelatin Solution   500-ml bottles containing 60 mg. of gelatin in 1 ml. of isotonic salt solution

DRUGS THAT STIMULATE THE FORMATION OF RED BLOOD CELLS AND HEMOGLOBIN

Anemias are caused by (1) hemorrhage, (2) accelerated destruction of erythrocytes, and (3) decreased rate of erythropoiesis, or a combination of any of these causes.

IRON-DEFICIENCY ANEMIA

Iron is a constituent of hemoglobin which is essential for the normal transportation of oxygen to the tissues. It is absorbed in the upper portion of the gastrointestinal tract, primarily the duodenum, and stored in the body as hemosiderin and ferritin. The body is able to conserve its iron very well, storing and reusing that which is released during the breakdown of the erythrocyte. It is estimated that the normal adult male loses only about 1 mg. per day. Dietary iron forms many insoluble compounds with various constituents; e.g., when the phosphorus content is increased, the amount of iron absorbed by the body is decreased. Recent studies indicate that normal subjects absorb approximately 10 per cent of the iron in the food they ingest.[1]

The most common cause of iron-deficiency anemia is chronic blood loss. Other less frequent causes include insufficient iron in the diet, impaired absorption, and increased requirements. Rarely is lack of dietary iron the primary cause of anemia; however, a poor diet in times when iron requirements are increased (as during growth, pregnancy, and lactation) may lead to anemia. Signs and symptoms include pallor, chronic fatigue, dyspnea, palpitations, anorexia, irritability, and menstrual disturbances.

While the underlying cause of iron loss must be found and corrected, the deficiency is treated with iron salts. The ferrous forms are used most widely as they are more readily absorbed than the ferric forms. Ascorbic acid, which increases the absorption of iron, may be given in combination with iron salts. A diet high in foods containing iron is also indicated. Most authorities agree that blood is seldom necessary in the treatment of iron deficiency as the body adjusts to the slow decrease in iron.[2]

IRON PREPARATIONS

There are many preparations of iron available for oral administration. Ferrous sulfate is the salt most widely used and is the least expensive. It is administered orally in doses of 300 mg. (200 to 600 mg.) three times a day in the form of tablets or a syrup. The dose of the syrup is 8 ml. (4 to 12 ml.) three times a day. Liquid oral preparations of iron should be drawn into the back of the mouth through a glass tube or straw in order to prevent the darkening of the teeth. Gastrointestinal irritation with nausea, diarrhea, or constipation may occur. If the drug is taken with or just after meals, these symptoms may be lessened. However, the amount of iron absorbed may also be decreased depending upon the composition of the diet and the acidity of the stomach and duodenum. While the patient is receiving iron therapy, his stools will be black.

Several organic preparations of iron, ferrous gluconate, lactate, succinate, fumarate, and chelated iron compounds have been introduced to lessen or prevent these side effects.

Preparations

Ferrous Gluconate Elixir, U.S.P.	
Ferrous Gluconate Tablets, U.S.P., B.P.	300 mg.
Ferrous Sulfate Elixir, U.S.P.	
Ferrous Sulfate Tablets, U.S.P., B.P., I.P.	200 and 300 mg.
Ferrous Sulfate Syrup, N.F.	40 mg. in 1 ml.

---

[1] Wintrobe, Maxwell: *Clinical Hematology.* Lea & Febiger, Philadelphia, 1961, p. 143.
[2] Harrison, T. R. (ed.) : *Principles of Internal Medicine*, 4th ed. McGraw-Hill Book Company, New York, 1962, p. 1280.

Chelated iron compounds are those in which the metal ions combine with an organic molecule to form a ring structure. They are usually soluble and nonionizable. **Iron-choline citrate complex, Ferrocholate (Chel-Iron, Ferrolip),** belongs to this group. It is well absorbed and produces a rapid and satisfactory response. It appears to have a particular advantage in the treatment of certain postgastrectomy patients because it is not as astringent as other compounds. The oral dose for adults and children over six is 40 to 80 mg. elemental iron three times a day; for infants and children under six, 12.5 mg. once a day. It is available in tablets containing 40 mg. iron, as a liquid containing 50 mg. in 5 ml., and as pediatric drops containing 25 mg. iron in 1 ml.

Parenteral iron (by injection) should be reserved for special uses: cases in which there is, for some reason, faulty absorption from the intestine; cases of ulcerative colitis; or some cases of late pregnancy, to ensure an adequate supply of iron for the unborn child.

Iron Dextran Injection, U.S.P. (Imferon) is injected intramuscularly for the treatment of iron-deficiency anemia in patients who cannot tolerate iron preparations administered orally. The oral administration is contraindicated in cases of impaired iron absorption and in gastrointestinal conditions such as ulceration or severe diarrhea.

After calculation of the patient's total iron need by the package chart, a test dose is injected the first day, followed by 0.5 to 5 ml. daily or every other day until the required amount is administered.

Side Effects. Occasional transient allergic reactions such as urticaria and headache have been noted. Excessive overdosage may cause hemochromatosis.

Preparation

Iron Dextran Injection, U.S.P.   2- and 5-ml. ampuls and 10-ml. vials
                                     containing 50 mg. in 1 ml.
Trade name: Imferon

Saccharated iron oxide (Proferrin) and other colloidal preparations are used for intravenous or intramuscular injection. A recently introduced preparation, **iron-carbohydrate complex (Astrafer),** is given intravenously. The initial dose is 1.5 ml. (30 mg.) followed by daily increases of 1 to 1.5 ml., with a maximum daily dose of 5 ml. This dose is continued until normal hemoglobin values are attained. The side effects of parenteral therapy include flushing of the face, warmth, palpitation, nausea and vomiting, hyperpnea, and precordial pressure.

Acute Poisoning with Iron. When taken in excessive amounts, oral or parenteral iron preparations may produce severe poisoning. Parents should be warned to keep all oral preparations out of the reach of children. Serious accidental poisonings and some fatalities have occurred in the United States and Great Britain when large quantities, particularly ferrous sulfate in sugar-coated tablets, have been consumed. The principal symptoms of poisoning are vomiting due to severe gastric irritation, pallor, and circulatory collapse. The blood pressure falls and there may be an acute phase of shock after a few hours. Death has occurred in many cases.

Treatment of Poisoning. Treatment is directed toward removing iron from the stomach and other parts of the body and combatting shock. Routine treatment is (1) to produce emesis, (2) to wash out the stomach with 1 per cent sodium bicarbonate solution, (3) to combat shock by administering oxygen, warmth, 5 per cent intravenous dextrose, plasma, and whole blood transfusions and pressor agents, (4) to prevent pneumonia and other infections by giving antibiotics, and (5) to remove excessive iron from the body by the administration of desferrioxamine-B, a chelating agent, specific for iron.

Hemochromatosis, an inborn disease, in which iron is stored in large amounts both as ferritin and the abnormal pigment, hemoseridin, in the parenchymal tissues, particularly the liver and pancreas, is associated with such complications as cirrhosis of the liver, diabetes mellitus, and heart failure. Acute shocklike episodes may occur in patients with this disease.

Desferrioxamine-B, an iron-free compound, is obtained by the removal of trivalent iron from ferrioxamine-B, a complex isolated from *Streptomyces pilosus.* It has a marked specificity for iron which it removes from ferritin and transferrin but not from hemoglobin. It forms a soluble, nontoxic complex (ferrioxamine) which is eliminated by the kidneys. After treatment, patients with hemochromatosis may excrete 20 to 50 mg. of iron daily in the urine. In patients with iron overload there is a considerable increase in iron excretion whether the drug is given intramuscularly or intravenously, but the intravenous method is more effective. Oral administration may block absorption of food iron which may be important in the treatment of iron overload.

Therapeutic Uses. There are three conditions in which desferrioxamine is valuable in rendering iron nontoxic and removing it by way of the urine.

1. Acute iron poisoning in children who have ingested ferrous sulfate tablets and in parenteral overdosage.
2. Acute shocklike episodes in hemochromatosis.
3. Treatment of primary and secondary hemochromatosis.

Dosage and Methods of Administration. The intramuscular or intravenous dose is 1 to 1.2 Gm. daily. It may be given intramuscularly in doses of 400 to 600 mg. each twice a day or by intravenous drip in physiological saline or 5 per cent dextrose. In many cases 400 to 600 mg. daily may be sufficient. The oral dosage is 600 mg. twice a day. In acute poisoning 8 to 12

Gm. may be given by gastric tube in addition to intramuscular or intravenous injection.

Preparation

Deferoxamine

Trade name: Desferal

PERNICIOUS ANEMIA

Pernicious anemia, or vitamin B_{12}-deficiency anemia, is a chronic disease that was invariably fatal before the introduction of liver therapy. The condition is characterized by a *defective formation* and *maturation* of red blood cells and occurs in the later years of life (it is rarely seen before 40 years of age). The symptoms are pallor, weakness, sore tongue and mouth, achlorhydria (lack of hydrochloric acid in the stomach), dyspepsia, itching, dyspnea, a reduction in the number of red blood cells, and megaloblastic *macrocytosis*. Serious changes occur in the *dorsal columns* of the spinal cord, which cause diminution or loss of the position sense of the feet and legs, tingling in the hands and feet (paresthesias), dizziness, psychoses, peripheral neuritis, and incoordination of movement. The onset is gradual, and the first complaints are chronic fatigue, glossitis, and achlorhydria. The administration of vitamin B_{12} completely prevents the blood changes and causes a remission of symptoms.

In 1926, Drs. G. R. Minot and W. P. Murphy introduced the feeding of liver in large amounts to pernicious anemia patients and demonstrated its effectiveness in relieving the symptoms. At first up to 400 Gm. were added to the patient's daily diet. Later, liver extracts, or concentrates, were made available for oral or parenteral use. The parenteral administration of liver was necessary only once every week or, in some cases, every three weeks. The use of liver concentrates was very successful, and it was not until 1948 that their antianemic principle was isolated and identified as vitamin B_{12}. Subsequently, when this product became commercially available, it largely replaced liver extracts in the treatment of pernicious anemia. Therefore, liver preparations are no longer included in the U.S.P. Such liver preparations as are recognized by the N.F. are recommended for use as vitamin supplements and hematopoietics.

It is interesting to note that the theory concerning the antianemic mechanism of the human body which was proposed by Dr. W. B. Castle in 1929 is still generally accepted. In simplest terms, this theory postulates that an *extrinsic factor*, now identified as vitamin B_{12}, which is available in common foods such as meats, liver, fish, and eggs, interacts with an *intrinsic factor* secreted by the stomach. The complex attaches to the intestinal mucosa, primarily the ileum. Vitamin B_{12} is released from the intrinsic factor and is transported across the intestine into the blood. Part of this process appears to be enzymatic. Vitamin B_{12} is stored in the liver until required. Therefore, a deficiency in either the *intrinsic* or the *extrinsic factor* will cause pernicious anemia. Since vitamin B_{12} is effective in microgram doses, it seems probable that its function is as a coenzyme.

Cyanocobalamin, U.S.P. (Vitamin B_{12}), B.P., I.P.

Cyanocobalamin, a red crystalline substance containing cobalt, is obtained from liver. It is also produced by certain microbial organisms, with cultures of *Streptomyces griseus* and *S. aureofaciens* being the important commercial sources. Cyanocobalamin exhibits all the antianemic activity of liver extract when injected in persons with pernicious anemia; therefore, vitamin B_{12} has almost completely replaced liver extract because the injection is painless, small uniform doses are readily available, and it is less expensive. The potency of cyanocobalamin preparations is determined spectrophotometrically.

Dosage and Method of Administration. The usual intramuscular dose of cyanocobalamin is 1 mcg. daily, preferably in amounts of 10 or 15 mcg. at appropriate intervals. In uncomplicated pernicious anemia, a dose of 15 mcg. is given once or twice a week until remission of symptoms occurs, then a maintenance dose of 15 mcg. every other week. In pernicious anemia with neurological symptoms, a dose of 15 to 30 mcg. is given once or twice a week until remission occurs, then a maintenance dose of 15 mcg. every other week. This is replacement therapy, similar to insulin in the treatment of diabetes mellitus; it is generally necessary to administer these drugs throughout life to maintain normal blood values. The deficit of the intrinsic factor is never restored. In sprue, a dose of 15 to 30 mcg. is administered once or twice a week, then a maintenance dose of 15 mcg, once a week to prevent relapse. In nutritional macrocytic anemia, a single dose of 15 mcg. is given; it may be necessary to give 15 mcg. at two-week intervals to prevent relapse.

Orally administered vitamin B_{12} with intrinsic factor produces satisfactory responses if given in five times the intramuscular dose. The intrinsic factor enhances the absorption of vitamin B_{12}. However, after periods varying from six months to two or three years, hematological relapses occur. The blood count begins to fall, and macrocytosis reappears. There is good evidence that an acquired refractoriness to certain intrinsic factors occurs and that they no longer increase the absorption of vitamin B_{12}. This takes place more frequently in some preparations than in others. This therapy, which leads to so many relapses, is unsatisfactory and unpredictable. It is therefore unwise to prescribe the oral preparations when the parenteral administration of the drug is completely reliable and dependable. The oral preparation has been deleted from the U.S.P.

No toxic reactions in man have been observed from overdosage with vitamin B_{12}.

Folic acid and ascorbic acid are also involved in blood formation and, consequently, are often administered with vitamin B_{12}.

Other Uses. Cyanocobalamin is used in nutritional macrocytic anemia resulting from a deficiency of vitamin B_{12}, tropical and nontropical sprue, growth acceleration in retarded children, and chronic type of drug poisoning such as with gold salts in arthritis.

Patients receiving vitamin B_{12} need to be taught the proper technique for preparing an intramuscular injection. Utilization of the thigh muscles allows them to give their own injections.

Preparation

Cyanocobalamin Capsules and Tablets	25 and 50 mcg.
Cyanocobalamin Injection. U.S.P., B.P.	300 mcg., 1 mg., and 10 mg. in 10 ml.; 900 mcg. and 3 mg. in 30 ml.

Trade names: Berubigen; Betalin; Bevatine; Beridox; Bexii; Cobione; Crystamin: Dodecabee; Dodex; Hemomin; Normocytin; Rametin; Rubramin; Redisol; Sytobex; Vitamin B_{12}

Hydroxocobalamin, B.P. (Hydrovit)

Hydroxocobalamin (Hydrovit) is closely related to cyanocobalamin (vitamin B_{12}). It is now believed that cyanocobalamin is an artifact of isolation procedures and that hydroxocobalamin is the true form of the vitamin in the body. It is absorbed more slowly and causes a more prolonged action. Less frequent injections are necessary. It is used in pernicious anemia and complications and other conditions for which cyanocobalamin is indicated.

Preparation

Hydroxocobalamin Injection, B.P.	Ampuls containing 500 and 1000 mcg.

Trade names: Hydrovit, Alpha Redisol

Folic Acid, U.S.P., B.P., I.P. (Pteroylglutamic Acid)

Folic acid, a potent nutrition factor (member of vitamin B complex) found in liver, beef, yeast, dark-green vegetables, such as spinach and kale, and cauliflower, was isolated in 1945. It is essential for the growth of *Lactobacillus casei* and a number of bacterial species. It is also an important factor in nucleoprotein metabolism and is an essential factor in the proper production of red blood cells in man. A deficiency of folic acid in man causes megaloblastic erythrocytopoiesis and marked hyperplasia of the bone marrow. The changes are reversible; hence the administration of folic acid causes the return of the blood picture to one of normoblastic regeneration. If the deficiency is severe, granulocytopenia, diarrhea, and death may result.

Physiological Actions. The role played by folic acid as an essential nutrient to bone marrow seems to occur after it is converted to an active form, folinic acid (Leucovorin). This reaction, which occurs in the liver, appears to be initiated by ascorbic acid; hence vitamin C, orange juice, or some other food containing vitamin C is included with folic acid therapy.

It is believed that folinic acid is the same as the "citrovorum factor," which is the factor (not present in the vitamin B complex) essential to the growth of cultures of *Leuconostoc citrovorium*. The refined liver extracts are a good source of this substance.

Therapeutic Uses

1. In nutritional macrocytic anemias of pregnancy and total gastrectomy.
2. In puerperium anemia associated with intestinal disease such as strictures or fistulas.
3. In sprue.

There is a prompt and excellent recovery when folic acid is administered in macrocytic anemias and sprue. It is sometimes given with vitamin B_{12} in the treatment of pernicious anemia. This use is not contraindicated, but it is unwarranted. Folic acid should never be administered alone in pernicious anemia.

Dosage and Methods of Administration. Folic acid is administered orally and subcutaneously. The usual oral or intramuscular dose is 10 mg. (5 to 20 mg.) daily. It is so readily absorbed from the gastrointestinal tract that parenteral administration does not offer any advantages. When folic acid is administered orally, there are generally no untoward effects.

Preparations

Folic Acid Injection, U.S.P.	15 mg. in 1 ml.
Folic Acid Tablets, U.S.P.	5 mg.

Trade names: Folacin; Folacide; Folate; Folvite

Other Drugs

Vitamin B_{12} with Intrinsic Factor Concentrate, N.F., a mixture of vitamin B_{12} with suitable preparations of mucosa of stomach of domestic animals used for food, is more readily absorbed from the gastrointestinal tract than vitamin B_{12} alone. The dose is 1 N.F. unit (oral) daily. The mixture is available as capsules and tablets, each containing $\frac{1}{3}$ or $\frac{1}{2}$ unit. (Trade names: Bevidoral; Bexitab; Bifacton; Biopar; Intrinase.)

DRUGS AFFECTING THE COAGULATION OF BLOOD

Drugs are available to increase (coagulants) or decrease (anticoagulants) the coagulation of blood. They produce these effects by hastening or retarding the normal processes that cause the formation of fibrin from its precursor, fibrinogen.

Although the mechanism of blood coagulation is not yet completely understood, it is thought that there are basically three steps in the process.

1. Activation of thromboplastin	Injured tissue + several coagulation factors → thromboplastin
2. Conversion of prothrombin to thrombin	Thromboplastin + prothrombin calcium → thrombin
3. Formation of fibrin	Thrombin + fibrinogen → fibrin Fibrin + formed elements → clot

BLOOD COAGULANTS

Vitamin K enters the body in the diet and is carried to the liver where it is used in the synthesis of prothrombin. Bacteria and bilesalts improve its absorption. If there is a deficiency of vitamin K, the prothrombin level of the blood is low and the coagulation time of the blood is prolonged. This was demonstrated by Dr. H. Dam, of Copenhagen, in 1929, when he produced a fatal hemorrhagic disease in chicks which were fed an inadequate diet; the disease was prevented or cured by the administration of a substance found in hog liver and alfalfa. The pure chemical substances were later isolated by Dr. E. A. Doisy from alfalfa (vitamin K) and sardine meal (vitamin K_2). Both vitamins elevate the prothrombin level in man.

Vitamin K is a fat-soluble, water-insoluble vitamin, the absorption of which is dependent upon the presence of bile salts. In biliary obstruction or liver disease, or following the destruction of the absorbing surface of the intestine, vitamin K deficiency and hypoprothrombinemia may result.

A synthetic analog of the K vitamins is also very effective in raising the prothrombin level in man. This compound, which is called *menadione*, is used clinically.

Phytonadione, U.S.P.; Phytomenadione, B.P. (Mephyton, Konakion)

Phytonadione is a nearly odorless, viscous liquid that produces more prompt and more prolonged effects than the vitamin K analogs. It is dependable in reversing anticoagulant-induced hypoprothrombinemia to safe levels, not only if bleeding is only potential but also if it has actually occurred. An adequate intravenous dose will stop bleeding in three to four hours and produce a normal prothrombin level in 12 to 14 hours.

Dosage and Method of Administration. For anticoagulant-induced hypoprothrombinemia, the intravenous or oral dose is 20 mg. (0.5 to 100 mg.). For hypoprothrombinemia from other causes, the dose varies with the severity of the condition. Phytonadione is available as an emulsion, which is mixed with a suitable diluent such as Water for Injection, U.S.P., or isotonic salt solution before injection.

Prothrombin time should be checked regularly so that prothrombin can be balanced properly between levels protecting the patient from intravascular clotting, on one hand, and pathological bleeding, on the other.

Preparations

Phytonadione, Aqueous Colloid Suspension	1-ml. ampuls and 5-ml. vials containing 10 mg. in 1 ml.

Trade name: Aquamephyton

Sterile Phytonadione Emulsion, U.S.P., B.P.	10 and 50 mg. in 1 ml.; 1 mg. in 0.5 ml.
Phytonadione Tablets, U.S.P., Phytomenadione Tablets, B.P.	5 mg.

Trade names: Mephyton, Konakion (synthetic form)

Vitamin K Analogs

There are a number of synthetic naphthoquinone derivatives that produce vitamin K activity. These are called vitamin K *analogs*. Some of them are water soluble.

Menadione, U.S.P., I.P.; Menaphthone, B.P. This is a yellow crystalline powder that is not very soluble in water. The usual dose is 2 mg. (1 to 2 mg.) daily.

Preparations

Menadione Capsules, N.F.	1 and 2 mg.
Menadione Tablets, U.S.P.	2 mg.

Menadiol Sodium Diphosphate, U.S.P. This is a prothrombogenic substance that is available for parenteral administration. The usual oral and parenteral dose is 5 mg. (4 to 75 mg.) daily.

Preparations

Menadiol Sodium Diphosphate Injection, U.S.P.	5 and 10 mg. in 1 ml.; 75 mg. in 2 ml.
Menadiol Sodium Diphosphate Tablets, U.S.P.	5 mg.

Trade names: Synkavite; Kappadione; Thylokay

Menadione Sodium Bisulfite, N.F.; Menaphthone Sodium Bisulphite. B.P. Menadione sodium bisulfite is water soluble and is available for parenteral administration. The intravenous and subcutaneous dose is 2 mg. (0.5 to 2 mg.; up to 100 mg. as an antidote to coumarin antagonists) daily.

Preparations

Menadione Sodium Bisulfite Injection.   2.5, 5, and 10 mg. in 1 ml.; 72 mg. in
   N.F.   10 ml.
Menaphthone Sodium Bisulphite Injec-
tion, B. P.

Trade name: Hykinone

Therapeutic Uses

1. In obstetrics. A deficiency of vitamin K in the newborn may result from a deficiency of the vitamin in the mother's blood. This may cause hemorrhagic diathesis in the infant, which may be prevented by the administration of 10 mg. of menadione daily to the mother one or two weeks before delivery.

2. Prophylactically to the infant to prevent or combat hemorrhagic diathesis. Menadione in oil (0.5 mg. in 0.5 ml.) is administered in drops.

3. To prevent hypoprothrombinemia when the bowel is being "sterilized" for gastrointestinal surgery.

4. In obstructive jaundice, hepatic disease, and hemorrhagic states associated with chronic diarrhea or ulcerative colitis. Menadione is administered in doses of 2 to 5 mg. four times a day.

5. To prevent hypoprothrombinemia. Menadione is administered with salicylates when they are used in large doses in rheumatic fever or arthritis.

6. To control hemorrhage in overdosage with bishydroxycoumarin.

Vitamin K and its analogs can be given either orally or by injection. Parenteral administration is necessary when the drug cannot be absorbed from the gastrointestinal tract. When giving such a drug, the nurse must be aware of the patient's prothrombin time. If it is increased, there may be bruising or oozing of blood at the site of injection, which may be minimized by the application of pressure for a period of a minute or more.

Fibrinogen (Human), U.S.P.

Fibrinogen is the blood plasma clotting factor. It is a sterile fraction of normal human plasma, dried from the frozen state. It is available in 1- and 2-Gm. amounts. This must be reconstituted with water for injection prior to injection. The intravenous dose is 2 Gm. (2 to 6 Gm.). It is used in certain surgical procedures for restoring plasma fibrinogen to normal levels and as an adjunct in treating certain hemorrhagic complications resulting from the absence of fibrinogen in the blood.

Carbazochrome Salicylate (Adrenosem Salicylate, Adrestat)

This preparation is used for the systemic control of capillary bleeding and oozing and also for the prevention of abnormal capillary permeability and fragility. The dose is expressed in terms of the adrenochrome content. The oral adult dose is 1 to 5 mg. four times a day. The adult intramuscular dose is 5 mg. every two hours. Toxicity is minimal. It is available as an injection containing 130 mg. in 1 ml. (representing 5 mg. of adrenochrome semicarbazone), as a syrup containing 65 mg. in 1 ml. (representing 2.5 mg. of adrenochromsemicarbazone), and tablets of 25 and 65 mg. (representing 1 and 2.5 mg. of adrenochromsemicarbazone).

This preparation is used to counteract the anticoagulant effect of heparin overdosage or where hemorrhage is caused by trauma or surgery in heparinized patients. A solution containing 10 mg. in 1 ml. is diluted with isotonic saline or 5 per cent dextrose to give a final concentration of 1 mg. in 1 ml. The intravenous dose is 1 ml. for each 100 U.S.P. units of heparin over a 10- to 15-minute period.

Sodium Estrone Sulfate (Premarin)

This is a conjugated estrogenic substance (see p. 611) that is used to control spontaneous hemorrhage or that which occurs during surgery. No undesirable side effects have been observed. The intravenous adult dose is 20 mg. For children the intravenous or intramuscular dose is 5 to 10 mg. It is available in vials containing 20 mg. in 5 ml. A sterile diluent containing 0.5 per cent phenol is provided.

Tolonium Chloride (Blutene, Toluidine Blue O)

Tolonium reduces the tendency to bleeding in certain hemorrhagic conditions associated with excessive heparinoid substances in the blood. It is used in the treatment of idiopathic uterine bleeding: menorrhagia or hypermenorrhea (abnormally profuse or prolonged menstruation) and menometrorrhagia (excessive and prolonged menstruation and intermenstrual bleeding). The usual oral dose is 200 to 300 mg. daily.

Preparation

Tolonium Chloride Tablets   100 mg.
                    Trade name: Blutene

HEMOSTATICS

Hemostatics are substances applied locally to stop bleeding. The hemostatics most often used are absorbable gelatin sponge, oxidized cellulose, and thrombin.

Absorbable Gelatin Sponge, U.S.P., B.P. (Gelfoam)

Absorbable gelatin sponge is a sterile, absorbable, water-insoluble gelatin-base sponge that is used to control capillary bleeding. It is generally moistened with thrombin solution. The sponge may be left in place after closing the incision and will be absorbed in four to six weeks without scar formation.

Oxidized Cellulose, U.S.P., B.P. (Hemo-pak, Oxycel)

Oxidized cellulose is an absorbable gauze or cotton that is useful when applied to the tissues from which blood is oozing. It is absorbed in about two to seven days and may be allowed to remain in the wound after closing the incision. Its action depends upon the formation of an artificial clot by cellulosic acid. Oxidized cellulose is useful in controlling bleeding in surgery of the liver, pancreas, spleen, kidney, thyroid, or prostate. It should not be used as a surface dressing except to control hemorrhage, since cellulosic acid inhibits the growth of epithelial tissue.

Thrombin, N.F., B.P.

Thrombin, a sterile protein obtained from human or bovine plasma, is applied locally to control capillary bleeding during operations. It may be applied as a dry powder or dissolved in normal salt solution.

Preparation

Thrombin Topical (Bovine, N.F.; Human, B.P.)   Vials containing 1000 and 5000 N.I.H. units

ANTICOAGULANTS

Useful in prolonging the coagulation of the blood, anticoagulants do not dissolve already existing clots but rather serve to prevent the formation of new thrombi. The objective in anticoagulant therapy is to prolong the clotting time two to three times the normal or decrease the prothrombin activity 15 to 20 per cent of normal. Sodium citrate, heparin, bishydroxycoumarin, ethyl biscoumacetate, and phenindione are the anticoagulants most frequently used in clinical medicine.

Patients receiving anticoagulants need to have close medical supervision. The dosage, which varies greatly from person to person, is based upon the laboratory studies of the patient (clotting time for heparin, prothrombin activity for others). When anticoagulant therapy is begun, each dose should be individually ordered following consideration of the results of the most recent laboratory study. After the patient becomes regulated on his individual maintenance dose, the studies may be done less frequently. When the need for anticoagulation is immediate, heparin is the drug of choice, while if long-term therapy is desired, one of the oral preparations is usually given. Initial therapy may consist of heparin and a synthetic preparation given together, after which heparin is discontinued as the action of the synthetic preparation begins.

The therapeutic uses of anticoagulants include:

1. To prevent clotting of blood during transfusions.
2. To prevent or treat thromboembolic phenomena such as:
   pulmonary embolism,
   thrombophlebitis,
   venous thrombosis,
   gangrene of extremities,
   thromboangiitis obliterans,
   rheumatic heart disease with atrial fibrillation,
   myocardial infarction,
   cerebral thrombosis and embolism,
   sudden peripheral arterial occlusion,
   after vascular surgery,
   after trauma to major vessels.
3. During use of extracorporeal circulation.

Anticoagulants should not be given if the patient has any concurrent condition which may lead to hemorrhage such as blood dyscrasias with bleeding tendencies, wounds with open raw surfaces, ulcerative gastrointestinal diseases, recent surgery of the brain or spinal cord, vitamin K and C deficiencies, and subacute bacterial endocarditis. Since the liver and kidney both play an important part in the detoxification of these drugs, their use is contraindicated in patients with hepatic and renal insufficiency.

Hemorrhage is the symptom of overdosage which all anticoagulants present. It may vary from microscopic oozing to massive, uncontrollable bleeding. For this reason any nurse who has contact with a person receiving anticoagulant therapy must be aware of the many possible ways hemorrhage may present itself. Among the more frequent ways bleeding is observed are changes in the color of the urine indicating hematuria, changes in the color of the stool indicating melena, bleeding from the gums on brushing of teeth or eating coarse foods, bruising at the site of injection or on slight trauma, petechiae, hematemesis, and epistaxis.

If a patient is placed on long-term anticoagulant therapy, he needs to understand the purpose of the treatment as well as the risks involved. He also needs to recognize the signs of hemorrhage and report these to the physician if they occur. It is also suggested that the person receiving long-term therapy carry a card indicating this as well as the name and telephone number of his physician.

The patient must understand that he must not miss a dose of his anticoagulant and that he must have his prothrombin activity tested routinely as the amount of medication ordered is based upon the prothrombin determination. He must also be aware that in any situation where there is a possibility of bleeding, as in dental extractions or surgery, the persons involved should be notified of his anticoagulant therapy so that complications may be prevented.

Sodium Heparin, U.S.P., B.P., I.P.

Heparin sodium is a mixture of active principles that prolong the clotting time of blood. It is a white or light-colored amorphous powder prepared from livers or lungs of domestic animals used as food by man. In the presence of blood plasma, both in vivo (in the body) and in vitro (shed blood), heparin antagonizes the activation of prothrombin to thrombin and so prolongs the clotting time of blood. It will not dissolve clots already formed but will inhibit the formation of thrombi, which can be produced by mechanical or chemical injury to the intima (innermost coat of the blood vessels) of the veins. Therapeutic doses that prolong the clotting time do not affect the bleeding time, which limits the danger of profuse bleeding from accidental injuries. The action of heparin is prompt and transient, since it is rapidly inactivated by enzymes in the blood and liver.

Overdosage may cause bleeding from the mucosa and open wounds. This action may be checked by transfusions. Protamine sulfate inactivates heparin and may be administered intravenously as an antidote in doses of 50 mg. The dose may be repeated as required.

Therapeutic Uses

1. To prevent postoperative thrombi (clots in the veins).

2. To prevent recurring thrombosis in thrombophlebitis and pulmonary embolism.

3. To initiate rapid anticoagulant action in vascular surgery and other procedures.

4. To prevent clotting during extracorporeal circulation.

Dosage and Methods of Administration. Heparin is inactive orally and is generally administered intravenously or by single injection or intravenous drip. The usual intravenous dose is 5000 U.S.P. units (5000 to 30,000 units). The intramuscular dose for the repository form is 20,000 units (20,000 to 40,000 units) every 12 to 24 hours. For continuous intravenous drip, 10,000 to 20,000 units are added to 1000 ml. of a 5 per cent sterile dextrose or isotonic salt solution, and the flow is started at about 20 drops a minute.

It has been found that when heparin therapy is stopped suddenly, there is a possibility of thrombi formation due to the rapid decrease in the clotting time. For this reason, it is suggested by some authorities that the dosage of heparin be gradually reduced over two or more weeks before discontinuation. During this period of time the patient should be ambulated if possible in order to prevent new thrombi formation. If ambulation is impossible, then active or passive movement or muscle-setting exercises should be carried out as the condition of the patient permits.

Preparations

Sodium Heparin Injection, U.S.P.; Injection of Heparin, B.P., I.P.	10-ml. vials containing 10,000 and 50,000 units; 4-ml. vials containing 40,000 units
Heparin Sodium Injection, U.S.P. Repository Form	1-ml. cartridges containing 20,000 units and 40,000 units in 2 ml.

Trade names: Depo-Heparin; Liquaemin Sodium; Panheparin; Pularin

Bishydroxycoumarin, U.S.P.; Dicoumarol, I.P.

In both Canada and the United States hemorrhagic manifestations were noted in cattle eating improperly cured silage. Dr. K. P. Link isolated a pure crystalline material, a coumarin derivative, from spoiled sweet clover, which was responsible for this condition. Later he synthesized the material, and it is now marketed under the name Dicumarol.

Bishydroxycoumarin is a white crystalline substance that is readily absorbed from the gastrointestinal tract; hence it is administered orally. The drug's principal action, which occurs only in vivo, is to prolong the clotting time of blood. It is believed that bishydroxycoumarin depresses the activity of the liver in its formation of prothrombin and thus diminishes the prothrombin level of the blood. There is no damage to the liver in therapeutic doses. The action of bishydroxycoumarin builds up slowly, and there is a latent period of 24 to 48 hours followed by a maximum decrease in the prothrombin time for three to five days, whereupon the effect diminishes. It is advisable to check the prothrombin time daily during the administration of the drug, at least until the individual is regulated, then less frequently after the patient is taking a maintenance dose.

Bishydroxycoumarin can be used alone or with heparin to prevent thrombus formation. It will not dissolve a clot already formed, but it will prevent further extension of the clot. It is used prophylactically when the need is indicated. Bishydroxycoumarin is contraindicated in bleeding from any cause, hepatic disease, or impaired kidney function.

Therapeutic Uses

1. For postoperative thrombophlebitis.
2. In pulmonary embolism.

3. In acute embolic and thrombotic occlusion of the peripheral arteries.

4. For coronary occlusion, in the acute phase and as a prophylactic.

5. For prevention of postoperative vascular thrombosis, especially coronary and cerebral.

Dosage and Methods of Administration. The usual initial oral dose is 200 to 300 mg. daily and 100 to 200 mg. daily thereafter, according to prothrombin determinations. If the prothrombin time reaches 30 to 35 seconds, the dosage should be reduced to 50 to 100 mg. daily. If the time is increased, the drug should be discontinued until the prothrombin time returns to 25 seconds or less. The drug is then given in doses of 50 to 100 mg. If hemorrhage occurs, an intravenous dose of 50 to 100 mg. of menadione sodium bisulfite is given slowly or a dose of 250 to 500 mg. of menadione is given orally. Transfusions of whole blood are also indicated.

Preparations

Bishydroxycoumarin Tablets, U.S.P.	25, 50, and 100 mg.
Bishydroxycoumarin Capsules, N.F.	50 and 100 mg.

Trade name: Dicumarol

Ethyl Biscoumacetate, N.F. (Tromexan Ethyl Acetate)

Ethyl biscoumacetate is a synthetic oral anticoagulant that is related to bishydroxycoumarin, although it is absorbed and excreted more rapidly than that drug. The initial dose of 1.2 Gm. for the first 24 hours is usually adequate. The maintenance dose is 150 to 900 mg. daily. The actions, uses, and contraindications are the same as for bishydroxycoumarin.

Preparation

Ethyl Biscoumacetate Tablets, N.F.	150 and 300 mg.

Trade names: Tromexan; Tromexan Ethyl Acetate; Pelentan

Sodium Warfarin, U.S.P., B.P. (Coumadin, Prothromadin)

This coumarol derivative is used for the prevention and treatment of intravascular clots. It maintains a predictable, relatively smooth, sustained hypoprothrobinemia for 12 to 24 hours. The side effects are excess bleeding from cuts and internal bleeding with overdosage. The oral or intravenous dose is 50 mg. (25 to 50 mg.), then 5 to 10 mg. daily in accordance with prothrombin determinations.

Preparations

Sodium Warfarin for Injection, U.S.P.	75 mg.
Warfarin Sodium Tablets	5, 10, and 25 mg.

Trade names: Coumadin; Prothromadin; Marevan; Panwarfin

Newer Coumarin Derivatives

These derivatives, acenocoumarol and phenprocoumon, are used for the prophylaxis and treatment of intravascular clotting, postoperative thrombophlebitis, pulmonary embolism, and acute thrombic and embolic occlusion of the peripheral arteries. The side effects are a hemorrhagic tendency, fever, rash, and a lowered white blood cell count.

Acenocoumarol (Sintrom). The oral dose on the first day is 16 to 28 mg.; on the second day, 8 to 16 mg. The maintenance dose is 2 to 10 mg. daily. It is available in 4-mg. tablets.

Phenprocoumon (Liquamar). Heparin sodium, 200 mg. in aqueous solution, is given intramuscularly with seven phenprocoumon tablets orally; 18 to 24 hours later, 200 mg. of heparin sodium intramuscularly with three to four tablets of phenprocoumon orally are given. Usually three to four doses of heparin are adequate, and then the patient may be maintained with phenprocoumon tablets orally. Tablets of 3 mg. are available.

Phenindione Derivatives

Phenindione, B.P. (Danilone, Hedulin). This is a synthetic oral anticoagulant that acts more promptly than bishydroxycoumarin and is effective in smaller doses. Therapeutic levels are obtained in 18 to 24 hours; the maximum effect occurs in 28 hours and lasts about 48 hours. The urine is colored orange by this agent. Adrenal bleeding and blood dyscrasias have also been reported.

Dosage and Method of Administration. The initial oral dose is 200 to 300 mg., of which half is given in the morning and half at bedtime. The average maintenance daily dose is 25 to 100 mg., given in the same manner as the initial dose. The drug is rapidly eliminated; hence untoward effects are seldom encountered.

Preparation

Phenindione Tablets, B.P.   50 mg.
   Trade names: Danilone; Dindevan; Eridone; Hedulin; Indon

Diphenadione, N.F. (Dipaxin), is closely related to phenindione and similar in action and uses to bishydroxycoumarin. It has a more potent and prolonged action. Its initial dose is 20 to 30 mg. followed by 10 to 15 mg. on the second day. The average daily maintenance dose is 3 to 5 mg. Prothrombin time determination should be made prior to treatment and daily until an effective maintenance dose is attained. Tablets of 1 and 5 mg. are available.
Anisindione (Miradon) is a new member of this group. The oral dose on the first day is 300 mg.; on the second day, 200 mg.; on the third day, 100

mg. The usual maintenance dose is 75 to 100 mg. (25 to 250 mg.) daily. Tablets of 50 mg. are available.

Bromindione (Halinone), a phenindione derivative, is a useful and very potent anticoagulant with minimal side effects. It is used for both short-term therapeutic and long-term prophylactic therapy. An initial oral dose of 12 to 18 mg. induces therapeutic anticoagulation in 28 to 34 hours. The drug is not administered in the second day. Treatment is resumed on the third day. The usual maintenance dose is 2 to 5 mg. daily. Drug action persists for three to ten days after the last dose. As with other oral anticoagulants, the usual precautions and laboratory controls must be observed. There is need for individualization of doses in accordance with the patient's response. In cases of overdosage, vitamin K_1 is an effective antidote, orally and parenterally.

Preparation

Bromindione Tablets   1, 2, and 5 mg.
Trade name: Halinone

Fibrinolysin (Plasmin) (Actase, Thrombolysin)

Fibrinolysin, a proteolytic enzyme, occurs in the blood in the form of a precursor, profibrinolysin, which is slowly inactivated by cell fragments and streptokinase (see p. 769). It causes the breakdown of a number of proteins including fibrinogen and fibrin and may release histamine. Fibrinolysin (human) is prepared for clinical use by the action of streptokinase on profibrinolysin (plasminogen) isolated from human plasma.

Side effects include fever, which frequently occurs, and allergic reactions such as rash, urticaria, and edema at times have been observed.

Fibrinolysin is used with anticoagulants to limit or dissolve fresh clots in thrombophlebitis, phlebothrombosis, and pulmonary embolism. Pain, inflammation, and edema are relieved.

The intravenous daily dose is 50,000 to 500,000 units given over a period of one to six hours. The dose may be repeated on one to three subsequent days. The powder is dissolved in 10 ml. of water and added to an intravenous infusion of dextrose.

Preparation

Fibrinolysin (human)   Vials containing 50,000 units
Trade names: Actase, Thrombolysin

Summary

In summary, there are two types of anticoagulants: the short acting and long acting. Hypoprothrombinemia may be maintained for long periods with small doses of the long-acting drugs. The advantage of using a short-acting anticoagulant is that the drug is rapidly eliminated if hemorrhage should occur. The synthetic anticoagulants may be given with heparin. In all cases, individual attention must be given to dosage and the effect on the coagulability must be adequately followed.

DIAGNOSTIC AIDS—BLOOD

Congo Red Injection

Congo red injection is a sterile solution of the aniline dye Congo red in water for injection. It is used as a diagnostic aid (e.g., in amyloidosis). The usual intravenous dose is 100 to 200 mg.

Preparation

Congo Red Injection   10 ml. containing 100 mg.

Evans Blue Injection, U.S.P.; Azovan Blue, B.P.

Evans blue injection is a sterile solution of the diazo dye Evans blue in water for injection. It is a diagnostic agent for the estimation of blood volume. The dye combines firmly with plasma albumin and leaves the circulation very slowly. In normal persons, the mixing of the dye is complete in nine minutes; in patients with congestive heart failure, 15 minutes may be required. A sample of blood is withdrawn, and the dilution of the dye in the blood is compared colorimetrically with the plasma of the patient before injection. This gives a quantitative indication of the volume of total circulating plasma.

Therapeutic Uses. The determination of the blood volume is important in detecting impending shock and as a guide to the amount of plasma or other fluids to be used to avoid inadequate or excessive dosage. Evans blue injection is used to determine blood volume in the pre- and postoperative management of chronically ill or debilitated patients.

Dosage and Method of Administration. The patient is fasted (to avoid lipemia), and the drug is administered intravenously. The intravenous dose is 25 mg. of dye in 5 ml. of a 0.5 per cent solution, diluted further with 1 to 2 ml. of isotonic sodium chloride solution. Before its administration, about 10 ml. of blood are withdrawn; 10 or 15 minutes after injection, another 10 ml. of blood are withdrawn for testing.

Preparation

Evans Blue Injection, U.S.P.   Ampuls containing 22.6 mg.

REVIEW QUESTIONS

1. *What substances are needed in the emergency treatment of shock? How do they benefit the patient?*
2. *When should whole blood be used in the treatment of shock, of anemia? When is it contraindicated in these two conditions?*
3. *Discuss the need for iron in health and disease. Express the range of dosage in number of grains.*
4. *Discuss the clinical picture and the cause of pernicious anemia.*
5. *Describe the roles of folic acid and vitamin B$_{12}$ in pernicious anemia.*
6. *What is the mode of action of menadione? In what conditions is it useful?*
7. *What nursing action needs to be taken when a patient is receiving vitamin K?*
8. *Compare and contrast heparin and bishydroxycoumarin including action, usual dosage, method of administration, duration of effect, and side and toxic reactions.*
9. *What drugs are given to counteract the effects of heparin and of coumarin type of drugs?*
10. *What laboratory test is used to determine the dosage of heparin and of bishydroxycoumarin?*
11. *What knowledge should the patient who is receiving long-term anticoagulant therapy have concerning his drug?*
12. *For what purposes are Congo red injection and Evans blue injection used?*

REFERENCES

Bowman, H. W.: "Clinical Evaluation of Dextran as a Plasma Volume Expander," *J.A.M.A.*, **153**:24, 1953.

Cecil, Russell L., and Loeb, Robert F. (eds.): *A Textbook of Medicine*, 11th ed. W. B. Saunders Company, Philadelphia, 1963.

Guis, John: *Fundamentals of General Surgery*, 2nd ed. The Yearbook Publishers, Chicago, 1962.

Harrison, T. R. (ed.): *Principles of Internal Medicine*, 4th ed. McGraw-Hill Book Company, New York, 1962.

Wintrobe, M. M.: "Blood Dyscrasias," *Am J. Nursing*, **60**:496, 1960.

————: *Clinical Hematology*, Lea & Febiger, Philadelphia, 1961.

————: "Principles in the Management of Anemias," *Bull. New York Acad. Med.* **30**:6, 1954.

BLOOD TRANSFUSIONS

Adriani, John: "Venipuncture," *Am. J. Nursing*, **62**:66, 1962.

Crouch, M. L., and Gibson, S. T.: "Blood Therapy," *Am. J. Nursing*, **62**:71, 1962.

Fuerst, E. V., and Wolff, L. V.: *Fundamentals of Nursing*. J. B. Lippincott Company, Philadelphia, 1956, pp. 452–59.

Harmer, Bertha, and Henderson, Virginia: *Textbook of the Principles and Practice of Nursing*, 5th ed. The Macmillan Company, New York, 1956, pp. 716–59.

McClaughey, R. L.: "Transfusion Reactions," *M. Clin. North America*, **46**:551, 1962.

Mervine, Charles K., and Schechter, D. C.: "The Prevention and Treatment of

Blood Transfusion Reactions," *The New Physician,* **11**:1, 1962.
Mollison, P. L.: *Blood Transfusion in Clinical Medicine,* 3rd ed. F. A. Davis Co.
Philadelphia, 1961.

IRON-DEFICIENCY ANEMIA

Adams, B. M.: "Iron Deficiency Anemia and Its Therapy," *Ped. Clin. North
America,* **8**:139, 1961.
Annotations: "Treatment of Iron-Deficiency Anaemia," *Brit. M. J.,* **2**:812, 1959.
Committee on Toxicology: "Accidental Iron Poisoning in Children," *J.A.M.A.,*
170:676, 1959.
Gubler, C. J.: "Absorption and Metabolism of Iron," *J.A.M.A.,* **123**:87, 1956.
Hagedorn, A. B.: "The Diagnosis and Treatment of Iron-deficiency Anemia," *M.
Clin. North America,* **40**:983, 1956.
Hayhoe, F. G. J.: "Iron Preparations for Anaemia," *Brit. M. J.,* **1**:1195, 1960.
Moore, C. V., and Dubach, R.: "Metabolism and Requirements of Iron in the
Human," *J.A.M.A.,* **162**:197, 1956.
Pritchard, J. A.: "Anemia in Obstetrics and Gynecology; An Evaluation of
Therapy with Parenteral Iron," *J.A.M.A.,* **175**:154, 1961.
Swan, H. T.: "Treatment of Iron Deficiency with Ferrous Fumarate," *Brit. M. J.,*
2:782, 1959.

IRON POISONING

Bannerman, R. M., and Callender, S. T.: "Effect of Desferrioxamine and D.T.P.A.
in Iron Overload," *Brit. M. J.,* **2**:1573, 1962.
Moeschlin, Sven, and Schnider, Urs: "Treatment of Primary and Secondary Hemo-
chromatosis and Acute Iron Poisoning with a New, Potent Iron-Eliminating
Agent (Desferrioxamine-B)," *New England J. Med.,* **269**:57, 1963.
"Today's Drugs, Treatment of Poisoning—2," *Brit. M. J.,* **2**:993, 1964.

PERNICIOUS ANEMIA

Annotations: "Oral Treatment of Pernicious Anaemia," *Brit. M. J.,* **2**:554, 1959.
Bethel, F. H.; Castle, W. B.; and Conley, C. L.: "Present Status of Treatment of
Pernicious Anemia," *J.A.M.A.,* **171**:2092, 1959.
Bull, F. E.; Campbell, D. C.: and Owen, C. A., Jr.: "The Diagnosis and Treatment
of Pernicious Anemia," *M. Clin. North America,* **40**:1005, 1956.
Glass, G. B. J.: "Applicability of Hydroxocobalamin as a Long-Acting Vitamin
B_{12}," *Nature, London,* **189**:138, 1961.
Reisner, E. H., Jr.; Weiner, L.; Schultone, M. T.; and Henck, E. A.: "Oral
Treatment of Pernicious Anemia without Intrinsic Factor," *New England J.
Med.,* **253**:502, 1955.
Special Article: "Present Status of Treatment of Pernicious Anemia," *J.A.M.A.,*
171:2092, 1959.
Suhrland, L. G., *et al.*: "Failure of Oral Therapy in the Maintenance of Pernicious
Anemia," *A.M.A. Arch. Int. Med.,* **104**:411, 1959.

ANTICOAGULANTS

Griffith, G. C.: "Anticoagulants in Cardiovascular Disease," *J. Am. Geriatric Soc.,*
2:719, 1954.

Marple, C. D., and McIntyre, M. J.: "Anticoagulant Therapy and Nursing Care," *Am. J. Nursing,* **56**:875, 1956.
Olwin, J. H.: "Principles of Anticoagulant Therapy and Their Application," *M. Clin. North America,* **39**:1, 1955.
Olwin, J. H., and Koppel, J. L.: "Anticoagulant Therapy," *Am. J. Nursing,* **64**:107, 1964.
Seaman, A. J.: "p-Bromindione: A Long-Acting Oral Anticoagulant," *J.A.M.A.,* **177**:712, 1961.
Sherry, S.; Fletcher, A. P.; and Alkjaersig, N.: "Fibrinolysis and Fibrinolytic Activity in Man," *Physiol. Rev.,* **39**:349, 1959.
Singer, M. M.; Fisch, S.; and DeGraff, A. C.: "Study of Bromindione, A New Anticoagulant," *J.A.M.A.,* **179**:150, 1962.

32

Drugs Acting on the Heart

Drugs may act on the heart in several ways. They are used clinically for the following purposes: (1) to slow or quicken the rate; (2) to correct or modify abnormal rhythms (arrhythmias); and (3) to increase the output by strengthening the contraction.

In general, there are two main conditions in which cardiac drugs are employed: (1) in treating heart failure and (2) in controlling arrhythmias.

CARDIAC DECOMPENSATION

Functioning as a pump, the heart propels blood through the arterial vessels to all parts of the body in order that the need of the cells for food, oxygen, and removal of waste products may be met. The body's need for blood varies greatly (sleep, extreme exercise), and the heart is able to increase its output accordingly in order to maintain an adequate circulatory rate. This potential for increase in functioning is known as cardiac reserve.

The mechanisms which are used to increase cardiac output include:

1. Increase in the heart rate.
2. Dilatation of the heart (an increase in the amount of blood in a chamber causing stretching of the myocardium which in turn produces stronger contractions—Starling's law).
3. Hypertrophy of the heart (increase in the size of the myocardial fibers).

Normally these mechanisms are used only when there is increased cellular need, e.g., during physical or emotional stress. However, when the heart is damaged, they are used to compensate for the damage during normal activity and thus the cardiac reserve is decreased. With severe anatomical or physiological alterations such as stenosed or insufficient valve, hypertension, or myocardial damage there is a point beyond which these mechanisms are not able to maintain effective heart action. This is known as cardiac decompensation. In a decompensated state the heart is unable to accept and pump to the arteries all of the blood that is presented to it from the veins, and the amount of blood that it does eject with each contraction of the ventricle is inadequate to meet the cellular needs of the body.

525

Many of the signs and symptoms a patient with cardiac decompensation presents are related to the congestion of blood in the veins and capillaries. As the venous pressure increases, engorgement of superficial veins and enlargement of the liver occur. Subcutaneous and pulmonary edema, ascites, and pleural effusion are all caused by fluid leaving the capillaries due to the increase in the venous pressure. Cyanosis which sometimes occurs is also related to the congestion of blood in the veins. As a result of the increased venous pressure the circulation time is slowed so that more than the normal amount of oxygen is removed from the blood and used by the cells. This causes an increased amount of carbon dioxide to be taken into the blood, which accounts for the bluish color of the skin and mucous membranes.

Cardiac decompensation is also known as congestive heart failure owing to the signs and symptoms which indicate congestion. It is not a disease but rather a complication of an underlying cardiac defect. The primary drug used in the treatment of congestive heart failure is one extracted from a plant of the digitalis group. If correctly used, a drug of this group will usually restore much functioning strength to the weakened heart muscle. Other drugs that are utilized, such as morphine, diuretics, and sedatives, assist in relieving symptoms but do not affect the heart directly.

ARRHYTHMIAS

The rate and rhythm of the normal heart is under the control of the sinoatrial (SA) node, a mass of neuromuscular tissue found in the right atrium. This node generates electric impulses at the rate of about 60 to 90 per minute in the adult and sends these impulses out across the adjacent atrial muscle in concentric waves, causing the atria to contract and thus empty their blood into the ventricles.

Part of the impulse traveling through the atrial musculature arrives at the atrioventricular (AV) node, which is located at the entrance of the electrical pathway to the ventricles. Once through the AV node, the impulse passes on down a special group of muscle fibers in the interventricular septum known as the *atrioventricular bundle*, or the bundle of His, which divides into two branches, one to each ventricle. Thus the impulse finally reaches the ventricular muscle. The impulse sweeps through the muscle fibers of the two ventricles simultaneously, causing them to contract in unison.

The SA and AV nodes receive autonomic innervation from both the parasympathetic (vagus nerve) and the sympathetic (accelerator nerve) systems. The function of the vagus is to slow not only the rate of impulse formation of the SA node but also the rate of transmission through the AV node, while the acceleration of the heart rate is under the control of the sympathetic fibers.

The electrical events and the anatomical structures involved in each contraction of the heart are shown in Figure 15. At the right of the diagram there is shown one complete cardiac cycle of the electrocardiogram (ECG). Each deviation of the ECG from the base line (P, Q, R, S, and T) represents the electrical activity of the heart that can be picked up by metal plates held against the skin of the body.

The P wave occurs as the electric impulse from the SA node spreads over the atria causing them to contract. Recession of this wave indicates relaxation of the atria. The impulse then passes through the AV node, down the AV bundle and bundle branches, and over the Purkinje network to the muscle fibers of the ventricles causing them to contract. The time required for the passage of the electric impulse from its inception in the SA node to the ventricular musculature is about one eighth to one fifth of a second. This may be measured upon the ECG and is known as the *P-R interval.*

The QRS complex indicates contraction of the ventricles. The duration of the QRS complex, representing the time between the activation of the first and last of the ventricular fibers, is less than one tenth of a second in normal hearts. Thus, all parts of the two ventricles receive the signal to contract (the electric impulse) practically simultaneously. At the beginning of the T wave, parts of the ventricular muscle, now relaxed, begin to repolarize themselves, and by the end of this wave virtually all fibers are poised electrically in such· a way as to be ready for the next excitation wave when it arrives from the SA node. The actual speed of conduction in the various tissues and pathways is given in the figure in millimeters per second.

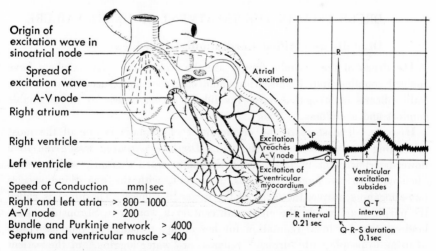

Fig. 15. Diagram showing the conduction system of the heart. Impulses are initiated at the sinoatrial node. As the wave of excitation travels through the conduction system, its relation to a tracing of a normal electrocardiogram is shown. (From Stackpole, C. E., and Leavell, L. C.: *Textbook of Physiology.* The Macmillan Company, New York, 1953.)

Any deviation from the orderly sequence described above is a disturbance of rhythm or an arrhythmia, and will cause changes in the ECG. These arrhythmias may be classified into two categories: (1) those caused by a disturbance in the impulse formation and (2) those caused by a disturbance in the impulse conduction. An example of the former is atrial fibrillation, one of the more common arrhythmias. In this situation there are no coordinated contractions or relaxations of the myocardium of the atria; rather there are rapid (about 400 per minute), irregular, uncoordinated contractions which cause the atria to quiver. The AV node is unable to handle this large number of impulses per minute so that only one out of every two to four impulses reach the ventricles. This in turn causes a rapid (100 to 200 per minute) ventricular rate. Many of the ventricular contractions are ineffective due to the very short diastolic period; so the apical pulse may be more rapid than the radial since only the effective contractions will cause a radial pulse.

An example of a disturbance in impulse conduction is atrioventricular block (heart block). Transmission of the impulses from the atria are either delayed or completely stopped at the AV node. If the impulses are completely blocked, then the ventricles respond to the AV bundle below the block beating independently of the atria at a slow rate.

Various drugs are used to correct arrhythmias. Those that act directly on the heart, such as quinidine, procainamide, digitalis, and isoproterenol (Isuprel), are discussed in this chapter. Other drugs are discussed in Chapters 29 and 38.

DRUGS USED IN THE TREATMENT OF HEART FAILURE

Digitalis and Allied Cardiotonic Glycosides

The drugs of the digitalis family are the most useful. Its members have enabled countless individuals, who would otherwise have succumbed to their failing hearts or struggled on as invalids, to live for decades in reasonable comfort and usefulness.

History.　The story of the development of digitalis is one of the most interesting in pharmacology. The name *Digitalis purpurea* was given to a flower-bearing plant in 1542, using the Latin word *digitalis*, which means "belonging to the finger" (*digitus*, a finger), with the qualifying species name meaning purple, the color of the finger-like flower. The plant is called the purple foxglove. In the eighteenth century a woman in Shropshire, England, acquired a local reputation for her ability to cause an increased flow of urine in people with "dropsy" (edema, or "water logging," of the patient with heart failure). Her medicine contained 20 different herbs. A noted physician, Dr. William Withering, heard of this concoction and its effects. He was able to purchase its formula from the owner, who had kept it a family secret for many years.

Because the concoction was known to produce nausea and vomiting, attention was focused on the digitalis ingredient, for it had long been known that this plant had been used to produce vomiting. Dr. Withering began in about 1775 to study the action and dosage of digitalis leaf preparations in cardiac failure. At first he thought that their action was upon the kidney because of the increased urinary flow and consequent loss of weight. We now know that this action is almost entirely upon the heart and insignificantly upon the kidneys.

Digitalis Leaf and Glycosides.   The leaves of *Digitalis purpurea* and other digitalis plants contain chemical substances known as glycosides. These are called *cardiotonic glycosides* because they stimulate the heart. They are characterized by the linkage of a sugar molecule, with a specific steroid molecule responsible for the action. The sugar portion of the molecule increases solubility and enables the glycoside to be fixed in the heart muscle.

In the leaves of *Digitalis purpurea* there are three principal cardiotonic glycosides. These are: (1) digitoxin, (2) gitoxin, and (3) gitalin. The other important digitalis species from which we derive glycosides for clinical use is *Digitalis lanata*. The cardiotonic glycosides contained in its leaves are called *lanatosides;* these are also three in number and are labeled A, B, and C. From lanatoside C there is derived another useful glycoside known as digoxin. All the glycosides mentioned above, with the exception of gitoxin, are used in clinical medicine.

In summary, the following digitalis preparations are in use: (1) whole leaf (from both purpurea and lanata), (2) digitoxin, (3) gitalin, (4) digoxin, and (5) lanatoside C.

Other Plants Containing Cardiotonic Glycosides.   *Strophanthus gratus* contains an active glycoside known as ouabain (G-strophanthin). From *Strophanthus kombé* a similar glycoside (K-strophanthin) is derived. Both these strophanthins are extremely rapid in action and are used in cardiac emergencies when minutes count. They are more freely used in Europe than in the United States. They must be administered intravenously and may be given in a dose of 0.6 mg., followed in two or three hours by 0.3 mg. and by 0.25 mg. every six hours for the first day and then 0.25 mg. every 12 hours. The physician usually orders a digitalis preparation as early as possible in order to maintain more conveniently the improvement provided by the rapidly acting strophanthin.

Urginea maritima, a plant known as squill, contains cardiotonic glycosides that are available commercially under the names urginin and scillaren. Still other plants, including the lily of the valley, and a poison obtained from certain species of toads have a tonic action on the heart, but they are not employed clinically.

Pharmacology of the Cardiotonic Glycosides. The digitalis glycosides enumerated above are responsible for the action of digitalis. If given alone, in purified form, each of the glycosides has the same general action. In the United States, digitoxin is used considerably more than the other glycosides. It has now been available for more than a decade, and the U.S.P. preparation is a mixture of glycosides containing 60 per cent or more of digitoxin. Thus it is not pure digitoxin like the French *digitaline Nativelle*. Its dose, as would be expected, is far less than that of the whole-leaf preparations—in fact, it is only one thousandth of that of the leaf. One-tenth milligram of digitoxin has approximately the same activity as 0.1 Gm. of the whole leaf.

The several cardiac glycosides vary in their onset and duration of action. At one end of the scale are certain strophanthins, which exert an appreciable effect in a matter of minutes, but which are rather rapidly destroyed in the body, so that at the end of an hour or two, little effect remains. At the other extreme are the whole-leaf preparations and digitoxin, which take six or more hours to achieve the maximal effect, but which are slowly eliminated and thus continue to exert an influence for two or three weeks. The other preparations—lanatoside C, digoxin, and gitalin—are immediate in their time of action.

The Response of the Heart to Digitalis. The manner in which the cardiotonic glycosides accomplish improvement in heart action is somewhat complicated. There are three primary actions:

1. An *inotropic* effect on the heart musculature (myocardium), increasing tone and the strength of contraction.

2. Stimulation of the vagus, both direct and reflexly, to produce slowing of the heart.

3. Depression of the conducting mechanism, causing a slowing down of the conduction of impulses from the atria to the ventricles.

The most important action is the strengthening of the heart musculature (myocardium). The digitalized fibers contract more vigorously and more completely than untreated fibers of a failing heart. The result is an increase in the amount of blood propelled at each contraction of the ventricles. The failing ventricles are usually distended, fatigued, and incapable of completely emptying at the time of contraction. After digitalization, they empty themselves more completely with each systole. In diastole (the rest period beween ventricular contractions) the atria, also strengthened by digitalis, are able to pump more blood into the empty ventricles. The exact mechanism by which digitalis increases the force of myocardial contraction is unknown, but it seems to be associated with a more efficient utilization of oxygen.

A less important but definite manner in which heart action is improved is the slowing of the rate of contraction. This has been called the *vagal action*. It is partly direct (effect on the center of the vagus) and partly reflex (effect on the myocardium plus the effect on receptors of the carotid body). This vagal branch of the parasympathetic nervous system sends some of its fibers to the heart for the purpose of slowing its rate when such action is needed. The action of digitalis through the vagus may be reflex, beginning with the circulatory improvement that results from the myocardial action of the glycosides, as described in the foregoing paragraph.

The arrhythmia *atrial fibrillation* may exist with no appreciable embarrassment or impediment to the circulation. If so, the heart is maintaining compensation even in the presence of this abnormal rhythm. The atria may be fibrillating at a rapid rate, perhaps 200 to 500, and the ventricles at a variable rate of 80 to 140 irregular contractions per minute. When failure accompanies this arrhythmia, and decompensation is present as described earlier, digitalis usually produces dramatic improvement and may completely restore compensation. In such failure, the ventricular rate is usually higher, up to 190. This excessive and wasteful rate contributes to heart fatigue and is usually easily reduced by digitalis and similar glycosides. The atrial rate is also slowed, although fibrillation may continue.

Through their depressant action on the AV node, the cardiac glycosides cause the ventricles to respond to fewer impulses reaching this node from the fibrillating atria. The dosage can be adjusted to bring the ventricular and pulse rates down to normal ones, 60 to 80. Excessive doses may depress these rates to 40 or 50, an undesirable condition. The slowing of the rate contributes to the increase in efficiency by allowing greater time for resting between beats (the diastolic period). Nutrition of the heart muscle, including oxygen requirements and removal of waste products, is improved. The ventricles can receive more blood in the longer diastole and can therefore propel more blood during systole. In some cases, digitalis causes reversion of the fibrillation to normal rhythm.

Other Responses of the Decompensated Heart to Digitalis. The size of the decompensated heart is nearly always larger than that of the compensated heart. Digitalis decreases the diastolic size of the organ and increases its output. Circulation is thus accelerated, and the distended veins are relieved of their excess of blood. The organs congested with excess blood are decongested, and edematous fluid in the organs or legs is gradually reabsorbed into the blood and excreted by the kidneys. The volume of urine excreted is thereby increased. Many pounds of weight may be lost from the water-logged body in which cardiac decompensation has been present for a long time. The lungs are usually congested with excess blood in heart failure, partly accounting for shortness of breath. This condition, causing pulmonary edema and cyanosis, is also reversed by digitalis. In terminal stages of heart disease. digitalis may fail to restore or maintain compensation.

Absorption and Excretion.   Digitalis preparations may be absorbed from the gastrointestinal tract in as few as two hours. The principal glycoside, digitoxin, is completely absorbed, and the oral and intravenous doses are the same. The glycosides accumulate in the body and then undergo a rather uniform rate of degradation. Their fate in the body is not completely under· stood.

Methods of Administration.   The digitalis preparations are given orally except in emergencies when they are injected intramuscularly or intravenously. The manner of regulating digitalis medication is much more exact and of a different nature than is that of most other drugs. There is an initial requirement for an adequate amount of cardiac glycoside in order to build up the necessary amount in the heart, which may be given at once or over a period of several days. This is known as the *digitalization* dose. Once the heart is digitalized, only a small daily *maintenance* dose is given in order to replace the amounts that are eliminated or destroyed.

Both initial digitalization and maintenance require rather critical dosage. The range of correct amounts is a narrow one. Too little of a digitalis preparation results in less than optimal cardiac improvement, and too much gives rise to toxic effects. The initial and maintenance doses are given in Table 35.

Effects of Overdosage with Digitalis.   The cardiotonic glycosides are capable of slowing the heart rate to an undesirably low one. The average maintenance dose of digitoxin may be too little for an occasional patient, yet too much for others. If, to a given individual, too large an amount of either a glycoside or whole-leaf preparation is administered, the pulse rate will be slowed excessively. Because of this, the pulse should always be taken before any digitalis preparation is administered. If the radial pulse is below 60, the apical pulse should be counted and both rates reported to the physician. The drug should be withheld until otherwise ordered. If the patient is in atrial fibrillation, the apical-radial pulse may be taken before the drug is given. The drug should be discontinued for a few days, and when the heart rate has increased to a satisfactory one, the daily dose may be resumed. It should be given in a moderately less amount, however, in order not to depress the heart rate again.

Low levels of potassium in the blood due to an inadequate diet, disease, or drug therapy (thiazide or mercurial diuretics, corticosteroids, or ammonium chloride) promote the action of cardiac glycosides and may contribute to digitalis toxicity. Patients on long-term therapy should be instructed to include in their diets foods which are high in potassium such as orange juice and bananas. When potassium deficiency is a contributory or causal factor, the administration of potassium salts is indicated (see p. 642).

Calcium is essential for the proper functioning of cardiac glycosides. How-

Table 35

Dosage and Onset and Duration of Action of Cardiotonic Glycosides

Preparation	Dose for Initial Digitalization* Oral†	Dose for Initial Digitalization* Intravenous	Daily Oral Maintenance Dose	Time of Action Onset	Time of Action Duration
Powdered Digitalis, U.S.P. (B.P., I.P.)	1.5 Gm. (1 to 2 Gm.)	—	100 mg. (100 to 200 mg.)	3-4 hr.	14-21 days
Digitalis Tincture, N.F. (I.P.)	10 to 15 ml.	—	1 ml.	3-4 hr.	14-21 days
Digitoxin, U.S.P. (I.P.)	1.0 to 1.5 mg.	1.0 to 1.5 mg.	0.05 to 0.2 mg.	Oral: 2-4 hr. I. v.: ½-2 hr.	14-21 days
Acetyldigitoxin (Acylanid)	1.0 to 2 mg.	—	0.1 to 0.2 mg.	8-10 hr.	9-12 days
Digoxin, U.S.P., B.P., I.P. (Lanoxin)	2.0 to 4.0 mg.	0.75 to 1.0 mg.	0.25 to 0.75 mg.	Oral: 1 hr. I. v.: 5-10 min.	3 days
Deslanoside, N.F. (Cedilanid D)	‡	1.6 (1.2 to 1.6 mg.)	‡	5-10 min.	2-3 days
Lanatoside C, N.F., I.P. (Cedilanid)	8 mg.	—	1 mg.	Variable	2-3 days
Ouabain, U.S.P., I.P.	‡	up to 0.5 mg.	‡	3-10 min.	1-3 days
K Strophanthin	‡	—	‡	3-10 min.	1-3 days
Gitalin, U.S.P.	4.0 to 8.0 mg.	—	0.25 to 1.0 mg.	2-4 hr.	7-10 days

* Average dose for adults with congestive heart failure, not having received digitalis in the preceding two weeks.
† In divided doses at six- to eight-hour intervals, over a period of 12 to 24 hours, if urgency of case necessitates.
‡ Not employed orally.

533

ever, high calcium blood levels will potentiate their activity and cause toxic effects. Edathamil disodium (Endrate Disodium) is administered intravenously in doses of 3 Gm. to lower the calcium level in the blood. It is a chelating agent which binds calcium and is then excreted in the urine.

Overdosage may cause a variety of arrhythmias of the heart, as, for example, premature contractions, *bigeminal rhythm* (with the beats grouped in pairs), ventricular tachycardia, or complete heart block. It may also cause side effects in areas other than the heart. These often warn the physician, as does the slow pulse or irregular rhythm, that intoxication has occurred. They may include nausea, vomiting, loss of appetite, abdominal cramps, and visual disturbances. Objects may appear brighter than they actually are. Green objects, particularly foliage, may appear almost white.

A lethal dose of digitalis produces death by causing the heart to stop, this being preceded by atrial standstill, fibrillation of the ventricles, or other disturbances.

Therapeutic Uses

1. In congestive heart failure with or without atrial fibrillation.

2. In atrial fibrillation. Digitoxin and its congeners may convert to normal SA rhythm or may merely reduce an excessively rapid ventricular response rate to a comfortable and more efficient one.

3. In atrial flutter. Digitoxin may convert this to fibrillation, which may, upon discontinuance of the drug, be replaced by a normal rhythm or again by flutter.

Preparations

Digitalis Capsules, N.F.	60 and 100 mg.
Digitalis Tablets, U.S.P., B.P., I.P.	30, 60, and 100 mg.
Digitoxin Injection, U.S.P.	0.2 mg. in 1 ml.
Digitoxin Tablets, U.S.P., B.P.	0.1 and 0.2 mg.

Trade names: Crystodigin; Digitaline; Purodigin

Acetyldigitoxin Tablets	0.2 and 0.5 mg.

Trade name: Acylanid

Gitalin Tablets, U.S.P.	0.5 mg.

Trade name: Gitaligin

Digoxin Injection, U.S.P., B.P., I.P.	0.5 mg. in 2 ml.
Digoxin Tablets, U.S.P., B.P., I.P.	0.25 and 0.5 mg.

Trade name: Lanoxin

Deslanoside Injection, U.S.P.	2- and 4-ml. ampuls, 0.2 mg. in 1 ml.

Trade name: Cedilanid-D

Lanatoside C Tablets, N.F., I.P.	0.5 mg.

Trade name: Cedilanid

Ouabain Injection, U.S.P.	0.25 mg. in 1 ml., 1- and 2-ml. ampuls

ANTIARRHYTHMIC AND ANTIFIBRILLATORY AGENTS

Quinidine Sulfate, U.S.P., I.P.; Quinidine Sulphate, B.P.

Quinidine and quinine are isomers occurring together as alkaloids in cinchona bark. Cinchona is a tropical tree whose powdered bark was long ago found to lower the fever in malaria. Quinine held a prominent place in this regard until the recently introduced synthetic antimalarials were developed (see Chap. 12).

A Dutch merchant, who used quinine while in malarious areas, found that the drug would also stop an irregularity of his heart. The specific arrhythmia, or disordered rhythm, present in this man was atrial fibrillation. He visited a noted Viennese physician, Dr. K. F. Wenckebach, in 1914, and demonstrated to him the controlling action of quinine on his cardiac irregularity. In 1918, quinidine, the dextrorotatory isomer of quinine, was found by Dr. W. Frey to be superior to quinine in the treatment of atrial fibrillation. Since that time quinidine has been widely used in this condition.

Pharmacological Actions.   Quinidine has a certain depressant activity on the myocardium, although it does not prevent it from contracting with normal strength. The depressant activity is more electrical in application, decreasing the number of times a given portion of myocardium can contract in a given period of time. In some way quinidine increases the *refractory period* that follows in the wake of a wave of contraction. We have seen that muscular contraction is immediately preceded and caused by an electric wave of excitation. In the brief period immediately following the contraction, an electrical neutrality exists, during which the muscle cannot again contract. This refractory period comes to a close automatically through certain biological readjustments within the muscle fiber, chiefly within its membrane wall. Following these adjustments, an electrical arrangement again exists, which will allow another excitation and contraction wave to occur. Ordinarily these biochemical changes occur in a fraction of a second. In the normal heart they are occurring with and following each heart beat. One can, with exercise, easily cause the heart to beat 120 times per minute, which, of course, means twice per second. We are thus dealing with a rapidly changing phenomenon.

In Atrial Fibrillation.   In the fibrillating atria, contraction waves pass over the atria several hundred times per minute. This is an undesirable rate and one to which the ventricles below cannot respond in kind. They do respond to more impulses than they normally receive; thus the rate is excessive and often irregular.

The rate of contraction is appreciably slowed by increasing the refractory period, making it impossible for a given segment of the atrial muscle to contract again, when stimulated. By careful control of the dosage, the accumulation of quinidine in the beating heart muscle can be adjusted to the amount required to eliminate the abnormal rhythm. The atria then resume their normal beating pattern in which one wave of excitation sweeps over their surfaces every second, or every two thirds of a second, causing them to beat in unison. Each atrium pumps blood into its respective ventricle and then rests until another excitation wave passes over and through it in due time.

Therapeutic Uses

1. In atrial fibrillation. It may terminate the fibrillation and restore normal rhythm more readily when the arrhythmia is not of long duration.

2. To establish normal rhythm in other conditions of cardiac irritability such as extrasystoles, tachycardia, and atrial flutter.

Dosage and Method of Administration. Schedules of administration vary among physicians. In order to detect any unusual sensitivity on the part of the patient, a test dose of 100 mg. is sometimes given before intensive therapy is started. If no untoward effects such as vomiting, perspiration, hives, purpura, or asthma occur in 6 to 12 hours, a dose of 200 mg. is given every four hours. When an attempt is made to treat atrial fibrillation, usually the quinidine dosage is increased gradually up to 600 mg. every two or three hours until conversion occurs or toxic symptoms are noted. Owing to its short action time, it is necessary that the drug be administered on a definite time schedule in order to maintain or increase the blood level required. Since the action of the drug changes the rate and rhythm of the heart, the pulse may be utilized as an index of its effectiveness; however, the ECG results are more accurate. If regular rhythm results, a maintenance dose of 200 mg. four times a day may be given for several days or weeks. No tolerance to the drug has been observed. In many cases, attempts to restore normal rhythm are fruitless and the drug must be abandoned.

Toxic Reactions. These effects may be caused by hypersensitivity to the drug or by overdosage. The symptoms include visual disturbances, ringing in the ears, vertigo, nausea, vomiting, abdominal cramps, and diarrhea. The more serious effects are respiratory depression and vascular collapse. Asthma, depression of breathing, and respiratory arrest may occur. Cardiac arrhythmias such as extrasystoles, ventricular fibrillation, and cardiac arrest due to heart block have been observed.

The treatment of these reactions is symptomatic. The drug must be stopped or dosage reduced. Artificial respiration as well as respiratory and circulatory stimulants are indicated. Quinidine therapy requires experience and close observation, including electrocardiographic monitoring.

Preparations

Quinidine Sulfate Capsules, N.F.	200 mg.
Quinidine Sulfate Tablets, U.S.P., B.P., I.P.	200 mg.

Two new preparations containing quinidine have been introduced for the treatment of cardiac arrhythmias. Their uses and side effects are the same as those for quinidine sulfate.

Approved and Trade Names	Dose	Preparations
Quinidine Gluconate (Quinaglute)	Orally: 2 tablets three or four times a day. Maintenance dose: 1 to 2 tablets every 10 to 12 hours	Dura-Tabs 330 mg.
Quinidine Polygalactu-ronate (Cardioquin)	Orally: 1 to 3 tablets initially. Maintenance dose: 1 tablet two or three times daily	Tablets 275 mg.

Procainamide Hydrochloride, U.S.P., B.P. (Pronestyl)

This derivative of procaine is useful for the treatment of certain ventricular and atrial arrhythmias and premature contractions. It has been used intravenously during surgery to control disturbances in rhythm. When given intravenously, it may cause lowering of blood pressure, owing to dilatation of blood vessels.

Dosage and Methods of Administration. The oral or intramuscular dose is 1 Gm. (500 mg. to 2 Gm.) four times a day.

Preparations

Procainamide Hydrochloride Capsules, U.S.P.	250 mg.
Procainamide Hydrochloride Injection, U.S.P., B.P.	1 Gm. in 10 ml.

Trade name: Pronestyl

Isoproterenol (Isuprel)

Isoproterenol is the drug of choice in the treatment of heart block and Adams-Stokes syndrome. It stimulates the SA node, the normal pacemaker of the atria, and accelerates the heart rate in severe bradycardia without increasing peripheral resistance. In addition isoproterenol enhances AV conduction, stimulates the ventricular pacemaker, and increases the ventricular rate.

The advantages of its use over other sympathomimetic amines are that it can be given sublingually and does not produce a rise in blood pressure nor does it cause ventricular fibrillation or tachycardia, which may occur with epinephrine. For dosage and preparations see page 462.

OTHER ANTIARRHYTHMIC AGENTS

Neostigmine has been used to arrest atrial tachycardia by stimulation of the vagus. The subcutaneous dose is 0.5 mg., or intravenous infusions may be required. Nausea and vomiting may be produced. Potassium deficiency may contribute to or cause arrhythmias, whereupon administration of potassium chloride may rectify the condition (see p. 642).

Slow cardiac arrhythmias, which may be as serious as rapid ones, are treated with certain sympathomimetic amines, such as ephedrine, epinephrine, and mephentermine, or with atropine sulfate. Sodium lactate infusions stimulate the heart and increase its rate, especially in Adams-Stokes attacks or when blood potassium levels are high.

REVIEW QUESTIONS

1. *In what ways may drugs affect the heart?*
2. *List the features that may be present in cardiac decompensation.*
3. *Discuss the actions of digitoxin and other digitalis glycosides in the treatment of decompensation.*
4. *Discuss the action of digitoxin in atrial fibrillation with an excessively rapid ventricular response rate.*
5. *Discuss the use of quinidine.*
6. *What are the fields of use of procainamide?*
7. *What are the dangers involved in the use of digitoxin and quinidine?*
8. *A patient receiving 0.2 mg. of digitoxin daily, to prevent the recurrence of heart failure, has a pulse rate of 48 to 56, with some intermittent irregularity. What may account for these findings?*

REFERENCES

CARDIAC PHYSIOLOGY AND FAILURE

Ashman, R., and Hull, E.: *Essentials of Electrocardiography*, 2nd ed. The Macmillan Company, New York, 1941.

Bing, R. J.; Danforth, W. H.; and Ballard, F. B.: "Physiology of the Myocardium," *J.A.M.A.*, **172**:438, 1960.

Blumgart, H. L. (ed.): *Symposium on Congestive Heart Failure*. The American Heart Association, New York, 1960.

Friedberg, C. K.: *Diseases of the Heart*, 2nd ed. W. B. Saunders Company, Philadelphia, 1956.

Luckey, E. H., and Rubin, A. L.: "The Correction of Hyponatremia in Congestive Heart Failure," *Circulation*, **21**:229, 1960.

Tocker, A. M.; Parmley, V. S.; Arbulu, A.; et al.: "Cardiac Resuscitation," *J. Kansas Med. Soc.*, **60**:443, 490, and 512, 1959.

DIGITALIS AND THERAPY OF CARDIAC FAILURE

Blumgart, H. L., and Zoll, P. M.: "The Clinical Management of Congestive Heart Failure," *Circulation*, **21**:218, 1960.

Friedman, M.; St. George, S.; and Bine, R.: "The Behavior and Fate of Digitoxin in the Experimental Animal and Man," *Medicine*, **33**:15, 1954.

Frohman, I. P.: "Digitalis and Its Derivatives," *Am. J. Nursing*, **57**:172, 1957.

Lown, B., *et al.*: "Digitalis and Atrial Tachycardia with Block," *Am. Pract. and Digest. Treat.*, **10**:2124, 1959.

Somlyo, A. P.: "The Toxicology of Digitalis," *Am. J. Cardiol.*, **5**:523, 1960.

Withering, W.: *An Account of the Foxglove and Some of Its Medicinal Uses: With Practical Remarks on Dropsy and Other Diseases.* C. G. J. and J. Robinson, London, 1785. Reprinted in *Medical Classics*, **2**:305, 1937.

THERAPY OF ARRHYTHMIAS

Bellet, S.: Current Concepts in Therapy. "Drug Therapy in Cardiac Arrhythmias, I.," *New England J. Med.*, **262**:769, 1960.

Friedberg, C. K.; Kahn, M.; Scheuer, J.; Bleifer, S.; and Dack, S.: "Adams-Stokes Syndrome Associated with Chronic Heart Block, Treatment with Corticosteroids," *J.A.M.A.*, **172**:1146, 1960.

Schwartz, S. P., and Schwartz, L. S.: "The Effects of Isuprel on Patients with the Adams-Stokes Syndrome During Normal Sinus Rhythm and Transient Heart Block," *Am. Heart J.*, **57**:849, 1959.

Smith, K. Shirley: "Drug Treatment of Disease: Cardiac Arrythmias," *Brit. M. J.*, **1**:628, 1960.

QUINIDINE SULFATE

Richardson, D. W.; Zee, M. E.; and Wyso, E. M.: "Maintenance Quinidine Therapy," *Am. J. Cardiol.*, **5**:417, 1960.

Sokolow, M.: "Some Quantitative Aspects of Treatment with Quinidine," *Ann. Int. Med.*, **45**:582, 1956.

Weisman, S. A.: "A Review and Evaluation of Quinidine Therapy for Auricular Fibrillation," *J.A.M.A.*, **152**:496, 1953.

PROCAINAMIDE HYDROCHLORIDE

Kayden, H. J.; Brodie, B. B.; and Steele, J. M.: "Procaine Amide—A Review," *Circulation*. **15**:118, 1957.

33

Drugs Acting on the Blood Vessels

Abnormal conditions affecting the arteries, arterioles, capillaries, and veins are many in number and variety. In the present chapter, we shall consider the drugs used in treating the following conditions: (1) angina pectoris, (2) coronary occlusion or insufficiency, (3) spastic arterial states, and (4) atherosclerosis.

Drugs may dilate arterioles by (1) direct action upon the smooth muscle of their walls or (2) interruption of the nerve impulses traveling to them from the vasoconstrictor center by way of the sympathetic nerves. Only the first of these methods is generally used in dilating the coronary arteries and arterioles which supply the heart muscle. Both methods are employed in the treatment of high blood pressure and in spastic arterial conditions of the hands, feet, and legs.

ATHEROSCLEROSIS

Atherosclerosis is a condition which affects primarily the large- and medium-sized arteries. Thickening of the intima due to the deposit of atheromatous plaques causes narrowing and even occlusion of the vessels. The underlying pathogenesis of atherosclerosis is not yet clearly understood. Probably the most widely accepted theory is that of a disturbance in the metabolism of lipids or lipoproteins. In relation to this theory, research has indicated that by reduction of the saturated fats in the diet, the cholesterol blood levels can be reduced. This has caused the development of many commercial products which contain polyunsaturated fats rather than the saturated ones. However, it cannot be said at the present time that a reduction of blood cholesterol will prevent atherosclerosis. Many other related areas are being studied including hormonal relationships, mechanical factors, and racial and hereditary aspects. Thus far there are no clinically used drugs which reverse or prevent the formation of atheromatous lesions.

The diseases associated with this condition cause more deaths in the United States than any other group of diseases. They include angina pectoris, coronary occlusion with myocardial infarction, cerebrovascular accidents, and peripheral atherosclerosis. Although they occur in different parts of the body, these diseases have the same pathogenesis and thus have common symptoms

540

related to the narrowing of the vessels. Pain, for instance, occurs when the needs of the muscle for oxygen are not met. This pain can be relieved by dilating the narrowed vessel or by decreasing the muscle's needs. Thus, rest and vasodilators are used in the treatment of all the diseases mentioned above.

If the vessel is completely occluded, death of the tissue occurs and inadequate functioning of the organ is seen. A vasodilator is used in this situation in the hope that subdivisions of another artery entering the deprived segment of tissue may be dilated and permitted to carry extra blood to nourish the affected area. By increasing the collateral circulation to the infarcted areas, the amount of permanent damage to the tissue may be decreased.

MEASURES FOR LOWERING BLOOD CHOLESTEROL

An effective but not a very extensively used agent for lowering blood cholesterol is nicotinic acid or niacin (a vitamin of the B complex; see p. 710). It causes flushing at first, but doses of 3 to 6 Gm. daily in divided amounts orally may be given for long periods of time with apparent safety and continued effect.

Another agent for the reduction of blood cholesterol is a 20 per cent suspension of beta-sitosterols (Cytellin), the sterols of certain plants. It is used in a dose of 15 to 30 ml. before meals. It is thought to suppress absorption of cholesterol from the intestines, but reports have been conflicting and it is not widely used.

Aluminum Nicotinate (Nicalex)

Aluminum nicotinate (Nicalex), an aluminum salt of nicotinic acid, is hydrolyzed slowly and uniformly in the gastrointestinal tract to nicotinic acid and aluminum hydroxide which provides a buffering action. The effectiveness of nicotinic acid in the treatment of hypercholesteremia has been well established. Aluminum nicotinate in doses of two to four tablets three times a day with or after meals provides the same therapeutic effects in reducing blood cholesterol levels with a markedly reduced incidence of annoying side effects such as flushing, itching, gastrointestinal distress, and nervousness associated with the administration of nicotinic acid. It should not be administered to patients with liver or gallbladder disease or peptic ulcer.

Preparation

Aluminum Nicotinate Tablets   625 mg. equivalent to 500 mg. nicotinic acid.

Trade name: Nicalex

Sodium Dextrothyroxin (Choloxin)

There are two isomers of thyroxin, levothyroxin and dextrothyroxin. Levothyroxin (see p. 674) is used for the treatment of hypothyroidism.

Dextrothyroxin is much less active in raising the metabolic rate. It reduces blood cholesterol levels and is used in the treatment of hypercholesteremia associated with arteriosclerosis and atherosclerosis, hypothyroidism, and other causes. The oral dose of 2 mg. given daily for 10 to 14 days may be increased to 4 mg. daily, if required.

Preparation

Sodium Dextrothyroxin Tablets   2 mg.
Trade name: Choloxin

NITRATES AND NITRITES

The organic nitrates and the inorganic and organic nitrites are vasodilator drugs which are used clinically. These drugs may be divided into two groups: (1) the rapidly and short-acting ones and (2) those with slow onset and prolonged activity. Among the first group are nitroglycerin (glyceryl trinitrate) and two drugs, amyl nitrite and octyl nitrite, whose vapors are inhaled. The pharmacological and other features of these agents are sufficiently similar that they are described for the entire group.

In contrast to the organic nitrates, which have a powerful relaxant effect on smooth muscle, the inorganic nitrates have no such action, even in many times the dose of the organic ones. The inorganic nitrates are simple salts of the same category as table salt and are excluded from the present discussion of organic nitrates and nitrites. Inorganic nitrites, on the other hand, have a relaxant effect on smooth muscle.

Pharmacological Actions. The nitrates and nitrites cause the smooth muscle of the blood vessel wall to relax in all arterioles and veins. They act directly on this smooth muscle. Thus the blood flows more readily through the dilated arterioles, and as a result, the blood pressure in the arteries falls. The sum of all arterioles in the body ordinarily acts as a control in the circulation of the blood. Arterioles can, by constriction, hold back some of the blood they otherwise allow to flow into the capillaries beyond. The aggregate of the capillaries constitutes a large reservoir with a volume far exceeding that of the arteries. The arterioles may be considered as a dam with a head of pressure on one side (the arteries) and a huge network (the capillaries) of tubes with a very low pressure on the other side.

It is by relaxing the arteriolar control that these agents cause the delivery of more blood to the overworked heart muscle. However, since this also happens throughout the circulation, the blood pressure falls. This ability to lower blood pressure is undesirable in most cases of angina, but we sometimes take advantage of this action in cases of hypertension.

The nitrates and the nitrites also relax the smooth muscles of the gastrointestinal tract, bronchioles, biliary tract, and urinary tract.

Routes of Administration and Rate and Duration of Response.
These drugs are all rapidly absorbed through the mucous membranes of the mouth, gastrointestinal tract, and lungs. The various preparations differ in rapidity and duration of response. The sublingual administration of nitroglycerin produces, in one to two minutes, effects that may last up to 30 minutes. Amyl nitrite and octyl nitrite, which are volatile liquids, are given by inhalation, and the effects are noted in a few seconds and last for five to ten minutes. Sodium nitrite is administered orally and is effective in 5 to 20 minutes, the duration of response being one to two hours. The responses obtained from the oral administration of the remaining nitrates occur in 15 to 20 minutes and last three to four hours. Some authorities do not consider the orally employed nitrates useful in angina.

Tolerance. The smallest effective dose of the nitrates and nitrites should be given at all times, especially in the beginning, since the desired therapeutic effects diminish with too frequent doses. Tolerance, which may be marked in the first two or three weeks, is lost rapidly. If the drug is discontinued for two or three weeks, the former initial dose is again effective. Therefore, when tolerance develops in nitrate or nitrite therapy, the drug can be discontinued. Some other vasodilator may be substituted for a few weeks, and then treatment with a nitrate or nitrite may be resumed with the smallest effective dose. Although tolerance may occur, these drugs are not habit forming. These factors should be explained to the patient so that he will not avoid or postpone needed use of the drug because of the fear of addiction.

Therapeutic Uses

1. In angina pectoris to relieve or prevent anginal pain. They are the most important drugs used for this purpose.
2. In biliary colic as an antispasmodic to relieve pain.
3. In bronchial asthma.
4. In cyanide poisoning.
5. For high blood pressure. The longer-acting organic nitrates are used in these conditions.

Side Effects. Among the undesirable features, a chief disturbance is the lowering of blood pressure. This sudden hypotension is variable in degree from mild to severe. It may be unnoticed by some patients, whereas it may be great enough to cause fainting in other individuals. Lightheadedness, dizziness, weakness, and similarly described feelings are caused by this lowering of blood pressure. Headache may be a pronounced symptom. It is frequently encountered until the patient's tolerance of the drug increases. When therapy with any of these drugs is begun, the patient should be informed of the possible side effects and encouraged to sit when he takes the drug.

Toxicity. Acute fatal poisoning with nitrates or nitrites is rare. However, large doses will produce circulatory collapse, which is characterized by flushing of the face and neck, headache, throbbing in the head, a marked fall in blood pressure, a soft, thready pulse, and fainting. Inadequate blood flow to the brain, when the pressure is very low, may be the cause of death. Methemoglobinemia would be contributory.

Methemoglobin Formation. Methemoglobin, in which the iron atom has been oxidized from the *ferrous* to the *ferric* state, may be produced by large doses of the nitrites; hence, the oxygen-carrying power of the blood may be reduced, resulting in hypoxia. This action, which is reversible, rarely occurs with therapeutic use of the drugs. The methemoglobinemia of the nitrites, etc., may be treated by the intravenous administration of methylene blue. One milligram of this dye per kilogram of body weight may be given intravenously in severe poisoning. Vitamin C (see p. 713) orally or intravenously may be used in less severe cases.

Amyl Nitrite, U.S.P., I.P. (Isoamyl Nitrite)

This organic nitrite is a volatile liquid. Upon inhalation it provides a rapid action of short duration and is used in the relief of acute attacks of angina. Amyl nitrite is sold in thin-walled glass ampuls enclosed in loosely woven fabric. The ampul is broken when needed and the vapor inhaled. Other people in the immediate vicinity may also inhale the drug and experience the side effects. The drug has a strong, unpleasant odor.

Nitroglycerin (Glyceryl Trinitrate), U.S.P.

Glyceryl trinitrate, popularly called *nitroglycerin,* is a triple nitrate of glycerin. It is considered the drug of choice in the treatment of angina. Patients are usually advised to carry the drug with them and take it as needed as soon as the pain begins, or one or two tablets may be taken before physical exertion or emotional strain to prevent attacks. Tablets of the drug may be placed under the tongue, where they are dissolved in the saliva and absorbed through the thin membrane of the floor of the mouth and the lower surface of the tongue. Within one to two minutes enough of the drug will have reached the blood and have been carried to the walls of the arterioles of the heart to begin relaxing them and to give relief from the pain. Within a few minutes after all the tablet is absorbed, the drug is metabolized and rendered inactive. The pain may not return immediately, and repetition of the dose will not be necessary. If the pain does return, or if it was only partially relieved and grows severe again, the dose may be repeated as soon as needed. The drug may be given every 15 minutes, if required.

The usual sublingual dose of nitroglycerin is 0.4 mg. with a range of 0.2 to

0.6 mg. up to ten times a day; however, the smallest effective dose should be used. Some patients can use a large number of tablets a day without headache or annoying fall in blood pressure and remain free from angina. The drug tends to deteriorate with age and in the presence of light. For this reason it is dispensed in dark bottles.

Preparations

Nitroglycerin Tablets, U.S.P.
Glyceryl Trinitrate Tablets, B.P. (I.P.)   0.3, 0.4, and 0.6 mg.
                    Trade names: Glonoin; Trinitrin; Trinitrol

Delayed-Release Tablets   2.5 and 5 mg.
                    Trade name: Nitroglyn

Other Organic Nitrates

Other organic nitrates are administered orally for a slower and more prolonged effect. Since the onset of the action of these drugs is slow, they are not effective in acute anginal attacks. At the present time their primary use is in the prevention of attacks. Tolerance to them may develop in a short period of time. Although these drugs are widely employed as prophylactic agents, their effectiveness is still questionable.

Preparations and Dosage

Erythrityl Tetranitrate (Cardilate, Eryth-rol, Tetranitrol)	15 to 60 mg. every four to six hours	Tablets: 15 and 30 mg.
Isosorbide Dinitrate (Isordil)	10 mg. four times a day	Tablets: 10 mg.
Mannitol Hexanitrate (Nitranitol)	15 to 60 mg. every four to six hours	Tablets: 15, 30, 32, and 60 mg.
Pentaerythritol Tetranitrate, B.P. (Angicap, Peritrate)	10 to 20 mg. every four to six hours	Tablets: 10 and 20 mg.
Triethanolamine Trinitrate (Metamine, Nitretamin)	2 mg. three times a day to 10 mg. twice a day	Tablets: 2 and 10 mg. (sustained release), 10 mg.

Dipyridamole (Persantin)

Dipyridamole (Persantin) is a coronary dilator unrelated to the nitrates. It is used in the treatment of coronary and myocardial insufficiency. In therapeutic doses, the drug does not affect the peripheral arteries and thus does not cause more widespread therapeutic effects such as the lowering of blood pressure. It may be used for long-term prophylaxis.

The side effects noted are headache, dizziness, nausea, vomiting, flushing, weakness and fainting. These are minimal and transient.

Dipyridamole is given orally or intravenously. The oral dose is 25 to 50 mg. two or three times a day before meals. The intravenous dose is 10 mg. once or twice daily.

Preparations

Dipyridamole Injection	10 mg. in 1 ml.
Dipyridamole Tablets	25 mg.

PAPAVERINE AND DIOXYLINE

Opium contains, besides the morphine-codeine group of alkaloids, an un-related group, the chief member of which is papaverine.

Papaverine Hydrochloride, N.F., B.P.

Papaverine has been found to have a relaxing effect on smooth muscle and is thus an antispasmodic drug. It has been used extensively in the belief that it would increase the blood flow through the arterioles as in angina and embolism. The usual intravenous or intramuscular dose is 30 mg. (30 to 60 mg.), although many authorities advise several times this amount. The value of papaverine in coronary artery disease is disputed.

Preparation

Papaverine Hydrochloride Injection, U.S.P., B.P., I.P.	1-, 2-, and 10-ml. ampuls containing 30 mg. in 1 ml.

Dioxyline Phosphate (Paveril)

Dioxyline is a synthetic drug that is closely related to papaverine and used for the same conditions. The usual oral dose is 200 mg. three or four times a day.

Preparation

Dioxyline Phosphate Tablets	200 mg.

Trade name: Paveril

OTHER AGENTS IN ANGINA PECTORIS

Since 1958 certain monoamine oxidase inhibitors (see p. 349) have been used for the relief of angina. The agents are now used as psychic stimulants in mental depressions, and some workers believe that elevation of the mood may cause patients with angina to be less aware of their discomfort and thus endanger the heart. Removal of the warning pain without increasing the blood flow is undesirable.

Various sedatives, such as phenobarbital, and tranquilizing drugs, such as the phenothiazines and reserpine, are used to relieve anxiety and nervous tension in persons with angina pectoris.

PERIPHERAL VASCULAR DISEASE

In certain diseases (for example, *Buerger's disease, Raynaud's syndrome*), the arterioles in the toes, feet, lower legs, or fingers are in a chronic or intermittent state of spasm. Pain, ulcerations, and other conditions ensue. The cause is often a greatly increased and sustained sympathetic vasoconstrictor tone. In thrombophlebitis, an inflammatory or infectious condition in certain veins wherein blood clotting occludes the vessel, relaxing drugs and procedures are indicated because spasm in the neighboring uninvolved veins is produced by the disease. Vasodilators are also used for frostbite of the feet and hands; trench foot or immersion foot, which were wartime conditions; and other spastic or thrombotic (clot-producing) and embolic conditions. An embolus is produced by the dislodgment and circulation of a clot to a distant location in the pulmonary or systemic arterial tree.

Drugs used in the treatment of the above group of vascular diseases are of three types, depending on the site of action. The most important group is that composed of adrenergic blocking agents (see Chap. 28). In addition, drugs that have a direct dilating action on the blood vessel wall and those which produce some vasodilation by an action upon the vasomotor mechanisms within the central nervous system are used.

ADRENERGIC BLOCKING AGENTS

The drugs most valuable in peripheral vascular disease at the present time are those that are capable of blocking the passage of nerve impulses from the ends of the vasoconstrictor sympathetic fibers to the smooth musculature of the arterioles. The chief members of this group are presented in Chapter 28. They are tolazoline, phentolamine, azapetine, and phenoxybenzamine.

OTHER VASODILATOR AGENTS

Nylidrin Hydrochloride, N.F. (Arlidin)

This is a sympathomimetic amine (see p. 461) that dilates the arterioles, especially in the skeletal muscles. It is used in the treatment of inadequate circulation of the limbs, eyes, and inner ear (in vertigo). The side effects observed are nervousness and palpitation. These are usually transient with continued use. The oral dose is 6 to 12 mg. three or four times a day. The intramuscular or subcutaneous dose is 0.5 to 1 ml. one or more times daily.

It is available as tablets (N.F.) of 6 mg.; in ampuls and vials containing 5 mg. in 1 ml. (Nylidrin Hydrochloride Injection, N.F.).

Isoxsuprine (Vasodilan)

This is also a sympathomimetic amine. It is used in peripheral vascular disease. It may relax the uterus in dysmenorrhea and threatened abortion. The side effects are the same as those for nylidrin. The oral dose is 10 to 20 mg. four times a day. The intramuscular dose is 5 to 10 mg. every four hours. Tablets of 10 mg. and an injection containing 5 mg. in 1 ml. are available.

Cyclandelate (Cyclospasmol)

This drug relaxes the smooth muscles of the blood vessels directly. The oral dose in peripheral vascular disease is 100 to 200 mg. four times a day. The side effects are nausea and vomiting. Tablets of 100 mg. are marketed.

Nicotinyl Alcohol Tartrate (Roniacol)

This drug also produces direct vasodilatation (see nicotinic acid, p. 710). The side effects are flushing and palpitation. The oral dose is 50 to 150 mg. three times a day after meals. Tablets of 50 mg. and an elixir containing 50 mg. in 5 ml. are available.

ADDITIONAL DRUGS

Alcohol is a well-known vasodilator although it is not ordinarily used as such in vasospastic states. Its pharmacological actions and uses are discussed in Chapter 22. Histamine, another vasodilator, and papaverine, dioxyline, and the nitrates are sometimes used. Reserpine or other *Rauwolfia* preparations may be useful, since they reduce peripheral sympathetic activities.

THE DRUG THERAPY OF MIGRAINE

Ergotamine Tartrate, U.S.P., B.P., I.P. (Gynergen)

Ergotamine, one of the alkaloids obtained from ergot, is produced by a fungus that grows on rye. It is one of the oldest drugs known to prevent the blood pressure–raising effect of epinephrine, but it is not ordinarily used for this purpose. It causes contraction of smooth muscle and is used in migraine by virtue of this action. Ergotoxine, which has the same actions as ergotamine, and other alkaloids of ergot are discussed on pages 602, 603. Ergotamine tartrate is a white crystalline powder.

Pharmacological Actions. *On the Blood Pressure.* A rise in blood pressure is produced by the intravenous injection of ergotamine, owing to its direct action on the smooth muscle of the arteries and arterioles.

On the Uterus. Ergotamine tartrate increases the tone and strength of uterine contractions and checks uterine bleeding. However, the drug has been replaced in obstetrics by ergonovine (Ergotrate). Its main use in medicine today is in the treatment of migraine.

Use in Migraine. Migraine is a periodic, excruciating headache which is often associated with emotional factors and which is accompanied by dilatation of cerebral arterioles and later by edematous swelling of their walls. Such a headache is usually on one side of the head and is often preceded by visual and gastric disturbances, such as nausea and vomiting. The pain may extend to the face, shoulders, neck, arms, and back. There is usually a sensation of throbbing in the head. The amplitude of contractions of the cerebral vessels is increased and pain is experienced. Ergotamine acts directly on the smooth muscle of the cerebral vessels and reduces the amplitude of contraction, thus reducing or abolishing the pain. The value of ergotamine lies in its constricting action on the dilated arterioles. Its usefulness is greatest at the beginning of the attack.

Dosage and Methods of Administration. The usual intramuscular dose of ergotamine tartrate is 0.25 to 0.5 mg., which may be repeated in an hour, if necessary. Relief is obtained in one-half hour in some cases. The usual dose is 2 mg. (1 to 6 mg.), followed by 1 mg. every half to one hour, if necessary, for five hours. The sublingual dose is 0.5 to 4 mg. An aerosol is available for inhalation. The absorption from this type of administration is very prompt. The patient should lie in a quiet, dark room.

The prophylactic use of ergotamine is not recommended, since ergotism or poisoning (p. 602) may result with continued use. The drug is contraindicated in vascular disease, hypertension, and pregnancy.

Preparations

Ergotamine Tartrate Tablets, U.S.P., B.P.	1 mg.
Ergotamine Tartrate Injection, U.S.P.; Ergotamine Injection, B.P.	0.5- and 1-ml. ampuls containing 0.5 mg. in 1 ml.
Ergotamine Tartrate Inhaler	9 mg. in 1 ml., 2.5-ml. vials
Cafergot Tablets	1 mg. of ergotamine and 100 mg. of caffeine

Trade names: Ergomar; Gynergen; Femergen; Medihaler-Ergotamine

Side Effects. These include nausea, vomiting, muscular weakness, leg pain, numbness, and paresthesias.

OTHER DRUGS USED IN THE TREATMENT OF MIGRAINE
Dihydroergotamine (D.H.E. 45)

Dihydroergotamine, which is obtained by hydrogenating (reducing) ergotamine, is also useful in the treatment of migraine. It is less toxic than ergotamine, and the incidence of side effects is less than with that drug. The usual intramuscular or intravenous dose is 1 mg. It may be repeated in one to two hours.

Preparation

Dihydroergotamine Injection   1-ml. ampuls containing 1 mg.

Serotonin Antagonist

Methysergide Maleate (Sansert) is used in the prophylactic treatment of vascular headaches including migraine and histamine headaches. The side effects are gastrointestinal disturbances and dizziness. The drug should be used with care in coronary artery disease and severe hypertension. Contra-indications to its use are pregnancy, peripheral vascular disease, and atherosclerosis.

The average daily dose is two to four tablets, preferably one tablet with each meal.

Preparation

Methysergide Maleate Tablets   2 mg.

Trade name: Sansert

Aspirin, phenacetin, and codeine are sometimes useful in mild attacks of migraine. Strong analgesics are occasionally required (see Chap. 15).

REVIEW QUESTIONS

1. *Describe the effects that glyceryl trinitrate may produce. How may it be administered? How often? In what doses? With what side effects? Which of these points should be discussed with the patient?*
2. *Of what advantages are amyl and octyl nitrites in angina pectoris? Is there any cumulative action of these or of nitroglycerin on repetitive use if the effects of each previous dose have nearly worn off before repeating doses?*
3. *Describe the effects of overdosage with organic nitrates and nitrites and of sodium nitrite, including methemoglobinemia. What treatment is available for the latter?*
4. *Name four adrenergic blocking agents, give their dosage, uses, and side effects (see Chap. 28). At what anatomical site do they act and what do they accomplish?*
5. *What are the actions and doses of cyclandelate, nylidrin, isoxsuprel, and trimethaphan?*
6. *Discuss the abnormalities in migraine attacks and the action of ergotamine tartrate and related agents in their treatment. Why must overdosage be carefully avoided?*

REFERENCES

Friedberg, C. F.: *Diseases of the Heart,* 2nd ed. W. B. Saunders Company, Philadelphia, 1956.

ATHEROSCLEROSIS

Ahrens, E. H.; Hirsch, J.; Peterson, M. L.; *et al.*: "Symposium on Significance of Lowered Cholesterol Levels," *J.A.M.A.,* **170**:2198, 1959.

Altschul, R.: "Nicotinic Acid and Cholesterol Metabolism," *G.P.,* **21**:115, 1960.

Altschul, R., and Hoffer, A.: "The Effect of Nicotinic Acid on Hypercholesterolaemia," *Canad. M.A.J.,* **82**:783, 1960.

Berge, K. G.; Achor, R. W. P.; Barker, N. W.; and Power, M. H.: "Comparison of the Treatment of Hypercholesteremia with Nicotinic Acid, Sitosterol, and Safflower Oil," *Am. Heart J.,* **58**:849, 1959.

Corday, E.: "Breakthrough on Cholesterol," *Med. World News,* June 17, 1960, p. 17.

Hashim, S. A.: "The Relation of Diet to Atherosclerosis and Infarction," *Am. J. Nursing,* **60**:348, 1960.

ANGINA PECTORIS

Chevalier, H., and Simon, J.: "The Management of Angina Pectoris," *Am. Heart J.,* **58**:120, 1959.

Editorial: "Drugs in Angina," *Brit. M. J.,* **1**:257, Jan. 23, 1960.

Editorial: "Iproniazide and Angina Pectoris," *Circulation,* **20**:1, 1959.

Fife, R.; Howitt, G.; and Stevenson, J.: "Iproniazid in Treatment of Angina of Effort," *Brit. M. J.,* **5174**:692, 1960.

Kowal, S. J.: "Emotions and Angina Pectoris," *Am. J. Cardiol.,* **5**:421, 1960.

Riseman, J. E. F.: Current Concepts in Therapy. "The Treatment of Angina Pectoris," *New England J. Med.,* **261**:1017, 1959.

Russek, H .I.: "Are the Xanthines Effective in Angina Pectoris?" *Am. J. Med. Sci.,* **239**:187, 1960.

NITRITES AND NITRATES

Brachfeld, N.; Bozer, J.; and Gorlin, R.: "Action of Nitroglycerin on the Coronary Circulation in Normal and in Mild Cardiac Subjects," *Circulation,* **19**:697, 1959.

Friend, Dale G., "Angina Pectoris Therapy," *Clin. Pharmacol. & Therap.,* **5**:385, 1964.

Plotz, M.: "The Treatment of Angina Pectoris with a New Prolonged Action Pentaerythritol Tetranitrate," *Am. J. Med. Sci.,* **239**:194, 1960.

Russek, H. I.; Urbach, K. F.; Doerner, A. A.; and Zohman, B. L.: "Choice of a Coronary Vasodilator Drug in Clinical Practice," *J.A.M.A.,* **153**:207, 1953.

Russek, H. I.; Zohman, B. L.; Drumn, A. E.; Weingarten, W.; and Dorset, V. J.: "Long Acting Coronary Vasodilator Drugs: Metamine, Paveril, Nitroglyn Coated Granules of Nitroglycerin) and Peritrate," *Circulation,* **12**:169, 1955.

CORONARY OCCLUSION

Biorck, G.: Editorial. "The International Study of Coronary Heart Disease," *Am. Heart J.,* **59**:3, 1960.

Gilchrist, A. R.: "Problems in Management of Acute Myocardial Infarction," *Brit. M. J.*, **5168**:215, 1960.

Russek, H. I.: "Role of Heredity, Diet, and Emotional Stress in Coronary Heart Disease," *J.A.M.A.*, **171**:503, 1959.

Yudkin, J.: Editorial. "Etiology of Cardiac Infarction," *A.M.A. Arch. Int. Med.*, **104**:681, 1959.

Peripheral Vascular Disease

Green, H. D.; Gobel, W. K.; Moore, M. J.; and Prince, T. C.: "An Evaluation of the Ability of Priscoline, Regitine and Roniacol to Overcome Vasospasm in Normal Man," *Circulation*, **6**:520, 1952.

Green, H. D., and Grimsley, W. T.: "Effects of Regitine in Patients, Particularly Those with Peripheral Arterial Vascular Disease," *Circulation*, **7**:487, 1953.

Samuels, S. S., and Shoftel, H. E.: "Use of a New Vasodilator Agent in Management of Peripheral Arterial Insufficiency," *J.A.M.A.*, **171**:142, 1959.

Wolf, G. A., Jr.: "Current Status of Therapy in Cerebral Accidents," *J.A.M.A.*, **172**:562, 1960.

Persantin

Kinsella, D.; Troup, W.; and McGregor, M.: "Studies with a New Coronary Vasodilator Drug: Persantin," *Am. Heart J.*, **63**:146, 1962.

Sansert

Abbott, Kenneth H.: "Clinical Studies on the Treatment of Vascular Headaches, A Further Report on Methysergide (Sansert)," *Bull. L.A. Neurological Soc.*, **27**:137, 1962.

Harris, M. C.: "Prophylactic Treatment of Migraine Headache and Histamine Cephalgia with a Serotonin Antagonist (Methysergide)," *Ann. Allergy*, **91**:500, 1961.

34

Drug Treatment of Arterial Hypertension

The term "hypertension" literally means abnormally high blood pressure. It indicates abnormal functioning of the circulatory system, as does low blood pressure. There are many known pathological conditions which result in an elevated arterial blood pressure such as hyperthyroidism, pheochromocytoma, adrenal cortical hyperfunction, rapidly expanding brain tumor, and coarctation of the aorta. When these disease states are treated, the elevated blood pressure returns to normal. However, there are also many persons who have arterial hypertension of unknown etiology. This condition is known as essential hypertension and tends to account for 90 to 95 per cent of all hypertensive cases. Although the cause is not completely understood, heredity, emotional factors, and various physiological conditions may play a major role in causing the increased blood pressure. If this syndrome is not treated, complications such as congestive heart failure, cerebral vascular accidents, kidney damage, and arteriosclerosis may develop. Therefore, a large number of drugs having different actions are employed in its treatment. These drugs will be presented in this chapter.

In order to understand why drugs are effective in the treatment of essential hypertension it is necessary to understand the factors which regulate arterial blood pressure, for it is upon these factors that the action of the various antihypertensive drugs is exerted.

Factors Affecting Blood Pressure. Blood pressure represents a ratio between the size of the cardiovascular system and the amount of blood in it and varies in accordance with the influences affecting either. Influencing factors may include:

1. Blood volume. Any change in the volume may directly modify the blood pressure; e.g., a decrease in volume from hemorrhage results in hypotension.

2. Cardiac output. An increase in the cardiac output (the amount of blood ejected by one side of the heart in one minute) will increase the volume of blood in the arterial vessels and thus elevate the arterial pressure particularly during systole.

553

3. Elastic properties of the walls of the large arteries. The aorta and other large arteries distend or stretch during systole and recoil or contract during diastole. When age or pathological changes cause a reduction in the elasticity of blood vessels, the lumens of the larger arteries fail to expand normally for the accommodation of increased amounts of blood during systole. Therefore, the systolic pressure is elevated. Conversely, during diastole inability of the vessels to recoil properly results in a larger chamber during a time when blood is not being pumped into the vessels. Consequently a lowered diastolic pressure is observed.

4. Peripheral resistance of the arterioles. Since the arterioles comprise a large part of the cardiovascular system, and hence contain a large portion of the blood volume, a relatively small change in the size of their lumen causes a considerable change in the arterial pressure, particularly during diastole. Several mechanisms are known to affect peripheral resistance.

   a. Autonomic innervation of the blood vessels.
      (1) Innervation of the smooth muscles of the arteries and arterioles by sympathetic nerve fibers.
      (2) The vasoconstrictor and vasodilator centers in the medulla.
      (3) Hormonal mediators such as epinephrine and norepinephrine.
   b. Other substances not related to the sympathetic system such as hypertensin, histamine, and serotonin, the functions of which are still obscure.
   c. The response of the individual to emotions and environment.

Normal Blood Pressure Values. The blood pressure of an adult is usually considered normal if it is between 90 and 140 mm. Hg. systolic and 60 and 90 mm. Hg. diastolic. These ranges are based on data collected during physical examinations of many persons. A slight increase beyond these limits does not warrant the pronouncement of high blood pressure to the patient. Treatment with blood pressure-reducing drugs is not necessary in all cases of hypertension as a satisfactory reduction in blood pressure is frequently observed as a result of conventional therapeutic procedures or removal of precipitating factors.

DRUG TREATMENT

Modern drug therapy in hypertension involves the use of a variety of drugs having different pharmacological actions. These drugs may be conveniently listed under the following categories:

1. Drugs acting on the central nervous system.
2. Drugs affecting the blood volume.
3. Drugs acting on the autonomic nervous system.
4. Drugs acting directly on the blood vessels.

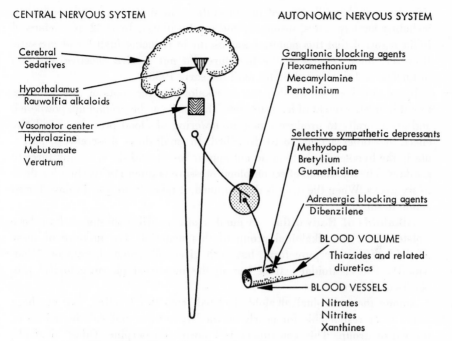

CENTRAL NERVOUS SYSTEM

Cerebral
Sedatives

Hypothalamus
Rauwolfia alkaloids

Vasomotor center
Hydralazine
Mebutamate
Veratrum

AUTONOMIC NERVOUS SYSTEM

Ganglionic blocking agents
Hexamethonium
Mecamylamine
Pentolinium

Selective sympathetic depressants
Methydopa
Bretylium
Guanethidine

Adrenergic blocking agents
Dibenzilene

BLOOD VOLUME
Thiazides and related
diuretics

BLOOD VESSELS
Nitrates
Nitrites
Xanthines

Fig. 16.   Sites of action of antihypertensive drugs.

Figure 16 indicates schematically the sites of action of various drugs useful in hypertension.

Drugs Acting on the Central Nervous System

Sedatives

General mild sedatives such as the barbiturates are used to reduce somewhat the mental and emotional factors involved in the maintenance of arteriolar tone. In many cases of hypertension physicians find that a satisfactory reduction of blood pressure is often obtained by the use of phenobarbital or other mild sedatives alone. When satisfactory control of blood pressure is not achieved by this means, then other types of drugs may be employed.

Rauwolfia and Its Alkaloids

Rauwolfia is the generic name of a plant, the many species of which grow in various parts of the world, usually tropical climates. In the United States the only species of this shrub that has been used clinically is *Rauwolfia serpen-*

tina. Its roots have been used for generations in India for many conditions, including anxiety states, insomnia, and mental illness. In 1942, physicians of India reported that this material was useful in reducing high blood pressure. However, these reports in the literature did not receive effective attention in Europe and the United States until the early 1950's.

It has now been shown that certain alkaloids in the roots of this plant are useful in the treatment of hypertension. The roots can be ground up, powdered, and given orally to produce a definite lowering of blood pressure, a sedative effect, and other actions to be described. In small doses these effects, particularly the hypotensive action, do not appear for several days, usually three to six days. The maximum effect on blood pressure is often not reached for three to six weeks. When the drug is discontinued, it takes from 3 to 14 days for its action to subside.

Alkaloids of Rauwolfia.   A number of crystalline substances have been isolated from the alkaloidal group of this material. The mixture of these alkaloids, in rather pure form, has been given the name alseroxylon (Rauwiloid). The alkaloidal extract has all the important pharmacological properties of the crude root.

Among the individual alkaloids isolated from this fraction, one has been found to be responsible for nearly all the hypotensive and sedative effects of the entire group. This constituent is known as reserpine. Other alkaloids, rescinnamine and deserpidine, have been isolated and found also to produce lowering of blood pressure.

Reserpine, U.S.P.   This alkaloid has been isolated and is now marketed in the United States under several trade names. Reserpine is found in other species of the *Rauwolfia* group.

Pharmacological Responses.   The action of reserpine whether given alone or as the whole-root preparation is probably mediated through:

1. The hypothalamus to produce sedation and relaxation.

2. The release of serotonin and norepinephrine from their storage sites in the central nervous system.

3. The vasoconstrictor or vasodilator centers, or both, and the cardiac rate-regulating centers in the hypothalamus. Through these centers, arteriolar tone is decreased, blood pressure is lowered, and the heart is slowed.

4. The interference with the storage of norepinephrine in nerve endings and blood vessels.

Therapeutic Uses

1. For neurogenic hypertension with tachycardia. It lowers the blood pressure; slows the pulse; and relieves anxiety, irritability, headache, palpitation, and dizziness.

2. In severe hypertension—as an adjunct with more powerful drugs to offset the side effects of other drugs. It is used in combination with *Veratrum viride*, hydralazine (Apresoline), and the ganglionic blocking agents.

3. In combination with thiazide or related diuretics in which case a better reduction in blood pressure is often obtained.

4. As a sedative and relaxant. This use is discussed on pages 341–43.

Side Effects. Patients often complain of stuffiness in the nose, some flushing of the skin, subjective tremors, diarrhea, and drowsiness, and a gain in weight while taking reserpine or the crude drug. Excessive doses may cause disturbed sleep, mental depression, and, occasionally, vertigo. Other serious side effects which are sometimes observed are the activation of a peptic ulcer and Parkinson-like syndrome. These effects disappear when the dosage is reduced or the drug is discontinued. Bradycardia and marked hypotension may occur during anesthesia when a patient is receiving one of the *Rauwolfia*-type drugs. If possible the drug should not be given two weeks before surgery.

Dosage and Method of Administration. The usual oral dose of powdered *Rauwolfia serpentina* is 100 to 150 mg. twice daily. The usual oral or parenteral dose of reserpine is 0.1 mg. two to three times daily. The drug should be taken with meals to decrease the gastrointestinal irritation. No evidence of tolerance has been observed. The drug may be given indefinitely unless side effects are noted.

Preparations

Rauwolfia Serpentina Tablets, N.F.   50 and 100 mg.
            Trade names: Raudixin; Raupena

Reserpine Tablets, U.S.P., B.P.   0.1, 0.25, 0.5, and 1 mg.
Reserpine Injection, U.S.P.   5 mg. in 2 ml.; 25 and 50 mg. in 10 ml.
            Trade names: Rau-sed; Reserpoid; Sandril; Serpasil; Serpiloid
Other names of *Rauwolfia* or reserpine preparations: Quiescin; Raubasin; Roxinoid; Serpina; Tranquilex

Deserpidine Tablets   0.1 and 0.25 mg.
            Trade name: Harmonyl

Syrosingopine, N.F. (Singoserp)

Syrosingopine is a chemically altered reserpine that has the same effects but is slightly less potent than *Rauwolfia* and produces less sedation in most patients.

Preparation

Syrosingopine Tablets, N.F.   1 mg.
            Trade name: Singoserp

Hydralazine Hydrochloride, N.F. (Apresoline); Hydrallazine, B.P.

Hydralazine hydrochloride is a potent hypotensive drug which reduces blood pressure by its action on the vasomotor center and by its dilating effect on blood vessels. It produces a marked decrease in peripheral vascular resistance, especially in the abdominal area and the lower extremities. An important action of this drug is that it does not decrease renal blood flow.

Side Effects.   A limiting factor in the use of hydralazine is the frequent headache that it produces, which may be quite severe. There often occurs an excitatory action upon the heart which increases its rate. The patient may complain of palpitation, shortness of breath on exertion, angina, headache, dizziness, and fainting. Numbness and tingling of the extremities, malaise, depression, disorientation, and anxiety may occur. On prolonged administration of large doses, joint pain resembling rheumatoid arthritis, or a condition resembling lupus erythematosus, may be produced. Occasionally the drug may have to be withdrawn and replaced by corticoid drugs or corticotropin (see Chap. 41).

Dosage and Methods of Administration.   The initial oral dose is 10 mg. four times a day. The maintenance dose is 10 to 100 mg. four times a day depending on the individual response. The intramuscular or intravenous dose is 20 mg. up to six times a day.

Preparations

Hydralazine   Hydrochloride   Injection,   20 mg. in 1 ml.
N.F.

Hydralazine Hydrochloride Tablets,   10, 25, 50, and 100 mg.
N.F.; Hydrallazine Tablets, B.P.

Trade name: Apresoline. (Nepresol is the trade name of a related compound of dihydralazine.)

Mebutamate (Capla)

Mebutamate, a compound chemically related to meprobamate, is a centrally acting blood pressure depressant which acts on the vasomotor center in a unique way to cause peripheral vasodilatation. Drowsiness and lightheadedness are occasional side effects. Patients should be warned of these, as operating machinery or driving a car may be hazardous when they occur.

Dosage.   Three or four doses of 300 mg. may be taken daily, before meals and at bedtime. Individual adjustment of the dose may be required.

Preparation

Mebutamate Tablets   300 mg.
Trade name: Capla

Veratrum Alkaloids

Two species of plants, known as *Veratrum viride* and *Veratrum album,* have been found to contain certain alkaloids which also lower the blood pressure and produce a slowing of the heart. A mixture of two alkaloids, protoveratrines A and B, has been isolated in pure form from *Veratrum album.* Alkavervir is a mixture of alkaloids obtained by selective extraction from *Veratrum viride.*

Pharmacological Actions. The veratrum alkaloids slow the heart through vagal stimulation and increase the cardiac output. They lower the blood pressure by inhibiting sympathetic nervous system tone, which results in a moderate vasodilatation, probably throughout the peripheral circulation. The mechanism by which the sympathetic system is inhibited is thought to be a potentiation of afferent stimuli to the central vasomotor regulating centers in the hypothalamus. The slowing of the heart rate can be pronounced with these drugs; however, this effect, if undesirably pronounced, can be treated with atropine.

The lowering of the blood pressure is more rapid in onset than with the *Rauwolfia* alkaloids. Blood pressure begins to fall within one or two hours after administration, reaching the minimum in three to four hours, then gradually rising.

Therapeutic Use. The veratrum alkaloids are used to lower blood pressure in mild, moderate, and malignant hypertension.

Side Effects. The side effects are substernal and epigastric burning, salivation, nausea, and vomiting.

Toxic Effects. In extreme overdosage, the following toxic effects may occur: slowing of the heart; excessive lowering of blood pressure, resulting in weakness and collapse (counteracted with ephedrine or phenylephrine); respiratory depression; constriction of the bronchioles; and respiratory arrest.

Contraindications. Veratrum products should not be used freely in patients suffering from cerebral vascular disease, coronary occlusion, renal insufficiency, or angina pectoris. Lowering of blood pressure in such individuals may be attended by complications or increase of damage already present.

Dosage and Methods of Administration. The veratrum alkaloids are administered orally and parenterally. The initial dose of protoveratrines A and B is 0.5 mg. four times a day; that of protoveratrines A and B maleate is 1.0 to 2.5 mg. daily in three or five divided doses; and that of alkavervir is 9 to 15 mg. daily in three divided doses. These doses are increased gradually within the limits of nausea. The intravenous dose of alkavervir is 0.15 ml. of a 0.04 per cent solution per 10 lb. of body weight; the intramuscular dose is 0.25 ml. of a 0.1 per cent solution with 1 per cent procaine hydrochloride per 50 lb. of body weight. A newer veratrum alkaloid preparation, cryptenamine, is given orally, 2 mg. two or three times daily, or intravenously, 1 mg. in 20 ml. of 5 per cent dextrose.

Preparations

Solution Alkavervir (Intravenous)	0.4 mg. in 1 ml.; 5-ml. ampuls
Solution Alkavervir with 1 Per Cent Procaine Hydrochloride (Intramuscular)	1 mg. in 1 ml.; 2-ml. ampuls
Tablets Alkavervir	2 and 3 mg.

Trade names: Veratrone; Vergitryl; Veriloid

Cryptenamine Tannate Tablets	2 mg.
Cryptenamine Acetate Injection	2 mg. in 1 ml.; 5-ml. ampuls

Trade name: Unitensin

Solution Protoveratrines A and B	0.2 mg. in 1 ml.; 10-ml. vials
Tablets Protoveratrines A and B	0.2 and 0.5 mg.

Trade name: Veralba

Tablets Protoveratrines A and B Maleate	0.5 mg.

Trade name: Provell Maleate

DRUGS ACTING ON THE BLOOD VOLUME

The "Thiazide" Diuretics

In 1957, chlorothiazide, a potent orally effective diuretic agent, was introduced. It is discussed in detail in Chapter 38. Its ability to lower blood pressure in hypertensive patients was soon observed. This effect is largely explained by its ability to cause increased excretion of sodium and chloride ions in the urine, with increased water excretion secondary to this salt loss. The blood volume (and interstitial fluid volume) is thereby decreased, causing a lowering in blood pressure in most hypertensive patients. However, in time, the blood volume returns to pretreatment value, or nearly so, yet blood pressure remains lowered. A number of derivatives of chlorothiazide possess a similar action in smaller doses (see Chap. 38). They may be adequate alone in mild degrees of hypertension but are best used with other hypotensive agents.

DRUGS ACTING ON THE AUTONOMIC NERVOUS SYSTEM

Ganglionic Blocking Agents

Ganglionic blocking agents block the ganglia of both the sympathetic and parasympathetic systems. Blockage of the ganglia of the sympathetic nerves which constrict blood vessels causes a fall in blood pressure. When these ganglia are blocked, the natural sympathetic reflexes are unable to constrict the arterioles in the lower extremities and abdomen, and pooling of blood in these areas occurs. Thus blood pressure is always lower in the upright position than when sitting or reclining. This possibly impairs the circulation to the brain, and as a result weakness and fainting may occur. Due to the unwanted blockade of the parasympathetic ganglia, many side effects such as constipation, abdominal distention, blurring of vision due to paralysis of accommodation, dryness of the mouth, and difficulty in micturition often occur. These side effects cause these drugs to be used less frequently than reserpine and the "thiazide" diuretics. However, their potency makes them valuable as adjuncts to other hypotensive agents when refractory or very severe cases are treated. They are rather dependable in malignant hypertension and in severe hypertensive crises.

The first ganglionic blocking agent used for oral medication in hypertension was hexamethonium chloride. This drug was used for the treatment of severe hypertension, but absorption was erratic and many severe side effects were encountered. Today it has been replaced largely by more reliable ganglionic blocking agents.

Mecamylamine Hydrochloride, U.S.P., B.P. (Inversine)

Mecamylamine is the most extensively used orally active ganglionic blocking agent. It is a secondary amine and is completely absorbed from the gastrointestinal tract. Oral doses of 2.5 mg. twice daily increased by 2.5 mg. at intervals of not less than two days, as required, have proved to be very satisfactory in the treatment of those patients with hypertension who respond to ganglionic blocking agents (a majority of patients). Maintenance dose is 25 mg. daily in three divided doses. The usual dose range is 2.5 to 60 mg. The dose must be individually determined within the above range. The duration of effect is longer and more consistent from day to day, and the side effects are less frequently encountered than with other ganglionic blocking agents.

Preparation

Mecamylamine Hydrochloride Tablets,   2.5 and 10 mg. B.P.

Trade name: Inversine, Nevasine

Pentolinium Tartrate, B.P. (Ansolysen)

This ganglionic blocking agent is about five times more potent than hexamethonium and the effects are more prolonged. It is used in the management of moderately severe, severe, and malignant hypertension.

Side Effects. The side effects are constipation, temporary cycloplegia, dry mouth, and frequent fainting due to low blood pressure on standing.

Dosage and Method of Administration. Pentolinium tartrate is given orally, subcutaneously, and intramuscularly. Each patient should be evaluated independently, and the dose must be accurately adjusted. The oral dose may range from 60 to 600 mg. per day. The initial dose should be as small as possible and increased gradually with constant observation of the patient. The initial parenteral dose should not exceed 3.5 mg. (2.5 to 3.5 mg.) and may be increased by 0.5 to 1 mg. until the desired response is obtained. The effective daily dose ranges from 30 to 60 mg. in appropriate divided doses.

Preparations

Pentolinium Injection, B.P.	10-ml. vials containing 10 mg. in 1 ml.
Pentolinium Tablets, B.P. (Scored)	20, 40, and 100 mg.

Trade names: Ansolysen; Pendine; Tensilest

Chlorisondamine Chloride (Ecolid Chloride)

Chlorisondamine chloride is similar to the foregoing ganglionic blocking agents in both action and side effects. It is approximately equivalent to pentolinium in potency. The oral dose is gradually increased as required from 10 mg. in the evening to as much as 200 mg. in several divided doses. One to ten milligrams are given subcutaneously or intramuscularly to lower blood pressure.

Preparations

Chlorisondamine Chloride Injection	5 mg. in 1 ml.
Chlorisondamine Chloride Tablets	10, 25, and 50 mg.

Trade name: Ecolid Chloride

Trimethaphan Camphorsulfonate, U.S.P., B.P. (Arfonad)

Trimethaphan camphorsulfonate is a short- and rapid-acting ganglionic blocking agent that produces vasodilatation and pools the blood in both the peripheral areas and the splanchnic system. It is used to produce controlled hypotension for surgery in very vascular areas in order to minimize bleeding. It is used in neurosurgery and peripheral vascular surgery. The drug is administered by intravenous drip. A 0.2 per cent solution is slowly infused at the rate of 3 to 4 ml. (0.2 to 5 ml.) per minute.

Preparation

Trimethaphan Camphorsulfonate Injection, U.S.P., B.P.	500 mg. in 10 ml. to be diluted before use

Trade name: Arfonad

Phenacyl Homatropinium Chloride (Trophenium)

This ganglionic blocking agent is used for the production of controlled hypotension during surgery. It reduces blood loss from capillaries and arterioles which are cut in making incisions and dissections. This agent should not be used with gallamine (p. 419) or thiopental (p. 305). Excessive fall in blood pressure should be countered by the careful use of a pressor agent such as levarterenol, phenylephrine, or others (pp. 454–57).

Dosage and Method of Administration. The contents of two ampuls (20 ml. or 1000 mg.) are diluted with 500 ml. sterile physiological saline or 5 per cent dextrose. The initial rate of the intravenous infusion should be 100 to 120 drops per minute with blood pressure determinations every 30 to 90 seconds. As the pressure declines, the rate of infusion may be decreased to 30 to 60 drops per minute. The systolic pressure is often maintained between 65 and 70 mm. Hg.

Preparation

Phenacyl Homatropinium Chloride Solution	10-ml. ampuls containing 50 mg. in 1 ml.

Trade name: Trophenium

Selective Sympathetic Depressants

Several new drugs have been developed that are useful in the treatment of hypertension mainly because they produce a depression of the peripheral sympathetic nervous system which is responsible for vasoconstriction and elevation in blood pressure. These drugs affect the synthesis, storage, and release of norepinephrine. They are methyldopa, pargyline, bretylium tosylate, and guanethidine. They bear some similarity to the *Rauwolfia* alkaloids insofar as peripheral inhibition of sympathetic tone is concerned.

Methyldopa

Methyldopa is structurally related to a substance (DOPA) involved in the synthesis of norepinephrine in the central and peripheral nervous system. It causes an inhibition of a decarboxylase enzyme which is needed for the synthesis of norepinephrine and serotonin. Hence, the main action of the drug is in inhibiting the formation of neurohormones which are involved in vasoconstriction. It is useful in the treatment of moderate to severe hypertension. Since the renal blood flow is not usually affected, it may be given to patients with impaired renal function. The drug is excreted primarily by the kidney so that patients with kidney damage may obtain satisfactory lowering of blood pressure with smaller amounts than usual.

Side Effects. The most frequently noted side effect is drowsiness, which occurs within the first three days of therapy. Other side effects which occur less often include: dryness of the mouth, nasal stuffiness, gastrointestinal disturbances, headache, skin rash, and postural hypotension with dizziness and lightheadedness. Lactation, breast enlargement, parkinsonism, arthralgia, and myalgia have also been reported.

Precautions. The drug has been observed to be hepatotoxic in some patients; thus it should not be given to persons with active liver disease. At the present time it is not recommended for use in pregnant women.

Administration.   Daily doses ranging from 500 mg. to 2 Gm. produce satisfactory blood pressure lowering. Therapy is initiated with 250 mg. three times a day for two days; then the dose may be increased or decreased by one or two tablets at intervals of two days. The usual intravenous dose is 250 to 500 mg. every six hours until satisfactory control is obtained. Then oral doses may be substituted.

Preparations

Methyldopa Tablets	250 mg.
Methyldopate Hydrochloride Injection	250 mg. in 5-ml. ampuls

Trade name: Aldomet

Pargyline (Eutonyl) is a monoamine oxidase inhibitor (see p. 349) which is an effective, long-acting hypotensive drug. It is said to lower both systolic and diastolic pressure. The full therapeutic effect develops slowly and is maintained for some time after the drug is discontinued. It is well absorbed orally and is excreted in the urine largely unchanged. It does not induce or aggravate depression.

The side effects and precautions in its use are the same as those listed for the monamine oxidase inhibitors (see p. 349).

Therapeutic Use.   It is recommended for use in moderate to severe hypertension.

Dosage and Method of Administration.   The initial oral adult dose is 25 to 50 mg. once a day for four days to three weeks or more. After the first two weeks the dose may be increased to 35 to 75 mg., if necessary. It should be reduced for geriatric patients and also if given with another antihypertensive drug.

Preparation

Pargyline Hydrochloride Tablets	10, 25, and 50 mg.

Trade name: Eutonyl

Bretylium Tosylate (Darenthin)

Bretylium tosylate prevents the release and action of norepinephrine at the postganglionic sympathetic nerve endings. It does not deplete the nerve endings of this sympathetic transmitter substance as does reserpine, but in some presently unknown manner it prevents the liberation of norepinephrine, by nerve impulses, from its bound form. Sympathetic activity and tone everywhere in the body are thus greatly reduced. As a result, arterioles held in constriction in hypertension are allowed to relax and blood pressure falls.

Bretylium does not reduce or block the actions of the circulating sympathomimetic hormones, epinephrine and norepinephrine, or other adrenergic drugs. Thus it is not an adrenergic blocking agent.

Side Effects.   These are the result of sympathetic blockade and include nasal stuffiness, pupillary constriction, irregularity of the heart, and postural hypotension with weakness, fatigue, and possible fainting. The drug has no known effects upon the central nervous system.

Dosage and Method of Administration. After oral doses of 100 to 300 mg., blood pressure may decline within one to three hours and may remain lowered for eight or more hours. Some patients have required 800 mg. every eight hours, and some are not benefited by the drug. Oral absorption is incomplete and variable. Dosage must be individualized and may be given at four- to eight-hour intervals. The ultimate place of bretylium in hypertension and peripheral vasospastic and thrombotic diseases is yet to be established, but a new approach is offered by this agent.

Preparation

Bretylium Tosylate Tablets   200 mg.
Trade name: Darenthin

Guanethidine Sulphate, B.P. (Ismelin)

Guanethidine also depletes the sympathetic nerve endings of norepinephrine, as does reserpine and other *Rauwolfia* preparations and syrosingopine. Unlike the latter group it does not remove serotonin from the body stores (platelets, brain, etc.). Neither does it deplete the brain of norepinephrine, as does reserpine. Guanethidine, like reserpine, is slow in onset of action. It is well absorbed orally, begins its hypotensive effect after 36 to 48 hours, and with continued medication reaches a maximum effect at about 72 hours.

Side Effects. Postural hypotension may produce the same effects as those described for bretylium. Diarrhea and bardycardia may occur, as well as other effects previously mentioned.

Dosage and Method of Administration. Guanethidine is given orally, in amounts varying from 25 mg. every other day to 150 mg. three times daily. Blood pressure is usually reduced markedly when the appropriate dosage is determined.

Preparation

Guanethidine Tablets, B.P.   10 and 25 mg.
Trade name: Ismelin

Adrenergic Blocking Agents

Phenoxybenzamine (dibenzilene), a long-acting adrenergic blocking agent, is occasionally used in the treatment of hypertension (see p. 468).

DRUGS ACTING DIRECTLY ON THE BLOOD VESSELS

Several types of drugs exert their action directly on the blood vessels. Occasionally they are used in the treatment of hypertension. They are: xanthine derivatives (see p. 639), nitrites (see p. 542), and nitrates (see p. 545).

Combinations of the Drugs.   One drug is seldom adequate unless the hypertension is mild. Combinations of two or more are more effective and may be administered separately or combined in the same tablet, capsule, or elixir. There is no antihypertensive drug that is effective for all persons. Various drugs and combinations may be tried until an effective lowering of the blood pressure is achieved. Many of the antihypertensive agents cause a decrease in blood flow. Therefore their use in patients with atherosclerosis is contraindicated as the blood flow of these patients is already compromised.

REVIEW QUESTIONS

1. *What abnormal situations in the body are present in hypertension as regards (1) sympathetic nervous outflow (2) arteriolar tone?*
2. *What is the upper limit of normal systolic and diastolic blood pressure? What factors may cause or contribute to the development of essential hypertension?*
3. *Discuss the means by which* Rauwolfia *alkaloids lower high blood pressure.*
4. *What are the side effects with reserpine (and* Rauwolfia*)?*
5. *How do the "thiazide" oral diuretic agents lower blood pressure?*
6. *What effects do ganglionic blocking agents have upon these parasympathetically innervated structures: Ocular lenses? Pupils? Salivary glands? Intestines? Urinary bladder?*
7. *What chief additional disadvantages do the ganglionic blocking agents possess? What are the tablet sizes of mecamylamine, chlorisondamine, and pentolinium?*
8. *What is the mode of action, in reducing blood pressure, of bretylium tosylate, guanethidine, veratrum alkaloids, hydralazine? What side effects may these agents produce?*
9. *A patient taking a drug to reduce her blood pressure feels well in bed and sitting in a chair. However, if she stands soon after taking her medicine, a feeling of fainting comes over her with momentary loss of vision, continued dizziness, and weakness. Why does this happen? What studies should be made, even by the nurse? Name all the drugs, by generic and trade names, which can cause this reaction.*

REFERENCES

Brest, A. N., and Moyer, J. H.: "Newer Approaches to Antihypertensive Therapy," *J.A.M.A.*, **172**:1041, 1960.

Dustan, H. P.; Page, I. H.; and Poutasse, E. F.: "Renal Hypertension," *New England J. Med.*, **261**:647, 1959.

Harington, M.: "Drug Treatment of Disease: Pharmacology of Hypotensive Drugs," *Brit. M. J.*, **1**:717, 1960.

RESERPINE AND SYROSINGOPINE

Barbour, B.; Irwin, G.; Yamahiro, H.; *et al.*: "The Use of Carbethoxysyringoyl Methylreserpate in Hypertension," *Am. J. Cardiol.*, **3**:220, 1959.

Yablonski, M. D.; Stockman, A. M.; Caliva, F. S.; and Lyons, R. H.: "Some Cardiovascular Effects of Reserpine," *Am. J. Med. Sci.*, **235**:639, 1958.

HYDRALAZINE

Dunsmore, R. A.; Dunsmore, L. D.; and Elias, Max: "The Use of Syrosingopine (SU-3118) and Hydralazine in Ambulatory Hypertensive Patients," *Am. J. Med. Sci.*, **239**:148, 1960.

MEBUTAMATE

Berger, F. M., and Margolin, S.: "A Centrally Acting Blood Pressure Lowering Agent (W-583)," *Fed. Proc.*, **20**:113, 1961.

CHLOROTHIAZIDE AND ITS DERIVATIVES

Bartels, C. C.; Evans, J. E.; and Townley, R. G.: "Hypertension: Survey of Treatment with Chlorothiazide," *Clinical Med.*, **7**:347, 1960.
Freeman, R. B.; Jenson, W. K.; and Gill, R. J.: "Hydrochlorothiazide Used Alone and with Other Hypotensive Agents in the Treatment of Arterial Hypertension: A Preliminary Report," *Am. Pract. & Digest. Treat.*, **10**:2147, 1959.
Montero, A. C.; Rochelle, J. B. III; and Ford, R. V.: "Use of Flumethiazide as an Adjunct to the Therapy of Hypertension," *New England J. Med.*, **260**:872, 1959.
Wilkins, R. W.: "New Drugs for Hypertension, with Special Reference to Chlorothiazide," *New England J. Med.*, **257**:1026, 1957.

GANGLIONIC BLOCKING AGENTS

Cottier, P. T.; Weller, J. M.; and Hoobler, S. W.: "Evaluation of Mecamylamine in the Treatment of Hypertension," *J. Lab. and Clin. Med.*, **50**:199, 1957.
Fennel, P. J.; Howland, W. S.; and Daniel, W. W.: "A New Ganglionic Blocking Agent for Induced Hypotension," *New York J. Med.*, **59**:2716, 1959.
Perkins, H. T.; Bogdonoff, M. D.; and Black, M. C.: "The Treatment of Hypertension with Trimethidinium Methosulfate in an Outpatient Clinic Group," *South. M. J.*, **53**:224, 1960.
Robertson, J. D.; Gillies, J.; and Spencer, K. E. V.: "The Use of a Homatropinium Derivative to Produce Controlled Hypotension," *Brit. J. Anaesth.*, **29**:342, 1957.

SELECTIVE SYMPATHETIC DEPRESSANTS

Council on Drugs: "A New Antihypertensive, Methyldopa (Aldomet)," *J.A.M.A.*, **186**:504, 1963.

PARGYLINE

Council on Drugs: "New Drugs and Developments in Therapeutics (Pargyline Hydrochloride [Eutonyl]," *J.A.M.A.*, **184**:887, 1963.

BRETYLIUM TOSYLATE

Boura, A. L. A.; Green, A. F.; McCoubrey, A.; Laurence, D. R.; Moulton, R.; and Rosenheim, M. L.: "Darenthin—Hypotensive Agent of New Type," *Lancet*, **2**:17, 1959.

Dollery, C. T.; Emslie-Smith, D.; and McMichael, J.: "Bretylium Tosylate in the Treatment of Hypertension," *Lancet*, **1**:296, 1960.

Genest, J.; Dufault, C.; Pigeon, G.; Davignon, J.; Biron, P.; and Trudel, J.: "Studies on a New Hypotensive Agent: Bretylium Tosylate," *Canad. M. A. J.*, **82**:872, 1960.

Lewis, J. A.: "Clinical Experience with Bretylium Tosylate," *Canad. M. A. J.*, **82**:877, 1960.

GUANETHIDINE

Frohlich, E. D., and Freis, E. D.: "Clinical Trial of Guanethidine Sulfate in Hypertension," *Clinical Med.*, **7**:363, 1960.

Leishman, A. W. D.; Matthews, H. L.; and Smith, A. J.: "Guanethidine: Hypotensive Drug with Prolonged Action," *Lancet*, **2**:1044, 1959.

Page, I. H., and Duston, H.P.: "A New, Potent Antihypertensive Drug," *J.A.M.A.*, **170**:1265, 1959.

VII DRUGS ACTING ON THE GASTRO-INTESTINAL TRACT

The functions of the gastrointestinal tract are (1) to convert complex foods in the diet into simpler substances that may be absorbed by the blood and used for nourishment by the body; (2) to propel the products of digestion to their point of absorption into the blood stream; and (3) to excrete waste materials. Chemical processes involving enzymes as well as digestive fluids of the proper pH for optimal enzyme activity are required for normal digestion. At times the presence of too much acid in the stomach may cause or contribute to gastritis or peptic ulcer. At other times a deficiency of acid may cause indigestion, flatulence, or colic. The rate of movement of the intestinal contents through the tract is influenced by many factors—character of the food eaten, variations in muscle tone, peristaltic activity, consistency of the fecal mass, emotional states, etc. When the normal rate of activity is retarded, constipation results; when the rate of expulsion of the contents is excessive, diarrhea occurs.

Drugs of many kinds are available for the control or detection of abnormal or diseased conditions in the gastrointestinal tract. They may be administered (1) to neutralize excessive acid in the stomach (antacids); (2) as replacement therapy when there is a deficiency of acid or enzymes (pepsin); (3) to stimulate the flow of bile; (4) to relieve flatulence and colic (carminatives); (5) to produce vomiting in acute poisoning (emetics); (6) to absorb poisons or toxins; and (7) as diagnostic acids in detecting abnormal or diseased conditions.

In addition, drugs may increase or decrease the motor activity of the intestines. Cathartics (laxatives and purgatives) increase peristalsis in a number of ways and produce evacuation of the bowels. Antidiarrheics decrease excessive bowel movement, and intestinal antiseptics are used to check the growth of bacteria.

569

35

Antacids, Digestants, Carminatives, Emetics, Adsorbents, and Diagnostic Aids

Gastric or Peptic Digestion. Hydrochloric acid (HCl) is produced by certain cells in the wall of the stomach and accumulates in the lumen of this organ for digestive purposes. Another substance, the enzyme pepsin, is manufactured by still other gastric cells. These two secretions constitute an excellent digestive mixture for the breakdown of protein foodstuffs. Ordinarily this is the normal situation in the stomach and is called "peptic digestion." The acid becomes so strong during the gastric phase of digestion that it could erode, by its dissolving action, an area of the skin upon prolonged contact. The stomach, however, under normal conditions is peculiarly immune to the powerful erosive or digestant action of its own juice. The first few inches of the duodenum are also bathed with the highly acidic stomach contents as they pass through the pyloric canal, which acts as a valve between these two parts of the tract. The membrane of the upper duodenum is likewise resistant to the erosive action of gastric juice.

Peptic Ulcer. Under certain conditions, a small area of the thin surface membrane of the stomach or duodenum may break down. The underlying connective tissue in the wall of the viscus (organ) is not nearly so resistant to the acid as the lining membrane. The gastric juice may eat away at the tissue and cause an open ulcer. This is termed a "peptic ulcer" because it is produced by "peptic digestion."

It now becomes highly desirable and often necessary to abolish the hydrochloric acid over a period of weeks in order to allow the ulcer to heal. The re-establishment of the completely intact lining membrane, with its natural immunity to strong acid, is the goal in therapy. In addition to temporary reduction or abolition of the acid, other agents and measures are usually employed. An antispasmodic is routine with most physicians (see discussion of this class of agents in Chap. 30). A general sedative, such as phenobarbital, a diet varying from milk and cream in the acute phase to merely selected bland items later, and possibly changes in environment constitute other phases of the treatment regimen.

570

Hyperacidity. This clinical term describes excessive production of hydrochloric acid The burning sensation, erroneously named "heartburn," may arise in an irritated stomach wall ("gastritis") or in the esophagus upon reflux of acid upward in this tube. The lining of the latter, unlike that of the stomach, does not have a natural immunity to acid and therefore is chemically irritated by the hydrochloric acid.

ANTACIDS

Often under conditions of hyperacidity and always in cases of peptic ulcer, *antacids* are indicated. Such agents either destroy the acid, wholly or in part, by neutralization, or absorb it, rendering it inactive. Neutralizers of acids are alkaline materials, or bases, which unite chemically with the acid. Strong bases, such as sodium hydroxide, cannot be used because they are too caustic themselves. Certain weak bases and other neutralizing agents are very useful.

Gastric antacids are divided into two classes: the systemic and the nonsystemic antacids. The systemic antacids are those that are readily absorbed from the gastrointestinal tract and which may produce changes in the pH of the blood and symptoms of alkalosis (e.g., headache, abdominal pain, nausea, and vomiting) if used in excess. Because of their effect on the pH of the blood they are seldom ordered in the treatment of patients with peptic ulcers; however, they are sometimes used by patients even though not prescribed by a physician. The nonsystemic antacids are not readily absorbed but produce their effects locally, either by neutralization of the acid, with the formation of neutral salts, or by physical adsorption of the acid, somewhat as a sponge absorbs water.

Systemic Antacids

Sodium Bicarbonate, U.S.P., B.P.

Sodium bicarbonate, commonly known as baking soda, is very soluble and is readily absorbed. It promptly neutralizes gastric acid, although this action is of short duration. It often causes gastric distention by the liberation of carbon dioxide, which is undesirable. Following the neutralization of the gastric contents with sodium bicarbonate, the rate of the secretion of hydrochloric acid is greater than if no alkali had been given. This is known as "acid rebound." The sodium bicarbonate ingested in excess of that required to neutralize the acid in the stomach passes into the intestine and is absorbed, whereupon the alkali reserve of the blood is increased. Following heart surgery utilizing extracorporeal circulation, sodium bicarbonate may be given to correct the acidosis which occurs if excess amounts of carbon dioxide have been removed from the blood by the pump-oxygenator. The usual dose is 2 Gm. (1 to 4 Gm.). The drug is administered in solution or tablets.

Preparations

Sodium Bicarbonate Tablets, U.S.P.	300 and 600 mg.
Compound Sodium Bicarbonate Tablets, B.P.	300 mg. sodium bicarbonate and oil of peppermint

Sodium Citrate, U.S.P., B.P., I.P

Sodium citrate, a readily absorbable antacid that does not liberate carbon dioxide, is an ingredient in many of the effervescent preparations commonly used for the alleviation of gastrointestinal distress. In its preparation, sodium bicarbonate and citric acid are mixed in the dry form. When this mixture is dissolved in water, carbon dioxide is liberated and sodium citrate is formed. After absorption, sodium bicarbonate is formed; consequently the ingestion of large amounts of sodium citrate may also produce alkalosis. The usual antacid dose of sodium citrate is 1 Gm. (1 to 3 Gm.) four times a day. Effervescent salts and tablets are available.

NONSYSTEMIC ANTACIDS

The nonsystemic antacids include compounds of magnesium, calcium, and aluminum. The magnesium compounds produce a laxative action (see p. 590). The calcium and aluminum compounds, on the other hand, have a constipating effect. For this reason, a calcium antacid may be alternated with a magnesium preparation, and combinations of aluminum and magnesium hydroxides in suspension (see p. 574) are available.

Magnesium Oxide, U.S.P.; Light Magnesium Oxide, B.P.

Magnesium oxide is a bulky white powder that slowly reacts with hydrochloric acid and is insoluble in water. Although the drug has a laxative action, it is used principally as an antacid, useful in some cases of gastric acidity accompanied by complications. Magnesium oxide is preferred to the carbonates, since carbon dioxide is not formed when acid is neutralized. It is administered in the form of a powder. The usual antacid dose is 250 mg.; the laxative dose is 4 Gm. The B.P. antacid dose is 300 to 600 mg.; the laxative dose is 2 to 4 Gm.

Milk of Magnesia, U.S.P.; Magnesium Hydroxide Mixture, B.P.

Milk of magnesia is an aqueous suspension of magnesium hydroxide containing approximately 8 per cent of the base. The usual antacid dose is 5 ml. The laxative dose is 15 ml. (5 to 30 ml.). Tablets containing the equivalent of one teaspoon of milk of magnesia are available.

Magnesium Carbonate, U.S.P.; Light Magnesium Carbonate, B.P.

This salt liberates carbon dioxide with the neutralization of hydrochloric acid. The usual antacid dose is 600 mg. The usual laxative dose is 2 to 4 Gm.

Magnesium Trisilicate, U.S.P., B.P.

Magnesium trisilicate is a long-acting antacid that becomes gelatinous in the presence of gastric juice and serves as an adsorbent for toxins. It is also useful as a protective agent for irritated and ulcerated mucosa of the gastrointestinal tract. The usual antacid dose is 1 Gm. (1 to 4 Gm.) four times a day. The drug is administered as powders or tablets. The B.P. dose is 300 mg. to 2 Gm.

Preparation

Magnesium Trisilicate Tablets, U.S.P.   500 mg.

Precipitated Calcium Carbonate, U.S.P.; Calcium Carbonate, B.P. (Precipitated Chalk)

Calcium carbonate reacts with the hydrochloric acid of the stomach to form calcium chloride with the production of carbon dioxide. It is used as an antacid in hyperacidity, gastritis, and gastric ulcer. The usual dose is 1 Gm. (1 to 2 Gm.) four or more times a day.

Preparation

Calcium Carbonate Tablets, N.F.   1 Gm.

Dried Aluminum Hydroxide Gel, U.S.P., B.P.; Aluminum Hydroxide Gel, U.S.P. (Alkagel, Al-U-Creme, Amphojel, Creamalin)

Aluminum hydroxide gel is a sweetened and flavored aqueous suspension of aluminum hydroxide equivalent to approximately 4 per cent aluminum oxide. It neutralizes the acid of the stomach, but it does not increase the pH sufficiently to prevent peptic digestion. It does not cause "acid rebound" nor does it produce alkalosis. The mild astringent and demulcent action of the drug produces a healing effect on the irritated or ulcerated mucosa of the stomach and intestines. It tends to increase the secretion of mucin.

Aluminum hydroxide gel is nontoxic because it is not absorbed. It is used as an adjunct in the treatment of peptic ulcer. The usual oral dose of the gel is 15 ml. (8 to 30 ml.) in a half-glass of milk or water four times a day.

In cases of severe pain, 1 part of gel may be diluted with 2 to 3 parts of water and administered by intragastric drip, slowly, giving 1.5 L. in 24 hours, or 30 ml. of the gel may be given every two hours alternating with 90 ml. of a mixture of half milk and half cream. The dose of the dried gel is 300 mg. (300 mg. to 5 Gm.) four times a day. It is administered in tablet form.

Preparations

Aluminum Hydroxide Gel, U.S.P.

Dried Aluminum Hydroxide Gel Tablets, 300 and 600 mg. U.S.P., B.P.

Trade names: Alocol; Alkagel; Al-U-Creme; Amphojel; Collumina; Creamalin

Magnesium and Aluminum Hydroxide Suspension

Magnesium and aluminum hydroxide suspension is a creamy white, flavored colloidal suspension of magnesium and aluminum hydroxide. It is an effective antacid which does not cause constipation and may be used for prolonged periods of time. The oral dose is two to four teaspoonsful or two to four tablets 20 minutes to one hour after meals and at bedtime.

Preparations

Magnesium and Aluminum Hydroxide in Suspension   400 mg. in 1 teaspoonful

Magnesium and Aluminum Hydroxide Tablets   400 and 800 mg.

Trade names: Aludrox, Maalox

Aluminum Phosphate Gel, N.F. (Phosphajel)

Aluminum phosphate gel is a 4 per cent aqueous suspension of aluminum phosphate. It is an antacid with astringent and demulcent properties. The usual dose is 15 ml. (15 to 30 ml.), alone or with water or milk, six times a day. It is used to relieve pain and hasten healing in peptic ulcer.

Oxethazine in Alumina Gel (Oxaine)

Oxethazine is a new topical anesthetic. It produces a more potent and prolonged anesthetic action on the mucous membranes than either cocaine or lidocaine. It also causes an antispasmodic action on smooth muscle. A 0.2 per cent concentration in aluminum hydroxide gel provides antacid and demulcent properties with local anesthesia of the mucosa. It is used in the treatment of gastritis, esophagitis, and irritable colon syndrome. The side effects noted are constipation, dizziness, drowsiness, or faintness. The adult oral dose is one to two teaspoonfuls four times a day and at bedtime. It is supplied in 12-oz. bottles.

Basic Aluminum Carbonate (Basaljel)

This is an aqueous suspension of an aluminum hydroxide carbonate complex containing 4.9 to 5.3 per cent aluminum oxide and 2.4 per cent carbon dioxide. This antacid is used to control gastric hyperacidity and as an adjunct in the treatment of peptic ulcer. The usual antacid dose is 4 to 8 ml. repeated when necessary.

Dihydroxyaluminum Aminoacetate, N.F. (Alglyn)

Dihydroxyaluminum aminoacetate is useful in the treatment of gastric acidity and peptic ulcer. It offers the same advantages as the aluminum hydroxide gel preparations. It is administered orally in doses of 500 mg. to 1 Gm. after meals and at bedtime.

Preparation

Dihydroxyaluminum Aminoacetate   500 mg.
Tablets, N.F.
        Trade names: Alglyn; Alzinox; Aspogen; Doraxamin; Robalate

Polyamine-Methylene Resin (Exorbin, Resinat)

Polyamine-methylene resin is a nonirritating anion-exchange resin that is insoluble and not absorbed. This drug can remove acids from solution by adsorption. It temporarily binds the gastric hydrochloric acid and carries it to the intestine, where it is slowly released. The resin is nontoxic and is eliminated unchanged from the gastrointestinal tract. The released acid is neutralized permanently by alkaline substances (chiefly sodium bicarbonate) in the bile and intestinal juices.

The recommended dose for the resin is 500 mg. to 1 Gm. every two hours for the relief of symptoms in peptic ulcer. It is administered orally in the form of a powder, capsules, or tablets. The powder is given with water or milk. Capsules or tablets (250 mg.) are the more convenient dosage forms.

DIGESTANTS

Digestants are substances that promote the digestion of foods in the gastrointestinal tract. Those commonly employed are hydrochloric acid, the enzymes of the stomach and the pancreas, and the bile and bile salts. With the exception of hydrochloric acid, their use in therapeutics is limited.

Hypochlorhydria, Achlorhydria, and Achylia Gastrica. The digestants are used for replacement therapy in deficiency states. *Hypochlorhydria* is a diminished secretion of hydrochloric acid in the stomach. *Achlor-*

hydria is the absence of hydrochloric acid in the stomach. If both acid and enzymes are absent, the condition is called *achylia gastrica*. Achylia gastrica occurs in carcinoma of the stomach, pernicious anemia, and other conditions.

HYDROCHLORIC ACID

Diluted Hydrochloric Acid, N.F.; Dilute Hydrochloric Acid, B.P., I.P.

Diluted hydrochloric acid is a 10 per cent aqueous solution of hydrochloric acid. It is administered in 5-ml. doses, well diluted with water, during or after meals, in hypochlorhydria, achlorhydria, and achylia gastrica. It is best administered through a glass straw to avoid injury to the teeth. The B.P. dose is 0.6 to 6 ml.

Glutamic Acid Hydrochloride, N.F. (Acidulin)

Glutamic acid hydrochloride, a white powder, is a combination of hydrochloric acid with glutamic acid which yields hydrochloric acid when added to water. Capsules are administered before meals and supply 0.6 ml. of diluted hydrochloric acid.

Preparation

Glutamic Acid Hydrochloride Capsules,   300 mg. N.F.

> Trade names: Achlor; Acidoride; Acidulin; Gastuloric; Glutan; Glutasin; Hydrionic; Muriamic

Betaine Hydrochloride (Normacid)

Betaine hydrochloride is available in tablets that contain betaine hydrochloride, pepsin, and methylcellulose. The mixture liberates hydrochloric acid slowly.

ENZYMES OF STOMACH AND PANCREAS

Pepsin, N.F.

Pepsin is a proteolytic enzyme that initiates the hydrolysis of protein food in the stomach. This enzyme is available in the form of transparent or translucent scales prepared from the glandular layer of the fresh stomach of the hog. It was formerly believed that a deficiency of pepsin caused digestive disturbances; consequently, the enzyme was administered to remedy this condition. It is now known that hypochlorhydria is the cause of most of these disorders and that pepsin is generally present in adequate amounts. In addition, it is also known that the proteolytic enzymes of the intestine may hydrolyze proteins. Therefore, pepsin is seldom used today as a digestant.

When it is given, the dose is 500 mg. taken after meals. Compound Pepsin Elixir, N.F. (Lactated Pepsin Elixir), is used as a vehicle for other drugs.

Pancreatin, N.F., B.P.

Pancreatin contains the enzymes of the pancreas—amylase, trypsin, and lipase. It is obtained from the pancreas of the hog or ox for use as an aid for duodenal digestion in sprue. The usual oral dose is 500 mg. Tablets containing 500 mg. of the drug are available.

PANCREATIC ENZYMES

Cotazym

Cotazym, a concentrated enzyme preparation, provides replacement of lipase in pancreatic enzyme deficiency characteristic of cystic fibrosis. Because it aids in the digestion of fats, it relieves steatorrhea, diarrhea, and flatulence and improves the patient's nutrition and strength. Three capsules are administered with each meal and one with each snack.

Preparation

Cotazym Capsules   300 mg.

BILE AND BILE SALTS

Bile is essential for the normal digestion of fats and the absorption of fatty acids. It is formed in the liver and flows to the small intestine through the hepatic and common bile ducts. The bile acids are absorbed from the intestine and are carried to the liver by the portal vein, whereupon they are re-excreted in the bile. Most of the actions of bile are due to the bile salts, sodium glyco-cholate and sodium taurocholate, which are essential for the optimal absorption of fat and fat-soluble substances such as carotene, vitamin A, vitamin D, and vitamin K. Bile has an antiputrefactive action and is mildly cathartic. In therapeutics, the most important actions are the stimulation of bile secretion (choleresis) and the promotion of absorption of fat and fat-soluble substances.

Bile and bile salts are used in the treatment of hepatic insufficiency, hepatic jaundice, cirrhosis of the liver, and biliary fistula and in cholecystography.

Cholic acid derivatives are more potent and less toxic than the natural bile salts.

Ox Bile Extract

Ox bile extract is very bitter and is administered in enteric-coated tablets or capsules (200 and 300 mg.) after meals.

Dehydrocholic Acid, N.F. (Decholin)

Dehydrocholic acid increases the secretion of bile and is used to increase the drainage of the bile ducts as well as to aid in the absorption of fat and fat-soluble vitamins in cirrhosis of the liver or steatorrhea. It is contraindicated in complete mechanical biliary obstruction. The usual oral dose is 500 mg. (250 to 500 mg.) three times daily after meals.

Preparation

Dehydrocholic Acid Tablets, N.F.   250 mg.

Trade name: Decholin

Sodium Dehydrocholate, N.F. (Decholin Sodium)

The actions and uses of sodium dehydrocholate are the same as dehydrocholic acid. It is administered intravenously as a 20 per cent solution. An injection of 5 to 10 ml. is given on the first day and is followed by 10 ml. on the next two days. Oral administration should replace intravenous therapy as soon as possible. Sodium dehydrocholate causes a bitter taste in the mouth when it is given intravenously. For this reason it is also used as a diagnostic agent for estimating the circulation time in the arm-to-tongue test.

Preparation

Sodium Dehydrocholate Injection, N.F.   500 mg. in 10 ml., 600 mg. in 3 ml.,
                                        1 Gm. in 5 ml., and 2 Gm. in 10 ml.

Trade name: Decholin Sodium

AMMONIA ANTI-INTOXICANTS

In severe liver disease ammonia may accumulate in the tissue fluids and blood leading to the production of hepatic coma. The amino acids, arginine and glutamic acids, reduce these elevated ammonia levels in the body. They are combined as a salt, arginine glutamate, or glutamic acid may be given as monosodium 1-glutamate or monosodium and monopotassium 1-glutamate. While no change in the status of the liver is produced, the blood ammonia levels are lowered. As a result, the individual's level of consciousness is improved.

The contents of a 100-ml. container of these drugs dissolved in 500 or 1000 ml. of a 5 per cent dextrose solution are given by intravenous drip over a period of one or more hours. The initial dose of 25 to 50 Gm. may be repeated after eight hours, if necessary. Severe cases may require repeated infusions for three to five days.

Preparations

Arginine Glutamate Injection	100-ml. bottles containing 13.5 Gm. 1-arginine and 12 Gm. 1-glutamic acid
Trade name:	Modumate
Monosodium 1-glutamate	100 ml. bottles containing 25 Gm. 1-glutamic acid and 170 meq. of sodium
Trade name:	Glutavene
Monosodium and monopotassium 1-glutamate	100-ml. bottles containing 25 Gm. 1-glutamic acid and 130 and 40 meq. of sodium and potassium, respectively
Trade name:	Glutavene-K

CARMINATIVES

Carminatives are drugs used to relieve flatulence and colic and to lessen griping. They are aromatic, mildly irritating, antiseptic volatile oils that check the formation of gas in the stomach and intestines, increase gastrointestinal motility and peristalsis, and aid in the expulsion of gas.

Peppermint Oil, U.S.P., B.P.

Peppermint is a volatile oil that is administered three times a day as peppermint water, in doses of 15 ml., or as peppermint spirit, in doses of 0.5 to 1 ml. in water or dispersed in sugar.

Ginger, N.F., B.P.

Ginger is administered as fluidextract of ginger, in doses of 0.6 ml., or as ginger ale. Other volatile oils, such as spearmint or anise, may be used for their carminative action.

EMETICS

Emetics (see p. 260) are drugs that are used to produce vomiting in cases of acute poisoning or alcoholic intoxication. The local emetics, which may be lifesaving, are administered with a large amount of water. The physician or hospital emergency room staff usually employs gastric lavage by tube to remove the poisonous material still remaining in the stomach. Systemic emetics such as apomorphine are rarely used now.

Household Remedies

Putting the finger down the throat and causing gagging is a very effective method to induce vomiting. Large amounts of tepid water will distend the stomach and also produce this effect. Two teaspoonfuls of salt or mustard are often added to the lukewarm water. Lukewarm tea is used in alkaloid poisoning.

Apomorphine Hydrochloride, U.S.P., B.P., I.P.

Apomorphine hydrochloride is a centrally acting emetic that produces vomiting a few minutes after subcutaneous injection. It is a derivative of morphine and is discussed on page 260. The subcutaneous dose is 5 mg. If vomiting does not occur in 15 minutes, the dose may be repeated. The B.P. subcutaneous or intramuscular dose is 2 to 8 mg.

Preparations

Apomorphine Hydrochloride Tablets,   5 mg.
N.F.
Apomorphine Hydrochloride Injection,   3 mg. in 1 ml.
B.P., I.P.

ADSORBENTS

Gastrointestinal adsorbents are finely divided inert powders that adsorb toxins and other substances on their extensive surfaces. They are used to adsorb (1) poisons, such as alkaloids, which have been swallowed (thus delaying their absorption until gastric lavage can be performed) and (2) toxins which cause diarrhea.

Preparations

Kaolin, N.F.; Heavy Kaolin, B.P.
Purified Animal Charcoal, N.F.
Attapulgite, Activated (Claysorb)

Gastrointestinal Tract Antiseptics

The use of the poorly absorbed sulfonamides in gastrointestinal tract infections is discussed on page 169.

Furazolidine, N.F. (Furoxone). This drug is used in the treatment of bacterial diarrheas and enteritis. It is active against a wide variety of bacteria, including intestinal pathogens of the genera Salmonella and Shigella. Concentrations a little greater than that required to inhibit growth are bactericidal. Upon oral administration the drug is partially absorbed and excreted in the urine. Some is presumably destroyed in the alimentary tract and the tissues. Furazolidine is being studied in the United States, Mexico, Great Britain, and India. The adult oral dose is 100 mg. four times a day. The dose for children is adjusted according to age or weight. Generally the normal bowel movement is restored in three to four days.

Preparations

Furazolidone Suspension	50 mg. in 1 tbsp.
Furazolidone Tablets	100 mg.

Trade name: Furoxone

DIAGNOSTIC AIDS FOR THE DIGESTIVE SYSTEM

DETERMINATION OF GASTRIC ACIDITY

Histamine Acid Phosphate, U.S.P., B.P.

Histamine acid phosphate is used as a diagnostic aid in suspected achylia gastrica or achlorhydria. See page 756 for the discussion of this agent.

Preparation

Histamine Phosphate Injection, U.S.P., B.P.	1-ml. ampuls containing the equivalent of 1 mg. of histamine

Betazole Hydrochloride, U.S.P. (Histalog)

This is an analog of histamine and can be used in its place as a diagnostic aid for determining gastric secretion. Betazole stimulates the secretion of hydrochloric acid without causing a significant fall in blood pressure and with only a slight increase in the pulse rate. The side effects are flushing, sweating, and in some cases headache. Urticaria and fainting seldom occur. The subcutaneous dose is 50 mg. (40 to 60 mg.). **Betazole hydrochloride injection, U.S.P.,** contains 50 mg. in 1 ml.

Quinine Carbacrylic Resin (Diagnex)

Quinine carbacrylic resin is used as an indicator for the estimation of gastric acidity without intubation. After oral administration, the quinine in the resin is replaced by the hydrogen ions of free hydrochloric acid that may be present in the stomach. About 1 per cent of the displaced quinine is excreted in the urine two hours after the administration of the resin. A stimulant to gastric secretion such as caffeine is given one hour prior to the administration of the resin. The urine voided during that hour is used as the control. Assay of the quinine content of urine specimens collected at the end of one- and two-hour periods determines the presence of hydrochloric acid in the stomach. This drug is useful in the diagnosis of gastric cancer and pernicious anemia, in both of which the gastric acid diminishes and may be absent.

The toxicity of quinine carbacrylic resin is low, but it is contraindicated in persons idiosyncratic to quinine and related drugs.

Dosage and Method of Administration. The single oral dose is 1 Gm. in the form of granules. Oral administration of caffeine and sodium benzoate stimulates gastric secretion.

Preparation

Granules Diagnex	Packet containing 2 Gm. of resin and capsule containing 250 mg. of caffeine and sodium benzoate

Azuresin, N.F. (Diagnex Blue)

This cation-exchange resin, with azure "A," a blue dye, bound to it, is given orally for the detection of free acid in the stomach. Hydrochloric acid, when present, liberates the dye from the resin. The dye is then absorbed into the blood and excreted in the urine, which may then be colored blue or bluish green. Urine samples are then analyzed, using *Diagnex Reagent,* a strongly acidic copper sulfate solution, which must *not be confused* with the powdered Diagnex Blue that the patient swallows. Two 250-mg. tablets of caffeine sodium benzoate, supplied in the package, are taken to stimulate gastric acid. Absence of acid (achlorhydria), or the presence of an abnormally small amount (hypochlorhydria) after attempted stimulation may signify a disease and require appropriate additional studies.

Preparation

Azuresin, N.F.	2 Gm.

Trade name: Diagnex Blue

Barium Sulfate, U.S.P.

Barium sulfate is a white, odorless, tasteless, bulky powder that is neither soluble in water nor absorbed; i.e., it passes through the gastrointestinal tract unchanged. The powder is much more impermeable to x-rays than are the tissues and is nontoxic in large doses; consequently it is used in x-ray studies of the gastrointestinal tract to locate abnormal conditions. For examination of the stomach, 300 mg. of barium sulfate are suspended in about 400 ml. of water and given orally. For examination of the lower bowel, 360 mg. of barium sulfate are suspended in 1500 ml. of water and administered rectally after one or more cleansing enemas.

RADIOPAQUE CHOLECYSTOGRAPHY

Radiopaque organic iodine compounds are excreted in the bile and concentrated in the gallbladder. These drugs cast a shadow upon x-ray films and are used for the visualization of the gallbladder in certain diagnostic tests. Persons allergic to iodine may have reactions to these compounds. Since the thyroid gland traps iodine, diagnostic thyroid tests (see p. 672) should be performed before the administration of these compounds.

Iodophthalein Sodium (Soluble Iodophthalein, Tetiothalein Sodium, Tetraiodophenolphthalein Sodium, Tetraiodophthalein Sodium, Iodeikon)

Iodophthalein sodium is a water-soluble, blue-violet powder containing 60 to 63 per cent iodine. It is administered intravenously. The intravenous dose of 2 Gm. (2 to 4 Gm.) is dissolved in 24 ml. of sterile distilled water and is administered in two doses at 30-minute intervals the morning of the examination. The intravenous injection may cause vertigo and nausea. The drug is contraindicated in myocardial insufficiency, nephritis, and jaundice.

Preparation

Iodophthalein Sodium	Vials containing 4 Gm.

Trade name: Iodeikon

Meglumine Diatrizoate (Gastrografin)

This water-soluble compound is administered in 76 per cent solution. For infants and children up to five years, the dose is 30 ml.; for older children, 60 ml.; for adults, 90 ml. For retention enemas, 240 ml. of a 76 per cent solution are diluted to 1000 ml.; for children, 90 ml. are diluted to 500 ml. The U.S.P. injection of this compound is available for the diagnosis of kidney or ureteral lesions (see p. 650).

Meglumine Iodipamide Injection, U.S.P. (Cholografin); Iodipamide Sodium Injection, N.F. (Cholografin Sodium)

These compounds are administered intravenously. They are well tolerated when administered slowly. Transient restlessness, nausea, vomiting, and pressure in the upper abdomen may occur, but severe reactions seldom occur. The intravenous dose of meglumine iodipamide injection is 20 ml. of a 52 per cent solution. The dose for iodipamide sodium is 40 ml. of a 20 per cent solution.

Preparations

Meglumine Iodipamide Injection, U.S.P.	52 per cent solution in 20 ml.
Iodipamide Sodium Injection, N.F.	4 Gm. in 20 ml.
Iodipamide Methylglucamine Injection, B.P.	

Trade names: Biligrafin, Cholografin, Endografin

Iodoalphionic Acid, N.F. (Priodax)

Iodoalphionic acid is a water-soluble compound. It is excreted mainly in the liver and concentrated in the gallbladder. The oral adult dose of 3 Gm. (1.5 to 12 Gm.) is administered in tablet form with several glasses of water, during or after a light fat-free evening meal. No food should be taken prior to the x-ray examination the following morning. Iodophthalein is contraindicated in nephritis and uremia.

Preparation

Iodoalphionic Acid Tablets, N.F.   500 mg.
Trade name: Priodax

Iopanoic Acid, U.S.P., B.P. (Telepaque)

Iopanoic acid is administered orally. It is promptly absorbed and produces dense shadows of the gallbladder with a single dose. There are seldom any undesirable reactions. The compound is contraindicated in acute nephritis and gastrointestinal disorders. The oral dose is 3 Gm. (2 to 6 Gm.).

Preparation

Iopanoic Acid Tablets, U.S.P., B.P.   500 mg.
Trade name: Telepaque

Ipodate Calcium and Sodium (Oragrafin)

Ipodate is an iodine-containing compound used for x-ray visualization of the gallbladder and other parts of the biliary tract. The calcium salt is available in a suspension and the sodium salt in capsule form. Each is given orally in a single dose of 3 Gm., followed by x-ray examination as scheduled by the roentgenologist.

Preparations

Ipodate Calcium   3 Gm. with 5 Gm. sucrose in 8-Gm. paper packet
Ipodate Sodium   500 mg. in capsules
Trade names: Oragrafin Calcium and Sodium

Iophenoxic Acid (Teridax)

This water-insoluble compound is administered orally. There are few incidences of side effects. The usual oral dose is 50 mg. per kilogram of body weight. Iophenoxic acid tablets, U.S.P., contain 750 mg.

LIVER FUNCTION TEST

Sulfobromophthalein Sodium, U.S.P.

Sulfobromophthalein sodium is a white crystalline, water-soluble compound that is used to test the function of the liver. It is administered intravenously in a 5 per cent solution. In normal individuals the compound is removed rapidly from the blood by the liver and is excreted in the bile. In impairment of liver function, the dye is removed much more slowly, and the amount of dye remaining in the blood is determined colorimetrically at various intervals following its injection. The administration intravenously of 5 mg. (2 to 5 mg.) per kilogram of body weight is followed in one hour by the estimation of the dye in the circulating blood. The retention of less than 6 per cent is considered normal. Impairment of liver function will cause a retention of 6 to 40 per cent or more of the dye.

Preparation

Sulfobromophthalein Sodium Injection,   3-ml. ampuls containing 150 mg.
U.S.P.

REVIEW QUESTIONS

1. *Explain the function of hydrochloric acid in peptic digestion.*
2. *What are some causes of peptic ulcer?*
3. *Name three types of drugs used in the treatment of this condition and indicate the place of each.*
4. *Define antacids. Describe the two types and give an example of each.*
5. *What is aluminum hydroxide gel? What are the advantages of its use in peptic ulcer?*
6. *What is cotazyme? For what purposes is it used clinically?*
7. *What is the action of ammonia anti-intoxicants?*
8. *Explain the use of organic iodine compounds in diagnostic tests.*
9. *Explain the use of a suitable dye in determining liver function.*
10. *What drug is used in the treatment of ammonia intoxication and hepatic coma? How does it act?*

REFERENCES

Adams, W. L.: "Critical Evaluation of Gastric Antacids," *Arch. Int. Med.*, **63**:1030, 1939.

Batterman, R. C., and Ehrenfeld, I.: "The Effect of Ambulant Treatment of Peptic Ulcer Syndrome: The Comparative Effectiveness and Constipating Action of Antacids," *Gastroenterology*, **9**:141, 1947.

Best, E. B.: "Pancreatic Replacement Therapy in Fibrocystic Disease: A

Preliminary Report Concerning a New Pancreatic Extract," *South. M. J.,* **53**:1091, 1960.

Deutsch, E., and Christian, H.: "Chronic Gastritis; Histological Criteria for Management and Medical Treatment with a Mucosal Anesthetic in Aluminum Hydroxide," *J.A.M.A.,* **169**:2012, 1959.

Hammarlund, E. R., and Rising, L. W.: "Comparative Study of the Buffering Capacity of Various Commercially Available Gastric Antacids," *J. A. Pharm. A.,* **38**:586, 1949.

Jankelson, O. M., and Jankelson, I. R.: "The Symptomatic Exaggerated Gastrocolic Reflex by an Oral, Topical Anesthetic (Oxethazine)," *Am. J. Gastroenterology,* **32**:719, 1959.

Rice, M. L., Jr.: "Efficacy of Dihydroxyaluminum Aminoacetate in the Medical Cure of Peptic Ulcer," *Am. J. Gastroenterol.,* **25**:74, 1956.

Rossett, N. E., and Rice, M. L., Jr.: "In Vitro Evaluation of the Efficacy of the More Frequently Used Antacids, with Particular Attention to Tablets," *Gastroenterology,* **26**:490, 1954.

36

Cathartics and Antidiarrheics

Constipation usually results from a combination of (1) an improper diet that leaves too little residue in the intestinal tract and is lacking in vitamins, (2) insufficient fluid intake, (3) nervous tension and worry, (4) lack of exercise, (5) failure to respond to normal defecation impulses, and (6) the abuse of cathartics. Proper food, sufficient fluid intake, freedom from worry, adequate exercise, and prompt response to the normal impulses for defecation will often remedy this condition. In other cases, the administration of laxatives as an adjunct to other measures is recommended.

CATHARTICS

Cathartics are drugs that are used to produce evacuation of the bowels. They may be classified, according to their action, as laxatives and purgatives. Laxatives produce few movements of the bowels and the stool is well formed. Purgatives cause frequent soft or liquid stools.

Cathartics may also be classified according to their mechanism of action. Some increase the bulk of the intestinal contents by the retention of water, whereupon the resulting mechanical pressure on the wall of the intestine stimulates peristalsis. Hydrophilic colloids such as agar and plantago seed retain water by imbibition and swell to form a gel. Saline cathartics either prevent the absorption of water from the intestinal tract or cause water to be drawn into the intestine by the phenomenon of osmosis. Because of this action the latter are often called *hydrogogue* cathartics.

Drugs such as mineral or vegetable oils are often used for their lubricating action. Likewise, there are many cathartics that irritate the mucosa of the intestinal tract and reflexly stimulate peristalsis and evacuation; examples of this type are cascara sagrada and senna. Neostigmine methylsulfate, upon injection, stimulates the cholinergic fibers to the intestines and increases peristalsis. Posterior pituitary solution, when injected, acts directly on the smooth muscle of the intestine and increases its muscular contraction. Both these drugs are used to relieve postoperative distention following abdominal surgery but are not used as cathartics.

587

Therapeutic Uses and Drugs of Choice

1. In food or drug poisoning—magnesium sulfate or castor oil.

2. To soften the stools in hemorrhoids and other disorders of the rectum and to prevent straining in various disease conditions—mineral oil, hydrophilic colloids (bulk cathartics), or cascara sagrada.

3. To remove irritating and infectious material from the intestinal tract, as in diarrhea and after the administration of some anthelmintics—saline cathartics and sometimes castor oil.

4. In edema to remove fluid from the tissues, as in nephritis and cardiac or cerebral edema—saline purgatives.

5. To prevent and treat constipation in the patient who is confined to bed or is on a restricted diet—bulk cathartics, mineral oil, or cascara sagrada.

Contraindications. Cathartics are contraindicated in disease conditions of the abdominal organs (peptic ulcer, appendicitis, gastroenteritis), and they should not be used in threatened intestinal hemorrhage, intestinal obstruction, or intussusception. During pregnancy or menstruation they should be used with great care because they may produce abortion or increased menstrual flow. Cathartics should be used sparingly in chronic constipation.

HYDROPHILIC COLLOIDS (BULK CATHARTICS)

The hydrophilic colloids are not absorbed and swell due to the absorption of fluid in the gastrointestinal tract. They are relatively nonirritating and nontoxic. The powdered forms should be mixed with water or fruit juice just before being taken because they become gelatinous very quickly.

Agar, U.S.P.

Agar is a dried hydrophilic colloid obtained from seaweed. It imbibes water and swells to form a mucilaginous mass that is soothing to the gastrointestinal mucosa. It increases the bulk and keeps the intestinal contents soft and moist. Agar is available as a powder or in the form of shreds. It may be administered with cereal or other food or in milk. The dose is 4 Gm. (4 to 16 Gm.) once or twice a day.

Plantago Seed, N.F. (Psyllium Seed)

Plantago seed, a small, dark seed containing a natural mucilage, absorbs water and increases the bulk in the intestinal tract, thereby producing a stool that is smooth and moist. Because of its demulcent action, plantago seed may be used in the presence of inflammation of the intestinal mucosa. The usual dose is 7.5 Gm. It is administered in fruit juice or water.

Plantago Ovato Coating (Konsyl)

Plantago ovato coating is a cream- to brown-colored granular powder prepared from the outer mucilaginous coating of blond psyllium seeds. It is a demulcent bulk laxative administered in doses of 5 to 10 Gm. three times daily in a glass of water or milk.

Psyllium Hydrophilic Mucilloid (Metamucil)

Psyllium hydrophilic mucilloid is a 50–50 mixture of the powdered mucilaginous portion of blond psyllium seeds and powdered anhydrous dextrose. It is a white- to cream-colored granular powder that swells in the presence of water to form a gel, thereby producing a soft, moist stool which has a soothing effect on irritated mucosa. The mixture is used in the treatment of some types of constipation and colitis and as an adjunct in the treatment of spastic colitis or irritable colon. The dose is 4 to 7 Gm. one to three times a day. The drug is stirred in water, milk, or fruit juice, and its administration is followed by an additional glass of water.

Preparation

Metamucil Powder

Methylcellulose, U.S.P. (Cellothyl, Methocel, Syncelose)

Methylcellulose is a hydrophilic colloid available in the form of tablets or a granular powder. Like the other cathartics of its class, it absorbs water and provides a lubricating action. Methylcellulose is administered with water and passes through the gastrointestinal tract in the form of a colloidal solution until it reaches the colon, where water is absorbed and a gel is formed. The dose is 1 Gm. (1 to 4 Gm.) in tablets or granules with water, one to four times a day. Later the dose may be reduced to 1 Gm. once or twice daily.

Preparations

Granules Methylcellulose
Tablets Methylcellulose   500 mg.
            Trade names: Cellothyl; Cologel; Methocel; Saraka; Syncelose

SALINE CATHARTICS (BULK CATHARTICS)

Saline cathartics are soluble salts that are only slightly absorbed and hence are retained in the gastrointestinal tract for some time. Because of their high osmotic pressure, they prevent the absorption of water out of the tract and also draw water from the tissues into the intestines. The bulk of the intestinal contents is increased, peristalsis is stimulated, and frequent fluid stools are rapidly expelled. Various salts of magnesium and the sulfates, phosphates, citrates, and tartrates of sodium and potassium are used as saline cathartics.

They produce a rapid action, particularly if taken well diluted, in the morning before breakfast. Catharsis results in one-half to four hours, depending upon the amount of fluid ingested with the drug.

The saline cathartics are used (1) in food poisoning, (2) with anthelmintics, and (3) in cerebral or cardiac edema to produce dehydration.

Preparations and Dosage

Magnesium Sulfate, U.S.P.; Magnesium Sulphate, B.P. (Epsom Salt)	15 Gm. (10–30 Gm.)—cathartic dose
Magnesium Citrate Solution, N.F.	200 ml.
Milk of Magnesia, U.S.P.; Magnesium Hydroxide Mixture, B.P.	15 ml. (5 to 30 ml.)—laxative 5 ml.—antacid
Magnesium Carbonate, U.S.P.	600 mg.—antacid
Light Magnesium Carbonate, B.P.	300 to 600 mg.—antacid
Magnesium Oxide, U.S.P.	250 mg.—antacid
Light Magnesium Oxide, B.P.	2 to 4 Gm.—laxative
Sodium Sulfate, N.F. (Glauber's Salt); Sodium Sulphate, B.P.	15 Gm. (well diluted)
Sodium Phosphate, N.F., B.P.	4 Gm.—laxative dose
Effervescent Sodium Phosphate, N.F.	10 Gm.
Potassium Sodium Tartrate, N.F.; Sodium Potassium Tartrate, B.P. (Rochelle Salt)	10 Gm.

LUBRICANT CATHARTICS

Mineral Oil, U.S.P.; Liquid Paraffin, B.P.

Mineral oil is a mixture of liquid hydrocarbons obtained from petroleum. It is indigestible and not absorbed; it acts as a mechanical lubricant and increases bulk in the intestinal tract by preventing the absorption of water. Mineral oil is used (1) to keep the stools soft in chronic constipation, (2) to reduce straining after rectal operations, and (3) in patients with hernia, hypertension, or cardiovascular accidents. The adult dose is 15 to 30 ml. once or twice a day usually given at night, often with fruit or as an emulsified preparation; in some cases, it is advisable to give the cathartic in divided doses between meals. Repeated administration over long periods of time may prevent absorption of fat-soluble vitamins and bile. When large doses are given, some of the oil may leak through the anal sphincter.

Liquid Petrolatum Emulsion, N.F.

Liquid petrolatum emulsion is a pleasantly flavored emulsion. There are many emulsions available that contain other laxative drugs such as phenolphthalein and cascara sagrada.

ANTHRACENE COMPOUNDS (IRRITANT CATHARTICS)

Rhubarb, cascara, aloe, and senna contain inactive glycosidal compounds which, when decomposed in the alkaline intestine, produce various anthraquinone derivatives such as emodin and chrysophanic acid. These metabolites, of which emodin is the most important, produce a cathartic action by irritating the mucosa of the intestinal tract.

Rhubarb, N.F., B.P.

Rhubarb is obtained from the dried roots of a plant grown in China and Tibet. This plant, however, is not the rhubarb that is used as a food in the United States.

Preparations and Dosage

Rhubarb Fluidextract, N.F.	1 ml.
Aromatic Rhubarb Tincture, N.F.	5 ml.
Compound Rhubarb Tincture, B.P.	

Cascara Sagrada, U.S.P., B.P., I.P.

Cascara sagrada is obtained from the bark of the tree *Rhamnus purshiana* (California buckthorn). It is one of the best laxatives available but is not suitable for strong purgative action. Its action is limited to the colon, and it is used in chronic or habitual constipation. Cascara does not lose its efficiency with repeated doses.

Preparations and Dosage

Aromatic Cascara Sagrada Fluidextract, U.S.P.; Cascara Elixir, B.P.	5 ml. (2 to 12 ml.)
Cascara Sagrada Fluidextract, N.F.; Cascara Liquid Extract, B.P.	1 ml. (2 to 4 ml.)
Cascara Sagrada Extract Tablets, N.F.; Cascara Tablets, B.P.	120, 200, and 300 mg.

Aloe, U.S.P.; Aloes, B.P.

Aloe is the dried juice of the leaves of a plant that grows in Africa and the West Indies. It contains aloin, a mixture of active principles which are chiefly glycosides. In the intestines these glycosides are decomposed, forming anthraquinone derivatives, which are the active cathartic agents. Aloin is the most irritating of all the emodin cathartics. The usual dose of aloe is 120 to 250 mg. It is available in the form of pills. Aloin is generally incorporated in pills containing other cathartics.

Senna, N.F.; Senna Leaf, B.P.

Senna is obtained from the dried leaves of *Cassia acutifolia* and *Cassia angustifolia*. It is an irritant cathartic that may produce considerable griping. Emodin is the cathartic principle.

Preparations and Dosage

Senna Fluidextract, N.F.	2 ml.
Senna Syrup, N.F.	8 ml.
Compound Senna Powder, N.F.	4 Gm.

OTHER IRRITANT CATHARTICS

Phenolphthalein, N.F., B.P.

Phenolphthalein is a white crystalline powder insoluble in water. When administered orally, it mildly irritates the mucosa of the large and small intestines and produces catharsis. A small amount of the drug may be absorbed and excreted in the bile and urine. Phenolphthalein is the active ingredient of many proprietary preparations. The dose is 60 mg. orally. The drug is a nontoxic substance, but in susceptible individuals a rash may appear and in some cases severe diarrhea is noted.

Preparation

Phenolphthalein Tablets, N.F., B.P.	60 and 120 mg.

Castor Oil, U.S.P., B.P., I.P.

Castor oil is a fixed oil obtained from the seeds of *Ricinus communis*. It is a distasteful, bland, yellow-colored oil that is hydrolyzed in the intestines to glycerol and ricinoleic acid. Sodium ricinoleate, which is then formed, is irritating to the mucosa of the small intestine. Liquid stools result in two to six hours. The dose of castor oil is 15 ml. (15 to 60 ml.). It is frequently given with fruit juice or in the form of an emulsion to mask its disagreeable taste. Castor oil is used in certain types of food and drug poisoning, acute constipation, and diarrhea caused by irritants and infections, as well as to initiate labor in obstetrics.

Preparations and Dosage

Castor Oil, U.S.P.	15 ml. (15 to 60 ml.)
Aromatic Castor Oil, N.F.	15 ml.

DETERGENT LAXATIVE

Dioctyl Sodium Sulfosuccinate, N.F. (Colace, Doxinate)

This compound, a "wetting" agent, is used as a nonlaxative fecal softener solely because it reduces surface tension of aqueous systems, just as do soap and detergents. It is bland, nonirritating, and free of side effects. A dose of approximately 100 mg. a day is sufficient to provide maximum softening of the stool. Additional amounts are usually ineffective; thus diarrhea is generally avoided. Dioctyl sodium sulfosuccinate is used to relieve chronic constipation and lower-bowel obstruction due to fecal impaction. The suggested oral dose for adults is 10 to 60 mg. daily; the dose for infants and children is 10 to 20 mg. A daily administration of 100 mg. in divided doses may be required for some adults.

Preparations

Dioctyl Sodium Sulfosuccinate Capsules 20, 50, 60, and 100 mg.
Dioctyl Sodium Sulfosuccinate Liquid 10 and 50 mg. in 1 ml.
(Oral)
Dioctyl Sodium Sulfosuccinate Syrup 4 mg. in 1 ml.

Trade names: Colace; Doxinate

CONTACT LAXATIVE

Bisacodyl (Dulcolax)

Bisacodyl is a contact laxative that acts directly on the mucosa of the large intestine, causing increased peristalsis without spasm or griping. There is little or no action on the small intestine. The drug is not absorbed and is free from toxic effects. The use of this preparation eliminates the necessity of giving enemas. This is timesaving for the nurse and lessens the discomfort to the patient. The drug is used preoperatively, postoperatively, in preparation for x-ray procedures, and in all types of constipation in adults and children. It is administered both orally and rectally. The oral dose is 10 mg., the rectal dose is 10 to 20 mg. For preoperative use, 10 mg. are given the evening before. If there is no satisfactory bowel movement, one or two suppositories may be inserted prior to the patient's going to the operating room.

Preparations

Bisacodyl Tablets 5 mg.
Bisacodyl Suppositories 10 mg.

Trade name: Dulcolax

ANTIDIARRHEICS

Diarrhea, a common symptom of gastrointestinal disease, is characterized by frequent evacuation of fluid stools with griping. It may be the result of eating contaminated food, bacterial or protozoal infections (see discussion of dysentery in Chap. 12, p. 166), or nervous hyperexcitability. Since diarrhea is often a defensive mechanism against irritating substances in the intestinal tract, it should not be checked until the cause is determined.

Antidiarrheics are substances used to check excessive bowel movements. The following groups of drugs are used:

1. Demulcents and astringents are used to lessen irritation and inflammation. Bismuth subcarbonate or bismuth subgallate in 4-Gm. doses, calcium carbonate, magnesium oxide, kaolin, and tannic acid preparations.

2. Carminatives are employed to lessen putrefaction and fermentation. Camphor and carbonated beverages.

3. Preparations of kaolin and pectin (e.g., Kaopectate and Pectosil) are used to absorb toxins or irritating substances. The dose is 15 ml. (one tablespoon) every three hours. Attapulgite is administered in doses of 2 or more Gm.

4. Intestinal antiseptics such as succinylsulfathiazole (Sulfasuxidine) or phthalylsulfathiazole (Sulfathalidine) are used when the enteritis is of bacterial origin. The dose is 2 Gm. every three hours.

5. Antispasmodic drugs such as paregoric, 4 ml.; papaverine, 100 mg.; belladonna tincture, 0.75 ml. in a glass of water; atropine sulfate, 0.5 mg.; dicyclomine (Bentyl) hydrochloride, 10-mg. capsules; or thiphenamil (Trocinate) hydrochloride, 100 mg., are used to decrease propulsive peristaltic waves in the colon.

6. Sedative drugs such as phenobarbital, 15 mg., are used when the diarrhea is due to hyperexcitability.

7. Analgesics such as codeine phosphate, 60 mg., or meperidine, 100 mg., are administered orally or hypodermically.

8. Resins are employed for adsorption of irritants.

Two new mixtures have been introduced for the treatment of diarrhea. They are diphenoxylate hydrochloride with atropine sulfate (Lomotil) and thihexinol methylbromide with polycarbophil (Entoquel, Sorboquel).

Diphenoxylate Hydrochloride and Atropine Sulfate (Lomotil)

Diphenoxylate hydrochloride is a synthetic pain-relieving drug. Its addiction liability is less than that of morphine and probably less than that of codeine.[1] Although it requires a prescription form in other countries, it is an exempt narcotic in the United States. An oral mixture of diphenoxylate and atropine is useful for the symptomatic relief of acute and chronic diarrhea. Side effects sometimes observed are drowsiness, dry mouth, nausea, and epigastric pain. The oral dose is 5 mg. three or four times a day. The maintenance dose may be as low as 10 mg. a day.

Preparation

Diphenoxylate Hydrochloride and Atropine Sulfate Tablets	Diphenoxylate hydrochloride 2.5 mg. Atropine sulfate 0.025 mg.

Trade name: Lomotil

[1] Fraser, H. F., and Isbell, H.: "Human Pharmacology and Addictiveness of Ethyl 1-(3 Cyano-3-Phenylpropyl)-4-Phenyl-4-Piperidine Carboxylate Hydrochloride (R-1132, Diphenoxylate)," *Bull. on Narcotics,* **13**:29, 1961.

Thihexinol Methylbromide and Polycarbophil (Entoquel, Sorboquel)

This is a mixture of polycarbophil, a hydrophilic gel, and thihexinol methylbromide, an anticholinergic agent, which decreases the motility of the gastrointestinal tract. It is useful in the treatment of mild diarrhea and irritable colon syndrome. When neomycin is added to the mixture, it is used in bacterial diarrheas caused by neomycin-sensitive organisms.

Side Effects.   There have been minor complaints of bloating. Dry mouth, mydriasis, and tachycardia occur infrequently and, in young children, flushing of the skin. The drug is contraindicated in patients with glaucoma or stenosis in any part of the gastrointestinal tract and in patients in whom tachycardia may be harmful.

Dosage.   The oral dose for older children and adults is one to four tablets or one tablespoonful of the syrup four times a day.

Preparations

Thihexinol Methylbromide Syrup	5 mg. in 1 tsp. (5 ml.)
Thihexinol Methylbromide Syrup with Neomycin	5 mg. with 50 mg. neomycin sulfate in 1 tsp.

Trade names: Entoquel, Entoquel with Neomycin

Thihexinol Methylbromide Tablets	15 mg.

Trade name: Sorboquel

ANTIFLATULENTS

Dexpanthenol (Cozyme, Ilopan, Motilyn)

Dexpanthenol is the alcohol derivative of pantothenic acid (see p. 712), one of the B complex vitamins. It is used in the correction and prevention of intestinal atony and abdominal distention, to relieve postoperative retention of flatus and feces, and to lessen the possibility of paralytic ileus. Dexpanthenol is administered intravenously or intramuscularly. The intravenous or intramuscular dose of 2 ml. (500 mg.) is repeated in two hours and again in 12 hours, if necessary. It should not be used with neostigmine or other cholinergic agents.

Preparation

Dexpanthenol Injection	1- and 2-ml. ampuls and 10-ml. vials containing 250 mg. per milliliter

Trade names: Cozyme, Ilopan, Motilyn

Methylpolysiloxane (Mylicon)

Methylpolysiloxane (Mylicon) is a defoaming agent which changes the surface tension of gas or air bubbles and causes them to coalesce. It is used to relieve flatulence by dispersing and preventing formation of gas pockets in the gastrointestinal tract. The gas is eliminated by belching or passing flatus. One tablet is taken orally after each meal and at bedtime.

Preparation

Methylpolysiloxane Tablets   40 mg.

Trade name: Mylicon

REVIEW QUESTIONS

1. *Name some of the causes of constipation.*
2. *What are cathartics?*
3. *Classify cathartics according to their mechanism of action. Give an example of each type.*
4. *List four therapeutic uses for cathartics.*
5. *Name some of the causes of diarrhea.*
6. *Name and define four types of drugs used in the treatment of diarrhea.*
7. *What is dexpanthenol? Name two clinical uses.*
8. *How does methylpolysiloxane act to prevent trapping of gas in the intestines?*
9. *What are the active substances used in the two mixtures administered to combat diarrhea?*

REFERENCES

Bargen, J. A.: "Use of Methylcellulose to Improve Function of the Bowel," *Gastroenterology*, **13**:275, 1949.

Bethea, O. W.: "The Use and Abuse of Purgatives," *Internat. M. Digest*, **24**:239, 1934.

———: "The Use of Cathartics," *J.A.M.A.*, **107**:1298, 1936.

Cornell Conferences on Therapy: "Management of Constipation," *New York J. Med.*, **41**:1959, 1941.

———: "The Rational Use of Cathartic Agents," *New York J. Med.*, **47**:387, 504, 1947.

Goldsmith, H., and Tignor, S.: "A Clinical Evaluation of d-Pantothenyl Alcohol," *Surgery*, **47**:663, 1960.

Hock, C. W.: "Observation of Use of Sorboquel in Chronic Diarrhea," *Am. J. Digest. Dis.*, **5**:971, 1960.

MacGregor, A. G.: "Purgatives and Laxatives," *Brit. M. J.*, **1**:1422, 1960.

McHardy, G. G.: "Inhibition of Intestinal Hypermotility with Thihexinol Methyl-bromide," *Am. J. Digest. Dis.*, **5**:962, 1960.

Pimparker, B. D., *et al.*: "Effect of Polycarbophil on Diarrhea and Constipation," *Gastroenterology*, **40**:397, 1961.

Rider, J. A.: "Intestinal Gas and Bloating: Treatment with Methylpolysiloxane," *Am. Pract. & Digest. Treat.*, **11**:52, 1960.

Rider, J. A., and Moeller, H. C.: "Use of Silicone in the Treatment of Intestinal Gas and Bloating," *J.A.M.A.*, **174**:2052, 1960.

Rutter, A. G.: "Bisacodyl, An Evacuant Drug," *Lancet*, **1**:1173, 1959.

Tainter, M. L.: "Methylcellulose as a Colloid Laxative," *Proc. Soc. Exper. Biol. & Med.*, **54**:77, 1943.

Van Derstappen, G., *et al.*: "Long Term Clinical Studies with R 1132, a New Constipating Drug," *Gastroenterology*, **39**:725, 1960.

Winkelstein, A.: "The Nature and Treatment of Chronic Constipation and Chronic Diarrhea," *M. Clin. North America*, **26**:787, 1942.

VIII DRUGS ACTING ON THE REPRODUCTIVE ORGANS AND KIDNEYS

A backward glance in the field of obstetrics, as in every field, reminds us of the serious difficulties faced by our ancestors who had few useful medicinal products. Puerperal infections probably accounted for most of the morbidity and maternal deaths during past centuries in which some type of operative assistance was practiced via the birth canal. Aseptic techniques and the anti-infective agents described in Section II have now virtually abolished perinatal infections as significant complications. Furthermore, prior to modern obstetrical practices, hemorrhage was an ever-present danger. After prolonged, difficult labor, especially with disproportion between fetal size and pelvic dimensions, breech presentations, or certain other abnormalities, the fatigued uterus, with its veins, venules, and capillaries exposed after expulsion of the placenta, was often unable to maintain sufficient muscular contraction to prevent the loss of excessive blood. Protracted weakness from anemia, or death, was the common misfortune of the women not benefited by uterine muscle stimulants.

Chapter 37 presents the oxytocic agents and something of their history. It also describes the use of the sex hormones and certain hormones of the pituitary gland. The employment of these materials in medicine is extensive. In the case of the sex hormones there has undoubtedly been unjustifiable overuse of these agents, but always in the hope that benefit would accrue to the patient, male or female.

In Chapter 38 substances that act upon the tubules of the kidneys, improving their function in the presence of disease, are discussed. Certain of these agents produce an outpouring of water and salt from the body, and with others, the excretion of uric acid is promoted. The first group, the diuretics, is useful in the condition known of old as "dropsy." "Water logging" of the legs or throughout the body is now termed edema, or if widespread and extensive, anasarca. The second group, which increases uric acid excretion, is of use in gout, which is characterized by higher blood levels of this normal excretory product.

599

Diagnostic agents for kidney studies are also included in Chapter 38.

Based on the fact that iodine effectively absorbs x-rays, certain organic compounds have been prepared which contain a maximal amount of iodine compatible with safety and which are excreted by the kidneys. After the administration of such a substance, highly important diagnostic features of the pelvic region can be recorded on film by the x-ray photographic technique. Other diagnostic agents are used to test the function of the kidney.

37

Drugs Acting on the Reproductive Organs

The normal female reproductive system is composed of the external genitalia, the vagina, the uterus, the fallopian tubes, the ovaries and their supporting tissues, and the mammary glands. The normal male reproductive system includes the testes, the epididymides, the ducti deferentes, the seminal vesicles, the prostate, the bulbourethral glands, and the penis. Knowledge of the anatomy and physiology of each of these systems is essential in understanding the action of drugs.

The uterus is a hollow muscular structure with abundant vascular, lymph, and nervous supplies. In addition to being the organ of menstruation, the uterus receives, retains, and nourishes the products of conception, expelling them at parturition.

The thick, muscular layer (the myometrium), making up the largest portion of the uterus, is composed of smooth-muscle fibers disposed longitudinally, vertically, and diagonally, thus forming a network. As the blood vessels are situated between these fibers, their contraction is a major hemostatic mechanism.

The uterine muscle contracts rhythmically with both pendular and peristaltic movements which are slight in nongravid women and vary with sexual activity. Although these movements are weak in early pregnancy, they increase in strength and frequency, reaching a peak at the time of delivery.

DRUGS ACTING ON THE UTERUS

Drugs affecting the uterus may be divided into three groups: (1) uterine stimulants, (2) uterine relaxants, and (3) sex hormones.

UTERINE STIMULANTS

Drugs that stimulate uterine contractions are called ecbolics or oxytocics. Those used most frequently are the ergot alkaloids and posterior pituitary extracts, although there are other drugs affecting uterine contractility. Discussion will be limited to these two groups which are used most often.

601

ERGOT AND THE ERGOT ALKALOIDS

Ergot

Ergot is the dried sclerotium (mycelium) of a parasitic fungus, *Claviceps purpurea*, which grows on infected rye and forms a purple, curved body which replaces the grain of rye.

Constituents of Ergot. The composition of ergot is very complex. It contains at least 12 alkaloids, a number of amines, acetylcholine, and some choline derivatives. The alkaloids used in clinical medicine are ergotamine (similar to ergotoxine), which is used in migraine headache (see discussion on pp. 548, 549), and ergonovine. The pharmacological actions of ergotamine and ergonovine are similar; however, the two agents differ in speed of action, effectiveness after oral administration, toxicity, and strength.

Pharmacological Actions. The main actions of ergot are on the smooth muscle of the uterus and its blood vessels. It produces a moderate and prolonged increase in the tone and rhythmical contraction of the uterus and constriction of the blood vessels. The gravid uterus is more sensitive to these drugs than the nongravid uterus and the parturient uterus is even more sensitive. Originally, extractive preparations of ergot such as the fluidextract and the wine of ergot were widely used. Now these preparations have been largely replaced by the alkaloid, ergonovine.

Ergonovine Maleate, U.S.P. (Ergotrate); Ergometrine Maleate, B.P., I.P.

Ergonovine maleate, a salt of the principal oxytocic alkaloid of ergot, is a white or faintly yellow powder soluble in water. Both ergotamine and ergonovine contract the muscles of the uterus; however, because ergonovine acts more forcibly and for a longer period of time, it is the drug usually used in obstetrics. Upon intramuscular, intravenous, oral, or sublingual administration, ergonovine contracts the uterus by a musculotropic action.

Therapeutic Uses of Ergonovine. The principal use of ergonovine is to prevent or check postpartum hemorrhage. To aid in uterine involution, the oral or sublingual dose is 0.2 mg. (0.2 to 0.5 mg.) every four hours for six doses. To sustain firm uterine contractions following delivery of the placenta, the intramuscular or intravenous dose is 0.2 mg. dissolved in water for injection. Some obstetricians prefer to make the injection just after the first shoulder of the infant is delivered. For all practical purposes, no untoward effects attend this use of ergonovine.

Ergot Poisoning. *Acute* toxic effects from ergot or its alkaloids are rare, although they may occur in cases of attempted abortion when large doses are taken. The symptoms are abdominal cramps, vomiting, diarrhea, rapid pulse, headache, mental confusion, and unconsciousness. Uterine hemorrhage and abortion may result from such overdosage.

Cases of *chronic* poisoning, or ergotism, are not uncommon, since these alkaloids are extensively employed in therapeutics. Such clinical poisoning is usually due to overdosage or certain disease states that increase the sensitivity to these alkaloids. The epidemic form of chronic poisoning caused by ingestions of contaminated grain is rare today, owing to improved agricultural procedures.

The gangrene in ergotism is caused by a prolonged constriction of the blood vessels and the filling of the blood vessels with a substance that blocks the circulation. Vascular stasis in the toes, fingers, hands, and feet causes drying and death of the tissues, whereupon the phalanges (or digits) and the joint break off with neither pain nor bleeding. Prolonged constriction of the retinal vessels causes blindness. Convulsions may also occur.

Treatment of poisoning is complete withdrawal of the drug and symptomatic therapy.

Preparations

Ergonovine Maleate Injection, U.S.P.;   1-ml. ampuls containing 0.2 mg.
Ergometrine Injection, B.P., I.P.
Ergonovine Maleate Tablets, U.S.P.;   0.2 mg.
Ergometrine Tablets, B.P., I.P.

Trade name: Ergotrate

Methylergonovine Maleate, U.S.P. (Methergine); Methylergometrine Maleate, B.P.

Methylergonovine maleate is a synthetic derivative of ergonovine. Its actions and uses are similar to those of ergonovine. However, it is more potent, its action is more prompt and more prolonged, the elevation of blood pressure is less, there is less uterine bleeding, and it is preferred in patients with preeclampsia and eclampsia. The oral and intravenous dose is 0.2 mg.

Preparations

Methylergonovine Maleate Injection,   1-ml. ampuls containing 0.2 mg.
N.F.; Methylergometrine Injection, B.P.
Methylergonovine Maleate Tablets,   0.2 mg.
U.S.P.

Trade name: Methergine Maleate

Sparteine Sulfate (Tocosamine)

Sparteine sulfate is used in the acceleration of the first and second stages of desultory labor and in the treatment of primary and secondary uterine inertia. The initial intramuscular dose is 150 mg. or 1 ml. If unsatisfactory stimulation occurs, the initial dose may be followed in an hour by 150 mg. Additional doses of 150 mg. may be given at one-and-one-half- to two-hour intervals until a total of four doses have been given. Contraindications are active heart disease, normal and forceful labor, cephalopelvic disproportion, previous abdominal deliveries, placenta previa, abruptio placentae, and other unusual obstetrical conditions.

Preparation

Sparteine Sulfate Injection   150 mg. in 1 ml.
Trade name: Tocosamine

THE POSTERIOR PITUITARY HORMONES

The pituitary gland is a small but important structure situated at the base of the brain. It consists of two lobes, the anterior and the posterior, and an intermediate part, the pars intermedia.

When an aqueous extract of the posterior lobe obtained from the glands of cattle and sheep is administered parenterally, it produces three responses: (1) stimulation of the uterine muscle (*oxytocic* effect), (2) promotion of water absorption by the kidney tubules (*antidiuretic* effect, discussed on p. 644), and (3) constriction of the peripheral blood vessels (*pressor* effect, discussed on p. 644). Two hormones account for all three actions.

The oxytocic principle *oxytocin* and the pressor and antidiuretic principle *vasopressin* have been separated from the dry posterior pituitary powder. The pure hormone oxytocin, which has been produced synthetically by Dr. Vincent du Vigneaud, has 150 times the activity of the original powder on the uterus and is devoid of the pressor response. Vasopressin has a pressor activity much greater than that of the posterior pituitary powder and has little action on the uterus.

Oxytocin and posterior pituitary injections increase the contractions of the uterus by acting directly on smooth muscle and are used to induce labor and to stimulate uterine contractions in prolonged labor. They may also be used in place of ergonovine, or in combination with it, to check postpartum hemorrhage after the delivery of the placenta.

Posterior pituitary injection and vasopressin have been used in the treatment of intestinal paresis (paralysis) following surgery and to raise blood pressure, and are still used in the treatment of diabetes insipidus (see p. 645).

Posterior Pituitary Injection, U.S.P., I.P.

Posterior pituitary injection is a sterile solution in water for injection of the mixed posterior pituitary hormones of domestic animals used as food by man. Its chief use in obstetrics is the prevention of postabortal or postpartum uterine atony. The main danger in its use is uterine rupture or fetal death due to anoxia. The usual subcutaneous or intramuscular dose is 10 U.S.P. units or less.

Preparation

Posterior Pituitary Injection, U.S.P.   10 units in 1 ml., 1-ml. ampuls, and 10-ml. vials

Trade names: Infundin; Pituitrin

Oxytocin Injection, U.S.P., B.P., I.P. (Pitocin)

Oxytocin injection is a sterile solution in water for injection of the water-soluble oxytocic principle from the posterior lobe of the pituitary of domestic animals. In human beings, its action is influenced by pregnancy, during which the sensitivity increases as the gestation advances.

The Induction of Labor. When pregnancy is at or near term, parturition may be initiated by (1) stripping of the fetal membranes, (2) amniotomy or artificial rupture of the fetal membranes, (3) administration of a purgative or an enema, and (4) administration of oxytocin.

Dosage and Methods of Administration. Before considering induction of labor, the doctor must first assess factors such as parity, duration of pregnancy, station of the presenting part, condition of the cervix, and presentation of the fetus. Oxytocin is generally administered by intravenous infusion with meticulous control of dosage and careful watching of the fetal heart tones. One method of intravenous administration is to thoroughly mix 10 units of oxytocin with 1000 ml. of 5 per cent dextrose in water with the rate of drip determined by the frequency, intensity, and duration of uterine contractions. The physician assumes full responsibility for the induction of labor and any subsequent complications. However, the nurse should be alert for signs such as rapid pulse, a rise or fall in blood pressure, fetal distress, prolonged uterine contractions, or a uterus that becomes hard and tender.

The intramuscular dose depends upon the stage of labor and ranges from 3 to 10 U.S.P. units. This method of administration is commonly used to shorten the third stage of labor and minimize blood loss.

Action. Rhythmic uterine contractions nearly always follow oxytocin-drip inductions. Between contractions, the uterine muscle is completely relaxed, thus permitting blood to circulate through the placenta.

Oxytocin is released into the blood stream by a reflex action during suckling of the infant and stimulates the smooth-muscle fibers of the lactiferous ducts. This stimulates the expression or ejection of milk from the lactating breasts and is part of the letdown reflex. It has no effect on the glandular system which produces the milk.

Preparation

Oxytocin Injection, U.S.P., B.P.   10 U.S.P. units in 1 ml., 0.5- and 1-ml. ampuls

Trade name: Pitocin

Oxytocin, Synthetic (Syntocinon)

Syntocinon is a pure synthetic oxytocin with properties identical to those of the oxytocic principle of the posterior lobe of the pituitary gland. Indications for intramuscular and intravenous use of this drug are: (1) therapeutic induction of labor, (2) stimulation of labor, (3) management of labor at the appearance of the anterior shoulder, (4) prevention and treatment of postpartum hemorrhage, and (5) postpartum atony.

For induction or stimulation of labor, 10 U.S.P. units of Syntocinon are mixed with 1000 ml. of 5 per cent dextrose in water and administered by intravenous infusion. Postpartum, a dosage of 2 units intravenously or 5 to 10 units intramuscularly is used. Contraindications for intravenous or intramuscular use are the same as those for oxytocin (Pitocin).

Oxytocin Nasal Spray (Syntocinon) prevents or relieves complications sometimes associated with lactation. In the nursing mother, one spray into one or both nostrils two to three minutes before nursing aids in the letdown reflex by relieving the pressure of the milk present in the breasts. In the nonnursing mother, one spray into one or both nostrils, as needed, quickly relieves pressure, discomfort, or pain in the presence of engorgement. Contraindications are negligible in postpartum use.

Preparation

Oxytocin Injection (Synthetic)   0.5- and 1-ml. ampuls containing 10 units in 1 ml.

Oxytocin Nasal Spray

Trade name: Syntocinon

UTERINE RELAXANTS

Indications for the use of uterine relaxants, which inhibit uterine contractions, are: (1) threatened abortion, (2) premature labor, and (3) reflex hyperactivity with frequent incoordinated contractions. Analgesics, sedatives, antispasmodics, and certain specific relaxants are the drugs commonly used.

Analgesics and Sedatives

Barbiturates, narcotics, tranquilizers, opiates, aspirin, and general anesthetics may reduce uterine activity. When these drugs are administered, their effect upon maternal and fetal respirations and uterine contractions must be considered.

Antispasmodics

Antispasmodics are agents that relieve muscle spasms. This group of drugs includes a number of depressants of the nervous system which decrease reflex activity (see p. 489).

Relaxin (Releasin, Cervilaxin)

Relaxin is a hormone produced by the corpus luteum during pregnancy. It is detectable in the blood and urine during the last two thirds of the gestation period. It virtually disappears quickly after delivery. The agent is obtained from the ovaries of pregnant sows, thus limiting its availability.

The chief site of action of relaxin is connective tissue, and since the cervix is chiefly connective tissue, it is conceivable that it may aid in cervical dilatation. Relaxation of the pelvic joints and dilatation of the ureters may also be attributed to this hormone.

At present experimental studies are being directed toward the effect of relaxin on uterine motility. It is not clear whether relaxin has the property to restrain uterine contractility thereby influencing uterine motility in pregnancy. It may prepare the birth canal for labor.

Side Effects. Since relaxin is a foreign protein, it may cause sensitivity reactions, ranging from chills and moderate allergic reactions to severe anaphylactoid shock. Skin testing is recommended in all cases prior to the use of the drug.

Dosage and Methods of Administration. Relaxin is administered intramuscularly and intravenously. For softening of the cervix in labor, doses of 40 to 120 mg. are recommended for intravenous drip, diluted to 250 or 500 ml. of saline or glucose solutions. The rate may be adjusted up to 8 ml. per minute. Intramuscularly, three doses of 40 mg. each on alternate hours, may be given. In dysmenorrhea, 20 mg. every four hours may be tried. Tenderness and swelling at the site of injection may also occur.

Preparation

Relaxin Solution (Injection)   20 mg. in 1 ml.; 1- and 2-ml. ampuls
                   Trade names: Cervilaxin, Releasin

Lututrin (Lutrexin)

Lututrin is a water-soluble extract of the corpus luteum obtained from the ovaries of the sow. When administered orally, this agent relaxes the uterus and increases its blood supply. It is used to prevent abortion and to treat dysmenorrhea. The initial oral dose for dysmenorrhea is 4000 to 6000 units, preferably before the onset of symptoms. This is followed by 4000 to 6000 units every three or four hours. The individual response varies; consequently, as many as 75,000 units may be given without untoward effects. The oral dosage schedules for threatened abortion and premature labor are 8000 units (four tablets) immediately; 6000 units (three tablets) in one hour; and 4000 units (two tablets) until contractions cease. A maintenance dose of 2000 units (one tablet) to 4000 units (two tablets) two to four times a day may be continued throughout pregnancy.

Preparation

Tablets Lututrin   2000 units of lututrin

Trade name: Lutrexin

HORMONES OF THE ANTERIOR PITUITARY

The anterior lobe of the pituitary gland is required for normal growth and sexual development, but it does not appear to be necessary for life. After removal of the gland, growth is arrested, sexual development is retarded, and atrophy of the adrenal cortex and thyroid gland occurs.

It is not known how many hormones are secreted by this portion of the gland, but at least seven extracts with a specific action have been prepared. It is believed that three of these affect the reproductive organs. In the female, the *follicle-stimulating hormone* (FSH) stimulates the growth and maturation of the graafian follicle and the production of estrogen and is responsible for changes in the first half or proliferative stage of the ovarian cycle. FSH in the male stimulates the cells of the seminiferous tubules and promotes the formation of spermatozoa. *Luteinizing hormone* (LH) or interstitial cell-stimulating hormone (ICSH) is active in the secretory stage of the ovarian cycle and promotes the growth of the interstitial cells in the follicle and the formation of the corpus luteum in the female. In the male LH stimulates the secretion of testosterone by the interstitial cells of the testes. A third hormone is *luteotropic hormone* (LTH), which causes the corpus luteum to become functional. This hormone is also referred to in the literature as the *lactogenic hormone*, which may influence mammary gland proliferation and secretion. A deficiency of the secretion of the gonadotropins during childhood causes *infantilism, adiposogenital dystrophy* or Froehlich's syndrome (abnormal development and function of the genital organs and excessive accumulation of fat), and cryptorchism (undescended testicles). Hyperactivity of gonadotropic hormones is the cause of sexual precocity (Cushing's syndrome), which accompanies certain tumors of the pituitary gland and adrenal cortex.

Clinical use of pituitary gonadotropic hormones is limited due to lack of their availability and increased incidence of allergic reactions.

CHORIONIC GONADOTROPIN

Chorionic gonadotropin is an anterior-pituitary-like gonadotropin produced by the placenta and found in the urine of pregnant women and animals. In the female, this gonadotropin is a single substance that is mainly luteinizing in action and neither stimulates the human ovary nor initiates follicle growth or the formation of corpora lutea. Its main action seems to be the prolongation of the secretory activity of the corpus luteum during early pregnancy. In the male, chorionic gonadotropin acts upon the interstitial cells of the testes, causing a secretion of androgens, which are responsible for the growth and development of the accessory sex organs, the prostate, seminal vesicles, and penis. It is obtained from the urine of pregnant women and is believed to be the substance responsible for positive pregnancy tests (Aschheim-Zondek, Friedman, and others).

Therapeutic Use. The principal use of chorionic gonadotropin is in the treatment of cryptorchism provided there is no anatomical obstruction to descent of the testicles. The usual intramuscular dose is 500 to 1000 international units two or three times a week. Long-continued injections may be dangerous; hence therapy should be discontinued after approximately eight weeks or upon the development of signs of precocious maturity. There is also some speculation as to the use of chorionic gonadotropin in the treatment of hypogonadism and functional uterine bleeding, but this is chiefly experimental.

Preparations

Lyophilized Chorionic Gonadotropin	10-ml. vials containing 5000 and 10,000 international units
Chorionic Gonadotrophin Injection, B.P.	Sterile solution

Trade names: Entromone; Follutein

Equine Gonadotropic Hormone

The blood serum of the pregnant mare is another source of the gonadotropic hormone, which stimulates ovarian growth and activity, ovulation, and also the activity of the testes. It is used in the treatment of menstrual disorders, cryptorchism, and sterility, and to stimulate development of secondary sexual characteristics. After the patient is tested for sensitivity to the serum, the substance is administered intramuscularly.

OVARIAN HORMONES

The ovaries secrete two hormones: estrogen, the follicular hormone secreted by the graafian follicle; and progesterone, the luteal hormone secreted by the corpus luteum. The production of these hormones is stimulated by the gonadotropins of the anterior pituitary.

Estrogens

The estrogens, a group of related substances that make up the follicular hormone, are responsible for the development of the sexual organs at puberty and the development and maintenance of secondary sexual characteristics. Estrogens cause thickening of the vaginal mucosa, hypertrophy of the myometrium, proliferation of the endometrium, development of the duct system of the breasts, and increase in the contractility of the uterus. Both natural estrogens and synthetic estrogens will have the same effect.

Side and Toxic Effects. The administration of natural and synthetic estrogens may cause mild effects such as nausea, vomiting, and diarrhea; skin rash; breast engorgement, tenderness of the nipples and areolar pigmentation of the nonlactating female. More severe symptoms such as calcemia, hypernatremia, with associated edema, endometrial hyperplasia, and premature closure of the epiphyses may develop. In the male, the hormone may cause gynecomastia and loss of libido. These symptoms are usually related to the dosage, potency, and route of administration of the drug. Some clinicians feel that estrogens may be contraindicated in women with a familial history of cancer since experimentation in animals has shown that estrogens can be carcinogens.

Therapeutic Uses. Estrogens are used to relieve conditions associated with this hormonal deficiency such as (1) symptoms of menopause, (2) senile vaginitis, (3) pruritus vulvae, (4) hyperactivity of the pituitary gland, (5) hypogenitalism in the female, (6) inhibition of lactation, and (7) as an adjuvant in the treatment of functional uterine bleeding. Large doses of estrogen are used in the palliation of local discomfort from prostatic carcinoma and its metastases as well as in the treatment of inoperable menopausal breast cancer.

Administration. Daily doses of estrogens should be taken at night so that the nausea, which usually develops, occurs while the patient is asleep. If the nausea is present upon awakening, it can be treated with dry food such as crackers, or a drug such as prochlorperazine (Compazine) may be given with the estrogen.

Preparations and Dosage

Estrone, N.F. (I.P.) (Theelin, Folliculin)	1 mg. (0.2 to 1 mg.) intramuscularly
Estrone Injection (I.P.)	1-ml. ampuls containing 0.1, 0.2, 0.5, and 1 mg.; 10 mg. in 10 ml.

Trade names: Estrugenone; Estrusol; Folestrin; Folliculin; Ketodestrin; Menformone; Œstrone; Thelestrin

Estradiol Benzoate, N.F.; Œstradiol Benzoate, B.P. (I.P.)	1 mg. (0.1 to 5 mg.) daily
Estradiol Benzoate Injection, N.F.; Œstradiol Benzoate Injection, B.P. (I.P.)	1-ml. ampuls containing 0.166, 0.33, 1, and 1.66 mg.; 10-ml. ampuls containing 3.33, 10, 16.6, and 33.3 mg.

Trade names: Benzestrin; Benzogynoestrol; Benztrone; Dimenformon; Gynformon; Oestrin; Ovocyclin B; Ovostab; Progynon B

Aqueous Estradiol Injection, N.F.	1-ml. ampuls containing 1 mg.
Estradiol Pellets, N.F.	10 or 25 mg.
Estradiol Dipropionate, U.S.P.	1 mg. (0.1 to 5 mg.) daily
Estradiol Dipropionate Injection, U.S.P.	1-ml. ampuls containing 0.1, 0.2, 0.5, 1, 2.5, and 5 mg.; 10-ml. ampuls containing 10 and 50 mg.

Trade names: Divocyclin; Ovocyclin P; Progynon DP. (The unesterified hormone is Glandubolin, Gynoestrol, and Oestroform.)

Ethinyl Estradiol, U.S.P.; Ethinyloestradiol, B.P., I.P.

Ethinyl estradiol is a partially synthetic estrogen. By injection it is as active as estradiol, and if administered orally, it is more active. The usual oral dosage range is 20 to 50 mcg. up to three times a day but varies greatly with the condition being treated. Menopausal symptoms can be controlled with a dose of 20 to 50 mcg. one to three times a day.

Preparations

Ethinyl Estradiol Tablets, U.S.P. (B.P.)	20 and 50 mcg.
Ethinylestradiol Elixir	0.006 to 0.03 mg. in 1 ml.

Trade names: Estigyn; Estinyl; Eston-E; Esticyclol; Hewoestrol; Lynoral;
Oradiol; Orestralyn
Synonyms: Ethidol; Ethin-oestryl (Oestryl)

Estradiol Cypionate, N.F.

Solutions of estradiol cyclopentylpropionate in vegetable oil, when injected intramuscularly, produce more prolonged estrogenic effects than similar solutions of estradiol benzoate or dipropionate. An intramuscular dose of 1 to 5 mg. administered weekly for two to three weeks and then every three to four weeks will produce maintenance effects.

Preparation

Estradiol Cypionate Injection, N.F.	1 mg. in 1 ml. and 5 mg. in 1 ml.

Estrogenic Substances, Conjugated

Conjugated estrogenic substances, an amorphous preparation containing naturally occurring water-soluble mixed estrogens (the principal estrogen of which is sodium estrone sulfate), is obtained from the urine of pregnant mares. The usual dose is 1.25 mg. daily (1.25 to 3.75 mg.) for the control of menopausal symptoms, vaginitis, and pruritus vulvae. For palliation of breast cancer, a daily oral dose of 30 mg. is recommended.

Preparations

Conjugated Estrogenic Substances Solution	0.16 mg. in 1 ml.

Conjugated Estrogenic Substances Tablets	0.3, 0.6, 1.25, and 2.5 mg.
Conjugated Estrogenic Substances Cream	1½-oz. tube containing 0.625 mg. estrogen in 1 Gm.
Conjugated Estrogenic Substances Powder for Injection	20 mg. with 5-ml. vial sterile diluent

Trade names: Amnestrogen; Conestron; Estrifol; Hormesteral; Konogen; Premarin

Piperazine Estrone Sulfate (Sulestrex Piperazine)

Piperazine estrone sulfate is administered orally in doses of 1.5 mg. daily. It is available as an elixir containing 0.3 mg. in each milliliter and as tablets containing 0.75, 1.5, and 3 mg.

SYNTHETIC ESTROGENS

Diethylstilbestrol, N.F.; Stilboestrol, B.P., I.P.

Diethylstilbestrol is one of the most widely used of a group of synthetic derivatives of stilbene that duplicate the actions of naturally occurring estrogens. The compound is relatively simple and inexpensive and, because it is readily absorbed from the gastrointestinal tract, is available orally as well as parenterally. The usual doses are 0.2 to 0.5 mg. daily for menopausal symptoms and senile vaginitis; 5 to 15 mg. daily to a total dose of 30 mg. for breast engorgement; 12 to 25 mg. daily for functional uterine bleeding; 15 mg. daily for cancer of the breast; 1 to 3 mg. daily or 10 mg. weekly for carcinoma of the prostate. If the dose is kept to a minimum, the possibility of untoward effects such as nausea, vomiting, and cramplike pains in the chest will be decreased.

Preparations

Diethylstilbestrol Tablets, N.F. (B.P.)	0.1, 0.25, 0.5, 1, 5, and 25 mg.
Diethylstilbestrol Injection, N.F.	1-ml. ampuls containing 0.5, 1, 2, 5, and 25 mg. in oil; also multiple-dose vials
Suppositories Diethylstilbestrol	0.1 and 0.5 mg.

Trade names: Clinoestrol; Cytren; Daes; Estromenin; Estromon; Estrostilben; Oestrostilben; Ovendosen; Pabestrol; Stibolum

Diethylstilbestrol Dipropionate, N.F.

Diethylstilbestrol dipropionate is administered intramuscularly in oil and is absorbed relatively slowly from the oil depot in the tissues. Although its concentration in the blood is lower than that of diethylstilbestrol, the effects are more prolonged, thus there is a decreased incidence of reactions such as nausea, vomiting, headache, and dizziness. Parenteral administration is two to five times as potent as oral administration. The intramuscular dose varies from 0.5 to 2 mg. two or three times a week in menopausal symptoms and senile vaginitis and up to 5 mg. once or twice daily for two to four days in carcinoma of the prostate and suppression of lactation.

Preparations

Diethylstilbestrol Dipropionate Injection, N.F.	10-ml. vials containing 500 mcg., 1, or 5 mg. in each milliliter
Diethylstilbestrol Dipropionate Tablets, N.F.	500 mcg., 1, 5, 25 mg.

Trade names: Pabestrol-D; Sinestrol; Synestrin

Promethestrol Dipropionate (Meprane)

Promethestrol dipropionate is similar in action to diethylstilbestrol. The initial oral dose for use in the treatment of menopausal symptoms is 1 mg. three times a day. The dosage is then gradually reduced to 1 mg. daily.

Preparation

Tablets Promethestrol Dipropionate	1 mg.

Trade name: Meprane Dipropionate

Hexestrol

Hexestrol is a compound that is closely related to diethylstilbestrol, although it is less toxic. The oral dose is 2 to 3 mg. daily for the relief of menopausal symptoms and senile vaginitis and 15 mg. one to three times daily for two or more days to suppress lactation. The parenteral dose is 1 mg. in oil three times a week.

Preparations

Hexestrol Tablets	1 and 3 mg.
Hexestrol Injection (in oil or other suitable solvent)	1-ml. ampuls and 20-ml. vials containing 1 or 5 mg. in 1 ml.

Chlorotrianisene, N.F. (TACE)

The average oral dose of chlorotrianisene in the treatment of menopausal symptoms, senile vaginitis, and pruritus vulvae is between 12 and 24 mg. daily for 30 to 60 days. In prostatic cancer a daily oral dose of 24 mg. is recommended. Postpartum breast engorgement is relieved with the administration of 12 mg. of TACE four times a day for seven days beginning eight hours after delivery.

Preparations

Chlorotrianisene Capsules, N.F.	12 mg. in corn oil
Solution Chlorotrianisene in Corn Oil	12 mg. in 1 ml.

Trade name: TACE

Dienestrol, N.F.; Dienoestrol, B.P. (Restrol)

This drug has fewer side effects and is less potent than diethylstilbestrol. Menopausal symptoms are relieved with a dose of 0.1 to 1.5 mg. daily. Larger doses may be necessary for the patient with mammary cancer.

Preparations

Dienestrol Tablets, N.F. (B.P.)	100 and 500 mcg., 10 mg.
Dienestrol Suspension for Injection	50 mg. in 10 ml.
Dienestrol Vaginal Cream	0.1 mg. in 1 Gm.

Trade names: Restrol, Synestrol

Methallenestril (Vallestril)

This is a newer estrogen. An oral dose of 6 mg. daily for three or four weeks suppresses menopausal symptoms and alleviates atrophic vaginitis. Menopausal osteoporosis may be relieved with 9 mg. daily for two weeks. In prostatic carcinoma, the dose is up to 20 mg. daily. In suppressing lactation, 40 mg. may be given daily for five days.

Preparation

Methallenestril Tablets	3 and 20 mg.

Trade name: Vallestril

Progesterone (The Luteal Hormone)

The ovarian hormones are concerned with characteristic uterine, ovarian, vaginal, and breast changes. Progesterone continues the proliferation of the endometrium induced by the estrogens for implantation and maintenance of the ovum if fertilization occurs. This hormone is essential for reproduction. It is secreted by the corpus luteum only through the third month of pregnancy but is produced in an increasing amount by the placenta. Progesterone stimulates the growth of mammary alveolar tissue, relaxes the smooth muscle of the uterus, and renders the uterus less sensitive to oxytocin and ergonovine.

Side and Toxic Effects. The administration of natural and synthetic progesterones may cause mild side effects such as vaginal spotting, irregular vaginal bleeding, nausea, and lethargy. Prolonged administration of large doses may produce more severe symptoms such as gastrointestinal disturbance, hypernatremia with associated edema and weight gain, headache, dizziness, oligomenorrhea, amenorrhea, congestion of the breasts, decreased libido, jaundice, and masculinization of the female fetus. Some clinicians feel that progesterone has carcinogenic properties and is contraindicated in women with a familial history of cancer.

Therapeutic Uses. Progesterones are used for functional uterine bleeding, primary and secondary amenorrhea, premenstrual tension, dysmenorrhea, endometriosis, threatened and habitual abortions, endocrine infertility, toxemia of pregnancy, afterpains, for ovulation control, and for tests for pregnancy. Experimentally, the drugs have been used in the treatment of cyclomastopathy, mastodynia, adenosis, cystic mastitis, and cervical cancer.

Progesterone, N.F., B.P., I.P. (Corlutone)

The progesterone used in therapeutics is prepared synthetically and is most effective when given by parenteral administration. Therapeutic parenteral doses are 10 to 25 mg. daily for functional uterine bleeding; 10 mg. daily for secondary amenorrhea; up to 25 mg. daily for dysmenorrhea and premenstrual tension; 2 to 20 mg. one to three times a week for habitual abortion; 5 to 50 mg. daily from the fifth to the twenty-fifth day of the menstrual cycle for ovulation control; 10 mg. daily for four consecutive days with withdrawal bleeding occurring within two to three days as a positive test for pregnancy; and 5 mg. daily increasing gradually to 20 mg. for six to nine months in the treatment of endometriosis.

Preparations

Progesterone Injection, N.F., B.P.	5 and 10 mg. in 1 ml.; 50 and 125 mg. in 5 ml.; 100, 250, and 500 mg. in 10 ml.
Sterile Progesterone Suspension, N.F.	25 mg. in 1 ml.; 100 and 250 mg. in 10 ml.
Progesterone Tablets, N.F.	10 and 25 mg.

Trade names: Corlutone; Gestone; Glanducorpin; Gonadyl; Gynolutin; Lipolutin; Luteomersin; Luteostab; Lutesterone; Lutocylin; Lutoform; Lutogyl; Lutren; Naluton; Neolutin; Progesterol; Progestin; Proluton

SYNTHETIC PROGESTERONES

Ethisterone, N.F., B.P. (Anhydrohydroxyprogesterone, Ethyl Testosterone, Pregneninolone)

Ethisterone is available for oral administration. The dose is 25 mg. (5 to 120 mg.) up to four times a day. Pro-Duosterone is a combination of 50 mg. of ethisterone and 0.03 mg. of ethinyl estradiol. It may be used to differentiate pregnancy from simple delay of menses. It is administered in a dose of three tablets daily for three days. Menses usually occurs within two to four days after the end of medication in the absence of pregnancy. If normal pregnancy exists, no bleeding occurs. Used alone, ethisterone has the actions and uses of progesterone.

Preparation

Ethisterone Tablets, N.F., B.P., I.P.   5, 10, and 25 mg.

Trade names: Lutocylol; Lutogyl Oral; Ora-Lutin; Pranone; Progestoral; Trosinone

Medroxyprogesterone Acetate, U.S.P. (Provera)

Medroxyprogesterone acetate is said to be 12 times as potent as ethisterone. The oral dose is 2.5 to 10 mg. for from five to ten days in amenorrhea.

Preparation

Medroxyprogesterone Acetate Tablets,   2.5 and 10 mg. U.S.P.

Trade name: Provera

Norethindrone; Norethisterone, B.P. (Norlutin)

This oral progestational agent is used in the same conditions as those described for the progesterones and may produce the same side effects.

Dosage. In order to produce anovulatory cycles in such conditions as amenorrhea, menstrual irregularity, excessive uterine bleeding, and dysmenorrhea, 5 to 20 mg. may be given daily from the fifth through the twenty-fourth day of the cycle. In habitual abortion, 5 mg. twice daily are given during the first five months or longer. In endometriosis, dosage is increased to 20 or 30 mg. daily. As a safe test for pregnancy, 10 mg. daily for three days will produce withdrawal bleeding within a few days only in the absence of pregnancy.

The acetate salt of this compound has approximately twice the potency of the base itself and need be given in but half of the above dosages.

Preparations

Norethindrone Tablets   5 mg.
Norethindrone Acetate Tablets   5 mg.

Trade names: Norlutin (the base), Norlutate (the acetate)

Hydroxyprogesterone Caproate (Delalutin)

This synthetic derivative of progesterone has the same action as natural progesterone except that it has longer duration. It is injected deep into the gluteal muscle and the usual dosage ranges between 125 and 250 mg. administered two days after ovulation and repeated each cycle as needed. In threatened or habitual abortion dosages of 250 mg. or more are given and repeated daily or weekly until two weeks before the expected date of delivery. For use in carcinoma of the endometrium see page 203.

Preparations

Hydroxyprogesterone Caproate (in   250 mg. in 2 ml.; 1.25 Gm. in 10 ml.
sesame oil)
Hydroxyprogesterone Caproate (in   1.25 Gm. in 5 ml.
ricinus oil)

Trade name: Delalutin

Oral Contraceptives

Derivatives of progesterone in combination with an estrogen are effective as contraceptive agents upon oral administration. They prevent ovulation by suppressing the gonadotropic hormones of the anterior pituitary. Suspension of ovulation continues as long as the drug is administered and until normal cycles are reinstituted upon cessation of treatment. By administering the drug from the fifth through the twenty-fourth day of the menstrual cycle an anovulatory cycle is produced and cyclic bleeding can be established monthly for long periods by repeating the process on schedule. Conception cannot occur in anovulatory cycles. These drugs do not impair subsequent fertility, and endocrine infertility can sometimes be reversed following their use with the creation of "rebound" fertility.

Side effects include nausea, headache, breakthrough bleeding, weight gain, and loss of increase of libido which disappear when therapy is stopped. Treatment should be discontinued if pregnancy intervenes because of the possibility of masculinizing the female fetus.

Norethynodrel with Mestranol (Enovid)

Dosage and Therapeutic Uses. For the establishment of anovulatory cycles, 5 and sometimes 10 mg. are given daily from the fifth through the twenty-fourth day, counting the first day of menstruation as the first day of the cycle. This is repeated in synchrony with the artificial rhythmic menses. In threatened abortion, 10 mg., two or three times daily, may be given until bleeding stops. In habitual abortion, 10 or 20 mg. daily may be given from the outset of pregnancy until at least the fifth month. In endometriosis the dose is increased to 40 mg. daily and continued for three to nine months.

Preparations

Norethynodrel Tablets (with mestranol 5 mg.
0.075 mg.)
Norethynodrel Tablets (with mestranol 10 mg.
0.15 mg.)
Trade name: Enovid

Other oral contraceptives used in the same manner as norethynodrel (Enovid) are norethindrone with mestranol and norethindrone acetate with ethinyl estradiol. One tablet is given daily for 20 days beginning on the fifth day and including the twenty-fourth day of the menstrual cycle.

Preparations

Norethindrone Tablets (with 0.06 mg. 10 mg.
mestranol)
Trade name: Ortho-Novum

Norethindrone Tablets (with 0.1 mg.   2 mg. mestranol)

Trade names: Ortho-Novum, Norinyl

Norethindrone Acetate Tablets (with   2.5 mg. 0.05 mg. ethinyl estradiol)

Trade name: Norlestrin

ANDROGENS

Androgens, substances which possess masculinizing activities, are responsible for the normal development and maintenance of spermatogenesis and the male sexual characteristics. These hormones are structurally similar to estrogens and some adrenal cortical hormones. In addition to their action on the reproductive system, androgens cause weight gain and act on the tissues to produce a positive nitrogen balance, increased protein anabolism, and decreased amino acid catabolism.

Therapeutically, androgens are used in the treatment of the following conditions in the male: primary hypogonadism, testicular hypofunction, eunuchism, Klinefelter's syndrome, male climacteric, and cryptorchism. In the female, the drug is used to treat menorrhagia, metorrhagia, premenstrual, functional dysmenorrhea, menopausal symptoms and endometriosis, and advanced inoperable cancer of the breast. Androgens given to both male and female, because of their anabolic activity, are used for tissue repair, paraplegia, protein depletion from corticosteroid therapy, delayed healing of fractures, debilitating conditions, decubitus ulcers, calciuria, postoperative states, chronic malnutrition, and osteoporosis.

Side Effects.   Those most often associated with androgen therapy are (1) oligospermia, (2) decreased ejaculatory volume, (3) priapism, (4) increased libido, (5) gastrointestinal upsets, (6) hypercalcemia, (7) jaundice, (8) virilization in the female, and (9) edema, if long-term therapy is employed. The drug should be used with caution in young boys as it may produce precocious sexual development and premature epiphyseal closure. Androgens are contraindicated in the treatment of prostatic carcinoma and in patients with liver damage.

Testosterone, N.F., B.P. (Androlin)

Testosterone is a hormone obtained from testicular extracts or prepared synthetically, the synthetic compound being available for clinical use. Therapeutic uses and side effects are the same as those mentioned above for androgens.

Although the hormone is active orally (in ten times the parenteral dose), the intramuscular injection of an oil solution is the preferred method of administration and is given in doses ranging from 10 to 50 mg., two to six times a week. Common dosages are: 25 mg. three times a week for several weeks to induce pubescence in eunuchoidism and for metrorrhagia; 10 mg. three times a week for constitutional symptoms and menorrhagia; 50 to 75 mg. for two to three days starting on the third or fourth postpartum day to decrease lactation and reduce breast engorgement; and 150 to 300 mg. weekly in divided doses for two months for a subjective response and five months for an objective response for palliation of breast cancer.

Preparations

Sterile Testosterone Suspension, N.F. (Aqueous Medium)	25 mg. in 1 ml.; 50 mg. in 1 ml.; 100 mg. in 1-ml. and 10-ml. vials
Testosterone Pellets, N.F. (Implants)	75 mg.

Trade names: Androlin; Andronaq; Andrusol; Malestrone; Mertestate; Neo-Hombreol; Oreton-F; Synandrol-F; Testandrone; Testobase; Testosteroid; Testrone; Testryl

Testosterone Propionate, U.S.P., B.P., I.P.

Testosterone propionate is made synthetically or obtained from the testes of the bull. The duration of androgenic effects is shorter than with testosterone. The therapeutic uses, side effects, and dosages are essentially the same as those mentioned for testosterone.

Preparations

Testosterone Propionate Injection, U.S.P.	25, 50, and 100 mg. in 1-ml. ampuls and 10-ml. vials
Testosterone Propionate Tablets, Sublingual	5 and 10 mg.

Trade names: Adronate; Masenate; Neo-Hombreol; Oreton; Perandren; Synandrol; Synerone; Testodet; Testoviron

Testosterone Cypionate, U.S.P.

Testosterone cyclopentylpropionate has a more prolonged androgenic effect than does testosterone. It is administered intramuscularly at intervals of 7 to 14 days in doses ranging from 10 to 50 mg. (up to 150 mg. weekly).

Preparation

Testosterone Cypionate Injection, U.S.P.	1-ml. vials containing 100 mg. 10-ml. vials containing 50 or 100 mg. in 1 ml.

Testosterone Enanthate, U.S.P.

The intramuscular dose for this androgen is 100 to 200 mg. every two to four weeks depending on the condition being treated.

Preparation

Testosterone Enanthate Solution in Oil,   1- and 5-ml. vials containing 200 mg.
U.S.P.   in 1 ml.

Trade name: Delatestinyl

Methyltestosterone, U.S.P., B.P., I.P.

The responses to testosterone and methyltestosterone are the same. Methyltestosterone is available for oral and buccal administration. The oral dose is 10 mg. (10 to 40 mg.) up to 100 mg. as a neoplastic suppressant three times a day; the buccal dose is 5 mg. (5 to 20 mg.) up to four times a day.

Preparation

Methyltestosterone Tablets, U.S.P., B.P.   5, 10, and 25 mg.
Trade names: Glossosterandryl; Oreton-M; Metundren; Neo-hombreol-M; Oraviron

Fluoxymesterone, B.P. (Halotestin, Ultandren)

Fluoxymesterone has all the actions and uses of the foregoing androgens but is more potent. It is used in oral doses of 15 to 30 mg. daily for mammary cancer and 2 to 20 mg. daily according to requirement and tolerance.

Preparation

Fluoxymesterone Tablets, B.P.   2, 5, and 10 mg.
Trade names: Halotestin; Ultandren

Dromostanolone Propionate (Drolban)

This steroid has weaker androgenic effects than testosterone but is used like the latter for inhibiting the growth of breast carcinoma. It is masculinizing; hence, dosage and duration of treatment may be limited. Three intramuscular injections of 100 mg. per week may be given for as long as tolerated and effective.

Preparation

Dromostanolone Propionate Solution   10-ml. vials containing 100 mg. in 1 ml.
(Oil)

Trade name: Drolban

ANABOLIC ANDROGENS

Norethandrolone, B.P. (Nilevar)

This androgenic steroid is used principally for its anabolic activity and to produce a positive nitrogen balance, accomplishing this with less than the normal degree of masculinization. If administered in high doses for prolonged periods of time, the drug may cause virilization, fluid retention, and liver damage with or without jaundice. For this reason, norethandrolone is used with caution for periods not exceeding three months. Contraindications are the same as those for androgens.

The average daily dose is 20 to 30 mg. daily for short periods up to three months. In children, 0.5 mg. per kilogram of body weight is recommended.

Preparations

Norethandrolone Tablets, B.P.	7.5 and 15 mg., 15 mg. with 15 mg. phenobarbital
Norethandrolone Injection	Ampuls containing 30 mg.

Trade name: Nilevar

OTHER ANABOLIC ANDROGENS

Nandrolone (Durabolin)	I.m.: 25 mg. weekly	Solution in oil, 25 mg. in 1-ml. in 5-ml. vials
Nandrolone Decanoate, B.P. (Deca-Durabolin)	I.m.: 50 to 100 mg. every three or four weeks	Solution in oil, 50 mg. in 1-ml. ampuls
Methandrostenolone (Dianabol)	Orally: 5 to 20 mg. daily for 3 weeks, and up to 10 mg. daily thereafter	Tablets, 5 mg.
Oxymetholone (Androyd)	Orally: 2.5 to 10 mg. t.i.d.	Tablets, 2.5 and 10 mg.
Stanozolol (Stromba, Winstrol)	Orally: 2 mg. t.i.d.	Tablets, 2 mg.

DRUGS THAT RELIEVE DYSMENORRHEA

Dysmenorrhea is one of the most common gynecological complaints in women of all ages. The chief symptoms are (1) sharp or steady abdominal pain, (2) abdominal distention, (3) painful breasts, (4) nausea and vomiting, (5) premenstrual tension, and (6) depression and irritability. These symptoms may appear as early as a week or ten days before the onset of the menstrual period, but characteristically appear 24 to 48 hours prior to the menses and persist for a varying time thereafter. Treatment of dysmenorrhea consists of good posture, exercise, proper hygiene, regular hours, good diet, and medications, if necessary.

Before menstrual bleeding, an increase in circulating progesterone may cause water retention thereby initiating complaints such as low-back pain, increased body weight, enlarged breasts, and headache. The combination of these symptoms is referred to as premenstrual tension. It may be effectively treated with diuretics and occasionally with sedatives or tranquilizers.

In the management of mild dysmenorrhea lututrin may be given every six hours with the onset of symptoms. Atropine, belladonna, and phenobarbital may be given in moderate doses. Aspirin, 300 to 600 mg., may be useful, or aspirin may be given in combination with phenacetin, caffeine (Empirin, Anacin, see p. 284), with ephedrine (as in Midol), or amphetamine (as in Edrisal), or with phenobarbital, 30 mg., three times a day. Sometimes a combination of 30 mg. of phenobarbital and 60 mg. of codeine three times a day may be required. Bed rest is often necessary, and the application of heat to the lower abdomen may be helpful. When these medications fail to relieve symptoms, a more severe case of dysmenorrhea is being dealt with. In more severe cases, estrogens and progesterone may be administered.

Since it has been postulated that causes of dysmenorrhea are reduced blood supply to the uterus and nonrhythmic uterine contractions, it seems logical that the vasodilator isoxuprine and lututrin may be indicated.

ORAL TRICHOMONACIDE

Metronidazole (Flagyl) is used in the treatment of leukorrhea and vaginitis associated with *Trichomonas vaginalis*, flagellate protozoa, present in the vaginal tract. An occasional cure but only temporary symptomatic relief has been afforded, in most cases, with the many topical drugs available (see p. 745). Treatment with metronidazole topically often causes an immediate apparent cure (relief of symptoms and disappearance of trichomonads). Vaginal therapy alone with this drug is not more effective than other topical methods, but when administered orally, the drug is superior to any agents available for topical use. Combined therapy with metronidazole (oral and vaginal) may control leukorrhea more quickly than oral therapy alone.

No evidence of toxicity has been noted. Side effects which have occurred infrequently are furring of the tongue, mild nausea, and a burning sensation of the vulvae. The drug is contraindicated in blood dyscrasias. The oral dose is 250 mg. three or four times a day for ten days. The vaginal dose is 500 mg. (vaginal insert) morning and evening.

Preparations

Metronidazole Tablets	250 mg.
Metronidazole Vaginal Insert	500 mg.

Trade name: Flagyl

REVIEW QUESTIONS

1. *What is ergot? What are the actions and uses of products obtained from it? What synthetic derivative of an ergot alkaloid is available and how does it differ in its actions from the naturally occurring parent substance?*
2. *What physiological effects are produced by injections of posterior pituitary extracts? Discuss the use of oxytocin.*
3. *List the anterior pituitary hormones and mention their chief effects in health and in diseases associated with them.*

4. *Briefly describe the hormonal and organic events of the menstrual cycle.*
5. *What are the composition and actions of chorionic gonadotropin? What are practical sources of gonadotropic hormone? What is the use of these materials?*
6. *Name all estrogens that are administered orally and give their dose.*
7. *Discuss the uses of estrogens.*
8. *Discuss the actions and uses of progesterone, its synthetic substitutes, and lututrin.*
9. *Discuss the uses of the new, orally active progestational agents in gynecology and obstetrics.*
10. *What side effects may they produce and what are their dosage schedules?*
11. *Of what uses are the androgens?*
12. *Breast malignancies beginning long after menopause may be treated with both estrogens and androgens. Why should androgens alone be used before menopause for this condition?*
13. *Name the androgens and the mode of administration of each.*
14. *Review the discussion of nitrogen retention as it relates to protein building and list the masculinizing side effects which the androgens and newer agents may produce when they are being used for anabolism.*
15. *List the conditions in which accelerated protein synthesis is desired and give the dosage of oxymetholone and stanozolol.*
16. *Discuss the action of oxytocin in ejaculating milk from the breast and the practical features in using this hormone of the posterior pituitary as a nasal spray.*
17. *If persistent uterine bleeding occurs during the twenty-sixth week of pregnancy, what measures may be required for removing the threat to the pregnancy? What agents may be employed and at what doses?*

REFERENCES

Eastman, Nicholson J., and Hellman, Louis, M.: *Williams Obstetrics*, 12th ed. Appleton-Century-Crofts, Inc., New York, 1961.
Parsons, Langdon, and Sommers, Shelton C.: *Gynecology*. W. B. Saunders Company, Philadelphia, 1962.
Reid, Duncan E.: *A Textbook of Obstetrics*. W. B. Saunders Company, Philadelphia, 1962.

ERGOT AND OXYTOCIN

Huntingford, P. J.: "Prophylactic Ergometrine," *Brit. M. J.*, **2**:1071, 1959.
Theobald, G. W.: Oxytocic Agents," *Brit. M. J.*, **5170**:413, 1960.

RELAXIN

Sands, R. X., and Stone, M. L.: "Relaxin, a Review of Clinical Progress," *Lancet*, **2**:32, 1959.

ANTERIOR PITUITARY AND ESTROGENS

de Alvarez, R. R., and Smith, E. K.: "Physiological Basis for Hormone Therapy in the Female," *J.A.M.A.*, **168**:489, 1958.
Council on Drugs: "Androgens and Estrogens in the Treatment of Disseminated

Mammary Carcinoma Retrospective Study of Nine Hundred Forty-four Patients,"
J.A.M.A., **172**:1271, 1960.

PROGESTINS

Abramson, D.: "Clinical Observations on the Use of 17-Ethinyl-19-Nortestosterone in Repeated and Threatened Abortions," *Ann. New York Acad. Sc.*, **71**:759, 1958.

Cook, H. H.; Gamble, C. J.; and Satterthwaite, A. P.: "Oral Contraception by Norethynodrel," *Amer. J. Obst. & Gynec.*, **82**:437, 1961.

Council on Drugs: "Norethindrone (Norlutin)," *J.A.M.A.*, **169**:1193, 1959.

Kistner, R. W.: "The Use of Steroidal Substances in Endometriosis," *Clin. Pharm. and Ther.*, **1**:525, 1960.

Pincus, G.; Garcia, C. R.; Rock, J.; *et al.*: "Effectiveness of an Oral Contraceptive," *Science*, **130**:81, 1959.

Pincus, G.; Rock, J.; *et al.*: "Fertility Control with Oral Medication," *Am. J. Obst. & Gynec.*, **75**:935, 1958.

Southam, A. L.: "A Comparative Study of the Effect of the Progestational Agents in Human Menstrual Abnormalities," *Ann. New York Acad. Sc.*, **71**:666, 1958.

Tyler, E. T.; Olson, H. J.; Wolf, L.; Finkelstein, S.; Thayer, J.; Kaplan, N.; Levin, M.; and Weintraub, J.: "An Oral Contraceptive. A 4-Year Study of Norethindrone," *Obstet. Gynec. (N. Y.)*, **18**:363, 1961.

Swyer, G. I. M.: "Progestins and Their Clinical Uses," *Brit. M. J.*, **1**:121, 1960.

Wilkins, L.: "Masculinization of Female Fetus Due to Use of Orally Given Progestins," *J.A.M.A.*, **172**:1028, 1960.

ANDROGENS

Bishop, P. M. F.: "Male Sex Hormones," *Brit. M. J.*, **5167**:184, 1960.

Buckle, R. M.: "Fluoxymesterone," *Brit. M. J.*, **1**:1378, 1959.

Goldenberg, I. S., and Hayes, M. A.: "Hormonal Therapy of Metastatic Female Breast Carcinoma. II, 2a-Methyl Dihydrotestosterone Propionate," *Cancer*, **14**:705, 1961.

ANABOLIC AGENTS

Berkowitz, D.: "The Treatment of Post-Gastrectomy Weight Loss with Two New Anabolic Agents," *Clin. Res.*, **8**:199, 1960.

Sobel, J.: "Clinical Study of Nandrolone Phenpropionate," *Clinical Med.*, **7**:481, 1960.

Szujewski, H. A.: "Nandrolone Phenpropionate, a New Palliative Agent in the Management of Mammary Carcinoma," *Amer. Pract. and Digest Treat.*, **10**:2157, 1959.

OXYTOCIN NASAL SPRAY

Friedman, E. A.: "Direct Measurement of Milk Ejection Pressure in Unanesthetized Lactating Humans," *Am. J. Obst. & Gynec.*, **80**:119, 1960.

Stewart, R. H.: "The use of Synthetic Oxytocin in Nursing or Non-nursing Mothers," *J.A.M.A.*, **175**:1071, 1961.

Menopause and Dysmenorrhea

Jeffcoate, T. N. A.: "Drugs for Menopausal Symptoms," *Brit. M. J.*, **5169**:340, 1960.

Jungck, E. C.; Barfield, W. S.; and Greenblatt, R. B.: "Chlorthiazide and Premenstrual Tension," *J.A.M.A.*, **169**:112, 1959.

Oral Trichomonacide

Roland, Maxwell: "Clinical Trial of Metronidazole, an Oral Trichomonacide," *J.A.M.A.*, **180**:242, 1962.

38

Drugs Acting on the Kidneys. Urinary Diagnostic Agents

THE KIDNEYS

The kidneys have the general and important function of maintaining a normal environment for the cells of the body as regards the water and dissolved substances that surround them. The substances absorbed from food, including water and many salts, and the many biochemical processes taking place in the body present the kidneys with the task of forming the urine as a means of excreting the excess of such substances and, by far, most of the waste products of metabolism. By so doing, *water and electrolyte balance* and certain other features of *homeostasis* are maintained.

Water, which constitutes more than two thirds of the body weight, is distributed in the body in three main compartments: the blood plasma; the interstitial fluid (fluid beween the cells); and the intracellular fluid (fluid within the cells), which is the largest compartment. The extracellular fluid (blood plasma, interstitial fluid) contains isotonic sodium chloride solution. The ingestion of 9 Gm. of table salt will hold 1 liter of fluid in the tissues. This proportion constitutes a solution of 0.9 per cent sodium chloride, which is practically isotonic.

The osmotic pressure of the electrolytes and the selective permeability of the cell membrane play an important role in maintaining water balance. The plasma proteins are essential in maintaining the blood volume and thus are important in controlling the water content of the tissues. Owing to their large size, these proteins cannot diffuse readily through the capillaries; thus by osmotic pressure they hold water in the blood.

During health the water content is very constant, whereas in certain pathological conditions there is a shifting of water balance. In cardiovascular and renal diseases, water and salts are retained in the body and excess fluid accumulates in the tissues, causing edema. In Addison's disease (of the adrenal cortex), the ability of the kidneys to retain sodium chloride is impaired; therefore this salt is excreted in the urine with large quantities of water, and dehydration results. Other conditions such as vomiting, diarrhea, hemorrhage, and excessive sweating produce generalized dehydration.

626

Dissolved Constituents of the Extracellular Fluid and the Blood Plasma. The extracellular water is in constant circulation in health, and certain dissolved substances are transported rather freely to and from the cells of the various organs and tissues. Among the more prevalent substances which pass across the capillary walls from the blood to the extracellular fluid compartment, or in the reverse direction, are oxygen; foods such as glucose, amino acids, and fatty acids; waste products, such as carbon dioxide, urea, and the water from metabolism of foods; and various salts. The latter include sodium chloride and sodium bicarbonate predominantly, and small amounts of potassium, calcium, and magnesium salts. Some of the salts are phosphates, chlorides, and sulfates.

Our diet contains salts of inorganic and organic acids and bases. These and the products of the metabolic activities of cells become ionized in the body fluids (see pp. 91–93). Some of these ions are normal constituents of the body fluids and cells. The usual concentration of each ion is fairly constant, but it varies among the different ions. When the plasma flowing to the kidneys contains ion concentrations in excess of those normally required, the excess is excreted in the urine. In this manner the kidneys assist in regulating the acid-base balance of the blood within the required narrow limits. The buffer systems in the blood, lymph, tissue fluids, and cells also aid in maintaining a physiological pH range of the blood between 7.3 and 7.5. The role of hormones in controlling the mineral or salt excretion is described on page 681.

The regulation of the normal total amount of water in the plasma and extracellular fluid is thought to be under the control of receptors in the hypothalamus which are sensitive to changes in osmotic pressure. This mechanism is mediated via the posterior pituitary gland as described on page 644. The regulation of all phases of the "internal environment" of the body, chemically and physiologically, is termed *homeostasis*. This must be accomplished within fairly narrow ranges, regardless of wide variations in the external environment.

Electrolyte and Fluid Balance and Homeostasis. In brief, the functions of the kidneys include: (1) the excretion of water and the end products of metabolism such as urea, uric acid, organic acids, and foreign substances; (2) the excretion of inorganic salts not needed by the body; (3) the maintenance of the osmotic pressure of the blood and tissues; and (4) the maintenance of the acid-base equilibrium of the blood. Adults usually consume from 5 to 15 Gm. of sodium chloride, 2 to 4 Gm. of potassium salts, smaller quantities of other salts, and 2 to 4 liters of water daily. More than half this water is excreted by the kidneys, more in cool weather than warm. The perspiration and feces, especially in diarrhea, are the chief additional avenues of excretion of water. The above intake of salt is approximately 20 times the daily requirement, our dietary habits thus oversupply our needs.

The formation of urine from the blood consists of glomerular filtration and tubular reabsorption. As the glomerular filtrate passes through the tubules, substances essential to the blood and tissues—water, glucose, salts, amino acids, and sodium bicarbonate—are reabsorbed. These compounds are called *threshold substances.* They must reach a certain concentration in the blood before they are excreted in the final urine flow. Other substances in the glomerular filtrate, such as potassium and urea, are not readily re-

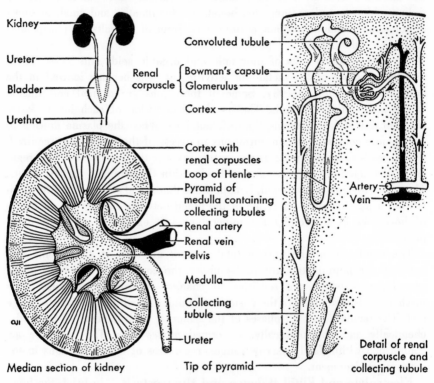

Fig. 17.   Excretory system of man. *Upper left.* Diagram of entire system. *Lower left.* Kidney in median section. *Right.* Relations of renal corpuscle tubules and blood vessels. *Solid arrows* indicate the path of the blood; *dotted arrows,* the path of excretion. (From Hegner, R. W., and Stiles, K. A.: *College Zoology,* 7th ed. The Macmillan Company, New York, 1959.)

absorbed by the tubules and are called *low-threshold* or *nonthreshold substances.* Thus K^+ in excess of the required amount are excreted in the urine. The proper K ion balance between the intracellular and extracellular fluids is essential for normal physiological functioning of the heart, enzyme, reactions, contractility of muscle, impulse transmission, and other action of the central nervous system. This balance may be displaced by excessive K^+

retention, i.e., hyperkalemia, or excessive K^+ excretion, i.e., hypokalemia. Either abnormality may cause serious symptoms even resulting in death. Because they are necessarily secreted in the urine *with water*, they may be used as diuretics.

The glomerular filtration rate is about 100 ml. per minute. About 99 ml. of the fluid are returned to the blood, and 1 ml. is secreted in the urine That which is not reabsorbed by the tubules is excreted as urine; therefore, by decreasing tubular reabsorption, more urine is excreted. Most of the diuretics (agents which increase the flow of urine) act by interfering with tubular reabsorption of sodium and chloride, and thus of water.

There are a number of other factors that affect the secretion of urine, such as the blood pressure, the amount of blood circulating through the kidneys, and the activity of the kidneys. Drugs that increase the blood pressure and improve the circulation as well as drugs that increase the activity of all cells also aid in producing urine formation when these factors are depressed.

Edema. The retention of fluid in the interstitial spaces in the body is known as edema. There are many causes of edema, such as inflammation, mechanical obstruction of lymph or return blood flow (clot formation, pregnancy, etc.), capillary injury, toxins, allergy, vasodilatation, and a number of specific diseases. Edema may occur locally in any area or it may be bilateral and involve the feet, legs, abdomen, and hands. To varying degrees, it may be considered "systemic," i.e., caused by general rather than local factors. The principal diseases associated with generalized edema are cardiac decompensation, renal disease (nephrosis and nephritis), liver disease, and toxemia of pregnancy (eclampsia). The corticosteroid drugs may cause edema.

Edema fluid is usually isotonic and hence contains sodium chloride. Drugs that suppress the reabsorption of sodium and chloride from the glomerular filtrate by the tubules, thus increasing the excretion of these ions, cause excretion of extra water because it is held in the forming urine by these ions. It is thus an obligatory accompaniment of the salt ions. Most of the diuretic agents produce their effects in this way.

In this chapter drugs producing diuresis, a hormone that suppresses urine flow, abnormalities of potassium metabolism, agents that inhibit the renal excretion of organic compounds, agents for combating kidney stone formation, and certain diagnostic agents of use in urological and renal diseases will be discussed.

DIURETICS

Classification of Diuretic Agents.   Drugs that increase the flow of urine are described in this chapter under the following classification: (1) the benzothiadiazine derivatives (the "thiazides"), (2) mercurial diuretics,

(3) miscellaneous synthetic diuretics, (4) xanthine diuretics, and (5) additional miscellaneous agents. The first group is the newest and most extensively used.

THE BENZOTHIADIAZINE DIURETICS

Chlorothiazide, U.S.P., B.P. (Diuril)

Chlorothiazide was the first of the group of benzothiadiazine or "thiazide" diuretics and is widely used as an orally effective substitute for the older mercurial compounds.

Pharmacological Actions.   Chlorothiazide and its congeners suppress the reabsorption of sodium and chloride by both the proximal and distal convoluted tubules. Since salt excretion is thus increased, extra water is carried along by the osmotic pressure of the salt ions, and diuresis results. The volume of urine output may be doubled or tripled until edema subsides. Potassium ions are also excreted in increased amounts but not to the extent of sodium and chloride. This is undesirable and may produce side effects. The loss may be overcome by the administration of potassium-rich foods (orange juice, etc.) or potassium salt.

There is a mild carbonic anhydrase inhibition, but this accounts for little of the diuretic effect and causes but little excretion of the bicarbonate ion from the blood. Acidosis is thus not a serious side effect. The potency of this group is approximately the same as that of the mercurial diuretics (see p. 634).

Absorption.   The thiazides are well absorbed from the alimentary tract. Diuresis begins within two hours after oral administration and persists for 6 to 12 hours after a single dose. Prolonged use does not usually produce refractoriness to this group.

Therapeutic Uses.   The thiazides are useful in most types of edema. After edema has been eliminated, continuation of one of these agents may maintain the patient edema free. Patients formerly requiring insipid low-salt diets for combating edema may be permitted somewhat increased amounts of salt for savoring the food.

The thiazides are extensively used in the treatment of hypertension since they decrease the blood volume and thus reduce the blood pressure (see p. 560). They are also recommended in premenstrual tension and dysmenorrhea in which there is usually water retention caused by the cyclic rise in estrogen and progesterone.

Side Effects.   Chlorothiazide and its congeners are well tolerated by the majority of patients. Relatively few serious reactions have been encountered, but a large number of side effects have occurred with extensive use. The effects upon fluid and salt ions (electrolytes) may become excessive. Thus excessive excretion of chloride in relation to sodium may cause retention of an excess of bicarbonate ions, with resultant alkalosis. Potassium loss may be greater in this situation but it may occur alone. In either case, low blood potassium levels cause increased sensitivity of the heart to digitalis. Digitalis toxicity upon the heart thereby increases and arrhythmias or heart block may ensue. The dosage of the thiazide must be decreased in electrolyte disturbances. Potassium chloride administration is indicated to replace both potassium and chloride ions. Caution is required with all patients receiving a thiazide, especially those with liver diseases.

Excessive reduction of sodium and potassium salts can produce weakness, hypotension, and other features of the "low-salt syndrome." These may include nausea, vomiting, epigastric distress, diarrhea, malaise, anorexia, paresthesias, muscle cramps, flushing, etc. Skin rashes with or without photosensitivity (to light) have occurred. Thrombocytopenia (platelet reduction), leukopenia, and agranulocytosis have occurred, although rarely. Inflammation in the parotid (salivary) glands has been observed, probably as a result of dehydration with decrease or cessation of flow of saliva. In the absence of adequate duct-cleansing action, bacteria may ascend from even the normal mouth to the glandular tissue and produce infection. Acute pancreatitis has also occurred, possibly as a duct-borne bacterial invasion from the duodenal flora or as a chemical effect of the drug. Liver impairment has also been reported.

An interesting additional and frequent side effect of this type of drug is a rise in uric acid in the blood and tissues. This waste product of nucleoprotein is normally constantly excreted by the kidneys. The thiazides apparently suppress tubular excretion of uric acid. Some patients receiving these drugs temporarily develop clinical gout with joint pains in the feet.

Dosage and Methods of Administration. Chlorothiazide is administered orally and its sodium salt intravenously. Adult dosage by both routes varies between 500 mg. and 1 Gm. once or twice daily. In hypertension the dose may vary from 250 mg. twice daily to 500 mg. three times daily. When chlorothiazide or any other diuretic is administered, the patient should be made aware of the expected action of the drug because a sudden increase in urine output can be quite frightening if the cause is unknown.

Preparations

Chlorothiazide Tablets, U.S.P., B.P.	250, 500 mg.
Chlorothiazide Sodium Powder (Injection)	500 mg., to be dissolved in 18 ml. or more of Water for Injection, U.S.P.

Trade names: Diuril, Diuril "Lyovac," Chlotride, Saluric

Hydrochlorothiazide, U.S.P., B.P. (Hydrodiuril, Esidrix, Oretic)

This analog of chlorothiazide is approximately ten times more potent than the drug discussed above. In general, it has the same mechanisms of action, uses, and side effects. It is said to cause less excretion of potassium for a given amount of sodium loss as compared with chlorothiazide. The oral dose is 50 mg. once or twice a day (25 to 100 mg. daily).

Preparation

Hydrochlorothiazide Tablets   25 and 50 mg.
    Trade names: Dichlotride; Direma; Esidrix; Hydril; Hydrodiuril; Hydrosaluric; Hydrozide; Oretic

Flumethiazide (Ademol)

This analog of chlorothiazide has approximately the same potency, uses, side effects, and dosage as the parent substance. To initiate diuresis and for the treatment of hypertension, daily doses of 500 mg. to 2 Gm. may be given orally, in divided amounts, until the effects become maximal. For maintenance, 250 to 1500 mg. daily are used.

Preparation

Flumethiazide Tablets   500 mg.
    Trade name: Ademol

Hydroflumethiazide, B.P. (NaClex, Saluron, Hydrenox)

This agent, an analog of hydrochlorothiazide, possesses the same degree of potency and usefulness and has the same side-effect potentials and dosage requirements. Clinical reports indicate that less potassium as well as less bicarbonate is excreted. Initial administration consists of 25 to 100, and occasionally 200, mg. daily, in divided doses. Appropriate reductions are made after optimal diuresis or blood pressure reduction has been effected.

Preparations

Hydroflumethiazide Tablets   50 mg.
Hydroflumethiazide Syrup   50 mg. in 5 ml.
    Trade names: NaClex; Saluron; Hydrenox; Di-Ademol; Rontyl

Bendroflumethiazide, Bendrofluazide, B.P. (Naturetin)

This "thiazide" derivative is similar in usefulness and side effects to each of the above diuretics, but it is considerably more potent. In addition, it has sufficiently prolonged action that one dose of 2.5 or 5 mg. (20 mg. initially) per day often suffices. Potassium loss is said to be less than with chlorothiazide and hydrochlorothiazide. Nevertheless, the foods relatively rich in this element, or potassium chloride tablets, may be required.

Preparation

Bendroflumethiazide Tablets   2.5 and 5.0 mg.
                Trade names: Naturetin; Neo-Naclex; Aprinox; Centryl

Trichlormethiazide (Naqua)

This agent is quite similar, in all respects, to benzydroflumethiazide. It is given in slightly smaller doses, 1 to 16 mg. daily, the average being 2 to 4 mg.

Preparation

Trichlormethiazide Tablets   2 and 4 mg.
                Trade name: Naqua

Methyclothiazide (Enduron)

This agent, similar to the other "thiazide" diuretics, has the same mechanism of action in causing diuresis. It is said to produce more sodium loss in the urine for a given amount of potassium loss than do some of the other members of the group.

Methyclothiazide is of some use in lowering hypertension. Side effects are no more frequent with this agent than with its congeners, and are less than with some. They are included in the discussion of side effects of chlorothiazide.

Dosage. The usual oral adult dose ranges from 2.5 to 10 mg., given once daily. The activity is greatest approximately six hours after medication with good maintenance for 24 hours.

Preparation

Methyclothiazide Tablets   2.5, 5 mg.
                Trade name: Enduron

Polythiazide (Renese)

Polythiazide is also a potent diuretic with a favorable sodium-to-potassium ratio. It is used in the same types of edema states as are the other agents: in congestive heart failure, renal edema, cirrhosis, and toxemia of pregnancy. It is also useful in hypertension. Its side effects are similar to those of chlorothiazide.

Dosage. Depending upon the degree of the edema present or of the hypertension, 1 to 12 mg. daily by mouth may be given initially. Patients can usually be maintained on 0.5 to 4 mg. daily.

Preparation

Polythiazide   1, 2, and 4 mg.
Trade name: Renese

Triamterine (Dyrenium) reduces the reabsorption of sodium in the renal tubules and promotes its excretion without loss of potassium. It is well absorbed orally and is excreted in the urine. The duration of the diuretic effect is about 12 hours. When given in combination with thiazide therapy, the diuretic and hypotensive effects are increased, and the risk of hypokalemia, which may occur with thiazide therapy alone, is reduced. Occasional side effects are nausea and vomiting, weakness, headache, dry mouth, and rash. Triamterine is a diuretic used in the treatment of edema and hypertension.

The adult oral dose is 100 mg. once or twice daily after meals.

Preparation

Triamterine Capsules   100 mg.
Trade name: Dyrenium

QUINAZOLINE DERIVATIVE

Quinethazone (Hydromox)

This drug is useful in all types of edema involving retention of sodium chloride and water. It is also useful in hypertension. The side effects occasionally seen are skin rash, nausea, weakness, and dizziness.

Dosage.   Quinethazone is given in a dose of 50 to 100 mg. orally once daily.

Preparation

Quinethazone Tablets   50 mg.
Trade name: Hydromox

MERCURIAL DIURETICS

Several organic mercurial compounds have been used as diuretics, beginning in 1920. Some exceed, when given parenterally, the oral potency of the thiazide derivatives. The introduction in 1957 of chlorothiazide greatly reduced the use of the mercurial diuretics because the latter are much less effective orally.

Pharmacological Actions.   The mercurial diuretics possess the same mechanism of action, the suppression of reabsorption of sodium and chloride, and thus cause loss of water, which must accompany the salt. This suppression, however, occurs only in the distal tubules of the kidneys. It results from the blocking of an enzyme, succinic dehydrogenase, by the mercurial compound. Potassium may be excreted in amounts greater than normal but not to the extent caused by the thiazides. Potassium loss is usually not a problem with the mercurial agents. Mercurial diuretics are well absorbed when given parenterally. However, they are absorbed less completely from the gastrointestinal tract.

The diuretic effect of the organic mercurials begins within a few hours after intramuscular or intravenous administration, reaches its peak in six to eight hours, and continues for perhaps a total of twenty-four. Because of this it is best to give the drug in the morning so that the patient's sleep will not be disturbed.

Theophylline, a xanthine diuretic, is combined with certain mercurial compounds to enhance their potency. Potency is also greatly enhanced by the prior administration of ammonium chloride.

Toxicity and Side Effects.   When the organic mercurials are given parenterally, local irritation such as the experience of a burning sensation occasionally accompanied by the formation of nodes at the site of injection may occur. Due to the differences in rate of absorption, these reactions take place more frequently after subcutaneous than after intramuscular injections. If the drugs are given orally, the dose must be increased, augmenting the possibility of systemic mercury poisoning. Gastrointestinal irritation may also occur, the symptoms of which include nausea, frequent bowel movements, abdominal pain, vomiting, and diarrhea. Although usually mild, the reactions may vary in severity.

Unlike the inorganic mercury compounds, the organic ones may usually be given repeatedly for prolonged periods without difficulty. Many and severe reactions may occur, however. Flushing, urticaria, itching, dermatitis, nausea, vomiting, fever, and suppression of white blood cell formation may occur as direct effects. High concentration may cause cardiac arrhythmias. With excessive excretion of salts, weakness, muscle pains, and shock may occur. Excessive or too prolonged administration may cause "mercurialism," or chronic mercury poisoning, as with inorganic mercury (see p. 776). These agents should be used with caution in kidney disease.

Therapeutic Uses.   The mercurials are used for the relief of edema of cardiac failure, in liver disease, and cautiously in nephrotic edema. They have been replaced largely by the thiazides (see pp. 630–33) for the continuous control of edema, but their potency upon parenteral administration makes them of greater value than the thiazides at times.

Mersalyl, N.F. (Salyrgan)

Mersalyl is the oldest organic mercurial diuretic in general use today, and one of the most potent. The usual oral dose is 160 mg. daily. The intramuscular dose of mersalyl and theophylline injection is 100 mg. once or twice a week.

Preparations

Mersalyl and Theophylline Injection, N.F.; Mersalyl Injection, B.P.	1- and 2-ml. ampuls containing 100 mg. of mersalyl and 50 mg. of theophylline in 1 ml.
Mersalyl and Theophylline Tablets	80 mg. of mersalyl and 40 mg. of theophylline

Trade names: Salyrgan-Theophylline; Mercugan

Meralluride, U.S.P. (Mercuhydrin)

Meralluride is administered intramuscularly, intravenously, or subcutaneously. However, the most efficient and safest method of administration is the intramuscular, the dosage for which is 1 ml. (equivalent to 39 mg. of mercury and 48 mg. of theophylline), with a range of 1 to 2 ml., once or twice a week.

Preparation

Meralluride Injection, U.S.P.	1- and 2-ml. ampuls and 10-ml. vials containing 39 mg. of mercury and 48 mg. of theophylline in 1 ml.

Trade names: Mercuhydrin; Mercardan

Mercaptomerin Sodium, U.S.P. (Thiomerin Sodium)

Mercaptomerin sodium is less irritating to the tissues at the site of injection and is less toxic to the heart than many of the other organic mercurials. The parenteral dose is 130 mg. (26 to 260.) in 1 ml. once or twice a week.

Preparation

Sterile Mercaptomerin Sodium, U.S.P.	Vials containing 1.4 and 4.2 Gm. of lyophilized powder

Trade names: Thiomerin; Diucardyn

Mercumatilin Sodium (Cumertilin)

The average daily oral adult dose of mercumatilin is 68 to 136 mg. One to one and one-quarter milliliters of the injection may be administered intramuscularly twice a week.

Preparations

Mercumatilin Tablets	68 mg. of mercumatilin (equivalent to 20 mg. of mercury)
Mercumatilin Sodium Solution	1- and 2-ml. ampuls and 10-ml. vials containing 132 mg. (equivalent to 39 mg. of mercury and 50 mg. of theophylline) in 1 ml.

Trade name: Cumertilin

Chlormerodrin (Neohydrin)

The oral dose of chlormerodrin is 18.3 mg. (equivalent to 10 mg. of mercury) to 73.2 mg. (equivalent to 40 mg. of mercury). The untoward effects are few; however, gastrointestinal symptoms occur in about 10 per cent of the patients. Chlormerodrin is the drug of choice as an orally administered mercurial diuretic.

Preparation

Chlormerodrin Tablets	18.3 mg. of chlormerodrin (equivalent to 10 mg. of mercury)

Trade names: Neohydrin; Merchloran

MISCELLANEOUS SYNTHETIC DIURETICS

Spironolactone (Aldactone)

Spironolactone is an antagonist of *aldosterone*, a steroid secreted by the adrenal cortex and first isolated in 1952. Aldosterone is by far the most potent adrenal hormone known to affect the renal excretion of sodium and potassium. It causes a decrease in the excretion of sodium and an increase in that of potassium when this is desirable. Aldosterone is secreted under the stimulatory influence of a hormone present in the pineal gland and in several areas of the brain. It is probable that this hormone, called *glomerulotropin*, is secreted under influence of sodium blood levels and of volume receptors that have yet to be located. These are sensitive to decreases in blood volume, as in hemorrhage, dehydration, or salt depletion, and result in aldosterone secretion with a decrease in water and sodium excretion.

Pharmacological Actions. Spironolactone prevents the sodium-retaining effect of aldosterone and thereby causes increased excretion of sodium and water and decreased excretion of potassium. Thus spironolactone is a diuretic and potassium-retaining drug. It is useful in edema and in preventing the potassium loss produced by the thiazide diuretics. It is reported that aldosterone is secreted in larger amounts during the use of the thiazides, as an attempt to counteract their sodium-excreting effect. The inhibition of aldosterone by spironolactone is thus a rational use of the latter with the thiazides (see pp. 630–33). These diuretics are thus made safer, since potassium loss can cause various side effects, including cardiac arrhythmias and weakness. When spironolactone has been used with the thiazides, a potentiation of their diuretic action has been reported.

Spironolactone has been found effective in reducing high blood pressure. This could be expected with a potent diuretic and sodium-excreting drug. However, preliminary investigations suggest still a further and unrecognized mechanism for reducing hypertension. Steroid agents similar to spironolactone will probably appear in the near future because of the novel, fundamental, and useful actions involved.

Dosage and Method of Administration. Spironolactone is given orally, in doses of 100 to 400 mg. daily, in divided amounts.

Preparation

Spironolactone Tablets   100 mg.

Trade name: Aldactone

Chlorthalidone (Hygroton)

Chlorthalidone causes sodium, chloride, and water loss, with some potassium loss that may have to be combated by the use of potassium replacement. This agent is being used for both diuretic and antihypertensive effects. The usual side effects associated with salt and potassium depletion may occur. White blood cell count may be lowered.

Dosage and Method of Administration. Chlorthalidone is administered orally in doses of 50 to 200 mg. daily or every other day. A single dose lasts up to two or three days.

Preparation

Chlorthalidone Tablets   100 mg.

Trade name: Hygroton

Acetazolamide, U.S.P., B.P. (Diamox)

This sulfonamide (not useful as an antibacterial agent) is a potent inhibitor of carbonic anhydrase, the enzyme that facilitiates the union of water and carbon dioxide to form carbonic acid. It also facilitates the reverse process. The compound suppresses the reabsorption of the bicarbonate ion by the kidney tubules from the glomerular filtrate. Thus sodium and potassium bicarbonate with the necessary water are excreted, and diuresis occurs. With the loss of these alkaline salts, systemic acidosis results, along with low blood potassium. These disturbances must be watched for and treated appropriately.

Therapeutic Uses. Acetazolamide has been used as a diuretic agent but has largely been replaced by the thiazide group, which does not produce acidosis. It has also been of some use in grand and petit mal epilepsy and in the treatment of glaucoma by decreasing the rate of formation of the aqueous humor.

Side Effects. Drowsiness and paresthesias over the face, arms, and legs often occur. Fatigue, excitement, intestinal disturbances, and thirst may also occur.

Dosage and Methods of Administration. Acetazolamide is administered orally. Its sodium salt may be given intravenously or intramuscularly. Dosage ordinarily varies between 250 and 500 mg. daily.

Preparations

Acetazolamide Tablets, U.S.P., B. P.	250 mg.
Acetazolamide Syrup	50 mg. in 1 ml.
Acetazolamide Sodium, U.S.P. (Injection)	500 mg. to be dissolved in Water for Injection, U.S.P., etc.

Ethoxzolamide (Cardrase)

This carbonic anhydrase inhibitor has the same uses and side effects as acetazolamide. It is administered orally in doses of 62.5 to 125 mg. daily.

Preparation

Ethoxzolamide Tablets   62.5, 125 mg.

XANTHINE DIURETICS

The three xanthine derivatives—caffeine, theophylline, and theobromine (see pp. 395–97)—produce diuresis by diminishing tubular reabsorption. Theophylline is the most powerful diuretic of this group; however, since the action of theobromine is more prolonged, it is the xanthine drug of choice for continued use. Theobromine is not readily absorbed when administered alone; therefore, it is marketed in combination with organic salts to increase its solubility and absorption.

The diuresis is not so prompt, dependable, or uniform as that produced by the previously described diuretics. The use of these drugs has decreased with the advent of the thiazide diuretics.

Preparations

Theobromine Sodium Acetate Tablets, N.F. (I.P.)	250, 500, 750 mg.
Theobromine Sodium Acetate Capsules, N.F.	100, 200 mg.
Theobromine Calcium Salicylate Tablets, N.F.	500 mg.
Theobromine and Phenobarbital (Theominal)	324 mg. (with 32 mg. of phenobarbital)
Theophylline Sodium Glycinate, Tablets, N.F.	150, 300 mg.
Theophylline Sodium Glycinate (Injection)	40 mg. in 1 ml.; 10- and 20-ml ampuls

Trade names: Glynazan; Glytheonate, Synophylate; Theoglycinate

Oxtriphyllin (Choline Theophyllinate, Choledyl) Tablets	100, 200 mg.
Dyphylline (Neothylline) Tablets	100, 200 mg.
Theophylline-Methylglucamine (Glucophyllin) Tablets and Suppositories	150 mg. (tablets), 500 mg. (suppositories)

ACIDOTIC DIURETICS

Ammonium Chloride, U.S.P., B.P.

Ammonium chloride is absorbed from the intestinal tract and is converted by the liver to urea and hydrochloric acid. A reduction in the alkali reserve of the blood occurs, and the urine becomes acid. The urea is excreted easily by healthy, but not by diseased, kidneys. The chloride is excreted with cations, mainly sodium, with the necessary amount of water from blood and tissues.

Ammonium chloride is given orally in daily doses of 4 Gm. to 12 Gm. in enteric-coated capsules. The lower range of dosage is preferred because the higher doses are not well tolerated. This salt is usually used with other diuretic agents, chiefly the mercurials, generally for several days before their parenteral injection, for potentiation of their effect.

Low Kidney Threshold Diuretics

Potassium Chloride, U.S.P., B.P., I.P., and Potassium Nitrate, N.F., B.P.

Potassium chloride and potassium nitrate are occasionally used as diuretics. The citrate and the acetate are also administered. The usual oral dose is 1 Gm., although as much as 12 Gm. are sometimes given. If the solution is used, it should be given with or after meals to prevent gastric irritability.

Solutions or enteric-coated tablets containing the salts are available.

Urea—Invert Sugar (Urevert)

Urea, the chief metabolic product of protein utilization in the body, is excreted by the kidneys as a low threshold substance. Normal kidneys are capable of excreting additional administered quantities and excrete additional water to accompany urea by virtue of its osmotic pressure. Urea is rarely used as a diuretic for ordinary purposes but is used to reduce intracranial, intraocular, and spinal fluid pressure. It is also used following prostate surgery as an internal irrigant thus decreasing the need for external bladder irrigations. It is available as a lyophilized sterile powder (90 Gm.) with 210 ml. of 10 per cent invert sugar (hydrolyzed sucrose) in which it is freshly dissolved before use.

Precautions and Contraindications. A 30 per cent solution of Urevert is hypertonic and irritating; therefore, venous thrombi may occur. If fluid extravasates, local irritation will result. Since the diuretic effect of urea is marked, a urethral catheter should be in place during and after infusion. Persons with marked liver disease and kidney dysfunction, dehydration, and active intracranial bleeding should not receive the drug.

Dosage and Method of Administration. This preparation is administered intravenously at a rate of about 6 ml. of the above solution per minute. For immediate effects in emergencies, 3 ml. per kilogram of body weight may be given.

Preparations

Lyophilized Urea	90 Gm.
Invert Sugar (Travert)	10 per cent, 210 ml.
(The above are freshly combined in solution)	

Trade name: Urevert

Osmotic Pressure Diuretics

Dextrose, sucrose, and sorbitol, when given in quantities that exceed the renal threshold, pass through the glomeruli and exert a high osmotic pressure in the tubules. They diminish water absorption and increase water excretion. Dextrose is the drug of choice among these agents.

Dextrose Injection, U.S.P., B.P., I.P.

Dextrose (glucose) is excreted by the kidneys usually when its concentration in the blood exceeds about 160 mg. per 100 ml. This is the usual threshold for blood sugar (glucose). The intravenous administration of solutions of 10 per cent concentration or more removes water from the blood and tissues.

Side Effects. Concentrations of 20 to 50 per cent are more effective than 10 per cent solutions but damage the veins in which administered. The dehydrating effect upon the endothelial lining may lead to constriction and to thrombosis.

Dosage. The complete volume available as listed below may be used in adults by intravenous drip.

Preparation

Dextrose Injection, U.S.P., B.P.	2.5, 5, and 10 per cent, 250-, 500-, and 1000-ml. bottles; 20 per cent, 500- and 1000-ml. bottles; 50 per cent in 50-ml. ampuls

Pyrimidine Derivatives

Amisometradine (Rolictin) and **aminometradine (Mictine, Mincard)** are moderately potent diuretics which are used to relieve edema in selected cases of moderate to severe heart failure. Nausea and vomiting have been reported.

The oral dose of amisometradine is 400 mg. three times a day with meals. The oral dose of aminometradine is 200 mg. one to three times a day.

Preparations

Amisometradine Tablets	400 mg.
	Trade name: Rolicton
Aminometradine Tablets	200 mg.
	Trade names: Mincard (new name for Mictine)

ABNORMALITIES OF POTASSIUM METABOLISM

Hypokalemia may result from decreased intake or absorption of K^+ as in inadequate diet, sprue, or diarrhea; or increased loss of K^+ in vomiting or severe diarrhea, renal failure, diabetic acidosis, administration of certain diuretics, and adrenocortical hormone therapy. The signs and symptoms include anorexia and nausea, muscle weakness, paralytic ileus, paresthesias of the limbs and feet, and cardiac arrhythmias and arrest. Potassium salts are used to remedy this deficiency.

Therapeutic Uses of Potassium Salts

1. Potassium deficiency associated with disturbances in electrolyte metabolism as in infantile diarrhea.

2. Oral potassium therapy routinely with modern diuretics and corticosteriod therapy to replace excretory K^+ loss.

3. With digitalis therapy to reduce toxicity and as treatment for digitalis intoxication.

4. As low threshold diuretics (see p. 640).

Side Effects.   Upon oral administration, potassium chloride may produce gastric irritation and vomiting. Other side effects are seldom noted when renal function is adequate. However, severe toxic effects such as muscular weakness, paralysis, bradycardia, decrease in blood pressure, and cardiac arrest may occur with intravenous infusions, especially when they are infused too rapidly.

Dosage and Methods of Administration.   Potassium salts are administered orally or by intravenous infusion. The usual dose is 20 to 40 mEq., but it varies, depending upon the severity of the deficiency. Oral administration is preferred.

Preparations.   Many salts of potassium are used, including the chloride, acetate, citrate, and bicarbonate.

Potassium Chloride is perhaps the most commonly used salt. It is available in tablets containing 300 mg. Since it causes gastric irritation, it is also marketed in enteric-coated tablets. For intravenous use it is available in ampuls containing 20 mEq. (1.5 Gm.) in 10 ml., and 30 mEq. (2.24 Gm.) and 40 mEq. (3 Gm.) in 12.5 ml. For intravenous administration the drug must be diluted with parenteral solutions such as isotonic saline or 5 per cent dextrose. Due to the possibility of potassium intoxication, the flow rate should be adjusted so that the patient receives no more than 10 to 20 mEq. per hour. Thus, if 20 mEq. of K^+ are diluted with 500 ml. of fluid, the rate of flow should not exceed 4 ml. per minute.

Potassium Triplex contains potassium acetate, bicarbonate, and citrate (15 mEq. in 5 ml.). The solution should be administered in fruit juice or broth.

Potassium Gluconate (Kaon) is available as an elixir and tablets. Each 15 ml. of the elixir contains 20 mEq. of potassium. Tablets supply 20 mEq.

Hyperkalemia.   The two most common causes of hyperkalemia are severe renal insufficiency and rapid intravenous infusions of potassium salts. It may also occur in adrenal insufficiency and with oral administration of the salts to patients with inadequate renal function. The signs and symptoms include muscular weakness, paralysis, bradycardia, decrease in blood pressure, and cardiac arrest.

Treatment

1. Intravenous calcium gluconate
2. Glucose and insulin
3. Cation exchange resins
4. Artificial kidney

ION EXCHANGE RESINS

In the intestinal tract these resins take up sodium and potassium ions in exchange for hydrogen ions, and the sodium or potassium is then excreted in the feces. They may be used in combination with a mercurial diuretic.

Side Effects. These resins may cause nausea and vomiting by local irritation and constipation by increasing the bulk in the gastrointestinal tract. Potassium deficiency may develop from overdosage. To prevent this, potassium salts may be administered. Serum calcium deficiency may also occur in which case calcium salts are indicated.

Dosage. These resins are administered orally in doses of 15 Gm. stirred into 150 to 200 ml. of water three times a day.

Carbacrylamine Resin (Carbo-Resin)

This preparation, a sodium-removing exchange resin, is used in the treatment and control of edema due to sodium retention associated with cardiac failure, cirrhosis of the liver, early stages of toxemia of pregnancy, and hypertension. It is contraindicated in patients with impaired kidney function and patients should be checked for acidosis and hyperpotassemia which may develop.

Preparation

Carbacrylamine Resins (powder)   8-Gm. packets
Trade name: Carbo-Resin

Sodium Polystyrene Sulfonate (Kayexalate)

This preparation, a potassium-removing exchange resin, is recommended for persons with hyperkalemia associated with oliguria or anuria due to acute tubular necrosis and shock or crushed kidney.

Precautions. Severe potassium deficiency may occur with overdosage. Toxic effects on the heart may occur during digitalis therapy.

Preparation

Sodium Polystyrene Sulfonate (powder)   1-lb. containers
Trade name: Kayexalate

PERITONEAL DIALYSIS SOLUTIONS

Peritoneal dialysis solutions utilize the peritoneum as a dializing membrane to remove toxic substances and metabolites from the body in the case of renal failure. These are hypertonic solutions containing Na, Cl, Mg, lactate, bisulfite ions, and varying amounts of dextrose. Potassium has been omitted since dialysis is often performed to correct hyperkalemia. This is a relatively safe, effective, and, at times, a vitally needed technique for the treatment of edema, hepatic coma, hypercalcemia, intractable edema, hyperpotassemia, uremia, and overhydrated or poisoned patients.

Precautions.   The most frequent complication is peritonitis. Other side effects are abdominal pain, restlessness, localized bleeding, abdominal distention, and shock which may respond to specific therapy.

Contraindications.   These include peritonitis, recent laparotomy, and very severe uremic symptoms which should be treated by hemodialysis with a disposable coil kidney.

Preparations

Dianeal Solution	Each liter of solution contains 140.5
Inpersol Solution	mEq. of sodium, 3.5 mEq. of calcium,
	1.5 mEq. of magnesium, 101 mEq. of
	chloride, 44.5 mEq. of lactate, and
	either 15 or 70 Gm. of dextrose.

THE ANTIDIURETIC PRINCIPLE OF THE POSTERIOR PITUITARY

Posterior Pituitary Injection, U.S.P. (Pituitrin)

Posterior pituitary injection is an aqueous extract of the posterior lobe of the pituitary body of cattle and sheep. It contains both *pressor* and *oxytocic* principles which are chemically very similar to each other. Its use in the prevention of postpartum uterine atony is described on page 604.

Vasopressin Injection, U.S.P. (Pitressin, Tonephrin, Tonitrin)

Vasopressin is a sterile aqueous solution for injection of the water-soluble *pressor and antidiuretic principle* of the posterior lobe of the pituitary body. Its antidiuretic action results from its facilitation of the reabsorption of water from the renal tubules. It constricts the blood vessels and causes a slight rise in blood pressure. It stimulates intestinal activity by a direct musculotropic action and, consequently, is sometimes used in postoperative intestinal stasis. Vasopressin increases the tone of the bladder musculature and is used in postoperative retention. The dose is 1 ml. intramuscularly every four hours. The most important use of vasopressin is in the treatment of diabetes insipidus.

Effect of Vasopressin in Diabetes Insipidus.   Diabetes insipidus is a rare disease probably associated with a degenerative change in the pituitary gland. Large volumes of diluted urine (5 to 20 liters) are excreted daily. This causes polydipsia (thirst) and tissue dehydration. Chills, tremors, nausea, vomiting, and headache are other symptoms resulting from water deprivation. If these are not treated, great volumes of water are ingested. The injection of vasopressin or its application to the nasal membranes in the form of a spray or as a powder will check the polyuria (excessive urine flow). The initial anuria (cessation of urine flow), which is caused by urethral spasm, lasts from 15 to 30 minutes. A somewhat normal rate of urine flow, resulting from increased tubular reabsorption, begins in one to two hours and lasts 12 hours or longer. The dose of vasopressin depends on the severity of the symptoms. In mild cases, 0.5 ml. every two or three days is adequate. In severe cases, the dose is increased to 1 ml. one to three times daily. Vasopressin tannate in oil is injected intramuscularly in doses of 0.3 to 1 ml. This drug is slowly absorbed, and the effects are prolonged for about 48 hours, making it the more useful agent.

Vasopressin therapy controls the symptoms of diabetes insipidus, but it does not produce a cure. It is replacement therapy and therefore must be continued indefinitely.

Preparations

Vasopressin Injection, U.S.P.	10 U.S.P. units in 0.5 ml.; 20 U.S.P. units in 1 ml.
Vasopressin Tannate in Oil	5 pressor units in 1 ml.

INHIBITORS OF TUBULAR TRANSPORT OF ORGANIC SUBSTANCES

The kidney tubules transport organic compounds from the blood to the tubular fluid (originally the glomerular filtrate) and thus into the urine, and from that fluid back into the blood. Both are normal functions of the tubules, depending upon the particular substances involved.

Probenecid, U.S.P., B.P. (Benemid)

Probenecid was found among a group of compounds made for the specific purpose of blocking the transport system in the kidney tubules which excretes penicillin. This was important when penicillin was scarce, but this antibiotic is now sufficiently plentiful and inexpensive that it is usually administered, without probenecid, in whatever doses are needed to produce desired blood levels and effects (see p. 106). This drug also blocks the excretion of p-amino-salicylic acid (PAS), which is used in tuberculosis (see Chap. 8), and phenol-sulfonphthalein (PSP), a dye used to test tubular function (see p. 650). The tubules are not damaged by probenecid. The excretion of other significant substances is not blocked by this drug.

Action in Gout.   Gout is a disease in which uric acid metabolism is disturbed and high levels are present in the tissues and blood. Deposits of urate crystals, called *tophi*, may form in various sites, as on the external ears and around joints. Probenecid and sulfinpyrazone block the enzyme system in the tubules that reabsorb uric acid present in the glomerular filtrate. By this means they cause the excretion in the urine of increased quantities of this waste product of purine metabolism.

In gout, more protein is converted to uric acid, rather than to urea, the normal metabolic end product. By diminishing the uric acid content of extracellular fluid and plasma, the severity of gout is decreased, and the symptoms and signs of the disease are reduced or abolished. Probenecid is known as a *uricosuric* drug because it causes increased secretion of uric acid in the urine.

A highly specific analgesic, colchicine, is also very useful in the treatment of the pain of gout, especially the acute attacks or exacerbations (see p. 695). It does not affect tubular function or uric acid blood levels.

Side Effects.   Probenecid may cause gastric irritation with nausea. Administration with meals reduces this, but the dosage may have to be reduced. Skin rash rarely occurs. Temporary increase in the symptoms of gout may occur when the drug is first begun.

Dosage and Administration.   For elevation of penicillin blood levels, 2 Gm. of probenecid are given orally daily, in divided doses. In gout, 500 mg. daily for one week, then twice or even four times daily, are required. Some physicians alkalinize the urine by administering sodium bicarbonate, thereby increasing the solubility of the increased uric acid being excreted and thereby reducing the possibility of urinary stone formation by the urates or uric acid.

Preparation

Probenecid Tablets, U.S.P., B.P.   500 mg.

Trade name: Benemid

Sulfinpyrazone (Anturan)

This uricosuric drug has the same actions, uses, and side effects as probenecid. It is given orally in doses initially of 50 mg. four times daily with food or milk, increasing to doses of 400 or even 800 mg. daily.

Preparation

Sulfinpyrazone Tablets   100 mg. (scored)

Trade name: Anturan

Phenylbutazone (Butazolidin)

This antiarthritic agent (see p. 692) is also a uricosuric agent with the same tubular inhibiting action as described for other members of this functional class.

Prevention of Urinary Calculi

Calculi, or "stones," may form in the drainage system of the urinary tract, grow in size, and cause hemorrhage, pain, and obstruction, and may be associated with infections. They may be composed of calcium salts, either phosphate, carbonate, oxalate, or urate, with magnesium and ammonium salts mixed in varying combinations.

Intestinal Phosphate Precipitation

Certain aluminum compounds that are primarily used as gastric acid-neutralizing agents (see Chap. 35) have the capacity to precipitate phosphate ions of foodstuffs in the intestines and cause their excretion in the feces. This may reduce greatly the amount of phosphate excreted in the urine. Thus phosphate stones may be prevented. Agents having this action are basic aluminum carbonate and aluminum hydroxide.

Urinary Acidification

The administration of urine acidifiers such as ammonium chloride (see pp. 639–40) and sodium acid phosphate may be useful in preventing the formation of calcium stones because the increased acidity of the urine makes calcium salts more soluble. Ammonium chloride is not advised for continued use, for it may lead to acidosis and even to increased urea blood levels in renal impairment.

The acid phosphate is preferred; the phosphate ion is not likely to precipitate in the urine in this form. Sodium acid phosphate may be administered in a dose of 0.6 Gm. four times daily. It should not be used in urinary infections caused by a urea-splitting organism.

An acidifying preparation for intravenous drip consisting of acid salts, anhydrides, and lactones is available under the name hemiacidrin (Renacidin). In acute situations, and with indwelling catheters that may become encrusted and plugged, a 10 per cent solution may be given, at the rate of 1 ml. per minute.

Hypercalcinuria Therapy

Sodium Phytate (Rencal) is used in the treatment of hypercalcinuria (with or without kidney stones) if and when it occurs in immoblized patients on a rigidly restricted calcium intake diet. It does not cause dissolution of existing stones or calcium deposits. It may also be used in vitamin D intoxication. It is contraindicated in hyperthyroidism or other conditions associated with metabolic disturbances of bone; in impaired cardiac or renal function; during pregnancy; and in pediatrics. It should not be taken with vitamin D or related preparations since these will increase urinary calcium excretion.

The oral dose of 4.5 Gm. suspended in a glass of cold water is taken three times a day with meals. Urinary calcium should be checked during its administration. With prolonged therapy, low serum levels of vitamin B_{12} may decrease urinary calcium; so 500 mcg. of this vitamin should be injected once a month.

Preparation

Sodium Phytate Granules   Packets containing 4.5 Gm.
Trade name: Rencal

Urinary Antiseptics

Nitrofurantoin, U.S.P., B.P. (Furadantin). This drug is related to nitrofurazone (see p. 745). It is effective, upon oral administration, in infections of the urinary tract, such as those caused by the genera *Proteus*, *Aerobacter*, and *Pseudomonas*. It is used in pyelonephritis, pyelitis, and cystitis caused by bacteria that are sensitive to it. The usual oral dose is 100 mg. (50 to 200 mg.) four times a day.

Preparations

Nitrofurantoin Oral Suspension, U.S.P.   100 mg. in 5 ml.
Nitrofurantoin Tablets, U.S.P., B.P.   50 and 100 mg.
Trade name: Furadantin

Methenamine Mandelate, U.S.P. (Mandelamine). This drug is a combination of two urinary antiseptics, mandelic acid and methenamine, which were once widely used. Methenamine mandelate is useful in the treatment of pyelitis, pyelonephritis, and cystitis. It is active against both gram-negative and gram-positive organisms and is sometimes effective when drug resistance to other agents occurs with certain otherwise susceptible strains. Untoward effects are seldom seen in therapeutic doses. The oral adult dose is 1 Gm. (250 mg. to 1 Gm.) four times a day. The drug is available in tablets containing 250 and 500 mg. (U.S.P.).

Phenazopyridine Hydrochloride (Pyridium)

Phenazopyridine (Pyridium) is administered orally for its analgesic and antiseptic effect in the urinary tract. Thus retention of urine due to spasm caused by pain is minimized. It may be given with other antibacterial drugs. The oral dose is 200 mg. three times a day after meals.

Preparation

Phenazopyridine Tablets   100 mg.

Trade name: Pyridium

Nalidixic Acid (NegGram) is a new synthetic compound with high antibacterial activity against gram-negative organisms such as *E. coli, Aerobacter, Klebsiella, Shigella, Salmonella,* and particularly *Proteus.* Gram-positive organisms are less sensitive. Disk sensitivity tests are recommended as a guide to bacterial sensitivity.

The drug is rapidly absorbed from the gastrointestinal tract, and 80 per cent is excreted, mainly in the urine, within the first eight hours as unchanged drug, a closely related compound, and conjugated derivatives.

Side Effects. The drug is well tolerated on prolonged treatment, even by patients with impaired kidney or liver function. The side effects, which are usually minor, are nausea, vomiting and other gastrointestinal disturbances, drowsiness, weakness, itching, rash, and urticaria.

Therapeutic Uses. Nalidixic acid is used extensively in the treatment of acute and chronic genitourinary infections caused by sensitive gram-negative bacteria.

Dosage and Method of Administration. The oral adult dose is 2 to 4 Gm. daily (500 mg. to 1 Gm. four times a day). A daily dose of 2 Gm. may suffice, but 4 Gm. daily for one to two weeks is recommended at the beginning of treatment, especially in chronic and severe infections, to minimize the development of bacterial resistance. Later the dose may be reduced to 2 Gm. daily. Proportionately less of the drug is given to children.

Preparation

Nalidixic Acid Caplets   250 and 500 mg.

Trade name: NegGram

Sulfonamides. The triple sulfonamides, sulfisoxazole and sulfadimethoxine, are useful urinary antiseptics. They are discussed on pages 167–69, 173–74.

Antibiotics. Penicillin, streptomycin, and the broad-spectrum antibiotics are useful in infections of the urinary tract. They are discussed under the individual drugs (see Index).

DIAGNOSTIC AGENTS

KIDNEY FUNCTION TESTS

In clinical medicine, the functional activity of the kidneys may be measured for diagnostic purposes. Two such tests give an approximation of activity by determining the ability of the kidneys to excrete a dye which has been injected intramuscularly or intravenously.

Phenolsulfonphthalein, U.S.P. (B.P.) (Phenol Red)

The patient is given 200 to 400 ml. of water prior to the administration of the dye. Then a 6-mg. (1-ml.) quantity of phenolsulfonphthalein is injected intramuscularly or intravenously. Specimens of urine are collected after 15 and 30 minutes and one and two hours after the intravenous injection of the drug. If the dye is given intramuscularly, the specimens are collected at different time intervals. The patient must completely empty his bladder for each specimen. Normally 80 per cent of the dye is excreted in two hours, 15 to 20 per cent of which is found in the first specimen. The specimens must be alkalinized before they are tested colorimetrically as phenolsulfonphthalein is colorless in acid urine. If the patient's urine is alkaline, then the specimens will be red. Since the results of the test are determined by the color of the specimen, false levels will be obtained if the patient is having hematuria or receiving drugs such as pyridium or acetyl sulfisoxazole (Azo Gantrisin) which also color the urine. Patients taking this test should not receive probenecid as it blocks excretion of the dye.

Preparation

Phenolsulfonphthalein Injection, U.S.P.   1-ml. ampuls containing 6 mg.

Sodium Indigotindisulfonate, U.S.P.; Indigo Carmine, B.P.

Sodium indigotindisulfonate is a diagnostic aid for renal function. The intravenous dose is 40 mg. (40 to 80 mg.). Sodium Indigotindisulfonate Injection, U.S.P., is a sterile solution in water containing 40 mg. in 5 ml.

Additional diagnostic measures of renal functional capacity are the mannitol clearance test, the urea clearance test, and the pitressin-concentration test.

VISUALIZATION OF THE URINARY TRACT

Intravenous injections of water-soluble organic compounds containing iodine are used to produce satisfactory roentgenograms for visualizing the urinary tract. These compounds, which are rapidly concentrated and excreted by the kidneys, are radiopaque, since the heavy iodine atoms block x-rays and produce shadows on the film. The substances thus outline the calyces, pelves, and ureters of the kidneys (as shown in Fig. 17, p. 628). These compounds may also be used for ureteral retrograde pyelography (direct injection into the renal pelvis by means of a ureteral catheter). They are called *urographic* (occasionally renographic) agents.

Sodium Diatrizoate Injection, U.S.P., B.P. (Hypaque Sodium)

Sodium diatrizoate is a very satisfactory urographic agent. By virtue of a high iodine content, clear visualization of the urinary tract is obtained, usually in good detail. There is a very low incidence of side effects.

A 50 per cent solution is used for excretory urography upon intravenous injection following an intravenous *test dose* of 1 ml. to rule out rare sensitivity. The dose employed is 20 to 30 ml. in adults. Crystals forming in the ampul or vial because of cooling may be redissolved by warming.

A 20 per cent solution in a dose of 6 to 10 ml. is used for retrograde urography in cases of renal impairment or of sensitivity. A 90 per cent solution is available for injection through a cardiac catheter directly into a chamber of the heart. Fifty or more milliliters are injected quickly (less than two seconds), and the x-ray exposure is made immediately, and perhaps repetitively, for visualizing the contour and openings of the chamber injected, of other chambers of the heart, and of the great vessels.

Side Effects. After intravenous administration of diatrizoate, side effects are absent or minor. Rarely, there may be, as with other organic iodides, certain severe reactions that cannot always be avoided by use of test doses. These are of two main types: (1) anaphylactoid reactions with respiratory difficulty, bronchial spasm, edema of the lips and eyelids, and giant urticaria; and (2) cardiovascular collapse with shocklike symptoms and signs. Oxygen is indicated in both types, an antihistamine agent (see Chap. 46) in the first and a vasopressor agent (see Chap. 27) in the second.

Preparations

Sodium Diatrizoate Injection, U.S.P., B.P. (50 per cent)	0.5 Gm. in 1 ml., 30-ml. ampuls; 20- and 30-ml. vials; and 1-ml. test vials
Sodium Diatrizoate Injection (20 per cent)	100-ml. bottles
Sodium and Meglumine Diatrizoate Injection (Hypaque-M, 90 per cent)	20- and 50-ml. vials (for angiocardiography)

Trade name: Hypaque

Additional Urographic and Angiocardiographic Agents

Several additional water-soluble organic iodine compounds are in use for excretory (intravenous) and retrograde urography and for visualizing heart chambers and blood vessels.

Preparations

Iodopyracet Compound Injection, N.F.	50 per cent, 20-ml. ampuls
Iodopyracet Concentrated (Injection) (for special angiocardiographic procedures)	70 per cent, 20- and 50-ml. ampuls

Trade name: Diodrast

Sodium Acetrizoate Injection, U.S.P., B.P.	70 per cent, 25- and 50-ml. ampuls 30 per cent, 25-ml. ampuls; 50 per cent, 25- and 40-ml. ampuls

Trade names: Urokon; Thixokon; Diaginol

Meglumine Diatrizoate Injection, U.S.P.	30 per cent, 50-ml.; 60 per cent, 25-ml.; 69.3 per cent, 20-ml.; 76 per cent, 20-ml.; 85 per cent, 50-ml. (ampuls or vials)

Trade names: Cardiografin; Gastrografin; Renografin

Sodium Diprotrizoate Injection, U.S.P.	50 per cent, 20- and 30-ml. ampuls

Trade name: Miokon

Methrodal Sodium, Injection, N.F.	20 per cent, 50-ml. bottles; 40 per cent, 50- and 100-ml. bottles (also with acacia 20 per cent, 10-ml. ampuls)

Trade name: Skiodan

Sodium Iodomethamate Injection, N.F.	10 and 15 Gm. in 20 ml.; 15 Gm. in 30 ml.; 37.5 Gm. in 50 ml.

Sodium Iodohippurate (I 131) (Radio-Hippuran Sterile Solution [I^{131}])

This agent contains radioactive iodine in an organic salt which is rapidly and selectively excreted by the kidneys. The radioactivity can be measured over each kidney with scintillation probes attached to a rate-meter and recorder. The functioning capacity of each kidney can thus be measured separately.

Dosage. This diagnostic substance is given intravenously in a dose of 0.3 microcuries (μc) per kilogram of body weight. The measurement requires about ten minutes.

Preparation

Sodium Iodohippurate (I 131) Injection	0.1-, 0.25-, and 0.5-mg. vials containing 1 to 10 μc as specially ordered

Trade name: Radio-Hippuran Sterile Solution (I^{131})

REVIEW QUESTIONS

1. *Chlorothiazide was the first of the "thiazides" to be used as a diuretic and antihypertensive agent. Which one or ones of the group are used most frequently in your hospital?*
2. *What are the mechanisms of action of chlorothiazide and other thiazides as diuretic agents?*
3. *What points should be included when you are teaching a patient about thiazide diuretics?*

4. *What advantages do flumethazide, hydroflumethazide, and benzydroflumethiazide have over the earlier thiazides?*
5. *Define the threshold value of a blood constituent.*
6. *Name as many threshold substances as you can. Explain the term "non-threshold."*
7. *Discuss the use and doses of a xanthine and of an acid-producing diuretic. What is the rationale for the use of dextrose and sucrose and of acetazoleamide?*
8. *How does spironolactone produce a diuretic effect and how does it affect sodium and potassium elimination from the body?*
9. *What advantages does spironolactone have in comparison with or in combination with the thiazides? How do you explain its action in lowering blood pressure?*
10. *What are the features of the actions of probenecid?*
11. *When preparing a patient for diagnostic urographic study, why is it necessary to determine his sensitivity to iodine?*

REFERENCES

Sawyer, Janet R.: *Nursing Care of Patients in the Urologic Diseases*. C. V. Mosby Company, St. Louis, 1963, p. 179.

WATER AND SALT METABOLISM

Leaf, A.: "Kidney, Water and Electrolytes," *Ann. Rev. Physiol.*, **22**:111, 1960.

BENZOTHIADIAZINES

Aronoff, A.: "Acute Gouty Arthritis Precipitated by Chlorothiazide," *New England J. Med.*, **262**:767, 1960.
Bryant, J. M.; Schwartz, N.; Fletcher, L., Jr.; Fertig, H.; Schwartz, M. S.; McDermott, J. D.; and Quan, R. B. F.: "Clinical Studies of the Antihypertensive Effects of a New Benzothiadiazine Diuretic," *Current Ther. Res.*, **3**:1, 1961.
Council on Drugs: "Chlorothiazide (Diuril)," *J.A.M.A.*, **169**:1191, 1951.
Dennis, E. W., and Ford, R. V.: "Hydroflumethiazide. The Clinical Pharmacology of a New Oral Diuretic," *Am. J. Cardiol.*, **5**:402, 1960.
Ford, R. V.: "Comparative Effects of Benzydroflumethiazide and Hydrochlorothiazide on Urinary Electrolyte Excretion," *Current Therap. Res.*, **2**:92, 1960.
———: "Clinical-Pharmacologic Investigation of Methyclothiazide, a New Oral Diuretic," *Current Ther. Res.*, **2**:422, 1960.
———: "Clinical-Pharmacologic Investigation of Polythiazide, a Potent Oral Diuretic Agent," *Current Ther. Res.*, **3**:320, 1961.
Goldberger, E.: "Benzothiadiazine (Thiazide) Diuretics," *Am. J. Cardiol.*, **5**:428, 1960.
Warshaw, L. J.: "Acute Attacks of Gout Precipitated by Chlorothiazide—Induced Diuresis," *J.A.M.A.*, **172**:802, 1960.

MERCURIAL DIURETICS

Leff, W. A., and Nussbaum, H. E.: "Chlormerodrin: Clinical Effectiveness and Absence of Toxicity in Congestive Heart Failure," *Brit. M. J.*, **1**:833, 1959.

Ray, C. T.: "Mercurial Diuretics: Their Mechanism of Action and Application," *A.M.A. Arch. Int. Med.*, **102**:1016, 1958.

MISCELLANEOUS DIURETICS

Beyer, K. H.: "Nonmercurial Organic Diuretics: Their Action and Application," *A.M.A. Arch. Int. Med.*, **102**:1005, 1958.

Duke-Elder, Sir S.: "The Diagnosis and Treatment of Simple Glaucoma," *Canad. M. Assoc. J.*, **82**:293, 1960.

Editorial: "Control of Aldosterone Secretion," *Brit. M. J.*, **2**:553, 1959.

Edmonds, C. J.: "An Aldosterone Antagonist and Diuretics in the Treatment of Chronic Edema and Ascites," *Lancet*, **1**:509, 1960.

Friedberg, C. K.; Taymor, R.; Minor, J. B.; and Halpern, M.: "The Use of Diamox, a Carbonic Anhydrase Inhibitor, as an Oral Diuretic," *New England J. Med.*, **248**:883, 1953.

Hoffman, F. G.; Zimmerman, S. L.; and Reese, J. D.: "Fatal Agranulocytosis Associated with Acetazolamide," *New England J. Med.*, **262**:242, 1960.

Hollander, W., and Chobanian, A. V.: "Antihypertensive Effect of Spironolactone (SC-9420) Steroidal Antagonist," *Circulation*, **20** (Part 2):713, 1959.

Moyer, J. H.: "Diuretics," *Am. J. Nursing*, **59**:1119, 1959.

Taheri, Z. E.: "Urevert in Cranial Trauma and Brain Surgery," *J. Internat. Col. Surg.*, **32**:389, 1959.

URINARY ANTISEPTICS

Barlow, A. M.: "Nalidixic Acid in Infections of the Urinary Tract," *Brit. Med. J.*, **2**:1308, 1964.

Diggs, E. S.; Prevost, E. C.; and Valderas, J. G.: "Treatment of Urinary Tract Infections in Obstetric and Gynecologic Patients with Nitrofurantoin," *Am. J. Obst. & Gynec.*, **71**:399, 1956.

Draper, John W., *et al.:* "Therapeutic Problems in Urinary Infections," *South. M. J.*, **57**:920, 1964.

Seneca, Harry: "Current Therapy of Infections of the Renal Excretory System," *J. Am. Geriat. Soc.*, **12**:1100, 1964.

URICOSURIC AGENTS

Bartels, E. C., and Matossian, G. S.: "Gout: Six-Year Follow-up on Probenecid (Benemide) Therapy," *Arth. and Rheum.*, **2**:193, 1959.

Reed, E. B.; Feichtmeir, T. V.; and Willett, F. M.: "Zoxazolamine—A Potent Uricosuric Agent," *New England J. Med.*, **258**:894, 1958.

Talbot, J. H.: "Gout and Gouty Arthritis," *Med. Sci.*, **6**:21, 1959.

RADIOPAQUE COMPOUNDS

Hoppe, J. O.: "Some Pharmacological Aspects of Radiopaque Compounds," *New York Acad. Sci.*, **78**:727, 1959.

Moore, T. D., and Mayer, R. F.: "Hypaque: An Improved Medium for Excretory Urography," *South. M. J.*, **48**:135, 1956.

Nesbit, R. M.: "The Incidence of Severe Reactions from Present Day Urographic Contrast Materials," *J. Urol.*, **81**:486, 1959.

Nordyke, R. A.; Tubis, M.; and Blahd, W. H.: "Use of Radioiodinated Hippuran for Individual Kidney Function Tests," *J. Lab. & Clin. Med.*, **56**:438, 1960.

IX DRUGS AFFECTING METABOLISM

The diseases of metabolism are an important and frequently encountered group. Among the metabolic disorders are malfunctioning of certain endocrine glands—the islet cells of the pancreas (diabetes mellitus), the adrenal cortex (Addison's disease), the thyroid gland (hyper- and hypothyroidism), and the parathyroids (tetany); vitamin deficiency states; and other conditions.

The greater portion of disorders involving disturbed metabolism are beyond the scope of this text because of the absence of specific drugs for use in correcting or modifying them; they are described in textbooks of medicine and endocrinology. In the chapters of this section we shall consider those agents which are useful in the management of the conditions listed above and of certain allied disorders.

39

Diabetes Mellitus. Insulin and Other Hypoglycemic Drugs

The hormone insulin, which regulates carbohydrate metabolism, is secreted by the islet cells of the pancreas. In 1889, Drs. Joseph von Mering and Oskar Minkowski removed the pancreas from dogs and produced the cardinal symptoms of diabetes, showing that the pancreas is the source of some substance that protects normal animals from diabetes mellitus. In 1922, Drs. Frederick Banting and Charles Best prepared an active extract from the pancreas which was effective in the treatment of diabetes. This substance was named insulin. In 1932, Drs. Bernardo Houssay and Alfredo Biasotte depancreatized dogs and kept them alive for 1 to 20 days with insulin. Then both lobes of the pituitary were removed. After recovery from this second operation, the diabetes, which was once severe, became mild, thus indicating that the pituitary plays an important role in carbohydrate metabolism. It has been demonstrated that certain adrenocorticosteroids also affect the metabolism of carbohydrates.

Action of Insulin.   The exact mechanism for the action of insulin is not completely understood. However, it is known that insulin (1) augments the peripheral utilization of glucose, (2) promotes the conversion of glucose to fat and glycogen, and (3) due to these actions, lowers the blood sugar level.

Deficiency of Insulin.   The basic factor in insulin deficiency is a failure in the oxidation of glucose which results in its accumulation in the blood. Since the need of the cells for this food is not being met, the glycogen stored in the liver and muscle is converted into glucose, depleting these reserves. Protein is also broken down to glucose, thus preventing it from being used in building and repairing tissues with consequent muscle wasting. However, the glucose obtained from these sources cannot be utilized; so there is an even greater elevation in the blood sugar level. When the blood sugar rises above the kidney threshold, glucose is excreted in the urine. The increase in solids (glucose) causes more water to be excreted by the kidneys, which in turn causes thirst. Therefore, the symptoms of hyperglycemia, polydipsia, polyuria, and glucosuria are seen. Since the carbohydrate in the diet is not

656

utilized, the person continues to experience hunger, and in an attempt to meet the nutritional needs of the cells, polyphagia occurs.

Normally the body obtains a small amount of energy from the breakdown of fat. When carbohydrate and protein cannot be oxidized, the amount of fat utilized increases. The intermediate products of fat oxidation (aceto-acetic acid, betahydroxybutyric acid, and acetone) are formed more rapidly than the body can oxidize them, resulting in their accumulation in the blood. The body tries to rid itself of these products. Since acetone is excreted by the lungs, the breath tends to have a fruity odor. Before removal by the kidneys, the acids are neutralized by sodium and other electrolytes from the buffer systems causing a decrease in the normal bicarbonate level in the plasma. The lowering of the pH of the blood which results is called acidosis. These are the signs and symptoms of uncontrolled diabetes mellitus.

Causes of insulin deficiency include the following:

1. Removal of the pancreas.
2. Inability of the beta cells of the islets of Langerhans to produce insulin.
3. Production of insulin antibodies.
4. Conversion of insulin into an inactive form.
5. Interference with the action of insulin at the cellular level.

Treatment of Diabetes Mellitus with Insulin.   One of the aims in the treatment of these patients is to correct the metabolic abnormality present. This must be done on an individual basis since in some cases, metabolic control may be obtained through diet regulation alone, while in others insulin or oral hypoglycemic agents are needed.

Insulin

Insulin is a highly purified extract of the pancreas of domestic animals: hogs, sheep, and cattle. It is so standardized that each milliliter contains either 40, 80, 100, or 500 units. Since there is a wide variation in the insulin requirements of persons with diabetes mellitus, there is no standard dose. The dose of insulin the patient receives is that amount which will maintain his blood sugar within normal limits. The amount of food required to main-tain the patient's normal weight and normal physical activity help determine this dose.

Standardization of Insulin.   Insulin is standardized by measuring its capacity to lower the blood sugar level of rabbits and also its capacity to produce hypoglycemic shocks in mice. A description of the official rabbit assay is given in the U.S.P. The potency of insulin is expressed in U.S.P. units, and the standard of comparison is the U.S.P. zinc insulin crystals reference standard.

Therapeutic Uses

Primary

1. To control the symptoms of diabetes mellitus.
2. In the treatment of diabetic coma and acidosis.

Occasional

1. For malnutrition in the nondiabetic. It stimulates the appetite.
2. In the treatment of schizophrenia.
3. In the treatment of acute alcoholism. The injection of insulin and glucose rapidly reduces the alcohol content of the blood and tissues.

Prolonging the Action of Insulin. From the clinical standpoint and that of convenience to the patient, it is important to reduce the number of injections to as few as possible and yet still maintain a normal blood sugar level. With ordinary insulin, the effects are rapid and transient, and frequent injections are required.

Many attempts have been made to prolong the action of insulin. In 1936, Professor H. D. Hagedorn demonstrated that when a solution of protamine (a substance prepared from the sperm or mature testes of salmon) is added to insulin, an insulin-protamine complex is formed. When this substance is injected subcutaneously, it is slowly absorbed and the lowering of the blood sugar is prolonged. Zinc added to insulin prior to combining it with protamine prolongs the action still further.

Types of Insulin Preparations. There are five types of insulin preparations. The basic action of all is alike. They all differ mainly in the time of onset of action and in the duration of the effect in lowering blood sugar. All preparations are available in 10-ml. multiple-dose vials that contain 40 or 80 U.S.P. units of insulin in each milliliter.

Unmodified Insulin. Unmodified insulin consists of Insulin Injection, U.S.P., B.P., or a clear aqueous solution of zinc insulin crystals. These are prompt-acting insulin preparations. (See Table 36, p. 659.) They are suitable for some cases of diabetes and are useful in diabetic coma and acidosis where rapidity of action is imperative. These are the only insulins which can be given intravenously.

Semi-Lente Insulin (Iletin). This preparation contains smaller particles of zinc insulin in suspension to give a total duration of effect of 12 to 16 hours. Its chief use is to modify lente insulin by shortening the duration of action.

Globin Zinc Insulin Injection, N.F., B.P. This intermediate-acting preparation is a clear solution modified by the addition of purified globin from beef hemoglobin. The action of this preparation is intermediate in time between that of regular insulin and protamine zinc insulin injections. The period of

Table 36

Type of Insulin	Time and Route of Administration	Onset of Action, hr. after administration	Peak of Action, hr. after administration	Duration of Action, hr.	Time When Glycosuria Most Likely to Occur	Time When Hypoglycemia Most Likely to Occur
Crystalline zinc	I.v. (emergency) 15 to 20 min. before meals Subcutaneously	Rapid, within 1 hr.	2 to 4	5 to 8	During night	2 to 4 hr. after administration
Semi-lente (amorphous zinc)	½ to ¾ hr. before breakfast Subcutaneously Never i.v.	Rapid, within 1 hr.	6 to 10	12 to 16	During night	Before lunch
Globin zinc	½ to 1 hr. before breakfast Subcutaneously Never i.v.	Intermediate, rapidity of onset increases with dose, within 2 to 4 hr.	6 to 10	18 to 24 also increases with dose	Before breakfast	3 P.M. to dinner
Lente (combination of 30% semi-lente and 70% ultra-lente)	1 hr. before breakfast Subcutaneously Never i.v.	Intermediate, within 2 to 4 hr.	8 to 12	28 to 32	Before lunch	3 P.M. to dinner
NPH (neutral protamine-Hagedorn) or Isophane	1 hr. before breakfast Subcutaneously Never i.v.	Intermediate, within 2 to 4 hr.	8 to 12	28 to 30	Before lunch	3 P.M. to dinner
Protamine zinc (PZI)	1 hr. before breakfast Subcutaneously Never i.v.	Slow acting, within 4 to 6 hr.	16 to 24	24 to 36+	Before lunch and at bedtime	2 A.M. to breakfast
Ultra-lente	1 hr. before breakfast Subcutaneously Never i.v.	Very slow, 8 hr.	16 to 24	36+	Before lunch and at bedtime	During night, early morning

its greatest activity extends from the sixth to the tenth hour after injection, and its effect almost disappears in 24 hours. (See Table 36, p. 659.)

Lente Insulin (Lente Iletin). Lente insulin is a sterile suspension, in buffered water medium, of insulin modified by the addition of zinc chloride. It contains approximately 70 per cent crystalline zinc insulin and 30 per cent amorphous zinc insulin. Lente insulin provides an antidiabetic action that is intermediate in time between that of unmodified (regular) insulin and protamine zinc insulin. (See Table 36, p. 659.) The time of action is so similar to that of isophane insulin that they may be used interchangeably. This preparation contains no foreign, modifying proteins; therefore, it does not produce sensitivity reactions that are attributed to globin or protamine. The container vial should be rotated and inverted several times to ensure uniform distribution of the suspended particles, but vigorous shaking should be avoided.

Isophane Insulin Injection, U.S.P., B.P. (NPH Insulin).   This intermediate-acting preparation is a sterile suspension in buffered water medium of insulin made from zinc insulin crystals modified by the addition of protamine in such a way that the solid phase of the suspension consists of crystals composed of insulin, protamine, and zinc. This type of insulin has a "time activity" best adapted to the requirements of the majority of patients. The active material is present in a finely divided, insoluble, milky-white precipitate. The time of onset and the duration of action of this type of insulin are intermediate between that of globin insulin and the slow, but prolonged, action of protamine zinc insulin. (See Table 36, p. 659.) It possesses the additional advantage of requiring only a single daily injection in the majority of cases without the necessity of an additional injection of unmodified insulin. The vial should be rotated so that the contents are evenly distributed before use.

Protamine Zinc Insulin Suspension, U.S.P., B.P.   This long-acting preparation is a suspension in buffered aqueous medium of insulin modified by the addition of zinc chloride and protamine. Protamine zinc insulin (often abbreviated PZI) is slowly absorbed exerting a hypoglycemic effect for 36 hours or longer. (See Table 36, p. 659.) It is a suspension and should be thoroughly mixed by rotation between the hands before use.

Ultra-Lente Insulin (Iletin). This preparation contains larger particles of zinc insulin in suspension to give a total duration of effect in excess of 36 hours. Its chief use is to modify lente insulin by prolonging its duration of action.

Factors Affecting Insulin Needs.   Muscular activity promotes carbohydrate metabolism even without insulin. Therefore, the physical activity of the diabetic is an important factor in determining the dosage of insulin. Even after this dosage has been established, the patient should be made aware of the fact that any unusual physical activity may result in a hypoglycemic reaction, in which event he should be prepared to either increase his carbohydrate intake or reduce the insulin dosage.

Fever, particularly resulting from noninfectious causes, reduces the insulin requirement. During an infection the insulin need of the diabetic patient increases. Therefore, in such cases increased insulin dosage is required to prevent acidosis. Anesthesia, also, increases the need for insulin. The reason for this is unknown.

Insulin Reaction. When there is an excessive amount of active insulin in the body, an extreme lowering of blood sugar occurs. This syndrome is referred to as hypoglycemic reaction, hypoglycemic shock, insulin reaction, insulin shock, or hyperinsulinism. It can occur if the individual has taken too much insulin, has had increased muscular activity, has vomited, or has skipped a meal. Poor absorption of the injected insulin or a change in the insulin needs may also be causes. The symptoms include: hunger, irritability, pallor, sweating, trembling, incoordination, and muscular weakness with staggering. As the blood level falls even lower, aphasia, vertigo, diplopia, disorientation, convulsions, unconsciousness, and even death may ensue. These symptoms are thought to be caused by the decreased amount of glucose and oxygen being utilized by the brain. Persons receiving modified insulin may not experience the symptoms described above. They may have only a headache and nausea before lapsing into unconsciousness. The symptoms may be rapidly relieved by the administration of orange juice, a lump of sugar, or candy. This condition may come on very suddenly; hence it is very important for the diabetic taking insulin to have some form of sugar readily available. These persons receiving modified insulin need, in addition to rapidly acting carbohydrates, some that are slowly digestible since their hypoglycemia may be prolonged and may reoccur. If the individual is unable to take the food by mouth, glucose should be administered intravenously or glucagon hydrochloride may be given parenterally (see p. 668). Persons with diabetes mellitus must be aware of the symptoms of an insulin reaction and take steps to correct it immediately as prolonged periods of hypoglycemia will cause irreversible brain damage.

Administration of Insulin. Insulin is administered subcutaneously. This method is satisfactory except for the discomfort and nuisance of repetitious injection. In emergencies unmodified insulin may be given intravenously. Insulin is not effective on oral administration because it is a protein that is broken down by the proteolytic enzymes produced by the pancreas.

Persons with diabetes mellitus who require insulin for satisfactory control of the disease should be taught how to administer it to themselves. They must utilize the same principles as does the nurse when giving a subcutaneous injection. Although the method of teaching may vary depending on the nurse-teacher and the patient, the content to be taught remains the same. This should include:

1. Need for insulin in diabetes mellitus and factors influencing this requirement.
2. Type of insulin used.
   a. Onset, peak, and duration of effect.
   b. Amount per milliliter—related to calibration of syringe.
3. Type of syringe used.
   a. Calibration.
   b. Color.
4. Technique of preparing and administering subcutaneous injections.
5. Sterilization technique and equipment needed.
   a. Heat (boiling).
   b. Chemical.
6. Sites for injection.
7. Need for and technique for urine testing.
8. Adverse reactions.
   a. Acidosis—causes, signs and symptoms, and treatment.
   b. Hypoglycemia—causes, signs and symptoms, and treatment.

Untoward Reactions

Allergic Reactions.   Erythemia, pruritus, and local swelling at the site of injection may occur occasionally. Generalized urticaria is less frequent but possible. Changing the brand of insulin or using that from the pancreas of a different animal may eliminate the hypersensitive reaction.

Local Subcutaneous Reactions.   When insulin is given in the same site constantly, fat hypertrophy (lipomatosis) or fat atrophy (lipodystrophy) may occur. Rotation of injection sites will prevent these reactions.

Insulin Resistance.   The failure of the body to respond to normal amounts of insulin occurs occasionally. The known causes of this condition include: endocrine abnormalities and the development of insulin antibodies. Very large amounts of insulin must be used to treat these patients. Usually the condition is temporary and the patient's normal response to insulin returns.

SYNTHETIC HYPOGLYCEMIC AGENTS

The use of orally administered drugs in the treatment of diabetes mellitus is a significant advance of recent years. In 1957, tolbutamide, the first agent effective for this purpose, was introduced into medical practice and is now very widely used. Though rare, hypoglycemic reactions may occur when these synthetic agents are used. The signs and symptoms are as previously described.

Tolbutamide, U.S.P., B.P. (Orinase)

Tolbutamide is a sulfonylurea derivative that is useful in diabetics whose disease began in adulthood, is of mild to moderate severity, and is rather stable.

Mechanism of Action.   The ability of tolbutamide to lower blood sugar appears to be through stimulation of the insulin-producing cells in the pancreas, probably causing a greater rate of insulin production and release. The blood sugar of normal animals is lowered by this agent, whereas it is not in depancreatized animals. There does not seem to be any action on the general body-tissue utilization of glucose, although some peripheral effects have been described.

Absorption and Fate.   Tolbutamide is rapidly absorbed from the alimentary tract and probably begins stimulation of the beta cells of the pancreas within an hour or two. The blood glucose concentration reaches the minimum value five to eight hours after a single moderate dose. Usually no greater hypoglycemic effect is obtainable with large amounts (over 3 Gm.) than with doses up to 3 Gm. The drug is oxidized in the liver over a period of 24 hours or less after single doses. Its metabolite is excreted in the urine.

Therapeutic Use.   Some diabetics are thin individuals who require insulin, since they quickly develop acidosis and ketosis. These are conditions produced by the burning of greater amounts of fats when carbohydrates are not being utilized for energy, in the absence of insulin. Such patients are *insulin deficient,* and sulfonylurea derivatives such as tolbutamide are not useful. These patients must be treated with insulin injections indefinitely.

Other diabetics who are or have been obese show no tendency to develop ketosis but merely have elevated glucose levels and glycosuria. These patients have become resistant to insulin. Plasma-insulin activity, indicating the amount and quality, has been found normal in this type of patient. Insulin resistance is apparently related to obesity. Weight reduction by suitable dietary measures and possibly by the use of appetite-reducing agents (see Chap. 23) often results in a return of blood sugar levels to normal.

In the latter type of case, often called *maturity-onset, stable, adult* diabetes, when weight reduction will necessarily be slow, as is usual in obesity, or when a normal blood glucose range is not reached with an appropriate diet, tolbutamide is indicated. If the response in lowered glucose blood levels is adequate, the drug may be continued. Maximal benefit may not occur for 1 to 16 weeks. Occasionally tolbutamide is useful with insulin when large doses of this hormone are required.

Juvenile diabetics are typically severe cases, requiring considerable amounts of insulin. They probably have nonfunctioning insulin-producing cells, and these cannot be stimulated by tolbutamide. Unstable or "brittle" types at any age are not suitable for tolbutamide therapy.

Side Effects.   Side effects occur in only about 3 per cent of cases. The most serious is hypoglycemia (see p. 661), but this is rare. Gastrointestinal upsets, weakness, headache, ringing in the ears, paresthesias, skin eruptions, and mild suppression of the white blood cell count may occur.

Dosage and Administration.   Usually, 2 or 3 Gm. are given orally the first day and 2 Gm. or less continued daily, reduced to as little as 0.5 Gm. daily as indicated by morning and fasting blood sugar determinations. When stabilized, the patient may need only occasional blood tests.

Preparation

Tolbutamide Tablets, U.S.P., B.P.   500 mg.
                         Trade name: Orinase

Chlorpropamide, B.P. (Diabinese)

Chlorpropamide is also a sulfonylurea derivative. It is more potent and longer acting than tolbutamide. The drug is scarcely metabolized, if at all, and is excreted far more slowly than tolbutamide. Whereas one half of an ordinary dose of tolbutamide is excreted or metabolized within four and one-half hours (the so-called half-life), it appears that the half-life of chlorpropamide in the serum is nearly eight times as long, or 35 hours. A cumulative effect is thus observed with daily administration of chlorpropamide. An oral dose appears in the blood within one hour, is maximal at two to four hours, and requires 96 hours for excretion of even 80 to 90 per cent of the total drug. The chief advantages in the use of chlorpropamide are (1) the lower dosage that is possible and (2) the fact that diabetic patients who cease to respond to one sulfonylurea will often respond to another. This suggests the development of tolerance to one drug without cross-tolerance to the other. The general utility and limitations described for tolbutamide apply to this new analog.

Side Effects.   Side effects thus far observed include loss of appetite, nausea, vomiting, abdominal discomfort, dizziness, headache, chest pain, tachycardia, weakness, skin rash, leukopenia, eosinophilia, lymphocytosis, decrease in blood platelets, and liver damage (with or without jaundice). Many of these reactions necessitate discontinuation of the drug, while the less dangerous ones may be controlled by lowering the dose.

Dosage and Method of Administration.   The initial single daily dose, best taken with breakfast, is usually 250 to 500 mg. This will cause increasing blood levels for three to five days, with a plateau thereafter that may be raised or lowered by alterations in subsequent dosage (as indicated by blood sugar levels). The maintenance dosage range may necessitate the use of 100 mg. to 1 Gm. Insulin may be required in addition to, or in place of, chlorpropamide.

Preparation

Chlorpropamide Tablets   100 and 250 mg.

Trade name: Diabinese

Acetohexamide (Dymelor)

Acetohexamide (Dymelor), another sulfonylurea, has the same uses and side effects as tolbutamide. The oral dose ranges from 250 mg. to 1.5 Gm. daily. Doses in excess of 1.5 Gm. are not recommended.

Preparation

Acetohexamide Tablets   500 mg.

Trade name: Dymelor

Phenformin (DBI, Dibotin)

Phenformin, a phenethylbiguanide introduced in 1959, represents a completely new chemical class of oral antidiabetic agents. It produces biochemical reactions different from those of the sulfonylureas; it effectively reduces elevated blood glucose levels in more types of diabetes than do the latter drugs, namely, in some cases of the *brittle* or unstable type, chiefly occurring or having begun in childhood, with wide spontaneous changes in severity and insulin requirements.

Mechanism of Action. The manner in which phenformin lowers blood sugar is not completely known, but it is active even when the pancreas is removed or the insulin-secreting cells are destroyed. It has been shown to increase the utilization of glucose by muscle tissue, to decrease its oxidation, to decrease the glycogen in the muscle and to inhibit cytochrome oxidase. It is thus apparent that this biguanide increases anaerobic glycolysis and inhibits oxidative phosphorylation.

Phenformin may be used alone, when adequate for control of diabetes, or with insulin in those *labile* (unstable) cases at any age which fluctuate markedly in insulin requirements. The latter are often made more constant, as well as lower, with the combination. This oral agent may also be used in combination with a sulfonylurea in certain cases.

Side Effects. Nausea, anorexia, vomiting, lassitude, weakness, diarrhea, an unpleasant metallic taste, and hypoglycemic reactions are easily caused by phenformin. Because of these reactions, especially nausea and vomiting, considerable care and patience may be required in adjusting the individual dosage. Reduction of dosage or withdrawal of the drug is required when side effects are severe. Liver, kidney, or bone marrow damage has not been seen.

Dosage and Method of Administration. Dosage must be individualized, beginning with low amounts, such as 25 mg. twice daily, and increasing

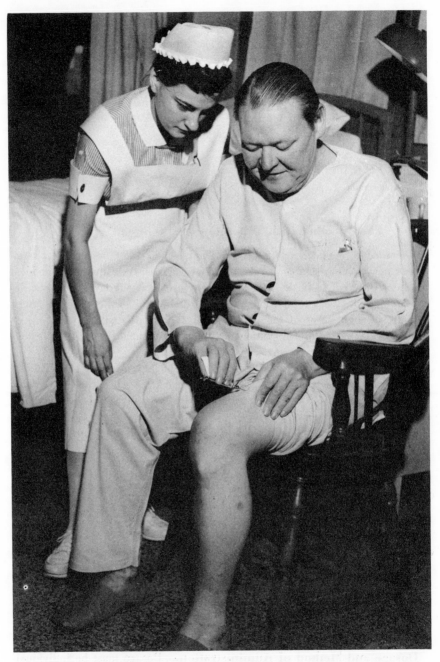

Fig. 18. Showing patient how to inject insulin. (*Courtesy of University Hospital, School of Nursing, and the Art Department, University of Maryland.*)

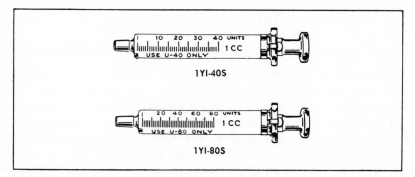

Fig. 19. Syringes used for insulin injection, showing the units in which they are calibrated. *(Courtesy of Becton, Dickinson and Company, Rutherford, N.J.)*

(if tolerated) by the same increments until blood glucose is reduced to satisfactory levels. Effective doses of phenformin are usually between 50 and 150 mg. daily, with a wider range of 25 to 300 mg. in rarer cases. From one to four weeks may be required for the appearance of blood glucose-lowering effects. Insulin, if already being administered, must usually be decreased and perhaps withdrawn, depending upon fasting glucose levels during the period of introduction of phenformin. Tablets of 25 mg. are available.

N,N-Dimethyldiguanide Hydrochloride (Glucophage)

This product, similar to but considerably weaker than phenformin, is available in Great Britain in 0.5-Gm. tablets. It is used for the oral treatment of cases of diabetes.

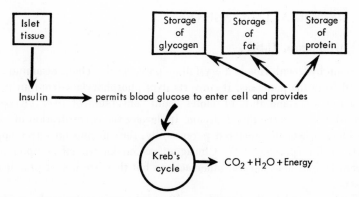

Fig. 20. Action of insulin. (Adapted from Krantz, J. C., and Carr, C. J.: *The Pharmacologic Principles of Medical Practice.* Williams & Wilkins, Baltimore, 1965.)

DIAGNOSTIC TEST FOR DIABETES

Tolbutamide Sodium Diagnostic (Orinase Diagnostic)

This solution is administered intravenously over a two- to three-minute period after proper preparation of the patient, and blood glucose concentrations at 20 and 30 minutes are compared with the preinjection, fasting value. In the normal, nondiabetic person, the substance causes a fast, progressive fall in blood glucose to approximately 50 per cent of the control value within 30 minutes. In diabetic patients, the glucose level usually falls by only 10 per cent. Depressions of the glucose concentration by 25 per cent within 20 minutes *may* indicate diabetes. This *tolbutamide tolerance test* is also useful in helping to diagnose the hyperinsulinism of pancreatic islet cell tumors. The test should be concluded with the oral administration of carbohydrate to restore the blood sugar to or near normal because some persons may become hypoglycemic. The drug is now known to facilitate the storage of glucose as glycogen in the liver.

Dosage and Administration. The 20 ml. of Sterile Water for Injection accompanying the 1.0-Gm. vial of tolbutamide powder (1.081 Gm. as the sodium salt) are used to dissolve the test dose with thorough shaking. The solution must be used within an hour and only if clear.

Preparation

Tolbutamide Sodium Diagnostic (as solution)	1.081 Gm., equivalent to 1.0 Gm. of the base; with 20 ml. Sterile Water for Injection, U.S.P.

Trade name: Orinase Diagnostic

HYPERGLYCEMIC AGENT

Glucagon, U.S.P.

Glucagon hydrochloride is a crystalline polypeptide (chain of amino acids) extracted from the pancreas. It converts liver phosphorylase from an inactive to an active state and thus promotes rapid conversion of liver glycogen to glucose which enters the blood stream. It elevates the concentration of glucose in the blood when administered parenterally, thus having an effect opposite that of insulin (pp. 657–62). Glucagon has no known effect upon muscle glycogen. It does have several other actions but they are not of practical significance.

Glucagon is used in the treatment of hypoglycemic states such as occur at times with insulin therapy in diabetes mellitus and in terminating the hypoglycemia after insulin shock therapy in psychiatry. Nausea and vomiting may occasionally be caused by glucagon and rare cases of hypersensitivity also occur.

Dosage and Administration. Lyophilized glucagon is dissolved in the accompanying solvent and given by subcutaneous, intramuscular, or intravenous injection in a dose of 0.5 to 1.0 mg. A patient who is unconscious because of hypoglycemia will usually awaken within 5 to 20 minutes following the administration of glucagon, but one or two additional doses may be required. Parenteral glucose may also be used or even required in an emergency. Some type of carbohydrate should at least be given orally to replenish liver glycogen and prevent further hypoglycemia.

Preparation

Glucagon Injection, U.S.P.
1 mg. with 49 mg. lactose as diluent and 1 ml. of Diluting Solution for Glucagon 10 mg. with 140 mg. lactose and 10 ml. of Diluting Solution for Glucagon

REVIEW QUESTIONS

1. Discuss the etiology of diabetes mellitus and list the principal features of the disease.
2. Describe, with regard to their duration.of action, the different forms in which insulin may be administered.
3. In what types of cases of diabetes is tolbutamide of some use? To what extent do you consider that it "substitutes" for insulin?
4. What is the principal mechanism of action of tolbutamide and chlorpropamide? Does phenformin share this mechanism?
5. Compare the side effects of the foregoing three drugs.
6. Discuss the dosage regimen with these agents.
7. The control of an obese diabetic of 48 years of age is not being maintained with 40 units of protamine zinc insulin each morning. Discuss the measures that could possibly bring the disease under control.
8. If a patient asks you (in his own words) why he had polyphagia, polydipsia, polyuria, and itching of the skin before his diabetes was treated, what would be your explanation to him of each of these symptoms?
9. In a patient just started on insulin, what are the symptoms indicative of hypoglycemia for which you would be on the alert? What instructions would you give him about the prevention and treatment of hypoglycemia?

REFERENCES

DIABETES

Beaser, S. B.: "Diabetes Mellitus," *New England J. Med.*, **259**:525, 1958.
————: "Oral Treatment of Diabetes Mellitus," *J.A.M.A.*, **187**:887, 1964.

Goodman, J. L.: "Clinical Discussion: Management of Uncomplicated Diabetes Mellitus," *Metabolism*, **4**:446, 1955.
Levine, Rachmiel: "Diabetes Mellitus," *Clin. Symposia*, **15**:119, 1963.
Martin, Marguerite M.: *Diabetes Mellitus, A Handbook for Nurses*. W. B. Saunders Company, Philadelphia, 1960.

INSULIN

Abel, J. J.: "Crystalline Insulin," *Proc. Nat. Acad. Sc.*, **12**:132, 1926.
Hauntz, E. A.: "Clinical Evaluation of *Lente* Insulin in One Hundred Nine Diabetic Patients," *J.A.M.A.*, **159**:1611, 1955.

ORAL ANTIDIABETIC AGENTS

Duncan, L. J., and Baird, J. D.: "Compounds Administered Orally in the Treatment of Diabetes Mellitus," *Pharmacol. Reviews*, **12**:91, 1960.
Feature: "Current Concepts in Therapy—Hypoglycemic Agents for Oral Administration," *New England J. Med.*, **262**:80, 1960.
Nabarro, J. D. N.: "Treatment of Diabetes Mellitus—Hypoglycaemic Agents Other Than Insulin," *Brit. M. J.*, **1**:1466, 1959.

TOLBUTAMIDE

DeLawter, De W. E., and Moss, J. M.: "Tolbutamide," *Am. J. Nursing*, **58**:1106, 1958.
Wilson, S. M., and Dumm, R. L.: "Tolbutamide on Trial," *Am. J. Nursing*, **58**:1108, 1958.

CHLORPROPAMIDE

Brown, G.; Zoidas, J.; and Spring, M.: "Hepatic Damage During Chlorpropamide Therapy," *J.A.M.A.*, **170**:2085, 1959.
Council on Drugs: "Chlorpropamide (Diabinese)," *J.A.M.A.*, **172**:57, 1960.
Greenhouse, B.: "Clinical Experience with Chlorpropamide," *Ann. New York Acad. Sc.*, **74**:643, 1959.
Rothfield, E. L.; Goldman, J.; Goldberg, H. H.; and Einhorn, S.: "Severe Chlorpropamide Toxicity," *J.A.M.A.*, **172**: 54, 1960.
Schumacher, O. P.; Fee, B. A.; McCullagh, E. P.; and Kovacs, L. L.: "Chlorpropamide, a New Drug for Diabetes Mellitus: Clinical Studies," *Cleveland Clin. Quart.*, **26**:12, 1959.

PHENFORMIN

Council on Drugs: "Phenformin Hydrochloride (DBI)," *J.A.M.A.*, **172**:702, 1960.
Feature: "Current Concepts in Therapy—Hypoglycemic Agents for Oral Administration. II," *New England J. Med.*, **262**:297, 1960.
Pomeranze, J.; Mouratoff, G. T.; Gadek, R. J.; and King, E. J.: "Phenethylbiguanide, a New Orally Given Hypoglycemic Agent," *J.A.M.A.*, **171**:252, 1959.

GLUCAGON HYDROCHLORIDE

Bondy, P. K., and Cardilla, L. R.: "The Effect of Glucagon on Carbohydrate Metabolism in Normal Human Beings," *J. Clin. Investigation*, **35**:494, 1956.

Elrick, H.; Witten, T. A.; and Arai, Y.: "Glucagon Treatment of Insulin Reactions," *New England J. Med.*, **258**:476, 1958.

TOLBUTAMIDE SODIUM DIAGNOSTIC

Fajans, S. S., and Conn, J. W.: "An Intravenous Tolbutamide Test as an Adjunct in the Diagnosis of Functioning Pancreatic Islet Cell Adenomas," *J. Lab. & Clin. Med.*, **54**:811, 1959.

Kaplan, N. M.: "Tolbutamide Tolerance Test in Carbohydrate Metabolism Evaluation," *Arch. Int. Med.*, **54**:212, 1961.

ACETOHEXAMIDE (DYMELOR)

Field, J. B., and Tyroler, S. A.: "Clinical Evaluation of Acetohexamide, a New Sulfonylurea Agent," *Diabetes*, **11**:74, 1963.

Raddin, R. S., *et al.*: "The Use of Acetohexamide in Stable Diabetes Mellitus," *Metabolism*, **72**:311, 1963.

Weller, Charles: "Oral Hypoglycemia Agents," *Am. J. Nursing*, **64**:90, 1964.

40

Iodine and Thyroid Metabolism

The thyroid gland, located in the neck, secretes a colloidal substance, thyroglobulin, which is stored within the gland. Thyroxin and 1-triiodothyronine, the hormones of the gland, which contain large amounts of iodine, are released from thyroglobulin by an enzyme, thyroid protease. They are carried in the blood bound to two proteins but are released in the tissues where they regulate the metabolism of all cells. Thus these hormones are important in the regulation of the basal metabolic rate. Thyroxin is present in much larger amounts. It is believed that it is converted to 1-triiodothyronine, the least plentiful but more powerful hormone, and in this form is utilized at the cellular level. It appears that 1-triiodothyronine enters the cells more readily than thyroxin.

The production of the thyroid hormones is under the influence of the thyrotropic hormone (TSH) from the anterior lobe of the pituitary gland. There is a check and balance operating between this hormone and the thyroid hormones circulating in the blood. TSH stimulates the thyroid gland, causing it to secrete more hormones into the blood. High concentrations of thyroid hormones in the blood inhibit the release of TSH; low concentrations increase the secretion of TSH. Thus, normally, a smooth regulation exists. The anterior pituitary is under the influence of the brain; hence, stress and perhaps other factors can lead to overproduction of TSH and, through it, of the thyroid hormones.

DIAGNOSTIC TESTS FOR THYROID FUNCTION

There are four tests that may be used to determine the activity of the thyroid gland.

1. The basal metabolism test (BMR), which is the measurement of the oxygen consumption during complete rest after a fasting period of 10 to 14 hours.

2. Measurement by means of a Geiger counter of the amount of radioactive iodine taken up by the thyroid gland after the administration of a known quantity.

3. Chemical determination of the concentration of protein-bound iodine (PBI) in the blood.

672

4. The TSH test, which involves comparisons of the radioactive iodine test and the PBI value before and 24 hours after the administration of a single intramuscular injection of TSH. This test can distinguish between inadequate anterior pituitary influence on the thyroid and primary dysfunction of the gland itself.

IODINE DEFICIENCY AND ENDEMIC GOITER

Thyroxin contains about 65 per cent iodine and triiodothyronine has somewhat less. If insufficient iodine salts are present in the diet or water, the normal amounts of the hormones cannot be produced. A prolonged deficiency reduces the concentration of the hormones in the blood, and as a result the secretion of thyrotropic hormone is increased, which in turn causes hypertrophy and hyperplasia of the thyroid. This enlargement of the gland, often visible and marked, is known as endemic or simple goiter. If iodine is supplied in the diet, the acini of the glands fill with colloid and the increase in size ceases. This resting stage of thyroid enlargement is called *colloid goiter*. Iodized table salt is a popular prophylactic measure against endemic goiter.

HYPOTHYROID STATES

Hypothyroidism results from a deficiency or lack of the thyroid hormones and is characterized by a slowing down of the metabolic rate causing a gradual retardation of physiological and mental functions. The symptoms vary according to the severity of the deficiency. This condition responds dramatically to the oral administration of the dried thyroid gland or one of its hormones.

Cretinism is a congenital form of hypothyroidism which occurs in the young child and is characterized by stunted growth and retarded mental development. All cells are biochemically abnormal, owing to the deficiency of the thyroid hormone. The skin is dry, the hair is coarse, and the tongue is thick. There are an imbecilic expression, a drawl in the speech, and a very low intellect. If thyroid is administered early (six months to one year), the child may be restored to normal development; but if administration is delayed longer, mental and physical retardation is irreversible. The drug must be administered throughout life; otherwise regression occurs very quickly.

Adult hypothyroidism may occur with or without myxedema. The basal metabolic rate is low, below -20 per cent; the hair is coarse and scanty; and there are a staggering gait, an impairment in the speech, tremors, muscular weakness, lethargy, loss of memory, and intolerance to cold. Myxedema is characterized by nonpitting edema, which causes the face and hands to appear puffy and swollen. The pulse is slow, and the heart may be enlarged. The patient is very sensitive to central nervous system depressants, especially morphine. With the administration of thyroid, the symptoms are relieved and the patient returns almost to normal. This is replacement therapy, and therefore the drug must be continued throughout life.

Thyroid, U.S.P., B.P., I.P.

Thyroid, which is a yellowish to buff-colored powder, is the dried, fat-free, *powdered thyroid gland* of domesticated animals used as food by man. The drug contains about 0.2 per cent iodine in organic combination and is assayed by virtue of its iodine content. It is effective upon oral administration and increases the metabolic rate of the body as a whole. There is a latent period before the effects are observed, and the maximum response is not observed for several days. The drug has a long action and produces cumulative effects when given daily. If it is withdrawn, the effects continue for several days or weeks.

Therapeutic Uses. Thyroid is used in mild hypothyroidism, cretinism, myxedema, obesity, certain skin conditions, and gynecological and obstetrical problems. The usual oral dose is 60 mg. (30 to 180 mg.) daily. Thyroxin, which is no longer an official drug, is administered intravenously in rare cases where thyroid is poorly absorbed.

Toxicity. Overdosage may cause hyperthyroidism the symptoms of which are palpitation, tachycardia, pain over the heart, nervousness, sweating, insomnia, tremors, and loss of weight. On decreasing the dosage the symptoms will subside in a week or two. However, thyroid is potentially dangerous in cardiac patients because it increases the work load of the heart.

Preparation

Thyroid Tablets, U.S.P., B.P.   15, 30, 60, and 120 mg.

Sodium Levothyroxine, U.S.P. (Synthroid)

This synthetic agent has the same actions and uses as thyroid tablets, for it is identical to the natural hormone thyroxin. It is several hundred times more potent than the powdered whole gland. Only about 50 per cent is absorbed orally. That which is absorbed from a single dose is present in the body for several weeks but is usually reduced to half of the original absorbed amount after one week. This factor can lead to a cumulative effect if excessive dosage is given daily. The toxic effects are the same as those for overdosage with thyroid.

Dosage and Administration. Sodium levothyroxine is administered orally in daily doses of 0.05 to 0.1 mg. daily, with adjustments every one to three weeks until the needs for thyroid replacement therapy are adequately met. These may vary between 0.02 and 1 mg., but are usually between 0.15 and 0.4 mg. daily.

Preparation

Sodium Levothyroxine Tablets, U.S.P.   0.05, 0.1, and 0.2 mg.

Trade name: Synthroid

Sodium Liothyronine, U.S.P. (Cytomel) (Levo-Triiodothyronine)

This agent, identical to one of the natural thyroid hormones (see p. 672), is prepared synthetically. It produces the same metabolic, therapeutic, and toxic effects as thyroid and thyroxin and may be used to replace these substances in the treatment of hypothyroidism. The onset of action is much more rapid, and its effects are of shorter duration. The rapidity of action is of distinct advantage when thyroid deficiency is severe. Liothyronine is about three to five times more potent than levothyroxine, described above.

Therapeutic Uses. Sodium liothyronine is used in the treatment of mild hypothyroidism, cretinism, myxedema, male infertility, and gynecological problems such as amenorrhea, premenstrual tension, and dysmenorrhea.

Dosage and Method of Administration. Sodium liothyronine is administered in single or divided doses. The initial oral adult dose is 5 mcg. daily. The dosage is increased by small amounts, at one- to two-week intervals, until a daily maintenance dose of 25 to 200 mcg. is reached. Smaller doses are recommended for children and geriatric patients.

Preparation

Sodium Liothyronine Tablets   5 and 25 mcg.

Trade name: Cytomel

Thyrotropic Hormone (Thyrotropin) (Thyroid-Stimulating Hormone, TSH) (Thyropar)

Thyrotropin is available as a sterile, lyophilized powder consisting of the highly purified thyrotropic principle of bovine anterior pituitary glands. Its stimulating action on the thyroid is useful for diagnostic (see p. 673) and therapeutic purposes.

Therapeutic Uses. Thyrotropin may be used to increase radioactive iodine uptake in the treatment of thyroid tumors, benign or malignant, or in thyrotoxicosis, and in some cases of thyroid inflammation.

Dosage and Methods of Administration. Thyrotropin powder is dissolved in sterile physiological saline solution (10 units per 2 ml.) and injected intramuscularly or subcutaneously. The usual dose is from 5 to 10 units for one to eight days.

Preparation

Thyrotropin (Injection, Lyophilized)   5 units in 5-ml. vial, 6 units in 10-ml. vial

HYPERTHYROIDISM

Hyperthyroidism is produced by overactivity of the thyroid gland, which may be due to a tumor of the thyroid or to its stimulation by the thyrotrophic hormone of the anterior lobe of the pituitary. Other terms for this condition include thyrotoxicosis, toxic goiter, exophthalmic goiter, and Graves' disease. The gland begins to swell and secrete a large amount of thyroxin. The metabolic rate increases, the pulse quickens, and the patient complains of feeling warm. Other symptoms are nervousness, restlessness, insomnia, sweating, muscular weakness, and emotional instability. In some patients there may be characteristic protrusion of the eyeballs (exophthalmos).

Hyperthyroidism may be treated by surgical subtotal thyroidectomy, x-rays, or antithyroid drugs. The antithyroid drugs are iodine and the iodides, radioactive iodine, thiourea, thiouracil, propylthiouracil, methylthiouracil, iothiouracil, and methimazole (Tapazole).

Iodine and Iodides

Iodine and the iodides were formerly used extensively in the treatment of thyrotoxicosis. After their administration the basal metabolic rate falls and there is a temporary remission of the symptoms of hyperthyroidism. The beneficial effects last only a few weeks, whereupon the symptoms reappear. These drugs are still used to prepare some patients for surgical removal of the major portion of the thyroid gland. Other drugs, to be described, are also employed in this situation; the iodides are used for one week prior to surgery because they decrease the vascularity (blood vessel network) of the gland, thus reducing bleeding when incised.

The iodides are usually administered in the form of *Strong iodine solution* (Lugol's Solution), which contains 5 per cent iodine and 10 per cent potassium iodide in aqueous solution or saturated solution of potassium iodide. Potassium iodide causes a metallic aftertaste and stimulates expectoration. The usual oral dose of either preparation is 0.3 ml. (0.1 to 1 ml.) three times a day diluted with water, milk, or orange juice. Iodine solution should be given through a straw placed behind the teeth so that it will not stain them.

Preparation

Strong Iodine Solution, U.S.P.	4.5 to 5.5 per cent solution of iodine in
Aqueous Iodine Solution, B.P. (Lugol's Solution)	9.5 to 10.5 per cent potassium iodide
Potassium Iodide Solution, N.F.	100 per cent solution

Radioactive Iodine

Sodium radio-iodide preparations contain a radioactive isotope of iodine (I 131). This isotope is obtained from a nuclear pile reactor and like all unstable isotopes undergoes constant change, termed *decay*. Within 8.08 days it has been reduced to one half its original radioactivity (*half-life*). Therefore, preparations of this salt are labeled with the date, the hour, and the radio-activity in microcuries or millicuries at the time of labeling.

Sodium iodide I 131 solution is a clear, colorless solution which contains I 131 and is suitable for oral or intravenous administration. Both preparations are used in the treatment of hyperthyroidism, thyroid tumor, or cancer and to determine the functional activity of the thyroid. Radioactive iodine is incorporated in the thyroxin molecule and is deposited in the colloid of the follicle. In carefully selected doses, the beta rays damage the thyroid without injury to the surrounding tissues. Smaller tracer doses, which are used to diagnose myxedema or hyperthyroidism, do not disturb thyroid function. Excessively large doses may damage surrounding structures, such as the parathyroids and trachea, or cause myxedema. After its administration, the basal metabolic rate falls and the symptoms of hyperthyroidism, such as tachycardia, palpitation, and irritability, disappear. Radioactive iodine is indicated in the treatment of severe toxic goiter or in recurring thyrotoxicosis after thyroidectomy. Radioactive iodine is administered orally in a half-glass of water or intravenously. The diagnostic dose is 1 to 100 microcuries. The therapeutic dose is 1 to 100 millicuries. The substance is present in the capsules in such a minute amount, absorbed on the inner surface of the capsules, that the capsule may appear to be empty.

Preparation

Sodium Iodide I 131 Capsules, U.S.P.	Size specified by the physician
Sodium Iodide I 131 Solution, U.S.P., B.P.; Sodium Iodide (^{131}I) Injection, B.P.	Concentration specified by the physician

OTHER ANTITHYROID DRUGS (GOITROGENS)

Thiourea, thiouracil, carbimazole, propylthiouracil, methylthiouracil, iothiouracil (Itrumil), and methimazole (Tapazole) depress thyroid function by blocking the synthesis of the thyroid hormones. This is accomplished by the prevention of the union of iodine with the amino acid tyrosine.

The decrease in circulating thyroxin and triiodothyronine results in an increased release of thyroid-stimulating hormone, TSH (see p. 672), which then causes an increase in the size of the thyroid gland itself. This is an attempt by the anterior pituitary to offset the diminished function of the thyroid. Because they produce enlargement of the thyroid, these antithyroid drugs are called *goitrogenic*, or goiter-producing, agents. At the present time these drugs are less frequently used for long-term therapy than previously owing to their toxic effects and the need for frequent medical follow-up.

Their principal use is for the production of a euthyroid state before surgery is performed. This prevents complications such as a thyroid crisis.

Propylthiouracil, U.S.P., B.P., I.P.

NB

Propylthiouracil is a synthetic powder, somewhat related chemically to the barbiturates, that depresses the basal metabolic rate. It does not inactivate thyroxin already formed but interferes with the formation of the hormone; consequently it requires several days to depress thyroid activity. Propylthiouracil is very useful in preparing a patient for thyroid surgery, as well as in treating patients in whom surgery is contraindicated.

The drug is rapidly excreted from the body; so the usual dose of 100 mg. (75 to 150 mg.) must be given every six to eight hours in order to maintain a satisfactory level in the gland. Otherwise, if a dose is missed, the effectiveness of the therapy is interrupted. After a few weeks the symptoms of hyperthyroidism may be completely arrested and the patient may avoid an operation. The combined use of propylthiouracil and potassium iodide appears to be more satisfactory in preparing the patient for surgery because the thyroid is not so *friable* and hemorrhagic as when propylthiouracil alone is used, and thus the gland may be removed more easily. In the preoperative control of the disease, 50 mg. of propylthiouracil and 5 to 10 minims of strong iodine solution three times a day are indicated.

Untoward Effects. Untoward effects are drug fever, leukopenia, skin rashes, and urticaria. The most serious complication is granulocytopenia. Patients should report to the doctor symptoms of sore throat, fever, head cold, and malaise. The patient's blood picture should be watched carefully. These untoward effects of propylthiouracil occur less frequently than with thiouracil. The drug is not contraindicated during pregnancy; however, the dosage should be kept as low as possible. Mothers receiving this drug should not breast-feed their infants so that the possible development of cretinism may be avoided.

Preparation

Propylthiouracil Tablets, U.S.P., B.P.   50 mg.

Methylthiouracil, U.S.P., B.P.

Methylthiouracil is a white crystalline powder that is only slightly soluble in water and organic solvents. The usual oral dose of this antithyroid drug is 50 mg. four times a day (150 to 250 mg. daily).

Preparation

Methylthiouracil Tablets, U.S.P., B.P.   50 mg.

Trade names: Methiacil; Muracil; Thimecil

Iothiouracil (Itrumil)

Iothiouracil is a white or light-yellow crystalline powder that is moderately soluble in water. This drug, which has the combined antithyroid activity of a goitrogen and an iodide, is given orally in doses of 50 to 100 mg. three or four times a day. The untoward effects are similar to those of propylthiouracil.

Preparation

Iothiouracil Tablets   50 mg.

Trade name: Itrumil

Methimazole, U.S.P. (Tapazole)

Methimazole produces actions similar to those resulting from the administration of propylthiouracil. However, methimazole is about 10 to 20 times more potent than propylthiouracil, and the duration of action is prolonged. The side actions are the same, although they are less frequent.

The usual oral dose is 10 mg. (5 to 20 mg.) every eight hours. After the remission of symptoms, which requires perhaps a month or two, a maintenance dose of 5 to 10 mg. daily may control the disease. This treatment may produce a cure; however, thyroidectomy is often performed after the symptoms of the disease are controlled.

Preparation

Methimazole Tablets, U.S.P.   5 and 10 mg.

Trade names: Tapazole; Mercazole

Potassium Perchlorate

This inorganic salt has proved in recent trials to be very useful in suppressing the overactive thyroid. It inhibits the iodine-trapping mechanism of the gland and therefore differs from the foregoing drugs in the site of action. It is recommended in daily divided doses of 1 Gm. It may produce rashes and agranulocytosis.

REVIEW QUESTIONS

1. Review the relationship of the anterior pituitary to the thyroid gland as a reciprocally functioning "axis."
2. Review the need for iodine in the body and the results of its deficiency in the diet and water.
3. What are the effects of thyroxin in the body?
4. What are the clinical pictures of excessive and of insufficient levels of thyroxin in the body?
5. What is the role of triiodothyronine believed to be?

6. *What differences do you see among the following drugs: thyroid (powdered gland), sodium levothyroxin, sodium liothyronine, and thyrotropin?*
7. *Discuss the use of sodium radio-iodide in diagnosing and treating thyroid disease.*
8. *How do ordinary iodide and iodine affect hyperthyroidism?*
9. *Name all other antithyroid drugs, and give their doses and general pattern of activity.*
10. *A woman with a large appetite continues to lose weight, is very tense, is nervous, must stay active, dislikes warm rooms, has trembling fingers, and looks continually frightened (prominent eyes). Explain the roles of the following, which could be involved in this case: the pituitary gland, the thyroid gland, PBI, BMR, general cellular oxidation, and an I 131 uptake test. How would you advise treating this case?*

REFERENCES

Asper, S. P., Jr., and Wiswell, J. G.: "Physiology and Treatment of Myxedema," *Am. J. Med.*, **20**:732, 1956.

Garrod, O.: "Drug Treatment of Disease: Thyrotoxicosis," *Brit. M. J.*, **1**:1123, 1960.

Hamolsky, M. W., and Freedberg, A. S.: "The Thyroid Gland," *New England J. Med.*, **262**:23, 70, 129, 1960.

Ibbertson, K.; Fraser, R.; and Alldis, D.: "Rapidly Acting Thyroid Hormones and Their Cardiac Action," *Brit. M. J.*, **2**:52, 1959.

Jefferies, W. McK.; Levy, R. P.; and Storaasli, J. P.: "Use of the TSH Test in the Diagnosis of Thyroid Disorders," *Radiol.*, **73**:341, 1959.

Nordyke, R. A.: "The Overactive and the Underactive Thyroid," *Am. J. Nursing*, **63**:66, 1963.

Solomon, D. S., and Dowling, J. T.: "Thyroid," *Ann. Rev. Physiol.*, **22**:615, 1960.

Spence, A. W.: "Thyroid Hormones," *Brit. M. J.*, **1**:706, 1959.

RADIOIODINE

Rubenfeld, S.; Lowenthal, M.; Kohn, A.; *et al.*: "Radioiodine in the Treatment of Hyperthyroidism," *A.M.A. Arch. Int. Med.*, **104**:532, 1959.

41

Adrenocorticosteroids and ACTH. Treatment of Arthritis

The adrenal glands, which are located above the kidneys, are composed of two parts: an outer portion, or cortex; and an inner part, or medulla. The medullary portion secretes epinephrine and norepinephrine, which were discussed on pages 450–55. The adrenal cortex secretes a number of hormones that are essential to life. Death results when this cortex is removed or severely impaired in diseased conditions unless exogenous hormones are administered. One of its most important functions is the regulation of mineral, carbohydrate, and water metabolism.

ADRENOCORTICOSTEROIDS

The adrenal cortex produces three main groups of hormones: the *glucocorticoids*, the *mineralocorticoids*, and sex steroids. The latter are of little consequence under normal circumstances. The glucocorticoids secreted are mainly hydrocortisone, cortisone, and some corticosterone. These have specific effects upon carbohydrate metabolism. They promote the conversion of some of the dietary protein to glucose and the deposition of glucose in the liver as glycogen. They also increase the response of the tissues to inflammation. Moreover, in severe inflammation glucocorticoids may be administered to supplement the endogenous hormones. They reduce the number of eosinophils circulating in the blood and suppress lymphoid tissue. They also have an effect on salt and water balance though not to the same extent as the mineralocorticoids. Cortisone, hydrocortisone, and numerous synthetic compounds of varying potency are available for clinical use.

Among the steroids, which regulate sodium, potassium, and water balance, are aldosterone and desoxycorticosterone. Aldosterone is of the greater physiological importance and potency. Its action as a sodium-retaining and potassium-excreting agent was briefly described on page 637. Occasionally the adrenal cortex or tumors of this tissue secrete larger amounts of this hormone, a condition known as *primary aldosteronism*. It is characterized by excessive secretion in the blood stream of aldosterone and by high sodium and low

681

potassium levels in the blood, although at times these levels may be normal. The symptoms noted are polyuria, polydipsia, muscular weakness, intermittent tetany, hypernatremia, hypokalemic alkalosis, and hypertension. The second mineralocorticoid, desoxycorticosterone, has long been available as the acetate salt for the treatment of adrenocortical deficiency disease. Aldosterone is not available for clinical use.

Hydrocortisone and other glucocorticoids are secreted under the influence of a hormone from the anterior pituitary gland known as adrenocorticotropic hormone (ACTH). These adrenal hormones are synthesized from cholesterol. When hydrocortisone is secreted in amounts greater than normal, or when it or synthetic gluco- or anti-inflammatory corticoids are administered, these substances decrease or abolish the elaboration of ACTH. The output of hydrocortisone by the adrenal is then curtailed. This check and balance mechanism was also seen with the thyroid relationship in the previous chapter. Aldosterone, on the other hand, is dependent upon and affected by ACTH to only a mild extent but mainly by the sodium concentration in the body fluids. When there is increased sodium in the blood, blood volume is increased by additional water which is drawn into the blood. "Volume receptors" in the hypothalamic area respond and are thought to cause the secretion of the hormone adrenoglomerulotropin, which then stimulates the cells of the adrenal cortex that elaborate aldosterone.

Addison's Disease. The adrenal cortex is a vital tissue and rarely deficient in its function, but when its progressive destruction occurs, the patient dies within a few years unless properly treated. This condition is known as Addison's disease and is usually caused by primary atrophy of this tissue (50 to 60 per cent) and by tuberculosis or fungi (40 to 50 per cent). Acute adrenocortical insufficiency may occur during meningococcal invasion of the blood stream which may cause fatal destruction of the cortex. Addison's disease is characterized by disturbances in carbohydrate and protein metabolism and salt and water balance. The symptoms noted are weakness, fatigue, loss of appetite and weight, vomiting, diarrhea, pigmentation of the skin, hypoglycemia, dehydration, dizziness, fainting, circulatory failure, and collapse. Since the loss of sodium is excessive, its level in the blood is low; on the other hand, potassium is retained resulting in an increased blood level.

Life may be maintained by the administration of desoxycortisone acetate (DOCA) or fludrocortisone, one of the more potent synthetic drugs, which can correct the sodium loss and potassium retention and thus lessen hypertension, muscular weakness, and dehydration. They have little effect on the abnormalities of carbohydrate and protein metabolism and do not prevent hypoglycemia. Therefore, cortisone is given at the same time for more complete replacement therapy.

Desoxycorticosterone Acetate Injection, U.S.P.; Deoxycortone Acetate, B.P.

Desoxycorticosterone is an adrenocortical hormone that has been made synthetically. It is administered parenterally in severe cases of Addison's disease because the hormone causes a retention of sodium and an excretion of potassium so that blood sodium and potassium levels are restored to normal. Water is retained, the plasma volume and interstitial fluid are increased, and the patient gains weight. The usual buccal dose is 2 mg. daily; the intramuscular dose is 1 (1 to 2) mg. daily; and the implantation dose, for which 75- and 125-mg. pellets are available.

Preparations

Desoxycorticosterone Acetate Injection (Oil), U.S.P.; Deoxycortone Acetate Injection, B.P.	1-ml. ampuls and 10-ml. vials containing 5 mg. in 1 ml.
Desoxycorticosterone Acetate Tablets, U.S.P.	2 mg.
Sterile Desoxycorticosterone Trimethylacetate Suspension, U.S.P.	25 mg. in 1 ml., 4-ml. vials
Desoxycorticosterone Acetate Pellets	75 and 125 mg.
Deoxycortone Implants, B.P.	

Trade names: Cortate; Cortiron; DOCA; Percorten

Fludrocortisone (Florinef)

Fludrocortisone may be administered orally, and its effects are more prolonged. For these reasons its use is preferred for maintenance therapy in the treatment of Addison's disease. It may be used alone or supplemented with cortisone. The usual oral daily dose is 0.25 to 1 mg. In addisonian crises the dose is 5 to 10 mg.

Fludrocortisone is used locally in the treatment of skin diseases. It is not administered systemically in the treatment of arthritis and related diseases because of its marked retention of sodium and water and the severe loss of potassium with the accompanying edema and hypertension.

Preparations

Fludrocortisone Acetate Tablets	0.1 and 1 mg.

Trade name: Florinef

Pharmacological Actions of Anti-inflammatory Steroids.   The term "anti-inflammatory steroids" is synonymous with the designation glucocorticoids. The latter emphasizes their chief physiological role, whereas the former is descriptive of their chief therapeutic use. There is no evidence that any of the diseases that are ameliorated by these steroids are associated with deficient adrenal secretion of hydrocortisone. These diseases are usually of unknown basic causes. The mechanisms by which the steroids affect them so favorably are unknown. The beneficial effects can be described, however. The side effects are to a great extent accounted for by the known physiological functions already discussed, merely carried to unphysiological degrees.

In general, the actions of these steroids in reducing inflammation of many types and in many tissues and structures are manifested by a reduction of the hyperemia, the edema, the increased growth of fibroblasts, and often the pain. Allergic reactions (see Chap. 47) are often reduced or abolished by these compounds. Fever, when present, is usually lowered, the erythrocyte sedimentation rate (if elevated) is usually reduced, and the weakness, aching, and general malaise associated with certain diseases are frequently replaced by a feeling of well-being (euphoria).

In diseases that are self-limited, such as a temporary allergy or a reaction to a chemical, infections, or other agents, the steroids may prevent significant symptoms and make the illness much milder. These drugs do not usually affect the etiological factors but merely suppress the manifestations of the disease. In certain diseases in which they are suppressive, the steroids[1] are contraindicated. Thus, in systemic bacterial infections, including pneumonia, tuberculosis, and typhoid fever, the immunological and other responses by which the body overcomes (or at least combats) the disease are jeopardized. Infections can thus become fulminating and lethal.

The importance of the protective action of the steroids stems from their ability to hold in abeyance cellular and tissue response to injury of various types—mechanical, chemical, hypersensitivity states, and antigen-antibody reactions. The drugs are thus only palliative, shielding, and not basically corrective or curing. The disease, if chronic, returns in its typical pattern and severity, and perhaps even aggravated, when steroid therapy is discontinued. Some conditions are cyclic, with natural remissions and exacerbations. The steroids are useful during the exacerbations and may not be needed in remissions.

Various types of stress, such as exposure to cold, deprivation of sleep, overwork, hypoxia, and those already discussed, cause the secretion of increased amounts of hydrocortisone. This agent and its synthetic congeners confer greater resistance to stress.

Therapeutic Uses of the Anti-inflammatory Steroids.   These agents are appropriate replacement therapy in *primary hypoadrenalism* (Addison's disease) and in *secondary hypoadrenalism* caused by hypopituitarism. In the former, desoxycorticosterone acetate may also be required for mineral control, especially in severe cases and in crises of the disease. These steroids are

---

[1] In this chapter only, the unmodified term "steroids" is restricted to the anti-inflammatory steroids or glucocorticoids. Other types of steroids are discussed in other chapters.

used to combat the virilizing (masculinizing) effects of congenital adrenal hyperplasia, through suppression of ACTH output.

They are also used for ameliorating or controlling the following diseases and conditions:

1. The collagen diseases, such as rheumatoid arthritis, acute rheumatic fever, disseminated lupus erythematosus, scleroderma, dermatomyositis, and periarteritis nodosa.

2. Gout or gouty arthritis.

3. Skin diseases, such as urticaria, angioneurotic edema, atopic dermatitis, exfoliative dermatitis, and pemphigus.

4. Allergic manifestations, such as hay fever, bronchial asthma, status asthmaticus, serum sickness, and drug hypersensitivity.

5. Eye conditions, such as uveitis, chloroiditis, iritis, and certain varieties of conjunctivitis.

6. Nephrosis in children.

7. Acute thyroid crisis and nonsuppurative thyroiditis.

8. Ulcerative colitis, regional ileitis, and sprue.

9. Idiopathic thrombocytopenic purpura, acute leukemia, and acquired hemolytic anemia.

10. Breast malignancy, for suppression of adrenal estrogenic substances via pituitary inhibition, or as replacement therapy when bilateral adrenalectomy is performed to eradicate this source of estrogens. Bilateral ovariectomy is always done prior to adrenalectomy in such cases, for the ovaries are usually a greater source of estrogen, which may stimulate certain breast malignancies.

11. Miscellaneous additional conditions of growing number.

Contraindications. Owing to a certain degree of sodium-retaining capacity possessed by the glucocorticoids, especially by hydrocortisone and cortisone (although much less than the strictly mineral corticoids), these agents and their derivatives are likely to be poorly tolerated in conditions complicated by heart disease, hypertension, or renal insufficiency. Diabetes mellitus may be worsened because blood glucose is raised by these anti-inflammatory steroids. Osteoporosis may be made worse by further demineralization of bone, for these agents cause increased breakdown of protein (catabolism), including that in bone matrix, with calcium loss. Convulsive disorders, treated peptic ulcers, and arrested (walled-off) tuberculous lung lesions may also be adversely affected.

Absolute contraindications include infections that cannot be controlled by chemotherapy, psychoses, severe psychoneuroses, active peptic ulcer, and herpes simplex of the eyes.

Side Effects and Cushing's Syndrome. Overfunctioning of the adrenal cortex occurs, although rarely, and is known as Cushing's syndrome.

Excessive levels of circulating glucocorticoids are produced and cause the many actions mentioned in the foregoing paragraphs. These are the same in general as those produced by continuous medication with these steroids in any of the diseases enumerated under the therapeutic uses above. The number and severity of side effects depend upon dosage and duration of treatment. Table 37 lists these side effects.

─────────────── **Table 37** ───────────────

Side Effects of the Anti-inflammatory Steroids

Fluid retention (edema)	Delayed wound and fracture healing
Facial rounding ("moon face")	Negative nitrogen balance
Increased fat deposits	Menstrual irregularities
Increased appetite; weight gain	Mental symptoms, euphoria or depression
Increased body hair growth with thinning of scalp hair	Neuritis
Acne and skin pigmentation	Accentuation of peptic ulcer
Ecchymosis, striae	Osteoporosis, fractures
Elevated blood pressure	Increased blood glucose
Tachycardia	Adrenal cortical insufficiency
Decreased resistance to infections	Increased coagulation time

Differences Among the Anti-inflammatory Steroids. Cortisone was the first of these steroids to be isolated from the adrenal cortex and was shown to have the major activities of the cruder adrenal cortical extract. It was synthesized and used first in rheumatoid arthritis (see below). Cortisone does not appear to be secreted into the blood from the cortex. Rather, its derivative hydrocortisone, which is about 20 per cent more potent, is now believed to be the form into which administered cortisone is changed in the body before it produces its various effects. Hydrocortisone was isolated from the gland about the same time as cortisone and was also synthesized and made available for medication. The actions of the two are practically, if not completely, identical.

SYNTHETIC ANTI-INFLAMMATORY STEROIDS

The newer synthetic derivatives that have become available are more potent and have less salt-retaining, edema-producing effects than the natural hormones. Side effects are identical.

Dosage and Methods of Administration. The various agents may be administered orally, intramuscularly, intravenously, or topically to the skin, the various mucous membranes, the eyes and directly into joints, bursae, etc. The systemic dosage depends upon the severity, the natural features, and the duration of the particular disease, but it should be the minimum that will provide an adequate but not necessarily complete suppression of the symptoms.

A dose of 80 to 100 mg. of cortisone daily may be administered initially in chronic, nonfatal conditions, such as rheumatoid arthritis or chronic asthma. In acute and severe disorders such as rheumatic fever, severe seasonal asthma, and certain blood dyscrasias, 200 to 400 mg. daily may be given initially. These doses are reduced daily until a minimum is reached which just controls the symptoms or other manifestations.

Approximately equal anti-inflammatory effects are produced by the following oral doses of the steroids:

Cortisone	25 mg.	Triamcinolone	4 mg.
Hydrocortisone	20 mg.	Fludrocortisone	1 mg.
Prednisone	5 mg.	Paramethasone	1.0 mg.
Prednisolone	4 mg.	Dexamethasone	0.75 mg.
Methylprednisolone	4 mg.	Betamethasone	0.6 mg.

The newer synthetic agents are considerably more potent than cortisone.

During the administration of glucocorticoids the secretion of ACTH is suppressed and the adrenal glands atrophy. As a result the production of the cortical hormones is diminished. A gradual decrease in the amount of steroid stimulates the production of ACTH causing the adrenal gland to secrete more endogenous hormones. If this is not done, symptoms of acute adrenal insufficiency will occur. The sodium content of the diet of a person receiving cortical steroids for long periods of time is usually reduced in order to prevent edema formation. The many side effects of these drugs must be observed since the steroids are not always discontinued when they occur. The severity of the disease is compared to the side effect. The steroid is not discontinued if the lack of it would be more harmful to the patient than the side effect. The side effect may be controlled with another drug; for example, insulin may be given to correct the hyperglycemia.

Patients on long-term steroid therapy who require surgical procedures will need increased amounts of the drug to handle the stress caused by surgery.

Preparations

Cortisone Acetate Tablets, U.S.P., I.P., Cortisone Tablets, B.P.	25 mg. (also 5, 10 mg.)
Cortisone Acetate Suspension, U.S.P. (Injection); Cortisone Injection, B.P.	25 mg. in 1 ml.; 10- and 20-ml. vials; 50 mg. in 1 ml.; 10-ml. vials
Cortisone Acetate Ointment, Ophthalmic	1.5 per cent
Cortisone Acetate Ophthalmic Suspension, N.F.	0.5, 2.5 per cent, 5-ml. bottles

Trade names: Anderson Cortelan; Cortisyl; Cortone; Cortogen; Synonym; Compound E

Hydrocortisone Tablets, U.S.P.	5, 10, 20 mg.
Hydrocortisone Injection, B.P.	5 mg. in 1 ml., 20-ml. vials; 50 mg. in 1 ml., 5-ml. vials
Hydrocortisone Ointment, U.S.P.; B.P.	1 per cent (also 2.5 per cent)
Hydrocortisone Cream (Topical)	0.5, 1, 2.5 per cent
Hydrocortisone Lotion (Topical)	0.5, 1, 2.5 per cent
Hydrocortisone Suspension (Oral)	2 mg. in 1 ml.
Hydrocortisone Tablets (Vaginal)	10 mg.
Sterile Hydrocortisone Acetate Suspension, U.S.P.; Hydrocortisone Acetate Injection, B.P.	25, 50 mg. in 1 ml., 5-ml. vials

Trade names: Cortef; Cortril; Hycortol; Hytone; Hydrocortone Synonym: Compound F

Hydrocortisone Sodium Succinate, U.S.P. (Powder, Injection)	100 mg.

Trade name: Solu-Cortef

Hydrocortisone Cyclopentylpropionate Suspension (Oral)	2 mg. in 1 ml.

Trade name: Cortef Fluid

Prednisone Tablets, U.S.P., B.P.	1, 2.5, 5 mg.

Trade names: Deltasone; Deltra; Meticorten; Paracort

Prednisolone Tablets, U.S.P., B.P.	1, 2.5, 5 mg.
Prednisolone Ointment, U.S.P.	0.5 per cent
Prednisolone Cream (Topical)	0.5 per cent

Trade names: Delta; Hydelta; Meticortelone; Meti-Derm; Paracortol

Prednisolone Acetate Suspension (Injection)	25 mg. in 1 ml., 5-ml. vials

Trade name: Sterane

Prednisolone Butylacetate Suspension (Injection)	20 mg. in 1 ml., 5-ml. vials

Trade name: Hydeltra-T.B.A.

Prednisolone Phosphate Sodium Lotion (Topical)	0.5 per cent
Ointment (Ophthalmic)	0.25 per cent
Ointment (Topical)	0.5 per cent
Solution (Injection)	20 mg. in 1 ml., 1-ml. ampuls
Solution (Ophthalmic)	0.5 per cent

Trade name: Hydeltrasol

Methylprednisolone Tablets	2, 4 mg.

Trade name: Medrol

Triamcinolone Tablets	1, 2, 4, 16 mg.

Trade names: Aristocort, Kenacort

Triamcinolone Acetonide Cream, Lotion, and Ointment	0.1 per cent

Trade name: Kenalog

Betamethasone Tablets	0.6 mg.

Trade name: Celestone

Paramethasone Acetate Tablets	1 and 2 mg.

Trade name: Haldrone

Dexamethasone Tablets	0.5, 0.75 mg.
Dexamethasone Phosphate Ophthalmic Solution	1 mg. in 1 ml., 5-ml. bottles
Dexamethasone Phosphate Ophthalmic Ointment	0.05 per cent, 3.5-Gm tubes

Trade names: Decadron; Deronil

Fludrocortisone Hemisuccinate Ophthalmic Solution	0.1 per cent (as the acetate equivalent)
Fludrocortisone Acetate Tablets	0.1, 1 mg.
Fludrocortisone Acetate Ointment	0.1, 0.2 mg.
Fludrocortisone Acetate Lotion	0.05, 0.1, 0.2 per cent

Trade name: Florinef

Dichlorisone Acetate Foam Aerosol	10-Gm. containers (18.75 mg. dichlorisone)
Dichlorisone Acetate Cream, 2.5 mg. per Gram	5-Gm. tubes containing 2.5 mg. per Gram

Trade name: Diloderm

Fluocinolone Acetonide Cream	15-Gm. tube, 0.025 per cent

Trade name: Synalar

Fluprednisolone Tablets	0.75 and 1.5 mg.

Trade name: Alphadrol

Flurandrenolone Cream and Ointment, 0.5 mg. per Gram	7.5- and 15-Gm. tubes containing 0.5 mg. per Gram

Trade name: Cordran

Adrenal Cortex Injection, N.F.

Adrenal cortex injection is a sterile solution of mixed natural adrenocortical hormones. The usual intramuscular or intravenous dose is 10 ml. (10 to 100 ml.), repeated as necessary. The solution is available in 10- and 50-ml. vials. Each milliliter is equivalent to 100 mcg. of U.S.P. Hydrocortisone Acetate Reference Standard.

ADRENOCORTICOTROPIC HORMONE (ACTH)

In 1946, Dr. J. R. Mote, using the method of Dr. C. H. Li, isolated a small quantity of the adrenocorticotropic hormone (ACTH) from the anterior lobe of the pituitary gland and made it available to the medical profession. Dr. G. W. Thorn found that it relieved symptoms of rheumatic fever and rheumatoid arthritis.

Corticotropin Injection, U.S.P.; Corticotrophin Injection, B.P. (ACTH Injection)

Corticotropin is a crystalline substance, obtained from the anterior lobe of the pituitary gland of domestic animals, that stimulates the adrenal cortex to secrete hormones such as hydrocortisone and related substances. The effects produced are due to the corticosteroids secreted by the adrenal cortex and are the same as those produced by the administration of cortisone or hydro-cortisone. Because its action depends on the functional integrity of the adrenals, corticotropin is of no value in Addison's disease except as a diagnostic agent. Corticotropin is not effective orally because it is destroyed by the digestive juices. Topical application is of no value, since the substance acts only on and through the adrenal glands.

Corticotropin is administered intramuscularly and intravenously. The dose is 10 to 100 U.S.P. units daily in four divided doses. The dose may be increased to 200 daily with caution, but it should then be reduced gradually to the smallest dose that can be used without symptoms, this amount being employed as a maintenance dose. Five to twenty U.S.P. units in 500 ml. of 5 per cent glucose or normal salt solution (if the patient is not on a salt-restricted diet) are given intravenously. When a repository form of the drug is administered, the activity persists for 18 to 24 hours.

Therapeutic Uses. Corticotropin is used in the treatment of gout, rheumatoid arthritis, rheumatic fever, lupus erythematosus, asthma, as well as eye and skin diseases, and most of the other conditions listed on page 685. The clinical uses are similar to those of the glucocorticoids which are generally preferred.

Contraindications. Corticotropin is contraindicated for long-term therapy in hypertension, mental disturbances, chronic nephritis, and congestive heart failure. The untoward effects are the same as for cortisone.

Preparations

Corticotropin Injection, U.S.P., Corticotrophin Injection, B.P.	10 U.S.P. units in 1 ml., 40 units in 2 ml., 100 and 200 units in 10 ml., and 200 units in 5 ml. (liquid form); 10, 25, 40 units (dry form)
Repository Corticotropin Injection, U.S.P.	40 U.S.P. units in 1 ml., and 200 and 400 units in 5 ml.

Trade names: Acthar; Acton; Corticotropin-Zinc; Solacthyl

DIAGNOSTIC AID FOR PITUITARY FUNCTION

Metyrapone (Metopirone)

This compound is used as a diagnostic test of the capacity of the anterior pituitary gland to secrete adrenocorticotropic hormone (ACTH). It prevents the production of glucocorticoids by the adrenal cortex. The decrease in their concentration in the body causes the outpouring of ACTH in an attempt to increase the production of the glucocorticoids. This is blocked by the diagnostic agent but certain precursors (compounds S and DOC) are produced in greater than normal amounts. Their detection by chemical tests on blood specimens indicates the degree of function of the ACTH-producing. cells of the pituitary.

Preparations

Metyrapone Tablets	250 mg.
Metrapone Ditartrate Solution	10-ml. ampuls containing 100 mg. in 1 ml. (43.8 mg. metyrapone base)

ARTHRITIS

Arthritis (hypertrophic and rheumatoid) is one of the oldest diseases known to man. There are about 11 million arthritics in the United States, and one out of ten cases progresses to crippling stages. This disease is character- ized by pain, stiffness, tenderness, and swelling in the joints, and immobility. The drugs used in the treatment of rheumatoid arthritis are the anti-inflamma- tory steroids, corticotropin, chloroquine, hydroxychloroquine, phenylbuta- zone, the gold salts, sodium salicylate and drugs to relieve pain, such as aspirin and codeine.

Rheumatoid arthritis is a disease of connective tissue, mainly of the synovial membranes, the periarticular surfaces, and the adjacent bone.

ANTI-INFLAMMATORY STEROIDS AND CORTICOTROPIN

In rheumatoid arthritis, the symptoms are sometimes quickly relieved by anti-inflammatory steroids and corticotropin. There are an increase in the appetite and a gain in weight, and the patient is brighter and more active. The steroids and corticotropin have an inhibitory influence on the inflammatory process, but they do not produce a cure. They fail to correct the deformities and structural changes that result from damage to articular cartilage and bone. The relief of symptoms is quickly noted and often maintained for long periods with uninterrupted therapy, but the effects last only as long as treat- ment is continued. The symptoms return when the drug is discontinued. If they return while therapy is maintained, larger doses or the addition of other measures may be indicated.

Chloroquine Phosphate, U.S.P., B.P. (Aralen Phosphate)

In recent years numerous reports have been published showing a consider- able value of certain antimalarial drugs in collagen diseases, among which are lupus erythematosus, rheumatoid arthritis, and spondylitis. The greater number of reported cases of arthritis have been treated with chloroquine phos- phate. Major improvement of signs and symptoms has been produced in a large number of cases. The drug is said to provide a greater degree of con- trol of the disease and a longer effect than has been seen with the adreno- corticosteroids or ACTH. It appears to affect the more basic pathology of the disease rather than to provide nonspecific anti-inflammatory action, as do the corticosteroids and ACTH. Results require several weeks for development, are usually maintained rather indefinitely, and persist for many months after discontinuing the drug. The mechanism of action is not known but may be related to a known inhibitory action on certain immunologic mechanisms or to other intracellular actions of the antimalarial drugs.

Dosage. The dosage now recommended in rheumatoid arthritis is 250 mg. per day in a single dose. Some physicians suggest 500 mg. daily. Side effects are reversible but may include skin reactions and other gastrointestinal symptoms, vertigo, headaches, blurring of vision, rare decrease in the white blood cell count, and depigmentation of the hair. A newer drug, hydroxychloroquine (Plaquenil), has been better tolerated by patients, appears equal or superior to chloroquine in effectiveness, and seems destined to become the drug of choice. It is given in a dose of 200 mg. (one tablet) up to five times daily.

The preparations and other details concerning chloroquine phosphate (Aralen) are given on page 212.

Phenylbutazone, B.P. (Butazolidin)

Phenylbutazone is a white or yellow crystalline powder soluble in water. It is a synthetic drug related to aminopyrine. Phenylbutazone is analgesic for muscle and joint conditions and is used especially in arthritis. Here it is effective in relieving pain, stiffness, and swelling and in increasing mobility. It is anti-inflammatory but not hormonal in action. Therapeutic effects should be obtained in a week if the drug is to be effective. As soon as the symptoms have been relieved, the dose should be reduced to a minimum to prevent the occurrence of serious untoward effects.

Phenylbutazone is given orally in doses of 300 to 600 mg. daily in divided doses. It is irritating to the gastric mucosa and therefore should be given with milk and crackers to prevent its contact with that tissue. The action of this drug in gout was described on page 646.

Contraindications. Phenylbutazone is contraindicated in peptic ulcer or dyspepsia. It causes sodium and water retention; hence it should not be used in congestive heart failure or hypertension. Since the drug may also produce agranulocytosis and other blood dyscrasias, examination of the blood, especially the white blood cells, should be made at frequent intervals. Skin rash and other side effects may occur.

Preparation

Phenylbutazone Tablets (Enteric   100 mg.
Coated)
                          Trade name: Butazolidin

Oxyphenbutazone (Tandearil)

This analog of phenylbutazone and one of its metabolites has anti-inflammatory properties similar to those of the parent compound. It is used in rheumatoid and osteoarthritis, acute gout, bursitis, tendon inflammation, acute superficial thrombophlebitis, and certain types of inflammation caused by infections. Side effects and cautions discussed in the text for phenylbutazone also apply to this derivative.

Dosage.   Initial daily dosage in adults ranges from 300 to 600 mg. in divided doses, with 100 to 400 mg. daily being used for maintenance.

Preparation

Oxyphenbutazone Tablets   100 mg.

Trade name: Tandearil

GOLD THERAPY

Gold salts have been used in the treatment of arthritis since 1907. They have some value for selected, carefully supervised cases of progressive rheumatoid arthritis that are not relieved by older and safer methods of treatment. Although corticotropin, cortisone, hydrocortisone, and now chloroquine are presently the drugs of choice in the treatment of arthritis, gold, in the form of gold and sodium thiosulfate, gold sodium thiomalate (Myochrysine), and aurothioglucose, is still used as an adjunct or as an alternative by some physicians. Gold sodium thiomalate appears to be the most generally used gold salt.

Gold Sodium Thiomalate, N.F.; Sodium Aurothiomalate, B.P. (Myochrysine); Other Gold Salts

Gold sodium thiomalate is a soluble salt containing 50 per cent gold in organic combination. In the treatment of arthritis, 10 to 15 mg. of the drug are injected intramuscularly to see if the patient is allergic to the drug. If not, 25 to 50 mg. are injected intramuscularly at weekly intervals until 500 to 2000 mg. have been administered. A minimum of two courses is usually given, with a 6- to 12-week interval, depending on how well the patient tolerates the drug. Gold salts are given in the gluteus maximus intramuscularly rather than in the arm or thigh as there may be a discoloration of the skin upon exposure to the sun.

The untoward effects with gold therapy are erythema, pruritus, stomatitis, and skin rash. Very serious reactions to gold salts are renal irritation, ulcerative enteritis, hepatitis and blood dyscrasias such as thrombocytopenia, agranulocytosis, and aplastic anemia. Because of the seriousness of these reactions, gold salts should be used very cautiously. Patients receiving these drugs should have frequent blood and urine studies performed. If any of the untoward effects occur, the drugs should be withheld.

Dimercaptopropanol (BAL) is useful in relieving the toxic effects of gold salts, perhaps by increasing their urinary excretion.

Preparations

Gold Sodium Thiomalate Injection, N.F.; Injection of Sodium Aurothiomalate, B.P.	1-ml. ampuls containing 10, 25, 50, and 100 mg. of gold sodium thiomalate, equivalent to 5, 12.5, 25, and 50 mg. of gold, respectively

Trade name: Myochrysine

Sterile Gold Sodium Thiosulfate, N.F.	1-ml. vials containing 10, 25, 50, 75, and 100 mg. (powder)
Aurothioglucose Injection, N.F.	10, 25, 50, and 100 mg. in 1 ml.

Trade name: Solganol

PAIN-RELIEVING DRUGS

Relief of pain in arthritis may be obtained with the salicylates, which have many effects in common with the adrenocorticosteroids. Aspirin has long been the drug of choice but is reported to be associated with chronic mild blood loss unless taken with meals. It is given orally in doses of 300 mg. with a range of 300 mg. to 1.2 Gm. three or four times a day. One milligram of menadione, or calcium succinate in doses of one half that of aspirin, is given to reduce hypoprothrombinemia. A combination of aspirin, phenacetin, and caffeine in a single tablet is available (A.S.A. Compound, Empirin, Falgos, A.P.S.) (see p. 284); a dose of one or two tablets is given three or four times a day. Heat, massage, and proper exercise may improve the circulation and the patient's comfort. Codeine phosphate, 30 mg., three or four times a day, may be taken with aspirin and the combination products when the pain is severe. These measures are sometimes recommended for lengthy trial before starting regimens of steroids, gold therapy, phenylbutazone, chloroquine, or hydroxychloroquine.

GOUT AND GOUTY ARTHRITIS

This condition was described on page 646 as a disorder of uric acid metabolism, with higher levels of this acid in the blood, joints, and other tissues. The uricosuric agents, probenecid, sulfinpyrazone, zoxazolamine, and phenylbutazone have already been discussed. The salicylates can double the excretion of uric acid at high doses such as 5 Gm. (75 grains) or more daily.

At least one experimental drug, DON, a leucine derivative, has been found to suppress the production of uric acid in patients with gout. Toxicity may preclude its widespread use, but other agents may be found that will be suitable for this specific activity.

The anti-inflammatory steroids and ACTH can control acute painful exacerbations of gout. Older agents, cinchophen and neocinchophen, were used for "mobilizing" uric acid but are seldom used now. One final and important drug is worthy of description: colchicine.

Colchicine, U.S.P., B.P., I.P.

Colchicine is an anti-inflammatory drug that is very prompt in relieving the agonizing pain in the acute attack of gout. It is more effective in the acute attack than in chronic gout. There is no adequate explanation for its action in this disease. The drug is not an analgesic and it does not change the renal threshold for uric acid, nor does it dissolve the tophi. In an acute attack the usual oral dose is 0.5 mg. every hour until the pain is relieved or signs of toxicity such as nausea, vomiting, and diarrhea appear. Usually six to eight doses are required. It has been found that the prophylactic use of colchicine will decrease the frequency and severity of acute attacks. Tolerance does not develop. Colchicine is often administered with aspirin or ACTH.

Other Actions of Colchicine. Colchicine stops mitotic cell division and has a greater specificity for cancer than for normal cells. Much work is being done at present to modify the drug to obtain a new substance that will make cancer cells more susceptible to x-rays.

Toxicity. Colchicine is irritating to the gastrointestinal tract, and in acute poisoning, the symptoms are severe abdominal pain, nausea, vomiting, and bloody diarrhea. There is marked capillary dilatation and shock may occur. The pulse is weak and rapid. The kidneys may be injured with resultant hematuria and oliguria (scanty urine). Death may result from paralysis of the respiration.

Long-continued administration of the drug may cause agranulocytosis, aplastic anemia, and peripheral neuritis.

The treatment of overdosage is symptomatic. Gastric lavage is indicated. Atropine and morphine are given to relieve pain. Artificial respiration and respiratory and circulatory stimulants are administered.

Preparation

Colchicine Tablets, U.S.P., B.P. (I.P.)   0.5 and 0.6 mg.

REVIEW QUESTIONS

1. *What are the actions of endogenous (internally secreted) hydrocortisone under normal conditions?*
2. *What are the actions of aldosterone and of desoxycorticosterone?*
3. *Discuss the various effects of exogenous (administered) ACTH, hydrocortisone, cortisone, or a newer derivative among the anti-inflammatory steroids.*
4. *Name as many diseases as you can which are amenable to the effects of these steroids.*
5. *Discuss the type of amelioration of diseases which these agents produce. Compare this general type with the specific curative feature in eradicating pneumonia with an antibiotic.*
6. *How many times more potent than cortisone are hydrocortisone, prednisone, prednisolone, methylprednisolone, triamcinolone, and dexamethasone? Make your own computations from the table of dosage equivalents on page 687.*

7. *What are the absolute contraindications of the use of the compounds mentioned in question 6?*
8. *What side effects may be produced in any use of these agents? What is Cushing's disease?*
9. *Name all the agents described in this chapter which could be reasonably used in the treatment of Addison's disease.*
10. *If you should develop rheumatoid arthritis with typical joint swelling, tenderness, mild fever, etc., how would you want your first episode treated? What would be the advantages and disadvantages of the many classes of drugs used in this disease?*
11. *Describe briefly the biochemical abnormality in gout and the mode of action of the following agents in this condition: salicylates (high doses), phenylbutazone, probenecid, sulfinpyrazone, colchicine, ACTH, prednisone or a congener, and DON.*
12. *What purpose does the inner, medullary portion of the adrenal glands serve (see Chap. 27)?*

REFERENCES

ACTH AND CORTICOSTEROIDS

Cope, C. L.: "Principles of Modern Steroid Therapy," *Brit. M. J.*, **1**:1583, 1959.
Council on Drugs: "The Use and Abuse of Adrenal Steroids," *J.A.M.A.*, **170**:951, 1959.
Dordick, J. R., and Bernstein, Z. L.: "Intra-Articular Administration of Triamcinolone," *New York J. Med.*, **59**:3393, 1959.
Feinberg, S. M.; Feinberg, A. R.; and Fisherman, E. W.: "Triamcinolone (Aristocort), New Corticosteroid Hormone," *J.A.M.A.*, **167**:58, 1958.
Frohman, I. Phillips: "The Steroids," *Am. Med. J.*, **59**:518, 1959.
Hollander, J. L.: "Clinical Use of Dexamethasone: Role in Treatment of Patients with Arthritis," *J.A.M.A.*, **172**:306, 1960.
Stresemann, E.: "The Dosage of Dexamethasone and Triamcinolone in Bronchial Asthma," *Lancet*, **2**:257, 1959.

ADDITIONAL ANTI-ARTHRITIS AGENTS

Council on Drugs: "Additional Uses of Chloroquine (Aralen) Phosphate," *J.A.M.A.*, **171**:1504, 1959.
Dall, J. L. C., and Keane, J. A.: "Disturbances of Pigmentation with Chloroquine," *Brit. M. J.*, **1**:1387, 1959.
Fuld, H., and Horwich, L.: "Treatment of Rheumatoid Arthritis with Chloroquine," *Brit. M. J.*, **2**:1199, 1958.
Ogryzlo, M. A., and Franklin, E. C.: "Rheumatoid Factor," *Bull. Rheum. Dis.*, **10**:207, 1960.
"Salicylates in the Treatment of Rheumatoid Arthritis" (editorial), *South. M. J.*, **49**:304, 1956.
Strauss, J. F.; Barrett, R. M.; and Rosenberg, E. F.: "BAL Treatment of Toxic Reactions to Gold," *Ann. Int. Med.*, **37**:323, 1952.
Weissmann, G., and Xefteris, E. D.: "Phenylbutazone Leukopenia," *A.M.A. Arch. Int. Med.*, **103**:957, 1959.

Young, J. P.: "Chloroquine Phosphate (Aralen) in the Long-Term Treatment of Rheumatoid Arthritis," *Ann. Int. Med.*, **51**:1159, 1959.

ANTI-GOUT AGENTS

Ferguson, F. C., Jr.: "Colchicine, I. General Pharmacology," *J. Pharmacol. and Exper. Therap.*, **106**:261, 1952.

Reed, E. B.; Feichtmeir, T. V.; and Willett, F. M.: "Zoxazolamine—A Potent Uricosuric Agent," *New England J. Med.*, **258**:894, 1958.

42

Calcium and Phosphorus Metabolism and Vitamin D

Calcium is present in the intracellular and extracellular fluids in a delicately regulated balance with sodium, potassium, and magnesium ions. Calcium ions are essential to the body for (1) growth and formation of bone and teeth, (2) clotting of blood, (3) skeletal and smooth-muscle contraction, (4) control of excitability of nerve centers, (5) maintenance of tonicity, rhythm, and contractility of the heart, (6) for selectivity permeability, and (7) as a constituent for intracellular cement. The average adult requirement of calcium is about 800 mg. daily. In children, and during pregnancy and lactation, more is needed. This amount is normally supplied in the diet. However, absorption from the intestinal tract depends upon a correct ratio of dietary calcium to phosphorus (2:1) and an adequate intake of vitamin D. An alkaline reaction or the presence of large amounts of fatty acids in the intestinal tract will decrease absorption. Calcium ions are excreted in the feces and urine.

Only a small portion of the calcium ingested orally enters the blood, where it is present both as calcium ions and nondiffusible (protein bound) calcium. Only the ionic form is physiologically active. The calcium level in the blood is maintained within certain permissible limits. The kidney plays an important role in maintaining this level by regulating the urinary excretion of calcium.

The greatest amount of calcium is found in the bone in the form of calcium phosphate and carbonate which is in dynamic equilibrium with that of the body fluids. An adequate intake of vitamins D and C and the functional integrity of the parathyroid glands are necessary for normal calcium metabolism.

Abnormalities in Calcium Metabolism. When there is an inadequate intake of calcium or during times of increased requirement, such as in infancy, the bones give up calcium ions to the blood. Even slight variations above or below the required amount of calcium ions in the blood (hypocalcemia or hypercalcemia) produce toxic signs and symptoms.

Hypocalcemia may be produced by hypoparathyroidism, severe vitamin D deficiency, or low calcium intake. It causes low calcium tetany, rickets in

698

infants, and osteomalacia in adults. The heart may stop in diastole due to the predominance of potassium ions.

The four small parathyroid glands, which are found closely associated with the thyroid gland located in the neck, play an important role in calcium-phosphorus metabolism. The removal or disease of these glands causes an immediate reduction in the calcium level in the blood and tissues. This reduction in calcium causes neuromuscular spasm and symptoms known as tetany. These symptoms are abolished by the injection of soluble calcium salts or an extract of the parathyroid glands. The parathyroid extract increases the serum calcium level by mobilizing calcium from the tissues and bones. Some investigators believe that this calcium mobilization is effected by increased urinary excretion of phosphorus.

CLINICAL TETANY

In adults, the symptoms of tetany are those resulting from nervous excitability and are largely confined to the hands and feet. Paresthesias in the extremities, muscle spasms, and, in severe cases, generalized convulsions may occur. Tachycardia and vascular spasm of the fingers and toes have been observed.

In infants, the disease is associated with calcium deficiency, rickets, severe gastrointestinal disturbances, and alkalosis. When spasms are more generalized, the condition is called *spasmophilia.*

Tetany is treated with the intravenous injection of 1 Gm. of calcium gluconate or another calcium salt. Simultaneously, parathyroid injection is administered intravenously. Vitamin D as well as a diet rich in calcium is also prescribed.

Parathyroid Injection, U.S.P.

Parathyroid injection is a sterile aqueous solution of the water-soluble hormone of the parathyroid glands. To relieve the symptoms of tetany, the intramuscular dose of parathyroid injection is 40 U.S.P. units (20 to 100 units) every 12 hours.

Preparation

Parathyroid Injection, U.S.P.   100 U.S.P. units in 1 ml., 500 units
                                        in 5 ml.

Trade names: Paroidin; Sodium Parathyroid Hormones; Solution of Parathyroid
                            Extract

CALCIUM SALTS

Calcium salts are specific for the emergency treatment of low-calcium tetany. In severe conditions the salts are administered intravenously. Milder symptoms or latent tetany may be controlled by oral administration. Calcium is primarily absorbed in the upper gastrointestinal tract in an acid medium, and at times hydrochloric acid may be given with it to promote absorption. When intravenous administration is necessary, calcium must be injected very slowly so that it may be well diluted, as large amounts in the blood will cause systolic arrest. Calcium salts are administered orally as antacids.

Calcium Chloride, U.S.P., B.P.

Calcium chloride is administered orally and intravenously in doses of 1 Gm. (1 to 2 Gm.) four times a day. The intravenous dose of 5 to 20 ml. of a 5 per cent solution is injected slowly, as it may be irritating to the veins. Care must be taken to see that none of the solution extravasates into the surrounding tissue, as this is very painful and may cause sloughing. Injections of calcium chloride cause peripheral vasodilatation and thus a fall in blood pressure may accompany its administration. Irritation of the gastrointestinal tract may also occur upon oral administration. Milk may be given with calcium salts.

Preparations

Calcium Chloride Injection, U.S.P.   1 Gm. in 10 ml.
Calcium Chloride Tablets

Calcium Gluconate, U.S.P., B.P., I.P.

Calcium gluconate is the calcium salt of choice. The oral dose is 5 Gm. (1 to 30 Gm.) three times a day. The intravenous or intramuscular dose of 1 Gm. (0.2 to 1 Gm.) is repeated daily. It is nonirritating to the gastrointestinal tract and the subcutaneous tissues.

Preparations

Calcium Gluconate Injection, U.S.P.,   1 Gm. in 10 ml.
B.P. (I.P.)
Calcium Gluconate Tablets, U.S.P.   500 mg and 1 Gm.
(I.P.)

Calcium Levulinate

Calcium levulinate is administered orally or intravenously. The adult oral dose is 4 to 5 Gm. three times a day, with each meal. The intravenous dose is 1 Gm. daily or on alternate days.

Preparations

Powder Calcium Levulinate   10-ml. ampuls containing 100 mg. in
Calcium Levulinate Injection   1 ml.

Other Calcium Salts

Calcium lactate and calcium carbonate are also employed in the treatment of low-calcium tetany. Both salts can be used only orally.

Dihydrotachysterol, U.S.P. (A.T. 10, Hytakerol)

Dihydrotachysterol is produced by the irradiation of ergosterol by ultraviolet light. Its action resembles that of the parathyroid hormone; i.e., it causes a mobilization of calcium by increasing urinary phosphate excretion. However, unlike the parathyroid hormone, dihydrotachysterol increases the absorption of calcium from the gastrointestinal tract. The drug is administered orally in doses of 1.25 mg. (0.625 to 6.25 mg.) daily for several days with oral calcium salts.

Toxicity. Symptoms of overdosage are hypercalcemia, loss of appetite, nausea, vomiting, renal calculi, and stupor. The symptoms disappear when the drug is discontinued.

Preparations

Dihydrotachysterol Capsules   0.625 mg. dissolved in oil
Dihydrotachysterol Solution (Oil)   1.25 mg. in 1 ml.
Trade names: A.T. 10; Hytakerol; Dichystolum; Tachystol; Calcamine (in oil)

Hypercalcemia may be caused by hyperparathyroidism (tumors of the parathyroid glands), hypervitaminosis D, physical immobilization, or the oral and intravenous administration of calcium salts. The signs and symptoms are anorexia, nausea, polyuria, headache, kidney stones, and tissue calcification. The heart may stop in systole. Initially an excess of calcium ions causes bradycardia, sinus arrhythmias, and various degrees of heart block. This action resembles that of digitalis.

Disodium Edetate (Endrate), a chelating agent (see p. 778), will remove calcium from the blood and tissues. It is used in hypercalcemia, corneal calcification, and digitalis poisoning for the removal of calcium. The dose of 50 mg. per kilogram (to a maximum of 3 Gm.) in 500 ml. of a 5 per cent dextrose solution is infused intravenously over three to four hours.

Toxicity. Hypocalcemia and a deposit of calcium in the kidney may result from the withdrawal of calcium from the blood and tissues.

Preparation

Disodium Edetate Solution   150 mg. in 1 ml. in 20-ml. ampuls
Trade names: Sodium Versenate, Endrate

For the prevention of urinary calculi and the treatment of hypercalcinuria, see pages 648–49.

PHOSPHORUS METABOLISM

Inorganic phosphorus in the diet, which averages about 1.5 Gm. daily, is the source of phosphate in the body. More is required for growing children and during pregnancy and lactation. It is slowly absorbed and circulates in the blood as dibasic and monobasic ions which are excreted mainly in the urine.

The phosphate ion performs a variety of functions in the body. It is essential for the formation of bone and teeth and for the regulation of calcium metabolism and the calcium ion level of the blood. It is used in the synthesis of phospholipids, nucleic acids, and membrane constituents of nerve and muscle tissues; a variety of coenzymes are also phosphorus compounds. The phosphate ions contribute to buffer systems throughout the body and phosphorylation is important in various processes involved in intermediary metabolism and energy transfer through high-energy phosphates such as ATP (see p. 94).

PHOSPHORUS DEFICIENCY

When there is a phosphorus deficiency due to inadequate phosphorus in the diet or a vitamin D deficiency, the bones fail to calcify. The control of calcium and phosphorus metabolism is dependent on adequate supplies of vitamin D.

Vitamin D

"Vitamin D" is the name applied to two or more fat-soluble substances that control the adequate utilization of calcium and phosphorus in the body. Two forms of vitamin D are available: calciferol, or vitamin D_2, which is one of the products of irradiated ergosterol; and vitamin D_3, which is obtained by the irradiation of 7-dehydrocholesterol. Other substances, upon irradiation, also have vitamin D activity. Vitamin D_2, vitamin D_3, and other products of irradiated ergosterol possess *antirachitic* properties. These vitamins promote the absorption of calcium ions from the intestines.

Pharmacological Actions.   With regard to phosphate metabolism, the principal action of vitamin D is to increase the inorganic phosphates in the blood. Vitamin D also causes tricalcium phosphate to be deposited in the bones. Both vitamin D and the parathyroid hormone produce hypercalcemia. However, the action of the hormone is at the expense of the bone, which is demineralized. Vitamin D increases the amount of calcium absorbed and diminishes urinary secretion. Spasmophilia, resulting from hypocalcemia, which is often associated with rickets, is cured with vitamin D.

Use of Vitamin D in Rickets.   Rickets is a disease of childhood associated with a lowered phosphate blood level that prevents ossification of the skeleton and thus causes a deformity of the bones. Vitamin D will obliterate the symptoms of the disease. The underlying cause of rickets and the mechanism of action of vitamin D are not clear. In rickets there are an increase in urinary excretion of phosphorus; a decrease in plasma phosphate; and an increase in the enzyme phosphatase, which is diagnostic of the disease.

The average curative dose of vitamin D in rickets is 1200 to 1500 units (30 to 37.5 mcg.) daily. The administration of the vitamin should be accompanied by adequate calcium and phosphorus in the daily diet. Exposure to sunlight is helpful. Prophylactic doses of the vitamin in infants are from 400 to 800 units daily.

Other Uses of Vitamin D.   Vitamin D is used in the treatment of osteomalacia in adults, during pregnancy and lactation, and to stimulate or accelerate healing of fractures.

Symptoms of Overdosage.   The early symptoms of poisoning are loss of appetite, nausea, vomiting, diarrhea, drowsiness, and headache. Later symptoms are calcium deposits in the kidneys and nephritis. Circulatory collapse may occur due to hypercalcemia, which increases the viscosity of the blood.

Ergocalciferol, U.S.P. (Vitamin D$_2$), Calciferol, B.P., I.P. (Drisdol)

Ergocalciferol is a crystalline vitamin D preparation obtained from the irradiation of ergosterol. It is used to fortify natural fish liver oils with vitamin D, or it can be dispensed in oil solutions to provide only vitamin D. The usual daily requirement is 400 units (10 mcg.). In rickets the dose is 1200 to 5000 units (30 to 125 mcg.), and in hypocalcemic tetany the dose is up to 200,000 units (5 mg.). Solutions in oil, capsules, and a solution in propylene glycol are available for oral administration.

Preparations

Ergocalciferol Capsules, U.S.P.	1.25 mg. (50,000 U.S.P. vitamin D units)
Ergocalciferol Solution, U.S.P.	0.25 mg. (10,000 U.S.P. vitamin D units) in 1 Gm. vegetable oil or in propylene glycol

Trade names: Drisdol; Davitin; Deltalin; Deratol; Diactol; Doral; D-Vatine; 'D' Vitamin; Entron; Hi-Deratol; Infron Pediatric; Sterogyl
Synonyms: Ergocalciferol; Vigantol

Cholecalciferol (Vitamin D$_3$), U.S.P.

Cholecalciferol is a crystalline compound prepared synthetically through the irradiation of 7-dehydrocholesterol. Its actions, therapeutic uses, and doses are similar to those of calciferol.

Concentrated Vitamin D Solution, B.P. (Viosterol in Oil)

Synthetic oleovitamin D is a solution of calciferol or activated 7-dehydrocholesterol in an edible vegetable oil. The daily requirement is 10 mcg. (400 U.S.P. units) of vitamin D. In rickets the dose is 30 to 37.5 mcg. (1200 to

1500 U.S.P. units), whereas in hypercalcamia it is 5 mg. (200,000 U.S.P. units).

Preparations of Vitamins A and D

Concentrates of fish liver oils and concentrates of vitamins A and D are used to make preparations containing both vitamins.

Oleovitamin A and D, N.F.; Concentrated Vitamins A and D Solutions, B.P. Oleovitamin A and D is either fish liver oil, or fish liver oil diluted with an edible vegetable oil, or a solution of vitamin A and D concentrates in either fish liver oil or an edible vegetable oil. The vitamins come from either natural or synthetic sources. The official preparation is used as a source of vitamins A and D and is equivalent in strength to Cod Liver Oil, N.F., and Concentrated Oleovitamin A and D Capsules, N.F., are also available.

Cod Liver Oil (Oleum Morrhuae), N.F. The usual oral dose is 4 ml. (4 to 16 ml.), containing 900 mcg. (3000 U.S.P. units) of vitamin A and 7.5 mcg. (300 U.S.P. units) of vitamin D.

Non-destearinated Cod Liver Oil, N.F. Non-destearinated cod liver oil contains in each gram not less than 850 U.S.P. units of vitamin A and not less than 85 U.S.P. units of vitamin D.

Halibut Liver Oil, N.F., B.P., I.P. The usual daily oral dose is 0.1 ml. (1.5 mg. [5000 U.S.P. units of vitamin A]). The N.F. capsules contain either 5000 or 25,000 units of vitamin A.

Burbot Liver Oil. Burbot liver oil has a potency of not less than 4880 U.S.P. units of vitamin A and not less than 640 U.S.P. units of vitamin D per gram. It is available as capsules.

Percomorph Liver Oil. Percomorph liver oil contains not less than 60,000 U.S.P. units of vitamin A and not less than 8500 U.S.P. units of vitamin D in each gram. Percomorph liver oil with other fish oils and viosterol is available as capsules that supply 5000 units of vitamin A and 700 units of vitamin D.

REVIEW QUESTIONS

1. *Discuss the function of the parathyroid glands. Discuss the syndrome of hypoparathyroidism with tetany. How can the condition be treated?*
2. *Name a few calcium preparations and their dosage.*
3. *What is the relationship of vitamin D to calcium metabolism and bone formation?*
4. *List as many preparations as you can which supply the vitamin D function and give their doses.*

REFERENCES

THE PARATHYROIDS

Bartter, F. C.: "The Parathyroids," *Ann. Rev. Physiol.*, **16**:429, 1954.

CALCIUM AND PHOSPHORUS METABOLISM

Cantarow, A.: "Mineral Metabolism," in Duncan, G. G. (ed.) : *Diseases of Metabolism*, 3rd ed. W. B. Saunders Company, Philadelphia, 1952, p. 260.

Hollinger, H. Z., and Pattie, C. J.: "A Review of Normal Calcium and Phosphorus Metabolism," *Canad. M. A. J.*, **74**:912, 1956.

Nicolaysen, R.; Eeg-Larsen, N.; and Malm, O. J.: "Physiology of Calcium Metabolism," *Physiol. Rev.*, **33**:424, 1953.

43

Vitamins Used in Therapy and Dietary Supplements

Vitamins are organic compounds present in minute amounts in natural foods. They are not, as a rule, synthesized by the animal body; rather, they must be supplied in the diet of man and animals for normal growth, development, nutrition, and maintenance of life. Many vitamins serve as integral parts (coenzymes) of enzyme systems that are essential for carbohydrate, fat, and amino acid metabolism and for the storage of metabolic energy in the compound adenosine triphosphate (ATP). ATP then, under the influence of coenzymes, releases this energy to the cells for many physiological activities such as muscle contraction and transmission of nerve impulses. Coenzymes also play an important part in reactions involving the utilization of amino acids and the synthesis of such compounds as epinephrine, thyroxin, and histamine.

Although the vitamins function physiologically as nutrients, they are often used in order to prevent and cure disease and in this sense may be classed as drugs.

In 1881, Dr. N. Lunin found that a diet consisting entirely of purified foods would not sustain life unless milk was added. What we now call "vitamins" were first named "accessory factors" (by Dr. Frederick Hopkins, in 1906) because, in addition to normal foods (carbohydrates, proteins, fats, minerals, and water), minute traces of these substances were found to be essential to health. Their lack or deficiency in the diet was discovered to cause deficiency diseases, which can be cured by their administration; the curative effects of specific diets in beriberi, scurvy, rickets, and night blindness are well known. Dr. Casimir Funk, an early worker in this field, believed that the antiberiberi factor he isolated from rice polishings was an *amine,* and he proposed the term *vitamine* to stress the fact that these substances were essential to life and not accessory factors. Later, when it was found that the amine group was not present in all the compounds, the name was changed to *vitamin.* Funk, a far-seeing scientist, suggested that many diseases result from the absence of these indispensable dietary factors. Modern medicine has substantiated his ideas.

Vitamin-deficiency diseases are widespread throughout the world, although they are rare in the United States. Subclinical deficiencies are even more prevalent, and these do occur frequently in the United States. They are found

706

in persons on a restricted diet or in whom abnormal conditions prevent adequate absorption. In conditions of stress (e.g., during pregnancy and lactation; in infants and growing children), in various diseases, and during comvalescence where larger amounts of vitamins are required, supplemental vitamin therapy is indicated. In old age, vitamin deficiency may occur because of poor appetite, refusal to eat a well-balanced diet, or an inadequate diet. There is general evidence that improved nutrition lengthens the useful and active period of a person's life, delays senility, and shortens the period of illness and convalescence.

The first classification of vitamins was made on the basis of solubility, and they were called *oil-soluble* and *water-soluble* vitamins. Then they were classified according to the disorders resulting from their deficiencies—for example, *antirachitic, antihemorrhagic,* and *antiscorbutic* vitamins. The next classification was based on priority of discovery, and different letters of the alphabet were assigned to the compounds as soon as they were described and isolated; names such as vitamin C and vitamin D are often used. The modern trend is to call these substances by their chemical names, such as thiamine (vitamin B_1) and ascorbic acid (vitamin C).

Many useful vitamins have been isolated from natural sources, and most of these have been synthesized and are available for clinical use. The potency of vitamin preparations is expressed in units. A unit is the biological activity of a specific quantity of a respective standard. These standards are made available by the United States Pharmacopeial Convention and the United Nations, and the U.S.P. and international units are identical in value. Man's daily requirement is generally expressed in milligrams of the pure substance, and the dose of most of the vitamins is given in milligrams or micrograms.

All vitamins work together to maintain optimal conditions of health in the body. A severe deficiency of one vitamin may interfere with the functioning of others. Therefore, multivitamin preparations containing a combination of a number of vitamins are often prescribed.

WATER-SOLUBLE VITAMINS

The water-soluble group of vitamins includes the vitamin B complex and vitamin C.

Vitamin B Complex

The vitamin B complex is a group of compounds that, although unrelated chemically, are often found together in food. The vitamins of this group discussed in this chapter are thiamine, riboflavin, nicotinic acid, pyridoxine, pantothenic acid, biotin, p-aminobenzoic acid, choline, and inositol. Biotin is the only substance not used in therapeutics. Two other members of this complex, folic acid and cyanocobalamin (vitamin B_{12}), both of which are concerned with the formation of red blood cells and are used in the treatment of anemia, are discussed in Chapter 31.

Thiamine (Vitamin B_1)

Thiamine is widely distributed in nature. It occurs in brewer's yeast, wheat germ, meat (pork), liver, milk, vegetables, and fruit. It is also prepared synthetically.

Thiamine plays an important role in the carbohydrate metabolism of all living cells. It is phosphorylated in the liver to form cocarboxylase, a coenzyme that is essential for the decarboxylation of pyruvic acid. When thiamine is absent in the diet, or when it is not absorbed, owing to various disease conditions, lactic and pyruvic acids accumulate in the brain, blood, and urine. It is probable that this impaired carbohydrate metabolism may be the cause of the nerve damage and other symptoms of thiamine deficiency.

Thiamine Deficiency. Beriberi is a metabolic disease that results from a lack or deficiency of thiamine in the diet. It is widespread in the Orient, but it is seldom seen in the United States except in chronic alcoholism. The symptoms of beriberi are multiple peripheral neuritis, cardiovascular changes, generalized edema, paralysis, and muscular atrophy. The heart enlarges, and death may result from heart failure. In certain parts of the Orient, a dramatic decrease in the incidence of the disease has resulted from spraying rice with thiamine chloride.

In the United States the disease occurs in a milder form (subclinical beriberi), the symptoms of which are loss of appetite, weakness, fatigue, dizziness, headache, irritability, muscular aches and pains, indigestion, sleeplessness, and mental depression.

Absorption and Excretion. Thiamine is readily absorbed from the gastrointestinal tract. The adult daily requirement is from 1 to 1.6 mg.; for children, 0.3 to 1.9 mg. Thiamine is not stored in appreciable amounts; consequently, deficiency symptoms may appear in 10 to 30 days. There are no known untoward effects with massive doses, since excessive amounts are excreted in the urine. Urinary excretion is used to determine the nutritional requirement and adequate absorption.

Dosage and Methods of Administration. Thiamine is usually administered orally. In the presence of persistent vomiting and diarrhea, it may be given subcutaneously or intravenously. The oral or subcutaneous daily therapeutic dose is 2 to 50 mg. A combination of B vitamins is sometimes more satisfactory than thiamine alone.

Therapeutic Uses. Thiamine is used in (1) beriberi, (2) polyneuritis caused by chronic alcoholism, (3) pregnancy and pernicious vomiting of pregnancy, (4) nervous disorders, (5) anorexia (loss of appetite due to vitamin B_1 deficiency), (6) cardiovascular manifestations of vitamin B_1 deficiency, and (7) irradiation sickness, to relieve nausea and vomiting.

Preparations

Thiamine Hydrochloride Injection, U.S.P.; Aneurine Hydrochloride Injection, B.P.	25 mg. in 1 ml.; 1 Gm. in 10 ml.; 3 Gm. in 30 ml.
Thiamine Hydrochloride Tablets U.S.P.; Aneurine Hydrochloride Tablets, B.P.	5, 10, 25, 50, and 100 mg.
Thiamine Mononitrate Tablets	3, 5, 10, and 25 mg.

Trade names: Anti-beri or Antineuritic Vitamin; Berocea; Betabion; Betalin; Betaxin; Bewon

Riboflavin (Vitamin B_2), U.S.P.; Riboflavine, B.P. (I.P.)

Riboflavin is an orange or yellow crystalline substance that is present in liver, yeast, leafy vegetables, and eggs and milk (the "protective foods"). The vitamin is also synthesized. It is converted in the tissues to riboflavin phosphate, which, in turn, combines with proteins to form *flavoproteins* (yellow enzymes). These latter substances play an important role in the oxidation-reduction reactions in cells. Hydrogen is removed from the substrate by a *coenzyme* (nicotinamide nucleotide) under the influence of dehydrogenase. The substrate in oxidized, and the coenzyme is reduced. The yellow enzymes, which are known as *transporting enzymes*, accept hydrogen from the coenzyme and thus become reduced. This reduced form can be oxidized spontaneously in the presence of oxygen to form hydrogen peroxide, which, in the presence of *catalase*, forms water. Thus, the substrate is oxidized, water is formed, and some oxygen is liberated in the process. The coenzymes and flavoproteins are then available for further oxidation-reduction reactions.

Riboflavin Deficiency.   A dietary deficiency of riboflavin causes *ariboflavinosis*. The typical symptoms in man are glossitis; visual fatigue; burning eyes; soreness and swelling of the eyelids; dermatitis; superficial fissures at the angles of the nose and mouth; and redness, swelling, and cracking of the lips (cheilosis). In rats, there are loss of hair, failure to grow, and development of cataracts. In dogs, the symptoms are loss of weight, vomiting, and diarrhea. Death may follow.

Absorption and Excretion.   Riboflavin is readily absorbed from the gastrointestinal tract; hence there is rarely need for parenteral administration. The vitamin is mainly excreted in the kidneys. It is nontoxic.

Dosage and Methods of Administration.   Riboflavin is usually administered orally. It may also be administered subcutaneously. The daily requirement is 2 mg. for adults and from 0.4 to 2.5 mg. for children. The therapeutic daily dose is 5 mg. (2 to 10 mg.) orally or subcutaneously. After severe burns, injury, or illness, the daily requirement may be increased five to ten times.

Therapeutic Uses.   Riboflavin is used in the treatment of ariboflavinosis and, with nicotinic acid or nicotinamide, in the treatment of pellagra.

Preparations

Riboflavin Injection, U.S.P.	50 and 100 mg. in 10 ml.
Riboflavin Tablets, U.S.P. (B.P.)	5 and 10 mg.
Solution Methylol Riboflavin	1-ml. ampuls and 10-ml. vials containing 10 mg. in 1 ml.

Trade names: Flavaxin; Hyflavin; Ovoflavin
Synonyms: Lactoflavin; Vitamin G

Niacin, N.F., B.P., I.P.

Niacin is obtained from yeast, liver, peanuts, meat, and rice. It is also made synthetically. The vitamin is converted in the body to nicotinamide, which is an essential part of the enzyme system concerned with hydrogen transport (oxidation) in the living cell. It is the functional group of two coenzymes: codehydrogenase I (NAD) and codehydrogenase II (NADP). These coenzymes accept hydrogen from certain metabolites and transfer it to flavoproteins.

Niacin Deficiency.   Niacin is an essential dietary constituent, a lack or deficiency of which will cause *pellagra* in man and *black tongue* in the dog. Both conditions may be corrected by the administration of the acid (niacin) or nicotinamide.

Pellagra occurs in areas where people ingest a great deal of corn in a very inadequate diet. The condition may be the result of faulty diet or poor absorption of the vitamin from the gastrointestinal tract. It is characterized by skin lesions on all exposed parts of the body, such as the hands, neck, and face. There is reddening of the skin followed by a rough, scaly, or ulcerated dermatitis. The mouth and tongue become red and sore. The mucous membranes of the nose, throat, and gastrointestinal tract become inflamed, and diarrhea and vomiting occur. There is loss of weight and strength. Nervous symptoms such as malaise, irritability, anxiety, confusion, and even dementia may result.

Pellagra is treated by the administration of niacin or niacinamide (nicotinamide). Thiamine and riboflavin are also indicated, since pellagra is a multiple-deficiency disease. A high-protein diet is important because of evidence that tryptophan, an essential amino acid, is converted to nicotinamide in the body. Severe pellagra, once very common in the southern area of the United States, has practically disappeared during the last few years as a result of better diets and increased scientific knowledge. The adequate daily requirement for either niacin or nicotinamide appears to be 20 mg. for adults and 3 to 19 mg. for children.

Absorption and Excretion.   Both niacin and nicotinamide are readily absorbed from the gastrointestinal tract. They produce the same effects in the body and form the same metabolites, which are excreted in the urine. Both substances are relatively nontoxic.

Niacin is a peripheral vasodilator and, as such, produces marked flushing of the face and neck and a mild, transient fall in blood pressure. It is sometimes used for this effect in migraine, arthritis, and angina pectoris. Niacinamide, which does not produce vasodilation, is preferred for parenteral administration in the treatment of pellagra.

Dosage and Method of Administration. These vitamins are generally administered orally. In severe illness and early convalescence the oral or subcutaneous dose is 50 mg. three to ten times a day. The maximum therapeutic daily dose is 500 mg. in divided doses. In supplementing diets, most multivitamin preparations contain 10 to 25 mg. in each capsule.

Therapeutic Uses. Both niacin and niacinamide are used in pellagra and, in combination with other vitamins, as a dietary supplement.

Preparations

Niacin Injection, N.F., B.P. (I.P.)	100 mg. in 10-ml. ampuls
Niacin Tablets, N.F., B.P.	25, 50, and 100 mg.
Niacinamide Injection, U.S.P.	100 mg. in 2 ml., 3 and 6 Gm. in 30 ml.
Nicotinamide Injection, B.P. (I.P.)	
Niacinamide Tablets, U.S.P., Nicotin-amide Injection, B.P.	25, 50, and 100 mg.

Trade name: Nicotamide

Pyridoxine Hydrochloride, U.S.P. (Vitamin B$_6$)

Vitamin B$_6$ is found in brewer's yeast, blackstrap molasses, liver, some vegetables, meats, and milk. It is concerned with protein and fat metabolism, especially the essential fatty acids. Pyridoxal, which appears to be the active form of the vitamin, combines with phosphoric acid to form phosphorylated pyridoxal. This phosphorylated sustance serves as a prosthetic group for enzymes that effect the removal of carbon dioxide from many amino acids and the transfer of amino groups from amino acids to keto acids. The daily requirement of pyridoxine, the form present in the vegetable foods and available by synthetic production, is thought to be 1 to 2 mg. daily.

Pyridoxine Deficiency. Pyridoxine deficiency has been observed in many animals, including man. The symptoms involve the skin as well as the central nervous and erythrocytopoietic systems. In man, lesions of the skin, similar to those occurring in riboflavin and nicotinic acid deficiency, have occurred a few weeks after initiating a diet poor in vitamin B to which daily doses of a pyridoxine antagonist have been added. The lesions do not respond to the administration of a vitamin B complex that does not contain pyridoxine but do clear up quickly upon the administration of pyridoxine. In a few clinical cases, pyridoxine-deficient infants have developed convulsions and hypochromic anemia.

Dosage and Methods of Administration. Pyridoxine is administered orally, intramuscularly, or intravenously. The oral and parenteral therapeutic dose is 5 mg. daily with a usual dosage range of 1 to 100 mg.

Therapeutic Uses. Pyridoxine is used as an adjunct in vitamin B deficiency and to control nausea and vomiting of radiation sickness and during pregnancy. The mechanism of this action is not clearly understood.

Preparations

Pyridoxine Hydrochloride Injection, 500 mg. and 1 Gm. in 10 ml. U.S.P.

Pyridoxine Hydrochloride Tablets, 10, 25, and 50 mg. U.S.P.

Trade names: Adermine Hydrochloride; Beadox Hydrochloride; Bedoxine; Hexabetalin; Hexavibex; Hexabione Hydrochloride

Pantothenic Acid

Pantothenic acid is widely distributed in nature and occurs not only in food but also as a constituent of the cells of animals, bacteria, and yeast. In its phosphorylated form, as a component of coenzyme A, it influences enzymatic acetylation as well as the rate of oxidation of pyruvic acid obtained from both carbohydrate and fat metabolism. It is essential in the diet and is needed for the growth of yeast and certain bacteria.

Dosage and Method of Administration. The vitamin is administered orally in the form of calcium pantothenate. The daily dose is 10 mg. In cases of severe illness and burns, the dose is 20 mg. (10 to 50 mg.).

Preparations

Calcium Pantothenate Tablets, U.S.P. 10 mg.

Biotin

Biotin, a substance present in egg yolk and liver, is essential to all cellular life. It is readily made by the intestinal bacteria. Biotin deficiency may be induced only by inhibiting the growth of all intestinal bacteria or by feeding diets containing excessive amounts of raw egg white. The protein avidin, which is present in raw egg white, forms a stable compound with biotin and prevents its absorption. At the present time biotin is not used in therapeutics

p-Aminobenzoic Acid, N.F. (PABA)

p-Aminobenzoic acid is an essential growth factor for chicks and certain species of bacteria. PABA deficiency has not been observed in man. It is used as an antirickettsial drug in doses of 10 Gm. Tablets of 500 mg. are available.

Choline

Choline is found in muscle and glandular meats—brain, liver, kidney, heart, tongue, sweetbreads—milk, and egg yolks. It is a constituent of lecithin, which is present in all living cells, and is used in the synthesis of acetylcholine and phospholipids. The methyl groups of choline are concerned with the transfer of methyl groups from one compound to another; consequently they play an important part in intermediary metabolism. A deficiency of choline in the diet of young growing rats may cause an excessive accumulation of fat in the liver and hemorrhagic conditions in the kidneys. The fatty livers may result from a decreased formation of phospholipids, compounds that are necessary for the transportation of fats in the body.

Therapeutic Uses. Choline is used (1) as a dietary supplement and source of choline in nutritional deficiencies, especially in persons exposed to certain industrial or medical hepatotoxic substances; and (2) in the treatment of liver diseases, particularly cirrhosis. It reverses fatty infiltration of the liver and prevents further destruction of cells.

Dosage and Method of Administration. Choline is administered orally, with large amounts of water, in divided doses totaling 2 to 3 Gm. daily. Its administration accompanies a high-protein, low-fat diet.

Preparations

Choline Dihydrogen Citrate Tablets, 500 and 600 mg. N.F.

Choline Dihydrogen Citrate Capsules, 250 and 500 mg N.F.

Trade name: Lipocholine

Inositol, N.F.

This vitamin is present in liver, kidney, meat, eggs, vegetables, fruits, and cereals. It is essential for the growth of yeasts, molds, and certain bacteria; for the growth of hair. It is used with choline and methionine in (1) fatty infiltration of the liver, (2) acute and chronic hepatitis, and (3) cirrhosis. The dose is 2 Gm. daily.

Ascorbic Acid, U.S.P., B.P., Vitamin C

Ascorbic acid was first isolated from lemons. It is also present in other citrus fruits (limes, oranges, and grapefruit), tomatoes, cabbage, berries, and green leafy vegetables, and is made synthetically. Ascorbic acid is essential in the formation and maintenance of the intercellular substances (e.g., the collagen of connective tissue and capillary walls; the matrix of bone, dentin, and cartilage). The normal daily requirement is approximately 70 mg.

Ascorbic Acid Deficiency. Only man, other primates, and guinea pigs suffer from a dietary deficiency of this vitamin. Other animals can synthesize ascorbic acid and therefore do not require it in the diet. A diet lacking in ascorbic acid causes a deficiency disease known as scurvy, which can be cured by the administration of the vitamin. Scurvy is seldom seen today, but many cases of subacute or latent scurvy occur in undernourished persons. The symptoms are sore, receding gums, sore mouth, defective and loose teeth, loss of weight, weakness and fatigue, pains in the joints, anemia, and small hemorrhages in the skin and mucous membranes. Scurvy may be observed in children during the first year of life. A deficiency of the vitamin may lead to the retardation of healing of wounds and bone fractures. Diseases such as peptic ulcer, tuberculosis, rheumatic fever, hyperthyroidism, and leukemia as well as pregnancy increase the requirement for ascorbic acid.

Dosage and Methods of Administration. The daily requirement for an adult is 75 mg.; for a child, 50 mg. The daily oral or subcutaneous therapeutic dose is 500 mg. (75 mg. to 1 Gm.). The vitamin may be administered orally or subcutaneously.

Therapeutic Uses. Ascorbic acid is administered (1) as a dietary supplement to infants and adults whose diet is inadequate or where there is impairment in absorption, (2) in the treatment of acute or subacute scurvy, (3) in infections of the gums and mouth caused by a diet deficient in vitamin C, (4) as part of the general supportive treatment of burns, (5) with procaine in various allergic conditions, (6) in peptic ulcer, and (7) to hasten wound healing after surgery.

Preparations

Ascorbic Acid Tablets, U.S.P., B.P. (I.P.)	25, 50, 100, 250, and 500 mg.
Ascorbic Acid Injection, U.S.P.	100 and 500 mg. in 2 ml., 500 mg. and 1 Gm. in 5 ml., 1 Gm. in 10 ml.

Trade names: Ascorbin; Cantaxin; Cebione; Cecon; Cevex; Cevalin; Cevaline; Cevimin; Ciamin; Vitacee

Synonyms: Antiscorbutic Vitamin; Cevitamic Acid

FAT-SOLUBLE VITAMINS

The fat-soluble group includes vitamins A, D, E, and K. Vitamin D is discussed on pages 702–4, and vitamin K is discussed on pages 510 and 512.

Vitamin A and Carotene

In 1913, Drs. E. V. McCollum and M. Davis discovered vitamin A, a yellow crystalline compound or viscous oil that is soluble in oil and insoluble in water. The vitamin is present in liver, egg yolk, butter, cheese, fish liver oil, and concentrates, which also contain vitamin D. It is isolated in the pure form from natural substances and is also made synthetically.

Vitamin A, in the form of its precursor, carotene, is widespread in nature, being found closely associated with chlorophyll in green leaves and in many fruits and vegetables such as carrots, yams, apricots, and yellow corn. Carotene is available in three isometric forms: alpha, beta, and gamma carotene. A related compound, the plant pigment cryptoxanthine, also yields vitamin A. These carotinoid pigments show vitamin A activity by virtue of their conversion into the vitamin during passage through the intestinal wall. Mineral oil diminishes carotene absorption. Vitamin A is assayed biologically, and the dose is given in units. The U.S.P. unit is the same as the international unit and is the number of micrograms that will produce the same growth and antixerophthalmic changes as 0.6 mcg. of beta carotene.

The fundamental metabolic action of vitamin A is not known, but it is essential in man not only to promote normal body growth and the proper development of bones and teeth but also to maintain the health and integrity of certain specialized epithelial cells such as the retina and the epithelial cells of the mucous membranes of the bronchi, sinuses, urinary tract, cornea and conjunctiva. Vitamin A plays a critical part in the process of vision. The light receptors of the eye (cones and rods) contain light-sensitive pigments that require the vitamin for their formation and functioning.

Vitamin A Deficiency.   A deficiency of vitamin A causes night blindness, xerophthalmia, drying and scaliness of the skin, and keratinization of the epithelial cells. The factors that cause a deficiency of this vitamin are improper diet, inadequate absorption in celiac disease, chronic ulcerative colitis, and steatorrhea.

Hypervitaminosis A.   Toxic effects may occur from an excessive intake of vitamin A. The signs and symptoms include subcutaneous swelling, particularly on the forearms which are painful and limit motion; excessive growth of bone tissue (hyperostasis) ; anorexia; pruritus; dry skin; bleeding fissures at the corners of the mouth; and sparse, course hair. The usual cause is excessive intake of vitamin A during prophylactic therapy

Dosage and Method of Administration.   The adequate daily requirement for vitamin A is 5000 U.S.P. units for adults and 1500 to 3000 U.S.P. units for children. Vitamin A, U.S.P., is either a fish oil or a solution of vitamin A concentrate from animal sources in an edible vegetable oil. The usual dose is 1.5 mg. (5000 U.S.P. units) daily. The therapeutic dose is 7.5 mg. (7.5 to 60 mg.) (25,000 to 200,000 U.S.P. units) daily. This vitamin is usually administered orally.

Therapeutic Uses.   Vitamin A is used in (1) the treatment of night blindness, (2) keratinization of epithelial cells, (3) retarded growth, (4) xerophthalmia, and (5) certain skin diseases.

Preparation

Vitamin A Capsules   1.5, 7.5, and 15 mg.
(Preparations containing both vitamin
A and vitamin D are listed on page
704.)

Vitamin E (Alpha Tocopherol)

Wheat germ oil is the richest source of vitamin E (the antisterility vitamin). It also occurs in other plant oils, such as cottonseed or peanut oil, and in lettuce, spinach, and watercress. There are at least three naturally occurring substances that have vitamin E activity: alpha, beta, and gamma tocopherols. Of these, alpha tocopherol, N.F., is the most potent and it has been synthesized.

Vitamin E appears to have no clinical value in the treatment of sterility, and its efficacy in the prevention of abortion is doubtful. Various preparations are described in the *National Formulary*.

MULTIVITAMIN PREPARATIONS

Multivitamin preparations are administered either as a supplement to a normal diet or as a therapeutic measure. They are indicated in conditions of subclinical malnutrition following secondary infections, vomiting, and diarrhea. They are also prescribed before and after operations, during an illness or convalescence, and during pregnancy and lactation, as well as in infancy and childhood. Many multivitamin preparations are on the market, some of which also contain minerals. Therapeutic vitamin preparations contain doses much larger than those intended for prophylactic medication. They are available in tablets and capsules, and in oil solution in dropping bottles for administration to infants and children.

Preparations

Decavitamin Capsules, U.S.P.; Decavitamin Tablets, U.S.P. — Each capsule or tablet contains not less than 1.2 mg. (4000 U.S.P. units) of vitamin A, 10 mcg. (400 U.S.P. units) of vitamin D, 70 mg. of ascorbic acid, 10 mg. of calcium pantothenate, 1 mcg. of cyanocobalamin, 50 mcg. of folic acid, 20 mg. of niacinamide, 2 mg. of pyridoxine hydrochloride, 3 mg. of riboflavin, and 2 mg. of thiamine hydrochloride or mononitrate

Hexavitamin Capsules, N.F.; Hexavitamin Tablets, N.F. — Each capsule or tablet contains 1.5 mg. of vitamin A, 10 mcg. of vitamin D, 75 mg. of ascorbic acid, 2 mg. of thiamine hydrochloride, 3 mg. of riboflavin, and 20 mg. of niacinamide.

PROTEIN HYDROLYSATES AND AMINO ACID PREPARATIONS

Amino acids, which are organic compounds essential for the synthesis of proteins in the body, are normally provided by the proteins in the diet. Protein deficiency, which is evidenced by a decrease in the level of plasma protein (hypoproteinemia), may be caused by inadequate protein in the diet. However, it may also occur as a result of (1) impaired digestion or absorption; (2) inadequate utilization, as in liver disease; (3) increased demand, as during growth and pregnancy; (4) increased metabolism, as in fever, infections, and hyperthyroidism; and (5) increased loss, through severe hemorrhage, extensive burns, and trauma.

PROTEIN HYDROLYSATES

Protein hydrolysate preparations are obtained by the acid or enzyme digestion of suitable proteins. They are available for oral or intravenous administration.

Therapeutic Uses

1. In hypoproteinemia associated with extensive burns, hemorrhage, trauma, infections, malnutrition, and severe gastrointestinal operations.
2. To promote healing of wounds in hypoproteinemia.
3. To protect the liver against certain hepatotoxic agents.

Protein Hydrolysate Injection

Protein hydrolysate injection is a sterile solution of amino acids and short-chain peptides to which dextrose is added to provide calories. The usual intravenous dose is 500 ml. (250 to 1500 ml.) of a 5 per cent solution.

Preparation

Protein Hydrolysate Injection, U.S.P.   5 per cent in 150, 250, 500, and 1000 ml.; 10 per cent in 500 ml.; 15 per cent in 100 ml.

    Trade names: Amigen; Aminosol; Hyprotigen; Parenamine; Travamin

Protein Hydrolysates (Oral)

These are available in powdered form, flavored or unflavored, and are administered with beverages or food. They are used in the diets of infants and children and to supplement the diet in the management of peptic ulcer. The dose is determined by the physician according to the weight, age, nutritional state, etc., of the patient.

Preparation

Protein Hydrolysates (Oral) Powder
> Trade names: Aminonat; Caminoids; Ketonil

AMINO ACID PREPARATION

Methionine, N.F.

Methionine is an essential sulfur-containing amino acid. It is useful in the prevention and treatment of liver damage due to poisoning with arsenic, chloroform, or carbon tetrachloride. It is also used in the treatment of shock and diseases of the liver. The daily oral dose of 3 to 6 Gm. is given as a supplement to a high-protein diet. It is contraindicated in severe liver damage.

Preparations

Methionine Capsules, N.F.	500 mg.
Methionine Tablets, N.F.	500 mg.

> Trade names: Meonine; Metione

REVIEW QUESTIONS

1. *What requirements must be fulfilled by substances qualifying for the name "vitamin"?*
2. *The water-soluble vitamins are depleted within days if the intake is stopped, as by severe accidents, disease, or poisoning. Name these vitamins and give the appropriate amounts that should be administered daily in intravenous fluids, by injection, or by mouth if practical.*
3. *Name and describe the conditions that are presented by patients having the various vitamin deficiencies.*
4. *Give for each vitamin, where covered in the text, the role played in the body and the chief sources where found.*
5. *What is the significance of each of the following to any life process and to any human abnormality or disease: biotin, choline, inositol, methionine, and cyanocobalamin (see Chap. 31, pp. 507–8)?*

REFERENCES

Bessey, O. A.: "Role of Vitamins in the Metabolism of Amino Acids," *J.A.M.A.*, **164**:1224, 1957.

Clausen, S. W.: "The Pharmacology and Therapeutics of Vitamin A," *J.A.M.A.*, **111**:144, 1938.

Elvehjem, C.: "Relation of Nicotinic Acid to Pellagra," *Physiol. Rev.*, **20**:249, 1940.

———: "The Vitamin B Complex" (Council on Foods and Nutrition), *J.A.M.A.*, **138**:960, 1948.

Goldsmith, G. H.: "Vitamin B Complex in Clinical Medicine," *South. M. J.*, **39**: 485, 1946.

Merck Manual, 9th ed. Merck & Company, Inc., Rahway, N.J., 1956.

Sebrell, W. H., and Harris, R. S. (eds.) : *The Vitamins.* Academic Press, Inc., New York, 1954.

Vitamin Manual. Upjohn Company, Kalamazoo, Mich., 1957.

Youmans, J. B.: "Deficiencies of Fat-Soluble Vitamins" (Council on Foods and Nutrition), *J.A.M.A.*, **144**:34, 1950.

————: "Deficiencies of Water-Soluble Vitamins" (Council on Foods and Nutrition), *J.A.M.A.*, **144**:307, 1950.

X DRUGS ACTING ON THE SKIN AND MUCOUS MEMBRANES

This section includes many different types of substances that are applied to the skin or mucous membranes including the eye, ear, and nose. Soothing substances are applied to irritated and abraded areas to protect them and also to alleviate itching. On the other hand, mild irritant drugs are used to stimulate healing, while strong irritants or caustics are used to destroy abnormal growths.

Many kinds of local antiseptics are available for preventing or stopping infection. These drugs may be used for their action on the skin or the mucous membranes of the body cavities and as antiseptics in the genitourinary and gastrointestinal tracts. Drugs are also applied locally to the skin to treat parasitic and fungous infections.

Drugs that cause local insensibility to pain (e.g., cocaine, procaine, and other synthetic local anesthetics) are discussed in Chapter 25 (pp. 423–37).

44

Protectives, Soothing Substances, Antipruritics, Astringents, Irritants, Counterirritants, Keratolytics, Escharotics or Corrosives

The skin is a complex structure that has many physiological functions, among which are: (1) protection of the underlying tissues, (2) regulation of body temperature through evaporation and radiation, (3) maintenance of water and electrolyte balance, (4) excretion of waste products, (5) metabolic activity such as activation of ergosterol by ultraviolet irradiation, and (6) sensory perception.

The mucous membranes line the body cavities and canals and are continuous with the skin. They secrete mucus, a watery fluid containing mucin (a glucoprotein) and inorganic salts, etc., which coats the surface and lessens irritation from food, foreign and waste material, and secreted substances. The functions of the mucous membranes are (1) protection, (2) support of all blood vessels and lymphatics, and (3) provision of a large surface for secretion and absorption.

Drugs applied to the skin or mucous membranes may exert local or systemic effects. Absorption through the skin takes place mainly through the lining of the sebaceous glands, which secrete sebum, an oily substance composed mostly of fat. In order for a drug to be absorbed upon local application to the skin, it is generally administered in an absorbable ointment base. On the other hand, aqueous solutions are absorbed from the mucous membranes because of their permeability and abundant supply of blood. Soluble substances, when placed in contact with the buccal mucosa (e.g., testosterone), put under the tongue (e.g., nitroglycerin tablets), or inserted in the rectum (e.g., aminophylline), have more rapid systemic effects and more complete absorption than when swallowed. Drugs may be applied for the following local effects: cleansing, alleviation of irritation (protective, soothing, or antipruritic action), production of mild irritation, and anti-infective and analgesic actions. Keratolytics are applied to the skin for the removal of excess horny layers, and escharotics or corrosives for the destruction of abnormal growths.

722

PROTECTIVES

Protectives are designed to cover the skin or mucous membranes in order to prevent contact with possible irritants. Collodions, demulcents, powders, lotions, and ointments may be used for this purpose.

Collodion, U.S.P. Collodion is made by dissolving nitrates of cellulose (pyroxylin) in an ether-alcohol solution. It has limited use as such, but when 3 per cent castor oil and 2 per cent camphor are added, it becomes flexible collodion.

Flexible Collodion, U.S.P., B.P. Flexible collodion is used to cover sutures in the scalp and skin and also to cover the blisters of herpes zoster (shingles). Solutions of plastics in volatile solvents are also used for this last purpose.

Dusting Powders. Dusting powders are used in the treatment of skin abrasions and itching of the skin. *Kaolin* (a native hydrated aluminum silicate), *purified talc* (a native magnesium silicate), and *cornstarch* are white soft powders that are frequently used. Medicated powders, such as *zinc stearate powder,* are made by incorporating the drug in the dry powder form into the dusting powder base.

SOOTHING SUBSTANCES

Demulcents. Demulcents are soothing agents, usually protective colloids of natural origin, such as egg white, milk, and gums. They are generally used to protect the mucous membranes and relieve irritation and are therefore a common constituent of lozenges and cough drops used to allay irritation of the mouth and throat. Milk, cream, egg white, and starch solution are used to protect or soothe the mucosa of the stomach when a corrosive poison has been swallowed. *Acacia* (gum arabic) and *gum tragacanth* are demulcent gums from which mucilages are prepared. They are also used in making emulsions. Demulcents are sometimes applied to the skin to allay the caustic action of poisons. Glycerin is also used as a soothing agent (see p. 393).

Emollients. Emollients are fatty or oily substances that produce a soothing effect when applied to the skin. They may be applied as oils or in the form of emulsions or ointments.

Ointments. Ointments are semisolid substances that contain oils or fats. They are used in dermatology as: (1) protective agents, to prevent contact with irritating substances and to prevent heat loss; (2) lubricating agents, to aid in the removal of crusts and scales and to prevent excessive dryness; and (3) vehicles for the incorporation of drugs used in the treatment of skin diseases.

Ointment bases may be classified into four types:

1. *Oleaginous Bases or Protective Ointments.* These are mixtures of hydrocarbons that are not miscible with water. They are most effective for the relief of dry skin. Petrolatum is one of the most frequently used ingredients in ointments. It may be used alone or in combination with other substances. Examples: Petrolatum, U.S.P.; and Plastibase.

2. *Water-in-Oil Ointment Bases.* Ointment bases of this type include:

a. ABSORPTION TYPE. These do not contain water but, upon the addition of water, form *water-in-oil emulsions.* Examples: Hydrophilic Petrolatum, U.S.P.; Anhydrous Lanolin, U.S.P.; Wool Fat, B.P.; Plastibase, Hydrophilic; Aquaphor.

b. WATER-IN-OIL EMULSION BASES. Droplets of water are dispersed in oil by means of emulsifying or dispersing agents. Oil, which is the continuous phase, is in contact with the skin and provides a protective oil film. These bases are used for lubrication and heat retention, and in the treatment of psoriasis. They increase the penetrability of drugs incorporated in them. Examples: Lanolin, U.S.P.; Hydrous Wool Fat, B.P.; Rose Water Ointment, N.F.

3. *Oil-in-Water (Water-Miscible) Ointment Bases.* Oil droplets are dispersed in water. Water, which is the external phase, is in contact with the skin. These bases are relatively greaseless and wash off readily; are cosmetically attractive and easily applied and removed; release medication readily and increase the penetrability of drugs. They are used for scalp preparations and for ointments to prevent sunburn. Examples: Hydrophilic Ointment, U.S.P.; Unibase; Neobase; Almay Emulsion Base.

4. *Water-Soluble Ointment Bases.* These bases are made from synthetic materials, the polyethylene glycols. The molecular weights of these substances range from 200 to 6000: those with molecular weights ranging from 200 to 700 are liquids; those with weights ranging from 1000 to 6000, solids (carbowaxes). By mixing of different members of this series, bases with the consistency of an ointment and which melt when applied to the skin may be prepared. The carbowaxes are miscible with water. When applied to the skin, they mix with the exudates. They are less occlusive than the absorption bases, do not stain linen or clothes, and do not deteriorate. These bases are compatible with almost all drugs used by the dermatologist, but may cause sensitization. Example: Polyethylene Glycol Ointment, U.S.P.

Other compounds belonging to this group are the *Tweens* and the *Spans,* which are dispersing agents.

Protective Ointments. Substances may be added to washable ointment bases for the following uses:

1. PROTECTION AGAINST WATER AND CHEMICAL AGENTS. Ointments containing silicone, which is chemically inert, form an invisible plastic-like film

that is not removed by water and is neither sticky nor greasy. They are occasionally useful in contact dermatitis, diaper rash, and decubitus ulcers. Examples: Covicone Cream; Silicote Ointment.

2. PROTECTION AGAINST ULTRAVIOLET LIGHT (SUNBURN). Salts and esters of p-aminobenzoic acid (PABA) absorb ultraviolet light. Titanium oxide, U.S.P., is an opaque substance that reflects light. It is applied as a 15 to 25 per cent ointment, as required. PABA ointment contains PABA and titanium oxide in a water-soluble ointment base. Skolex contains the propylene glycol ester of PABA in a water-soluble ointment base.

Anti-infective Ointments. There are many commercially available ointments containing antibiotics. They are useful in superficial infections, such as pyodermas.

Other medicated ointments are available for keratolytic and local anesthetic effects. They will be discussed later in this chapter. Coal Tar Ointment, U.S.P., and Coal Tar Solution, U.S.P., are employed locally in eczema.

Vegetable Oils. Olive oil, cottonseed oil, corn oil, etc., are emollient to the skin and mucous membranes. They are used as vehicles for many drugs. Theobroma Oil, U.S.P. (cocao butter, cocoa butter), a solid at room temperature, is used as a lubricant for massage and as a suppository base.

ANTIPRURITICS

Pruritus, or itching, is a common subjective symptom accompanying skin diseases or allergic manifestations. It is also associated with liver disease, blood dyscrasias, diabetes, gout, intestinal infestations, drug sensitiveness, and endocrine disturbances. Dietary, metabolic, and psychic factors are also included. The causes of this condition should be sought and treated appropriately. Because pruritus causes scratching, with possible abrasion of the skin, which may lead to inflammation and secondary infection, local remedies such as wet dressings, lotions, ointments, and powders are also indicated.

Wet Dressings and Compresses. The application of wet dressings and compresses to the skin is very useful in relieving itching, reducing inflammation, removing crusts and debris, and stimulating healing in the affected areas. *Hot wet dressings* may be applied to relieve pain and to treat secondary infections. Old bed linen or other soft cloths are soaked with water or medicated solutions and applied frequently. Plastic or wax paper may be placed over the dressing to retain the heat. *Cold wet dressings,* which cool the affected areas by the evaporation of water, are used to relieve itching and burning. These dressings may be covered with Turkish toweling, which allows evaporation. Water alone will often relieve itching.

The following solutions are frequently used as antipruritics:

1. Aluminum Acetate Solution, U.S.P. (Burow's Solution). This solution is diluted with 10 to 40 parts of water. It is used in acute inflammatory conditions, edema, and vesicular dermatoses.

2. Boric acid solution, 2 per cent solution. This is used in acute and subacute inflammatory conditions and in contact and atopic dermatitis. It is contraindicated in abraded or denuded areas.

3. Potassium permanganate 1:5000 to 1:10,000, is an antiseptic, astringent, and keratolytic; it is used in weeping, blistered, and denuded areas.

4. Normal salt solution.

5. Milk, starch, and oatmeal baths (Aveeno Colloid Oatmeal).

Lotions and Ointments. Lotions and ointments containing menthol are often used to produce a cooling effect. Simple ointments or protective oils will improve hydration of the skin by affording an occlusive covering. Phenol, 0.5 to 1 per cent in lotions or 1 to 2 per cent in cottonseed oil, is often used.

Drugs. Many antihistamines are administered locally and orally to relieve itching in allergic conditions (see Chap. 26). Preparations containing cortisone, hydrocortisone, and synthetic derivatives are also very effective (see Chap. 41). Local anesthetics are sometimes used but they may cause sensitization resulting in allergic reactions.

ASTRINGENTS

Astringents shrink swollen and inflamed tissues such as those of the mouth, throat, and intestinal mucosa. They act by precipitating the proteins on the surface layers of the skin and mucous membranes and by precipitating the proteins in the blood. Thus they extract water from the tissues, lessen secretions, and check bleeding.

They are classified into two groups (1) mineral astringents which include heavy metals which combine with the albumin of the tissues and form insoluble precipitates and (2) the vegetable astringents which depend upon the presence of tannic acid.

Tannic Acid. Tannic acid or tannins are complex principles found widely distributed in plants. Tannic acid is used (1) for topical administration in bed sores, weeping ulcers, and eczematous dermatoses, (2) for the symptomatic treatment of diarrhea especially in children, and (3) as an antidote in the form of strong tea in the treatment of poisoning because it precipitates numerous alkaloids, glycosides, and some heavy metals in the stomach. Dosage forms are the glycerite, the ointment, and the powder.

Hamamelis Water, N.F. (Witch Hazel Water, Witch Hazel Extract). This preparation is obtained by distilling with steam or water the bark and twigs of *Hamamelis virginiana.* It possesses astringent as well as sedative properties. It is used as a soothing lotion (1) for black eye, (2) for edema of the eyelids, (3) for skin irritations, (4) for superficial bleeding as in razor cuts and in epistaxis, (5) in obstetrics to relieve itching and pain of edema about stitches in the perineum, and (6) as an ointment in painful hemorrhoids. It may be applied locally undiluted to the area or in the form of hot compresses. The ointment is available for the treatment of hemorrhoids.

IRRITANTS

Drugs that produce mild irritation of the skin and mucous membranes are applied locally to an abraded or inflamed area of the skin or mucous membranes to stimulate or hasten healing.

Irritants produce reddening (rubifacient action) at the site of application by dilating the blood vessels and bringing more blood to the surface. If the drug is applied in too high concentration, or its period of contact is prolonged, vesication and corrosion may result. Vesication is caused by prolonged wide dilatation of the capillaries. The vessels become more permeable, and plasma escapes into the tissues (vesicant war gases). Permanent scarring may result from the action of irritant drugs that cause corrosion of the skin or mucous membrane.

COUNTERIRRITANTS

Counterirritants are drugs used to irritate the unbroken skin in order to relieve pain in the viscera (neuralgias, rheumatoid arthritis, bursitis, muscle pains). Heat, in the form of a hot-water bottle or an electric heating pad, is the most frequently used counterirritant. However, many drugs are used for this purpose. A few examples are Mustard Plaster, N.F.; Methyl Salicylate, U.S.P., B.P.; Iodine Tincture, U.S.P. (B.P., I.P.); Camphor Liniment, N.F. (B.P.); and Chloroform Liniment, N.F.

Counterirritants produce vasodilatation and rubefaction and a pleasant feeling of warmth. The local irritation resulting from a stimulation of the sensory nerve endings brings relief from pain, which originates in the viscera or muscles. Several theories have been offered to explain this action, but there seems to be no unanimity of opinion.

Methyl Salicylate, U.S.P., B.P. Methyl salicylate is a volatile oil that produces mild irritation when it is rubbed on the skin. The drug is absorbed and produces a general analgesic action also. It is usually administered in arthralgias and neuralgias.

KERATOLYTICS

Kerotolytics soften and loosen keratinized epithelium so that it can be removed with rubbing. They reduce excessive scaling and hypertrophy of the horny layer of the skin and tend to soften the skin and prevent the formation of more scales. These drugs are indicated in scaling, dry, subacute, and chronic inflammatory processes of the glabrous skin and scalp. They are used in the treatment of epidermophytosis, seborrheic dermatitis, chronic eczema, infections of the scalp, dandruff, corns and calluses, and fungal infections. Salicylic acid is the drug most often used. Other keratolytics are coal tar, pyrogallol, resorcinol, chrysarobin, and sulfur. They are applied in collodions, pastes, and ointments. The U.S.P. preparations containing salicylic acid are the collodion, which contains 10 per cent in flexible collodion; the ointment, containing from 2 to 10 per cent salicylic acid; the plaster; and benzoic and salicylic acid ointment (Whitfield's ointment).

ESCHAROTICS OR CORROSIVES

Escharotics are chemicals that produce necrosis, or the death of tissue. They are used to cauterize fissures and ulcers, destroy excessive granulation tissue and proud flesh, and remove warts. Liquid nitrogen and ethyl chloride destroy tissues by freezing.

Liquid Nitrogen.   Liquid nitrogen is available in vacuum bottles. The end of a cotton-tipped applicator is immersed in the liquid nitrogen, removed, and immediately applied to the wart until it freezes solid. After 12 to 24 hours, a vesicle develops at the base of the wart. When this involutes, the wart frequently sloughs off. Liquid nitrogen is much colder than dry ice and requires less time to destroy the wart.

Ethyl Chloride.   Ethyl chloride is sprayed on the tissues. It is used for the treatment of creeping eruption, in plaster planing, and prior to curetting warts.

Other Corrosive Substances.   Other substances that produce necrosis of tissue are:

1. Trichloroacetic acid, 25 per cent in water to full strength. Bichloroacetic acid may also be used.

2. Salicylic acid ointment, 5 to 10 per cent, in which concentration the ointment is keratolytic.

3. Silver nitrate, which is used in the form of an applicator stick to cauterize fissures and ulcers and to destroy excessive granulation tissue and proud flesh. The stick is moistened before use.

4. Liquefied phenol.

REVIEW QUESTIONS

1. *For what purposes are drugs applied to the skin and mucous membranes?*
2. *What are protectives? Name several.*
3. *List three uses for ointments in dermatology.*
4. *Discuss the use of wet dressings and compresses.*
5. *What drugs are used to remove warts?*

REFERENCES

Goodman, J. M.: "Liquid Nitrogen Therapy of Warts and Other Skin Lesions," *Canad. M.A.J.*, **82**:628, 1960.

Hadgraft, J. W., and Somers, G. F.: "Percutaneous Absorption," *J. Pharm. & Pharmacol.*, **8**:625, 1956.

Wurster, D. E.: "New Ointment Bases," *Am. Prof. Pharm.*, **18**:704, 1952.

45

Drugs Acting Locally on the Eye, Ear, and Nose

DRUGS ACTING LOCALLY IN THE EYE

For the discussion of the innervation of the eye and drugs used in the treatment of glaucoma and iritis see pages 446–48, 472.

Infections of the eye may be treated with local medications. The drugs used are anti-infective, anti-inflammatory, or local anesthetic agents. They are administered in aqueous suspensions, ointments, or small wafers or in suspension which causes the medication to remain in the eye for longer periods of time.

The surfaces of the conjunctiva are lubricated and cleansed by the tears which are secreted by the lacrimal glands. The principal salt, sodium chloride, is present to the extent of 0.7 per cent, and the pH of the tear ranges from 7.2 to 7.4. In various disease conditions the pH may vary from 5.2 to 8.3.

Aqueous suspensions instilled in the eye should be isotonic, adjusted to the pH of the tear and buffered. Suspensions of the detergent type include wetting agents which increase surface tension and spreadability and provide a longer surface contact. Benzalkonium is a fairly good antiseptic detergent. It tends to soften the cornea, and overuse may cause corneal edema. It is used in balanced salt solutions to aid in cleansing and application of contact lenses. Methylcellulose in 1 per cent solution increases the viscosity and keeps the drops in contact with the eye for eight to ten minutes after administration. It tends to lower surface tension and increases the absorption of the drug incorporated in the suspension. ISOPTO is the name applied to these ophthalmic preparations.

Ointments are generally prepared with a solid petrolatum base which provides an emollient and protective effect. They are applied when long action is desired, especially before going to bed at night.

Administration of Eye Medications. Solutions are instilled in the eye by drops. To instill the drops the head is tilted back; the lower lid is drawn down exposing the conjunctival sac; and the patient looks up. The medicine dropper is held parallel to the eye but not touching it. It should never be

730

held perpendicular to the eye as a sudden movement on the part of the nurse or the patient could force the dropper into the eye. The drops are instilled into the pocket created by the everted lower lid. The lid is closed gently to allow the solution to flow over the conjunctiva. An eye dropper should be used for only one patient if infections are to be prevented. In many hospitals they are sterilized between uses. A number of the drugs frequently used are available in plastic containers from which drops are expressed. These also should be used on an individual basis. Ointments are administered by placing a small amount on the everted lower lid as the patient looks up.

Corticosteroids such as cortisone, hydrocortisone, prednisolone, fludro-cortisone, methylprednisolone, dexamethasone, and triamcinolone are used for their anti-inflammatory or antiallergic actions. They are used to prevent heavy scarring, adhesions, or visual defects caused by prolonged irritation. They are contraindicated in ocular tuberculosis, herpes simplex, and fungal keratitis. They are available as suspensions or ointments.

The adrenergic agents such as ephedrine, phenylephrine, and epinephrine are used to produce decongestion and vasoconstriction. They are sometimes combined with other agents, i.e., ephedrine and prednisone in the preparation called Prednefrin.

The antibiotics such as neomycin, tetracycline, chloramphenicol, bacitracin, polymixin B, and erythromycin and the sulfonamides such as sulfacetamide, sulfamethazole, and sulfisoxazole diethanolamine, and the antiseptics such as zinc sulfate, boric acid, nitrofurazone, thiomersol, ammoniated mercury, and sodium propionate are used for their antibacterial and antifungal properties. Chloramphenicol is the only antibiotic which provides a good intraocular concentration upon systemic administration. Therefore, it is administered topically, orally, or parenterally.

Local anesthetics are instilled into the eye for the relief of pain due to pathology of the globe, a foreign body in the eye, exposure to a chemical blast, overexposure to light, or local manipulation of the surgeon. The drugs used are tetracaine, phenacaine, lidocaine, and proparacaine. For other preparations see the index.

Other drugs useful in the treatment of diseases of the eye are miotics (see p. 472), mydriatics (see p. 490), and cycloplegics (see p. 490). For a discussion of glaucoma and its treatment see page 472.

Idoxuridine (IDU)

Idoxuridine (IDU) is an antimetabolite which blocks the incorporation of thymidine into DNA. It is effective in the treatment of ocular herpes simplex which is caused by a virus which produces a dendritic ulcer on the surface of the cornea. The virus requires DNA for reproduction, and thymidine, an essential constituent, is closely related chemically to IDU. If IDU is present in sufficient concentrations and for long enough periods of time, it is incorporated into DNA instead of thymidine, and reproduction of the invading virus is inhibited.

The side effects which occur infrequently are irritation, pruritus, inflammation and edema of the eye or eyelids, and photophobia. Allergic reactions are rare.

Dosage and Administration. Initially one drop is instilled into the infected eye every hour during the day and every two hours at night. This dosage is continued until improvement is noted as evidenced by the absence of staining with fluorescein. The dosage may then be reduced to one drop every two hours during the day and every four hours at night until healing is complete.

Preparation

Idoxuridine Ophthalmic Solution	0.1 per cent in 15-ml. plastic dropping bottles

Trade names: Dendrid, Herplex, Stoxil

Alpha-Chymotrypsin

In selected cases alpha-chymotrypsin is irrigated in the eye to loosen the attachment of the lens and facilitate cataract extraction. Ampuls contain 750 units of lypholized enzyme which is dissolved in 10 ml.

DIAGNOSTIC AID, EYE

Antibiotics are used in the eye for the treatment of corneal abrasions and ulcers as well as conjunctivitis. Small abrasions often cannot be seen without the use of a material that stains the broken corneal membrane.

Fluorescein Sodium Solution, U.S.P.

Fluorescein sodium solution is a sterile solution for ophthalmoscopic purposes containing approximately 2 Gm. of fluorescein, 3 Gm. of sodium bicarbonate, and a suitable bacteriostatic agent in 100 ml. of purified water. It is applied topically to the conjunctiva and is used to demonstrate the depth of corneal lesions and to detect foreign bodies embedded in the cornea. Weak solutions, which do not stain the cornea, color with green fluorescence the ulcers or parts deprived of epithelium. Foreign bodies are surrounded by a green ring; loss of substance in the conjunctiva is indicated by a yellow hue; defects or diseased portions of the endothelium are also colored.

Preparation

Fluorescein Sodium Ophthalmic Solution, U.S.P.	2 per cent

DRUGS USED IN THE TREATMENT OF EAR INFECTIONS

Infections of the external and middle ears may be treated with local medication. Since it is impossible to reach the internal ear, it is necessary to administer drugs such as antibiotics or sulfonamides for otitis media or antimotion sickness drugs (see p. 377) for labyrinthitis either orally or parenterally.

The external ear is subject to the same type of infections as the skin. They may be caused by bacteria, fungi, or viruses. The drugs used are anti-infectives and anti-inflammatory agents. They are administered as drops or a pack gauze strip. Heat may be applied.

Hygroscopic vehicles such as glycerin or propylene glycol are used to soften, dehydrate, and cleanse the area for better penetration of the medication. Thonzium, a wetting agent, is often included to increase penetration and spreading of the drugs over the infected area. Acetic acid may be incorporated to restore the acid mantle of the skin which is normally pH 6 to 6.5.

Drugs used for their antibacterial or antifungal action are the antibiotics such as neomycin, polymixin B, tyrothricin, gramicidin, and colistin sulfate; the sulfonamides such as sulfisoxazole diethanolamine and sulfathiazole; and the antiseptics, thiomersol, undecylenic acid, sodium propionate, and benzethonium chloride. Antihistamines are administered for their antiallergic and antipruritic effects (see pyralamine [Neo-Antergan] and thonzylamine [Neo-Hetramine], p. 759). For their anti-inflammatory action the corticosteroids hyrdocortisone and fludrocortisone and the decongestants phenylephrine and ephedrine may be used. Urea liquefies purulent exudates and urea (carbamide) peroxide, 6.5 per cent in anhydrous glycerin (Debrox), combines cleansing and debridement action with a slow release of oxygen. Local anesthetics such as dibucaine, diperodon, lidocaine, and benzocaine (see Chap. 25) are administered for the relief of pain.

DRUGS ACTING LOCALLY ON THE RESPIRATORY TRACT

The entire respiratory tract is lined with ciliated epithelium. It begins at the lips and nostrils and extends through the sinuses, trachea, bronchial tubes, and alveoli. This membrane is covered by a blanket of mucus which is propelled by the cilia to the nasopharynx where it is expelled.

THE NOSE AND SINUSES

The purpose of the nose is to supply clean, moist air to the lungs. The blood in the mucous membrane and tissues gives off heat which warms the air and the mucus blanket which covers it, keeps it moist and traps foreign particles such as dust and bacteria which are then swept by the cilia to the nasopharynx. If the cilia and mucus blanket function normally, infection should not occur. The normal pH of mucus is acid (pH 5.5 to 5.6), which exerts a bacteriostatic action.

The pH of the nasal mucosa shifts to the alkaline side in the presence of allergy, trauma, infection, sudden change in temperature, or noxious gases. When this occurs, the action of the cilia slows or ceases and the blood vessels in the mucosa covering the turbinates become engorged causing edema of the mucus membrane. An increased blood supply to the area due to irritation raises the temperature locally. This, in addition to the edema, causes increased secretions which result in a runny nose and postnasal drip.

When inflammation of the nasal mucosa occurs, drugs are applied to restore the normal function of the nose. Aqueous solutions which are miscible with mucus and which do not interfere with the action of the cilia, a protective mechanism, should be used. In addition they should be isotonic and buffered to maintain a pH of 5.5 to 5.6. They are administered as (1) atomized vapors or drops (see p. 15), or (2) liquid or solid aerosols (see p. 16). Oily bases should not be used as they may be inhaled and may cause lipid pneumonia. They also inactivate the cilia.

Rhinitis and Sinusitis. In these conditions the adrenergic agents which are decongestants are very effective. They shrink the mucosa of the turbinates and start to restore the normal function of the nose. If they are used too often, they produce a rebound effect by stimulating the sympathetic nerves to the nasal mucosa and thus produce more swelling. The stronger the solution or drug, the greater the rebound.

Ephedrine sulfate in 1 per cent solution (0.5 to 2 per cent) in buffered salt solution is very effective. Phenylephrine (Neo-Synephrine) in 0.25 to 0.5 per cent solutions is also widely used. It causes less rebound than ephedrine but its duration of action is less. For other decongestants see page 463.

Corticosteroids (see p. 681) and antihistamines (see p. 758) are also used. Antiseptics are useless upon topical administration to the nose because they are ineffective and cause irritation and damage to the tissues, which are then less able to handle the infection. Astringents should not be used as they draw water out of the tissues and desiccate them.

REVIEW QUESTIONS

1. *What points should be included when teaching a patient about his eye drops?*
2. *What are the uses of fluorescein sodium solution?*
3. *In what diseases of the eye are adrenergic agents used? Corticosteroids? Why are their actions helpful?*
4. *How does IDU act in the treatment of herpes simplex?*
5. *Why is the action of ephedrine sulfate useful in rhinitis?*

REFERENCES

Editorial: "IDU in the Eye," *J.A.M.A.*, **188**:160, 1964.

Kaufman, H. E.: "Treatment of Ocular Herpes Simplex: Use of Corticosteroids and IDU," *South. Med. J.*, **57**:163, 1964.

Leopold, I. H.: "Anti-inflammatory Agents in Ophthalmology," *Am. J. Nursing*, **63**:84, 1963.

46

The Local Anti-infectives

The local anti-infectives include antibacterials, antifungal agents, and parasiticides. The antibacterials include disinfectants (bactericides), antiseptics (bacteriostatics), and antibiotics. No sharp distinction can be drawn between the disinfectants and antiseptics, and the terms are often used interchangeably. The antibiotics are either bactericidal, as in the case of the tyrothricins (pp. 154–55), or bacteriostatic, as exemplified by tetracyclines, etc. (pp. 147–52).

ANTISEPTICS

Antiseptics are chemical agents that are applied locally to the skin or mucous membranes to destroy or prevent the growth of bacteria or other pathogenic microorganisms. They may be classified as (1) salts of heavy metals, (2) halogens, (3) oxidizing agents, (4) phenol and related compounds, (5) surface-active agents (detergents and quaternary ammonium compounds), (6) dyes, and (7) miscellaneous drugs.

Mechanism of Action. The antiseptics may act in three ways: (1) coagulate proteins; (2) lower the surface tension of the solutions in which the bacteria are growing, which increases the penetrability of the plasmatic membrane of the bacteria and causes them to imbibe water; (3) react with certain enzyme systems in the bacteria and interfere with their normal metabolism.

Many drugs are toxic to all cell protoplasm and consequently are toxic to the tissues of the host as well as to the tissues of the bacteria. Others, which have an action more selective on the cells of the microorganisms than on the tissues of the host, may be used as antiseptics.

SALTS OF HEAVY METALS

The salts of heavy metals appear to react with certain chemical groups on the protein surfaces of the enzymes of bacterial cells. Very small amounts of silver and mercury salts kill bacteria.

Mercury Preparations

Compounds of mercury are used for the preparation of antiseptic and disinfectant solutions.

736

Mercury Bichloride, N.F.; Mercuric Chloride, I.P. Solutions of 1:1000 to 1:2000 are used for disinfection of dishes and utensils. They are irritating to the tissues and are seldom used on the skin or mucous membranes. They have limited germicidal action, which is decreased in the presence of proteins. Mercury bichloride tablets, large and small, are available to prepare a 1:1000 solution. One large tablet is dissolved in 500 ml. of water, or the small tablet is dissolved in 100 ml. The tablets are colored blue and must have a distinctive shape.

The soluble salts of mercury are very poisonous. They may be absorbed through the skin and consequently are a source of industrial poisoning. Acute poisoning may also result from the ingestion of mercury bichloride, which is corrosive to the mucous membranes of the alimentary tract and may cause vomiting and bloody diarrhea. It is excreted by the kidneys and may produce irreversible renal damage, which may result in death.

Other Preparations of Mercury. Two other mercury preparations used as antiseptics are Ammoniated Mercury Ophthalmic Ointment, U.S.P. (3 per cent), and Ammoniated Mercury Ointment, U.S.P., B.P. (5 per cent).

Organic Mercurials

The organic mercurials are less toxic and irritating than inorganic mercury.

Mercocresols (Mercresin). This combination of cresol derivatives and an organic mercurial possesses germicidal, fungicidal, and bacteriostatic properties. The undiluted 1:1000 tincture is applied to superficial wounds and to the ear, nose, and throat, and is used for preparation of the skin prior to surgery. Dilutions of 1:5 to 1:20 are used for irrigations and wet dressings.

Phenylmercuric Nitrate, N.F., B.P., I.P. (Merphenyl). Solutions or ointments are used topically, as prophylactic and therapeutic disinfectants of the skin, for superficial abrasions, wounds, and infections. An ointment and a solution, 1:500, are available.

Synthetic Derivatives of Mercury in Combination with Dyes

Merbromin, N.F. (Mercurochrome). Aqueous merbromin solutions have a weak bacteriostatic action when applied to the skin, mucous membranes, and wounds. A 2 per cent alcohol-acetone-water solution (Surgical Merbromin Solution, N.F.) is sometimes used as an antiseptic for the skin prior to surgery. Merbromin has been almost replaced by thimerosal (Merthiolate) and nitromersol (Metaphen).

Thimerosal, N.F. (Merthiolate). Thimerosal solutions are nonirritating when applied topically to the skin and mucous membranes and are antiseptic, germicidal, and fungicidal. Tincture of thimerosal is a 1:1000 solution of the drug in alcohol-acetone-water. It is applied to the skin preoperatively. A 1:1000 aqueous solution is used for the disinfection of instruments and for application to wounds and denuded surfaces. Thimerosal is incompatible with acids, salts of heavy metals, and iodine.

Nitromersol, N.F. (Metaphen). Nitromersol tincture is a 1:200 acetone-alcohol-water solution that is used for the disinfection of the skin prior to surgery. The 1:1000 aqueous solution is used for disinfection of surgical instruments and rubber goods; 1:2000, for the disinfection of the skin; and 1:5000, for urethral irrigations and gonorrheal infections of the eye.

Silver Preparations

The soluble salts of silver ionize in water to produce solutions that are astringent and antiseptic in high dilutions. They precipitate proteins and produce irritation. Silver nitrate is the salt most frequently used.

Silver Nitrate, U.S.P., B.P., I.P. When applied to the skin or mucous membranes, weak solutions of silver nitrate are astringent and strong solutions are corrosive. Silver Nitrate Ophthalmic Solution, U.S.P., is a 1 per cent solution, one to two drops of which may be instilled in the eyes of infants at birth to prevent gonorrheal ophthalmia. However, the recent trend is to use penicillin. rather than silver nitrate, for the prevention of ophthalmia neonatorum. Weaker silver nitrate solutions of 1:1000 to 1:10,000 are used for irrigation of the bladder or urethra in gonorrheal infections: 1:1000 kills bacteria rapidly, but may produce irritation; 1:10,000 is antiseptic. Solutions of 1:750 to 1:1000 are used as wet dressings. Five to ten per cent solutions are caustic and are used to check excessive granulation tissue.

Toughened Silver Nitrate, U.S.P., B.P. (Lunar Caustic). This is available in the form of sticks or pencils. Its use is discussed on page 728.

Colloidal Silver Preparations. Colloidal silver preparations contain silver, which is combined mostly with protein. Solutions of these preparations liberate silver ions slowly. Being astringents they draw water out of tissues, desiccating them. Thus they are basically harmful. It is impossible to prepare isotonic solutions. For these reasons, although available they are not recommended for use. Mild Silver Protein, N.F. (Argyrol, Lunargen, Silvol), contains 19 to 23 per cent silver.

Toxicity of Silver Salts. The silver salts do not produce acute toxicity even upon oral administration. Proteins and chlorides precipitate silver and prevent its absorption; hence egg white and sodium chloride are used as antidotes for the local corrosive action of these salts.

Continued topical administration of silver salts may produce chronic silver poisoning, or *argyria*. The salts are absorbed into the blood and deposited in the tissues of the body. The sunlight causes them to turn dark, and the skin becomes a slate-gray color. Argyria persists indefinitely, there being no known treatment.

Zinc Preparations

Salts of zinc are astringents and mild antiseptics and are used for these effects on the skin and mucous membranes. Zinc sulfate is used for instillation in the eye in conjunctivitis in 0.1 to 1 per cent solutions. For application to the skin, 4 per cent solutions are used.

Zinc oxide, an insoluble preparation, is incorporated in powders, ointments, and salves. It is used in skin diseases, impetigo, pruritus, and eczema.

Preparations

Zinc Oxide Ointment, U.S.P.	20 per cent
Calamine Lotion, U.S.P.	8 per cent calamine and 8 per cent zinc oxide
Phenolated Calamine Lotion, U.S.P., containing 1 per cent phenol	

HALOGENS

Iodine Preparations

Iodine is a nonmetallic element obtained from seaweed. When dissolved in a hydroalcoholic solution, it may be used as a disinfectant for the patient's skin preoperatively or as an antiseptic for abraded areas of the skin. Iodine stains the skin a dark-brown color. In high dilutions, it is mildly irritating. Strong solutions cause blisters and may even destroy the skin. Because of this action excess iodine should be removed with alcohol.

Iodine Tincture, U.S.P. (Mild Surgical Tincture of Iodine); Weak Iodine Solution, B.P. (I.P.). This is a 2 per cent solution of iodine and 2.4 per cent sodium iodide in 50 per cent alcohol. Iodine tincture penetrates the skin and is slightly absorbed. It retains its antiseptic action in the presence of serous exudates and fluids. Seventy per cent alcohol is generally used to remove excessive tincture after application to the skin. Strong Iodine Tincture, N.F., is 7 per cent.

Strong Iodine Solution, U.S.P. (Lugol's Solution); Aqueous Iodine Solution, B.P. (I.P.). This is a 5 per cent solution of iodine made soluble by 10 per cent potassium iodide. The solution is a deep-brown color. It is an antiseptic, although it is not generally used for that purpose. Rather, it is administered orally in the treatment of goiter, which is discussed on page 676.

Organic Compounds of Iodine. The organic compounds are fungicidal and amebicidal. Iodochlorhydroxyquin (Vioform) and chiniofon are discussed on page 219.

Chlorine Preparations

Chlorine is a nonmetallic element that occurs as a greenish yellow, very irritant gas. In high dilutions, chlorine and its compounds kill bacteria. It reacts with water to form hypochlorous acid, which is rapidly bactericidal, partly owing to its oxidizing action and partly owing to its action on the bacterial enzymes concerned with the metabolism of glucose. Chlorine preparations have been used for years as antiseptics, disinfectants, and deodorants. At the present time they are mainly used for purifying drinking water and the water in swimming pools.

Sodium Hypochlorite Solution, N.F. This is a 5 per cent solution of sodium hypochlorite. It is diluted ten times for germicidal use.

Diluted Sodium Chlorite Solution (Modified Dakin's Solution); Surgical Chlorinated Soda Solution, B.P. This is a 0.5 per cent aqueous solution of sodium hypochlorite. It is used as an irrigant for wounds and as a wet dressing. The solution is relatively unstable and should be freshly prepared. It is somewhat irritating to the skin.

OXIDIZING AGENTS

The following chemicals readily liberate oxygen when they come in contact with pus or organic material and thus are useful as antiseptic and cleansing agents.

Hydrogen Peroxide Solution, U.S.P., B.P. This is a 3 per cent aqueous solution of hydrogen peroxide. When applied to the abraded skin or mucous membranes, it liberates bubbles of oxygen. Oxygen destroys bacteria and produces antisepsis of the tissues. Hydrogen peroxide solution also acts as a mechanical cleansing agent and deodorant.

Potassium Permanganate, U.S.P., B.P. Potassium permanganate occurs as dark-purple crystals that are soluble in water. Dilute solutions of the compound are irritant, astringent, and deodorant, and liberate oxygen upon contact with organic matter. Bacteria are inhibited or destroyed by these dilute solutions. Potassium permanganate is used as an antiseptic on the mucous membranes in concentrations of 1:1000 to 1:5000. It is used also as a wet dressing. When the solutions turn brown, the compound is therapeutically inactive. The U.S.P. tablets contain 60, 120, 200, and 300 mg. (1, 2, 3, and 5 grains).

Sodium Perborate, N.F. Solutions of sodium perborate gradually decompose, thereby releasing oxygen. The drug is generally described as a powder, 1 teaspoon of which may be dissolved in a glass of water and used as a mouthwash. In contact with the mucous membranes, oxygen is rapidly liberated. Sodium perborate is widely used in the treatment of glossitis, gingivitis, and stomatitis. Sometimes the powder may be applied directly to the gums.

Metallic Peroxides. Some inorganic peroxides release hydrogen peroxide upon hydrolysis. Zinc peroxide is used for the disinfection and deodorization of wounds. Zinc oxide, which is astringent, remains at the site of application after the elimination of oxygen.

PHENOL AND RELATED COMPOUNDS

Phenol, U.S.P., B.P., I.P. (Carbolic Acid). Phenol was introduced into surgery by Dr. Joseph Lister in 1867, and at first it was extensively used. Its solutions are antiseptic, germicidal, or escharotic, depending on their concentration. Antiseptic solutions are toxic or irritating to the tissues of the host and therefore are seldom used today. One half to one per cent concentrations produce a mild local anesthetic effect and are added to oils or ointments to enhance their antipruritic effect. However, large areas of the body should not be exposed to prolonged contact with these preparations because phenol may be absorbed and produce systemic toxic effects.

Acute suicidal or accidental poisoning may occur occasionally from the ingestion of phenol. If large quantities are taken, the patient becomes unconscious and may die quickly of respiratory arrest. This may result from the sudden destruction of large areas of the mucous membranes, which produces collapse.

Preparations include Liquefied Phenol, U.S.P., B.P., and Phenol Glycerin, B.P.

Cresol, N.F., B.P., I.P. Cresol, which is a mixture of cresols, is three to ten times as active as phenol and is no more toxic. It is sparingly soluble in water; hence it is used in the form of an emulsion with soap and water (Lysol). The emulsion is used for the disinfection of excreta, instruments, and operating room equipment. Preparations include Saponated Cresol Solution, N.F., and Cresol with Soap Solution, B.P.

Resorcinol, U.S.P., B.P. Resorcinol is antiseptic and keratolytic and is used in the treatment of ringworm and various skin diseases. It is available in the form of ointments (Compound Resorcinol Ointment, N.F.) and lotions.

Hexylresorcinol, N.F., B.P. Solutions of hexylresorcinol have a low surface tension and a high penetrating ability, which accounts for their bactericidal action. A 1:1000 solution in glycerin and water (S.T. 37) is used as an antiseptic for the skin and mucous membranes. Hexylresorcinol was first introduced as a urinary antiseptic. Its use as an anthelmintic is discussed on page 236.

Thymol, B.P. An alcoholic solution (1 to 2 per cent) of thymol is an effective fungicide. It is also antiseptic. A crystal may be used to preserve urine specimens.

Hexachlorophene, U.S.P. (Gamophen, Septisol). This is a chlorinated diphenol which, when incorporated in soaps and synthetic detergents, exerts a bacteriostatic action on skin bacteria. Soaps and detergents containing hexachlorophene (see p. 742) must be used many times a day for some time to produce desirable effects. Preparations such as Hexachlorophene Liquid Soap, U.S.P., Dial soap, pHisoderm, and pHisoHex are available for many uses.

SURFACE-ACTIVE AGENTS

Surface-active agents are wetting agents that greatly decrease the surface tension of solutions, usually aqueous in character. The reduction in surface tension is responsible for the emulsifying, detergent, and penetrating properties of these substances. They aid water in emulsifying sebaceous secretions of the skin and hold bacteria and "solid soils" in suspension until they are rinsed off. The essential characteristic of these substances is that they contain polar, or hydrophilic, groups and nonpolar, or hydrophobic, groups. The anionic detergents ionize to form an hydrophilic group in the anion; the cationic detergents ionize to form an hydrophilic group in the cation.

Anionic Detergents

Soaps have been used for years as cleansing and weak antibacterial agents, but they are only effective against gram-positive organisms. Now available, however, are synthetic anionic detergents, which are more efficient and less irritating to the skin. Examples of these soap substitutes are pHisoderm and pHisoHex.

pHisoderm. This is a synthetic, soapless, sudsing detergent cream or white creamy emulsion. It is used as a soap substitute, especially where soap is contraindicated, as in eczema and other skin conditions. The detergent is available in three forms: (1) regular, for normal skin; (2) oily, for dry skin; and (3) dry, for seborrhea. It may be applied to the skin, scalp, and mucous membranes, and it may be used for the irrigation of open wounds. Its pH, a measure of acidity or alkalinity, is adjusted to that of the skin.

pHisoHex. This is pHisoderm with 3 per cent hexachlorophene. It is an antiseptic detergent that leaves an emollient and protective film at the site of application. It has a cumulative and persistent action when employed routinely and exclusively. pHisoHex is used for the preoperative preparation of the hands and arms of operating teams as well as the operative areas of the patients, and for cleansing mucous membranes and open wounds. It is also used prophylactically in skin and scalp infections. As an antiseptic detergent, a few drops are rubbed on the hands and arms, or 1 teaspoon or 1 tablespoon may be added to the bath water. For irrigation, 1 teaspoon or 1 tablespoon is added to 1 pt. of water. pHisoHex is available in 3-oz. refillable hand dispensers, 5-oz. squeeze bottles, and 1-gal. bottles.

Cationic Detergents

Quaternary ammonium compounds, which combine detergent action with pronounced antibacterial activity, are used in medicine as antiseptics. They are active against both gram-positive and gram-negative organisms. Soap inactivates these detergents and consequently must be removed before they are applied. Benzalkonium, benzethonium, and cetylpyridinium chlorides and Cetylcide are quaternary ammonium compounds that are often used as antiseptics.

Benzalkonium Chloride Solution, U.S.P., B.P. (Zephiran Chloride). This is a 1:1000 aqueous solution used in dilutions of 1:2000 to 1:10,000 for denuded areas and mucous membranes; 1:20,000 for bladder and urethral irrigations; and 1:40,000 for retention lavage of the bladder. Solutions of 1:5000 are applied as wet dressings to denuded areas. Instruments, rubber gloves, and tubes are sterilized and then stored in 1:750 solutions. Benzalkonium chloride has a prolonged germicidal effect when applied to operating room equipment. It also acts as a deodorant. Roccal is a 10 per cent solution (technical) for general disinfection.

Benzalkonium Chloride Tincture. This is a 1:750 alcohol-acetone-water solution used for disinfection of the unbroken skin as well as for superficial injuries and fungous infections.

Benzethonium Chloride, N.F. (Phemerol Chloride). A 1:1000 aqueous solution and a 1:500 tincture are used as germicides and antiseptics in cleansing wounds, lacerations, and infected areas of the skin. The aqueous solution is diluted to 1:5000 for use in the eyes and nose.

Methylbenzethonium Chloride, N.F. (Diaprene Chloride). This is used topically as an ointment containing 1 mg. per Gm.

Cetylpyridinium Chloride, N.F. (Ceepryn). Cetylpyridinium chloride is used as a local anti-infective. It is relatively nontoxic, nonirritating, and noncorrosive. It is applied topically to the intact skin in 1:100 to 1:1000 solution; 1:1000 for minor lacerations; 1:5000 to 1:10,000 to mucous membranes. Cetylpyridinium chloride is also marketed as a 1:1000 solution, U.S.P., as a 10 per cent solution, and as vaginal suppositories.

Cetylcide. This preparation is used for cold disinfection of instruments, rubber drains, and gloves from which soap has been rinsed. It is available in 10-ml. ampuls. The contents of an ampul are added to 1 qt. of water.

DYES

Certain dyes are used in medicine as antiseptics, antifungal agents, and wound-healing agents. They may be classified into three groups: (1) triphenylmethane dyes, (2) acridine dyes, and (3) azo dyes.

Triphenylmethane (Rosaniline) Dyes

Dyes in this group used medicinally are gentian violet, fuchsin, and brilliant green. The most useful of these drugs is gentian violet.

Gentian Violet Solution, U.S.P. (Methyl Violet, Crystal Violet). This is a 1 per cent solution of gentian violet in 10 per cent alcohol. It is used in moniliasis of the skin or mucous membranes, other superficial fungous infections, and certain pyodermas. It is applied with a cotton applicator to the involved areas twice a day. It is also used as an antiseptic dressing on wounds and the mucous membranes. The stain on the skin may be removed with aromatic ammonia spirit, and stains on cloth may be removed by washing. The use of gentian violet as an anthelmintic is discussed on page 237.

Carbol-Fuchsin Solution, N.F. (Castellani's Paint, Carfusin). This is an acetone-alcohol-water solution containing fuchsin, phenol, resorcinol, and boric acid. It is applied topically to superficial fungous infections twice a day.

Acridine Dyes

Proflavine Hemisulphate, B.P., and Acriflavine, N.F. These substances, which are derivatives of acridine, are active against gram-positive organisms. They are applied to open wounds as 0.1 per cent solutions and 1 per cent ointments, in which concentrations they are not irritating. Their tendency, upon continued administration, to retard the growth of granulation tissues limits their usefulness.

Azo Dyes

The azo dyes are useful in stimulating tissue proliferation and are employed in the treatment of wounds, chronic ulcers, and burns. They are administered in the form of 4 to 8 per cent ointments or oily solutions. Higher concentrations are irritating. Examples of these drugs are Scarlet Red, N.F., and Pyridium (see p. 649).

MISCELLANEOUS DRUGS

Alcohols

Alcohol (Ethanol, Ethyl Alcohol), U.S.P., B.P. (I.P.). Alcohol is widely used for disinfection of the skin prior to parenteral injections, venipuncture, and pricks to obtain blood.

Isopropyl Alcohol, N.F. This alcohol is slightly more antiseptic than ethyl alcohol. It may be used for the same local effects.

Boric Acid, U.S.P., B.P.

Boric acid is a weak antiseptic. Two per cent solutions are used for their soothing and weak antiseptic effect in the eyes and as wet dressings. A dusting powder (alone or diluted with starch or talcum powder) and a 10 per cent ointment are also used. Boric acid is still widely employed by the dermatologist; however, because accidental poisoning and death have resulted from internal administration, the pediatrician bars its use.

Preparations

| Boric Acid Ointment, N.F. | 10 per cent |
| Boric Acid Solution, N.F. | 4 per cent |

Nitrofuran Derivates

Nitrofurazone, N.F. (Furacin). Nitrofurazone has a wide antibacterial spectrum that includes both gram-negative and gram-positive organisms. It is applied topically to wounds, ulcerations, and burns which are contaminated with mixed infections. It is also useful in certain pyodermas. A 0.2 per cent aqueous solution (Nitrofurazone Solution, N.F.) is useful in the treatment of various eye, ear, and nose infections, the preparation of areas for skin grafting, and the treatment of osteomyelitis.

Nitrofurazone Ointment, N.F. (Furacin Soluble Dressing), contains 0.2 per cent nitrofurazone in a water-soluble ointment base. It is applied directly, or to dressings which are applied directly, to the infected area. Continued application of nitrofurazone may cause sensitization and allergic skin reactions.

Furazolidine, N.F. (Tricofuron). This drug is safe and nonirritating to inflamed tissues. It is used in the treatment of *Trichomonas vaginalis* vaginitis, and mixed trichomonal and monilial vaginitis. It is available as a 0.1 per cent powder and suppositories of 0.25 per cent.

Furazolidine and Nitrofuroxine, N.F. (Microfur, Tricofuron Improved), is administered intravaginally for trichomonal and monilial infections. It is available as 0.1 per cent powders and 0.25 per cent suppositories.

Triclobisonium Chloride (Triburon)

This is an antibacterial agent for use on the skin in burns, wounds, and various infections. It is used as a vaginal cream in *Trichomonas, Candida albicans,* and bacterial infections of the vagina. There are no side effects other than sensitization reactions, which are infrequent. The ointment is applied to the skin one to four times daily. The cream is introduced with applicators furnished. It is used nightly for two weeks. Ointments and creams contain 0.1 per cent.

ANTIFUNGAL AGENTS

Fungous infections in man may be divided into two types: (1) superficial infections of the skin, hair, nails, mucous membranes, and scalp; and (2) systemic mycotic infections. When fungi invade the nervous system and internal organs, they generally cause death (see p. 153). Systemic infections are rare in the United States.

Superficial infections do not endanger life, but they do cause disfigurations and extremely contagious diseases, which are often refractory to treatment.

The fungi do not invade living cells but, rather, the horny layers of the skin. This invasion may occur in any part of the body—the scalp, glabrous skin, groin, nails, or feet. The tissues react to the presence of the fungi by forming circular patches, scales, or crusts; hence one disease is often known as *ringworm*. Infections of the feet are commonly called *athlete's foot;* this is the most prevalent type and is found most often in the adult male. Scalp ringworm is essentially a childhood disease and is endemic to most of the major cities of the United States. For drugs used in treatment, see page 154.

The antifungal agents generally used are fungistatic. They are applied externally to the parts affected in the form of powders, ointments, and lotions. Hexachlorophene is sometimes added to the preparations to reduce the number of skin bacteria and thereby prevent secondary infections.

Triacetin (Enzactin, Fungacetin); Glyceryl Triacetate

Triacetin is an antifungal agent that liberates acetic acid slowly. It is applied topically in the treatment of superficial fungous diseases of the skin. No side effects other than sensitization reactions, which are infrequent, occur. Aerosols, powders, ointments, and liquids in concentrations of 25 per cent or more are applied to the skin. Preparations available are an aerosol (25 per cent), an ointment (25 per cent), a powder (33⅓ per cent), and a liquid containing 30 per cent in alcohol. The powder and aerosol may be used in shoes in epidermophytosis. (Rayon, nylon, and Dacron clothing should be protected.) Under the name of Vanay, a 25 per cent cream is available for application to the vagina at bedtime for the control of vaginal moniliasis.

Chlorquinaldol (Sterosan)

Chlorquinaldol (Sterosan) is applied topically in the treatment of gram-positive, mycotic, and mixed infections of the skin and minor wounds. It is used alone in the treatment of fungous infections of the scalp, nails, or skin or as an adjunct to griseofulvin therapy. Chlorquinaldol is marketed as a 3 per cent ointment or cream.

Chlordantoin (Sporostacin)

Chlordantoin (Sporostacin) is a potent, nonstaining, antifungal agent. It is applied locally as a lotion in monilial dermatitis or as a cream in vaginal moniliasis (candidiasis). Chlordantoin relieves symptoms promptly, usually in two days. The rate of cure is high, and a single course of treatment is, as a rule, adequate. It is available as a cream, lotion, or solution.

Fatty Acid Fungistatics

The long-chain fatty acids, which are normally present in the sweat and sebum, are used in the treatment of ringworm infections. They are nonirritating to the skin; nontoxic; and bacteriostatic (or bactericidal) as well as fungistatic (or fungicidal), which is fortunate because pathological bacteria tend to multiply in the inflamed skin. Three of these acids—undecylenic, caprylic, and propionic—are widely used in the prevention of athlete's foot (effective if used daily in powder form) and for glabrous skin infections.

Preparations

Undecylenic Acid, N.F., I.P., Undes-enoic Acid, B.P.	Marketed as a 1 to 10 per cent solution
Zinc Undecylenate Ointment, N.F. (Zincundecate)	20 per cent marketed as an ointment containing 5 per cent undecylenic acid and 20 per cent zinc undecylenate and as a powder containing 2 per cent undecylenic acid and 20 per cent zinc undecylenate

Trade names: Desenex; Undesol; Undex

Zincundesal Ointment	Mixture of 2 per cent undecylenic acid, 25 per cent zinc undecylenate, and 5 per cent salicylanilide in a carbo-wax base

Trade name: Salundek

Caprylic Compound	Mixture of 10 per cent sodium capry-late and 5 per cent zinc caprylate; marketed as an ointment and a powder

Trade name: Naprylate

Propionate Compound	Mixture of 10 per cent calcium pro-pionate and 10 per cent sodium pro-pionate in a water-miscible base

Trade name: Propion Gel

Propionate-Caprylate Mixtures	Mixtures of propionic and caprylic acids and their zinc, calcium, or sodium salts in varying proportions; marketed as an ointment, a powder, and a solution

Trade name: Sopronol

Methenamine undecylenate is used in elderly persons for skin infections of "devitalized limbs," particularly the toes of diabetics. It is dusted on the skin and between the toes. A powder is available.

OTHER ANTIFUNGAL AGENTS

Salicylanilide, N.F. (Ansadol, Salinidol). This mixture of salicylic acid and aniline is a powerful fungicide that is particularly useful in ring-worm of the scalp. Salicylanilide is available as an ointment containing 4.5 to 5 per cent. Because the drug is irritating to the skin, it should not be used is higher concentrations. This agent is sometimes employed in combination with fungistatics.

Diamthazol (Asterol Dihydrochloride). This drug is useful in all types of fungous infections. It is available as a 5 per cent ointment, powder, or tincture.

Coparaffinate (Iso-par). This drug is applied externally in mycotic infections of the hand and feet and in pruritus ani and vaginae. It is available as a 17 per cent ointment.

Benzoic Acid, U.S.P., B.P., I.P. This antifungal agent is essentially nontoxic and nonirritating. It is combined with salicylic acid in Whitfield's ointment.

Benzoic Acid and Salicylic Acid Ointment, U.S.P. (Whitfield's Ointment). This agent contains 6 per cent benzoic acid and 3 per cent salicylic acid.

Other Drugs. Salicylic acid, resorcinol, sulfur, gentian violet, and carbol-fuchsin are also used as fungistatic drugs. The quaternary ammonium detergents are mildly fungistatic.

PARASITICIDES

The common parasitic skin diseases are scabies, pediculosis, creeping eruption, and infections from chiggers and bedbugs. Scabies is caused by infestation of the skin with the mite *Sarcoptes scabiei*. The main symptoms are itching and scratching. Pediculosis is caused by the head, crab, and body louse.

The drugs most often used are benzyl benzoate, chlorophenothane, gamma benzene hexachloride (hexachlorocyclohexane), sulfur, and isobornyl thiocyanoacetate. The selective action of these drugs makes them very satisfactory substances for the treatment of scabies and pediculosis. They are toxic and should be used with great care. If ingested, they are poisonous.

Benzyl Benzoate Lotion, N.F.; Benzyl Benzoate Application, B.P. This is a mixture of benzyl benzoate with soap and isopropyl alcohol, a single application of which may cure a patient with scabies. It kills the larvae and mature forms; however, the eggs are more resistant. Repeated administration at short intervals may irritate the skin. Therefore, application should not be repeated in less than four or five days.

Chlorophenothane, U.S.P. (DDT); Dicophane, B.P. (I.P.). This drug is very useful in the treatment of scabies and pediculosis. It is available in the form of a powder (1 per cent DDT in talcum powder), a lotion, and an aerosol bomb (containing 3 per cent DDT). DDT is harmless to man, when properly used and if excessive inhalation is avoided. It is readily absorbed from oil solutions and ointments, and severe toxic effects and even fatalities have resulted. Therefore, oil solutions and ointments of DDT are contraindicated.

Benzyl Benzoate–Chlorophenothane Lotion (Enbin). This lotion is used in the treatment of pediculosis, whereas, for scabies, benzyl benzoate is adequate. Repeated applications of the lotion may cause sensitization, and in rare cases allergic skin reactions have been observed.

Gamma Benzene Hexachloride, U.S.P., B.P. (Hexachlorocyclohexane), U.S.P., B.P. (Gammexane, Gexane, Kwell, Lindane). This drug is used topically as a scabicide and pediculicide. Although it is highly toxic and is readily absorbed, it can be safely used as a lotion or ointment in concentrations up to 1 per cent, if prolonged or repeated application is avoided. A single application may be adequate; the drug should not be used more than twice.

Sulfur Ointment, U.S.P.; Ointment of Sulphur, B.P. Sulfur ointment has been used for many years, and still is one of the most effective scabicides. When it is applied to the skin, it not only destroys the parasites but also slightly checks the growth of bacteria. The drug softens the keratin, thereby facilitating penetration of the stratum corneum, into which the mites have burrowed.

Isobornyl Thiocyanoacetate (Lotion Bornate). An oil emulsion containing 5 per cent isobornyl thiocyanoacetate is used as a pediculicide. It is applied externally to the hairy surfaces of the body and allowed to remain for ten minutes, whereupon it is washed off with bland soap and water. The agent should not be applied more than twice.

SPECIAL SURGICAL MATERIALS

Tetrafluoroethylene Resin and Fiber (Teflon). This fibrous material is substituted for body tissue in the repair of arterial, aortic, cardiac, and other defects of various sizes. It is indestructible, possesses considerable strength, remains where it is placed in the body, and is associated with healing in a two- or three-week period. There is low tissue reactivity, as regards foreign-body reactions; and fibrin becomes adhered to the graft to produce a lining membrane.

Tetrafluoroethylene resin and fiber are available as knitted or woven tubes, mesh, and patches. The degree of porosity is selected according to the type of prosthesis, depending on the desirability for drainage (as in wound healing) or for a tight seal (as in open-heart surgery). Arterial and bifurcated aortic grafts, interlock mesh, and intracardiac patches are available.

Trade name: Teflon

Surgical Film and Adherent (Vi-Drape). This film is a soft, pliant plastic that may be sterilized and applied to the skin after the latter has been prepared for surgery (cleaned and disinfected). It is firmly attached by means of the special adherent. A sheet of the film may be applied to the operative site and the incision made through it. The film should extend far enough beyond the incision to protect the wound from bacteria on the skin or on the nonsterile draping material. It is especially useful in areas that are difficult to drape or to keep draped without shifting.

Trade names: Vi-Drape Film; Vi-Hesive Surgical Adherent

Vibesate Spray-on Plastic Bandage (Aeroplast). Vibesate is a solution that is sprayed on skin burns and wound edges where it quickly dries, leaving a protective, transparent, flexible, occlusive, plastic film. This film is inert biologically and chemically, nontoxic, nonsensitizing, and mildly bacteriostatic.

Certain abrasions, sutures or small wounds, burns, ulcerations, and other minor skin lesions can be covered with this film, following cleansing, disinfecting, and drying, without gauze, tape, or bandaging. Visual observation is possible without redressing. The film is peeled off when the area has healed, or when necessary. Used on the skin surrounding colostomies and draining wounds, this dressing protects contiguous areas from infection or erosion. Vibesate spray-on plastic bandage is available in 3-, 6-, and 12-oz. cans.

Trade name: Aeroplast

Methacrylate Resin Spray Dressing (Rezifilm). This spray-on liquid dressing is used in the same way and for the same skin conditions as vibesate. Neither spray should enter the eye or respiratory passages, or be used on second- or third-degree burns or for bleeding or granulating wounds. Methacrylate resin film is bacteriostatic and permits evaporation of perspiration. It is available in 2-oz. cans.

Trade name: Rezifilm

REVIEW QUESTIONS

1. *How do antiseptics act to produce their desired effects?*
2. *What are detergents? Give several examples. How do detergents produce their effects*
3. *Describe the care of instruments that are to be stored in benzalkonium chloride solution. What strength solution should be used?*
4. *Which of the mercury preparations may be used for skin preparation and in what strength of solution?*
5. *Name the precaution to be taken with instillation of silver nitrate 1 per cent solution. What strength solution should be used?*
6. *Give the precaution to be taken with the use of iodine tincture for skin antisepsis.*
7. *Name two types of fungous infections. What drugs are used in the treatment of these infections?*

8. *What drugs are used in the treatment of scabies and pediculosis? How are they administered?*
9. *Describe the features of artificial arterial prostheses.*
10. *What are the advantages in the use of a plastic film sealed to the skin, through both of which an incision may be made?*
11. *Describe vibesate and methacrylate resin spray dressing. In what form are they available? What are the conditions for which they are used and the advantages they offer?*

REFERENCES

Davis, B. D.: "Principles of Sterilization," in Dubos, R. J. (ed.) : *Bacterial and Mycotic Infections of Man*, 2nd ed. J. B. Lippincott Company, Philadelphia, 1952, pp. 707–23.

Davis, H. L. (ed.) : "Symposium. Mechanism of Evaluation of Antiseptics," *Ann. New York Acad. Sc.*, **53**:1, 1950.

Goodman, J. M.: "Liquid Nitrogen Therapy of Warts and Other Skin Lesions," *Canad. M. A. J.*, **82**:1, 1959.

Hardt, R. A.: "News from the Fungus Front," *Am. Prof. Pharm.*, **18**:792, 1952.

Rhoads, P. S.; Billings, C. E.; and O'Conor, V. J.: "Antibacterial Management of Urinary Tract Infections," *J.A.M.A.*, **148**:165, 1952.

Zintel, H. A.: "Asepsis and Antisepsis," *S. Clin. North America*, **36**:257, 1956.

Nitrofuran Derivatives

Diggs, E. S.; Prevost, E. C.; and Valderas, J. G.: "Treatment of Urinary Tract Infections in Obstetric and Gynecologic Patients with Nitrofurantone," *Am. J. Obst. & Gynec.*, **71**:399, 1956.

Mintzer, S.; Kadison, E. R.; Shales, W. H.; and Felsenfeld, O.: "Treatment of Urinary Infections with a New Antibacterial Nitrofuran," *Antibiotics & Chemother.*, **3**:151, 1953.

Special Surgical Materials

Adams, R.; Fahlman, B.; Dube, E.; Dube, F. J. C.; and Read, S.: "Control of Infections within Hospitals," *J.A.M.A.*, **169**:1557, 1959.

Adams, R., and Fraser, F.: "Plastic Skin Drapes," *Am. J. Nursing*, **59**:845, 1959.

East, W. M., and Muller, W. H.: "An Experimental Study of Resection and Replacement of the Superior Vena Cava," *Am. J. Surg.*, **99**:6, 1960.

Eisenberg, G. M., *et al.*: "Preliminary Studies of the Antibacterial Activity of a Plastic Spray Containing Tetramethylthiuramdisulfide Intended for Use on the Skin," *Antibiotic Med. & Clin. Therapy*, **7**:594, 1959.

Radigan, L. R., and Jontz, J. G.: "The Routine Use of a Spray-on Plastic Dressing in the Care of Surgical Wounds," *J. Indiana M. A.*, **51**:1521, 1958.

XI DRUGS USED IN THE TREATMENT OF ALLERGY. ENZYMES. TOXICOLOGY

In this section, several highly important but unrelated subjects are dealt with. The first chapter (Chap. 47) is concerned primarily with several types of drugs used in the prevention and treatment of allergy. Also discussed is another group of useful therapeutic agents: enzymes, taken from various living materials, purified, and administered by injection or inhalation.

The final chapter (Chap. 48) describes the problems of accidental and intentional poisoning, acutely and chronically acquired. Since the nurse is frequently the first professional person to see poisoning cases (e.g., in accident or emergency rooms, industrial clinics, wards, and homes), she must learn as well as possible the urgent features of management of poisoning. Much depends upon her training and proper actions before a physician arrives.

47

Drugs in Allergy. Enzymes in Therapy

ALLERGY

Approximately 10 per cent of the population in the United States is reported to possess some form of allergy. This is an altered and abnormal reaction of cells to various substances to which they are temporarily or continuously exposed. The alteration in the tissue reaction is perhaps always based upon a previous exposure or upon repeated exposures. The multitude of materials to which man can develop an allergy and the number of diseases caused or possibly caused by allergy make this subject a major problem.

A specific antigen-antibody type of reaction is involved in the allergic state. The antigen may be an ingredient of food, such as egg albumen or wheat protein. It may be a pollen from a plant, dander from a household or farm animal, wool, a bacterial substance, an ingredient of the injection-sting of an insect (which may be suddenly lethal), or almost any drug or chemical. The antibody is a complex protein that is produced by certain cells in response to the foreign material. This new specific protein remains a part of certain tissue cells or circulates in the blood. The involved tissue is the reacting target when the antigen, an inciting agent, is reintroduced to that tissue.

The tendency to develop allergy (frequently called hypersensitivity) is probably a hereditary matter, but the specific substances involved are environmental. Allergy of the respiratory tract comprises more than half of the allergy seen in medicine. There are many cases and types of allergy in which environmental antigens (allergens) cannot be demonstrated, e.g., urticaria (hives), asthma, and perennial rhinitis. Rheumatic fever and acute glomerulonephritis are quite probably hypersensitivity responses to streptococcal material. The collagen diseases listed on page 685 (lupus erythematosus, rheumatoid arthritis, etc.) are thought to be caused by autoimmune mechanisms or some type of hypersensitization. The body can apparently become sensitive to altered chemical materials that it produces itself.

The allergic diseases that are most prevalent are listed in Table 38. In all these disorders, cellular injury or reaction occurs when an antigen and its specific antibody interact. Thus, a variety of responses may follow. Smooth muscle may contract in an affected area, vessels may dilate, capillaries may

754

become more permeable, edema may be produced, glands may secrete excessively, and necrosis may occur, followed by fibroblastic invasion.

It has been reported that various substances are liberated in the body in the antigen-antibody reaction. Among these are histamine (chiefly), serotonin, acetylcholine, and heparin. Many allergy-type reactions produced experimentally may be blocked by a group of drugs known as *antihistamines*. Histamine injections produce certain phenomena similar to allergic reactions, and these can be prevented or abolished by these drugs. They have been extensively and successfully used in a number of the types of allergy.

─────────────────── **Table 38** ───────────────────

Some Allergic Diseases

Respiratory system
  Hay fever, pollinosis (seasonal)
  Perennial or vasomotor rhinitis
  Extrinsic bronchial asthma
    (inhalants, ingestants)
  Intrinsic or infectious asthma
    (antigens of resident bacteria)

Skin
  Contact dermatitis
    (plant substances such as poison ivy; various chemicals,
    animal danders, eczema)
  Atopic dermatitis
    Dermatitis from drugs and other ingestants such as foods

Blood vessels
  Urticaria (hives)
  Angioedema (usually called angioneurotic edema)
  Headache, including some migraine cases

Broad involvement
  Serum sickness
  Anaphylactoid shock

Bronchial Asthma.   When a reaction occurs in the bronchi, all the following effects are combined: muscular contraction in the tube wall, stimulation of the glands of the tubes with the production of a thick mucus, and swelling of the lining mucous membrane. As a result, breathing becomes difficult. This is known as bronchial asthma.

One type of asthma is said to be a psychosomatic disorder in which neurogenic impulses via the parasympathetic nerves to the bronchioles produce constriction in response to a subjective reaction to stress. The bronchodilators among sympathomimetic amines (see p. 461) and theophylline agents (pp. 764–65) are also used in asthma. Antihistaminic agents are of no value in neurotic asthma except through a sedative (or even a mild tranquilizing) action, which most of them possess.

Dermatitis.   This may be of two types.

1. *Contact Dermatitis.*   The offending agent touches the skin and produces a reaction in the epidermis, mainly at the point of contact. The common offenders are chemicals in industry, dyes, plastics, and, best known, poison ivy. This is an inflammatory-type reaction with the production of vesicles. If the cause can be determined, treatment is usually effectual. If not, the condition may resist therapy. Antihistaminics administered locally may be somewhat effective.

2. *Atopic Dermatitis; Infantile Eczema.*   This is thought to be hereditary. The offending agents are not in contact with the involved area and are thought to be in solution in the body fluid. Mental stress seems to be an important factor in many childhood and adult cases. Other allergies, such as asthma, are often present.

Urticaria.   This term is applied to itchy, localized wheals that result from capillary dilatation, with escape of fluid into well-defined areas of a given tissue such as the skin. They are similar in appearance to a mosquito bite and may vary greatly in size. The agent or material causing them is soluble and is carried by the blood stream to distant points. Thus, foods and drugs of many kinds are the offenders.

If an outpouring of fluid, as in urticaria, occurs in subcutaneous tissues, particularly the loose tissues of the lips and eyelids, large swellings occur and are termed *angioedema* or angioneurotic edema.

HISTAMINE

Histamine is found in nearly all plant and animal tissues, i.e., wherever protein is broken down. Most animal tissues contain a lethal amount of histamine in a combined or inactive form. However, no effect is produced until the substance is released in a free form into the body fluids as a result of certain stimuli.

Pharmacological Actions.   Histamine is not absorbed when taken orally; rather, it is destroyed in the intestinal tract by the enzyme histaminase. After injection, histamine produces a direct constricting action on certain smooth muscle, such as the bronchi, uterus, and intestines, as well as a powerful vasodilating action on the capillary bed.

Dilatation of the capillaries and arterioles produces flushing of the face, a fall in blood pressure, and an increase in skin temperature. Dilatation of the meningeal vessels, accompanied by an increase in cerebrospinal fluid, causes a severe headache, often called a "histamine headache."

Histamine stimulates all types of glandular secretions—gastric, duodenal, salivary, lacrimal, and nasal. An important effect in man is the stimulation of the gastric glands and an increase in hydrochloric acid in the stomach. Small amounts of histamine are injected as a diagnostic test to differentiate between nonspecific hypochlorhydria of the stomach and that caused by pernicious anemia.

If histamine, in diluted solution, is applied to the broken skin, the area first becomes blanched, then capillary dilatation occurs, whereupon a typical wheal is produced. The wheal is white and is usually surrounded by a "red flare." In susceptible individuals, a subcutaneous or intramuscular injection of 0.5 to 1 mg. of histamine will produce this same type of reaction over large areas of the skin.

The action of histamine is of short duration because it is rapidly destroyed, partly by oxidation and partly by histaminase.

Histamine Shock. Histamine shock resembles anaphylactic or traumatic shock. There is a profound fall in blood pressure, which is long lasting. Excessive dilatation of the small vessels permits the escape of fluid from the circulation into the tissues, and edema results. There is stasis of the blood in the capillary bed and poor venous return.

The toxic symptoms are rarely dangerous. They may be combated with stimulants and by restoration of the blood volume.

Uses of Histamine

1. *Diagnostic*

   a. To differentiate between transient hypochlorhydria and that caused by pernicious anemia.

   b. To test the capacity of the capillaries to dilate in certain peripheral vascular diseases.

   c. To diagnose pheochromocytoma.

2. *Therapeutic*

In certain conditions where histamine is thought to be a cause of the condition, namely: vasomotor rhinitis, "histamine headache," and other clinical entities. Minute but gradually increasing doses are administered for desensitizing to histamine.

Dosage and Method of Administration. Histamine is available as a phosphate and is supplied as a 3-mg. tablet that contains 1 mg. of histamine base, the active principle. The test dose used for the differentiation of non-specific hypochlorhydria and that caused by pernicious anemia is 0.3 mg., which is given subcutaneously. There is also a 1:1000 solution available for injection, which is given in the same dose as for testing.

Preparations

Histamine Phosphate, U.S.P.; Histamine Acid Phosphate, B.P. (I.P.) (Colorless Soluble Crystals)	0.3 mg. subcutaneously
Histamine Phosphate Injection, U.S.P.; Histamine Acid Phosphate Injection, B.P. (I.P.) (1:1000 Solution)	1 mg. of histamine base in 1 ml.

DRUGS USED IN THE TREATMENT OF ALLERGY

Drugs used in the prevention and treatment of allergy produce their beneficial effects in a number of ways. They may: (1) compete with histamine, (2) constrict the blood vessels, (3) relax the bronchi, (4) liquefy bronchial secretions, (5) modify tissue reactivity, or (6) produce sedation.

ANTIHISTAMINICS

Antihistaminics are stable, white, crystalline substances. Their salts are soluble in water.

Mechanism of Action.   Theoretically, histamine that has been released from the body cells or has been given by injection becomes attached to these body cells and thus causes a histamine reaction.

The body cells are thought to possess what are known as *receptors*, and it is with these that the histamine combines. The antihistaminics seemingly have this same ability. Consequently, when they are given therapeutically, they accomplish this first. Hence there are no free receptors left for histamine, and its action is blocked. Antihistaminics do not destroy histamine or combine with it chemically.

Effects Produced.   The antihistaminics, as a rule, produce sedation of the central nervous system. Large doses produce excitement and convulsions, and death may result from respiratory failure due to the convulsive seizures. They combat the fall in blood pressure, the urticaria, hives, and angioneurotic edema caused by histamine. They are not particularly useful as antispasmodic drugs.

Absorption and Fate.   The antihistaminics are readily absorbed from the gastrointestinal tract and therefore are generally administered orally. They are decomposed in the body by the liver, and the degradation products are excreted in the urine.

Therapeutic Uses

1. In a wide variety of allergic reactions, such as nasal allergies (particularly hay fever), vasomotor rhinitis, drug sensitization, serum reactions, "histamine headaches," pruritus, food sensitivity, and angioedema.

2. In asthma only when it is associated with hay fever or pollen sensitivity. They are not useful in the acute attack.

3. In irradiation sickness following exposure to x-rays.
4. In motion sickness (see pp. 379–80).
5. In Parkinson's disease (see p. 374).

Methods of Administration and Dosage Forms.   The antihistaminics are usually administered orally or topically. For oral administration, the drugs are available in tablets, capsules, and solutions such as elixirs or syrups. They may be given in combination with other drugs such as ephedrine, aminophylline, salicylates, stimulants, and in cough remedies. Ointments, creams, and lotions are available for local effects; however, these preparations are sometimes irritating, which limits their use. Sprays or aerosols are also used for their local effects.

Dosage.   There are at least 28 antihistaminic agents available and more than 200 combination products which contain an antihistamine. They vary widely in potency. Some are administered at three- or four-hour intervals because of short duration of activity. Others are longer acting, and some are prepared with slowly dissolving or slowly digested materials for providing prolonged activity, even to 12 hours.

Differences Among the Antihistamines.   In addition to simple potency comparisons, some antihistamines are found more suitable in certain patients or in certain conditions than in others. Trial of several may be made consecutively in chronic conditions. Furthermore, the side effects, principally drowsiness or sedation, may vary among the various agents. Diphenhydramine, doxylamine, and promethazine are reported to produce more sedation than others. Patient response also varies in this regard.

Toxicity.   Since these drugs are taken for long periods of time, the possibility of poisoning should not be overlooked. All these compounds have toxic potentialities, but they are relatively harmless in therapeutic doses. Most of the antihistaminics produce central nervous system depression, which is beneficial in some cases where calmness is desired. If the depression is marked and consciousness is blurred, accidents may occur, particularly among industrial workers operating machines, persons driving automobiles, and pilots of airplanes. Other side actions, which are minor and transient, such as dry mouth, nervousness, and irritability, may occur. Contact dermatitis and acute psychoses are observed at times. Anemia and agranulocytosis are rare. Severe toxic effects, such as convulsions and unconsciousness, may result in death.

Preparations and Dosages

Antazoline Phosphate Ophthalmic Solu-   0.5 per cent
tion, N.F.

Trade name: Antistine

Bromodiphenhydramine	Hydrochloride	25 mg. (25 to 50 mg.) three times daily
Bromodiphenhydramine Capsules	Hydrochloride	25 mg.
Bromodiphenhydramine Elixir	Hydrochloride	10 mg. in 4 ml.
Bromodiphenhydramine Steri-Vials	Hydrochloride	10 ml., 5 mg. in 1 ml.

Trade name: Ambodryl Hydrochloride

Brompheniramine Maleate, N.F.	4 mg. (up to 8 mg.) four times daily 12 mg. every 8 to 12 hours
Brompheniramine Maleate Tablets, N.F.	4 mg.
Brompheniramine Maleate Prolonged Action Tablets	12 mg.
Brompheniramine Maleate Elixir, N.F.	2 mg. in 5 ml.
Brompheniramine Maleate Injectable	10 and 100 mg. in 1-ml ampuls

Trade name: Dimetane
Synonym: Parabromdylamine

Carbinoxamine Maleate, N.F.	4 mg. three to four times a day 8 to 12 mg. two to three times a day
Carbinoxamine Maleate Tablets, N.F.	4 mg.
Carbinoxamine Repeat Action Tablets	8 and 12 mg.

Trade name: Clistin Maleate

Chlorcyclizine Hydrochloride, U.S.P.	50 mg. (25 to 100 mg.) up to four times a day
Chlorcyclizine Hydrochloride Tablets, U.S.P.	25, 50 mg.

Trade names: Di-Paralene; Perazil; Histantin (the base)

Chlorothen Citrate, N.F.	25 mg. (25 to 50 mg.) up to four times a day; parenteral, 10 mg. (5 to 10 mg.)
Chlorothen Citrate Tablets, N.F.	25 mg.

Trade name: Tagathen

Chlorpheniramine Maleate, U.S.P.	4 mg. (2 to 8 mg.) up to four times a day
Chlorpheniramine Maleate Tablets, U.S.P., B.P.	4 mg.
Chlorpheniramine Maleate Injection	10 mg. in 1-ml. ampuls; 100 mg. in 2-ml. ampuls
Chlorpheniramine Maleate Syrup	0.5 mg. in 1 ml.

Trade names: Chlor-Trimeton Maleate; Piriton; Teldrin

Clemizole Hydrochloride	20 mg. (10 to 40 mg. four times a day)
Clemizole Hydrochloride Tablets	20 and 40 mg.

Trade names: Allecur; Reastrol

Dexbrompheniramine Maleate	2 mg. four times daily
Dexbrompheniramine Maleate Tablets	2 mg.
Dexbrompheniramine Maleate Syrup	2 mg. in 5 ml.
Dexbrompheniramine Maleate Prolonged Action Chronotabs	4 and 6 mg. every 6 to 12 hours

Trade name: Disomer

Dextro-Carbinoxamine Tartrate | 2 mg. (2 to 4 mg. up to four times a day)

Dextro-Carbinoxamine Tartrate Tablets | 2 mg.

Trade names: Twiston; Rotoxamine

Dexchlorpheniramine Maleate, N.F. | 2 mg. three or four times daily or 6 mg. every 12 hours

Dexchlorpheniramine Maleate Tablets, N.F. | 2 mg.

Dexchlorpheniramine Maleate Dual Action Repetabs | 6 mg.

Dexchlorpheniramine Maleate Syrup, N.F. | 2 mg. in 5 ml.

Trade name: Polaramine

Dimenhydrinate, U.S.P. (Chloronautine) | 50 mg. (50 to 100 mg.) four times a day

Dimenhydrinate Tablets, U.S.P. | 50 mg.

Dimenhydrinate Solution | 50 mg. in 1 ml.; 5-ml. vials

Dimenhydrinate Syrup, U.S.P. | 3 mg. in 1 ml.

Trade names: Dramamine; Amosyt; Bontourist; Dramarin; Dramyl; Nautamine; Permitol; Suprimal

Diphenhydramine Hydrochloride, U.S.P., I.P. | 25 mg. (25 to 50 mg.) up to four times a day; intravenous, 50 mg. (10 to 50 mg.)

Diphenhydramine Hydrochloride Capsules, U.S.P. | 25 and 50 mg.

Diphenhydramine Hydrochloride Elixir, U.S.P. | 2.5 mg. in 1 ml.

Diphenhydramine Hydrochloride Injection, U.S.P. | 10 mg. in 1 ml., 10- and 30-ml. vials; 50 mg. in 1-ml. ampuls

Trade names: Benadryl Hydrochloride; Amidryl; Benapon; Benodine; Dabylen; Dimedrol; Restamin

Diphenylpyraline Hydrochloride | 2 mg. three or four times daily; 5 mg. every 12 hours

Diphenylpyraline Hydrochloride Tablets | 2 mg.

Diphenylpyraline Hydrochloride Prolonged Action Spansule | 5 mg. every 12 hours

Trade names: Diafen; Hispril

Doxylamine Succinate, N.F. | 25 mg. (12 to 25 mg.) up to four times a day

Doxylamine Succinate Tablets, N.F. | 12.5 and 25 mg.

Doxylamine Succinate Syrup | 1.25 mg. in 1 ml.

Trade name: Decapryn Succinate

Isothipendyl Hydrochloride | 4 mg. two to four times daily; 12 mg. (up to 24 mg.) twice daily

Isothipendyl Hydrochloride Tablets | 4 mg.

Isothipendyl Hydrochloride Prolonged Action Tablets | 12 and 24 mg.

Isothipendyl Hydrochloride Syrup | 4 mg. in 5 ml.

Trade name: Theruhistin

Methapyrilene Hydrochloride, N.F.	50 mg. (25 to 100 mg.) up to four times a day
Methapyrilene Hydrochloride Tablets, N.F.	25, 50, and 100 mg.
Methapyrilene Hydrochloride Elixir	6.67 mg. in 1 ml.

Trade names: Thenylene Hydrochloride; Histadyl Hydrochloride; Parathyn; Thenylpyramine; Semikon

Phenindamine Tartrate, N.F.	25 mg. (10 to 50 mg.) up to four times a day
Phenindamine Tartrate Tablets, N.F.	10 and 25 mg.
Phenindamine Tartrate Syrup, N.F.	2.5 mg. in 1 ml.

Trade name: Thephorin Tartrate

Pheniramine Maleate, N.F.	25 mg. four times a day
Pheniramine Maleate Tablets, N.F.	25 mg.
Pheniramine Maleate Elixir	1.88 mg. in 1 ml.

Trade names: Trimeton; Tripoton

Promethazine Hydrochloride, U.S.P., B.P., I.P.	25 mg. (6 to 50 mg.) up to four times a day; parenteral, 25 mg.
Promethazine Hydrochloride Injection, U.S.P.	25 mg. in 1 ml.; 250 mg. in 10 ml.
Promethazine Hydrochloride Syrup	1.25 mg. in 1 ml.
Promethazine Hydrochloride Tablets, U.S.P.	12.5 and 25 mg.

Trade name: Phenergan Hydrochloride

Pyrilamine Maleate, N.F.; Mepyra- mine Maleate, B.P. (I.P.)	25 mg. (25 to 50 mg.) up to four times a day
Pyrilamine Maleate Tablets, N.F.	25 and 50 mg.
Pyrilamine Maleate Syrup	2.5 mg. in 1 ml.

Trade names: Neo-Antergan Maleate; Anthisan; Neobridal; Paraminyl Maleate; Stangen Maleate; Statomin Maleate; Thylogan Maleate; Pyranisamine Maleate

Pyrrobutamine Phosphate, N.F.	15 mg. up to four times daily
Pyrrobutamine Phosphate Tablets, N.F.	15 mg.

Trade name: Pyronil

Thenyldiamine Hydrochloride, N.F.	15 mg. (15 to 30 mg.) up to six times a day
Thenyldiamine Hydrochloride Tablets, N.F.	15 mg.

Trade names: Thenfadil Hydrochloride; Thefanil

Thonzylamine Hydrochloride, N.F.	50 mg. up to four times a day
Thonzylamine Hydrochloride Tablets, N.F.	25, 50, and 100 mg.
Thonzylamine Hydrochloride Syrup	6.25 mg. in 1 ml.

Trade names: Neohetramine Hydrochloride; Anahist; Thonzylene

Tripelennamine Hydrochloride, U.S.P., I.P.	50 mg. (50 to 100 mg.) up to three times a day, 25 mg. parenterally
Tripelennamine Hydrochloride Tablets, U.S.P.	25 and 50 mg.

Tripelennamine Citrate, U.S.P.	50 mg. (25 to 75 mg.) four times a day
Tripelennamine Citrate Elixir	7.5 mg. in 1 ml.
Tripelennamine Hydrochloride	25 mg. in 1 ml. in 10-ml. vials

Trade names: Pyribenzamine; Azaron; Dehistin; Pyribenzoxal

Triprolidine Hydrochloride	2.5 mg. three times daily
Triprolidine Hydrochloride Tablets	2.5 mg.
Triprolidine Hydrochloride Syrup	1.25 mg. in 5 ml.

Trade name: Actidil

ANTIALLERGIC ANTIPRURITICS

Cyproheptadine (Periactin)

Cyproheptadine (Periactin) is a potent antagonist to both histamine and serotonin. It is recommended primarily for pruritic dermatoses. It is used in pruritus associated with angioneurotic edema, urticaria, dermatitis, drug reactions, poison ivy, sunburn, insect bites, pruritus ani and vulvae, neurodermatitis, and eczema. The oral dose is initiated with 4 mg. three or four times a day. The effect of a single dose lasts four to six hours, so it should be given three or four times a day for continuous relief. The principal side effect is drowsiness. Other side effects such as dry mouth, dizziness, jitteriness, nausea, and skin rash may occur infrequently.

Preparation

| Cyproheptadine Tablets | 4 mg. |

Trade name: Periactin

Trimeprazine (Temaril)

Trimeprazine (Temaril) is used orally to control itching. It antagonizes the action of serotonin and histamine. The side effects are, as a rule, mild. Drowsiness is noted. Blood dyscrasias and jaundice are rare. The oral dose is 5 mg. at bedtime and 2.5 mg. twice a day after meals. It is available as 2.5-mg. tablets and as a syrup containing 2.5 mg. in 5 ml.

Dimethpyrindene Maleate (Forhistal)

Dimethpyrindene (Forhistal) is effective in a large number of allergic and pruritic conditions, such as respiratory and ocular allergies, pruritus, and allergic dermatoses. The primary side effect is drowsiness. Other side effects which may occur infrequently are dryness of the mouth, nausea, diarrhea, insomnia, irritability, dizziness, and headache. The oral dose for adults and children over six years of age is one to two tablets one to three times daily; Lontabs, one in the morning and one in the evening, or 1 to 2 teaspoonfuls of syrup one to three times daily. Children under six should receive 0.3 to 0.6 ml. (0.25 to 0.5 mg.) of pediatric drops two or three times a day.

Preparations

Dimethpyrindene Pediatric Drops	30-ml. dropping bottle containing 0.5 mg. in 0.6 ml.
Lontabs	2.5 mg.
Syrup	1 mg. per 5 ml.
Tablets	1 mg.

Trade name: Forhistal

Methdilazine (Dilosyn, Tacaryl)

Methdilazine (Dilosyn, Tacaryl) is useful in the treatment of hay fever, rhinitis, bronchitis, and asthma. It is especially useful in relieving pruritus, contact dermatitis, and pruritus ani and vulvae. The adult oral dose is 8 mg. twice a day. Children receive 4 mg. twice daily. The primary side effect is drowsiness. It should be used with caution in patients receiving alcohol, analgesics, or sedatives, particularly the barbiturates.

Preparations

Methdilazine Syrup	4 mg. in 5 ml.
Methdilazine Tablets	8 mg.

Trade names: Dilosyn, Tacaryl

VASOCONSTRICTORS

Vasoconstrictors, which include epinephrine, ephedrine, and other sympathomimetic amines, are among the most effective agents in the symptomatic treatment of allergy. They constrict the blood vessels and decrease the exudation of fluids in the tissues responsible for the symptoms. Certain of these drugs are also good bronchodilators. The most potent drug of this group, epinephrine, is used in asthma and angioneurotic edema (see p. 452).

BRONCHODILATORS

Sympathomimetic Amines

The bronchodilator group of sympathomimetic amines (see p. 461) includes the most potent agents of this class and the most widely used drugs for relief in asthma.

Aminophylline

Among the bronchodilator drugs free of vasoconstrictor action, aminophylline (theophylline with ethylenediamine) has been one of the most useful.

Aminophylline has long been used in asthma. In this condition, the smooth muscle cells encircling the bronchioles are contracted, narrowing the air passages that lead to and from the alveoli. In some cases, all or part of the encroachment upon the air passage may be caused by swelling of the inner lining, the bronchial epithelium, and of the entire wall of the bronchioles. There are many causes for this condition (allergy, bronchitis, and psychosomatic illness). Relaxation of these encircling muscle fibers usually allows much better air flow in and out of the alveolar spaces. The rapid and labored breathing of the asthmatic is thus relieved, at least in part.

Aminophylline is most effective when it is administered intravenously; it is less effective rectally; and it is least effective orally. The usual oral dose is 200 mg., with a range of 100 to 200 mg. three times a day; the usual intravenous dose is 500 mg. with a range of 250 to 500 mg., up to three times a day; and the rectal dose is 500 mg. (250 to 500 mg.), up to twice a day. In anaphylactic shock, aminophylline is given to supplement epinephrine therapy.

LIQUEFIERS OF BRONCHIAL SECRETIONS

The bronchial glands may secrete a large amount of tenacious mucus, and bronchial obstruction resulting from the accumulation of this thick, viscid mucus or mucopurulent exudate is a serious problem in the treatment of respiratory diseases. The obstruction may involve a lobule, a lobe, or an entire lung and may cause atelectasis, emphysema, or infection beyond the obstruction. These conditions may require prolonged medical treatment or even surgical removal of the infected tissue. Therefore, it is very important to remove secretions before obstruction of the airway and its potential complications occur.

The inhalation of steam and vapors has been used for many generations. "Croup kettles" or tents, funnels, etc., have been employed. Compound Tincture of Benzoin is an old and popular aromatic material which is added to boiling water for this purpose. Vaporizers and nebulizers have been introduced for producing true aerosols with the particles small enough to remain in the air current. Water and various solutions are used in this way. Alevaire and Tergemist have the following desirable physical properties: (1) droplet size, (2) detergency, and (3) liquify secretions in the pulmonary tree. They are nebulized and inhaled as required to loosen and detach thick secretions. Some enzymes are useful in thinning bronchopulmonary secretions by a digestive action.

The above measures aid in coughing up secretions and constitute an *expectorant* action. Other expectorants in use for systemic medication are ammonium chloride, potassium iodide, guaiacol, and ipecac.

ENZYMES USED AS DRUGS

An enzyme is a biochemical catalyst that has the specific property of causing chemical changes to take place within an organism. Enzymes of many types are present in the body for the purpose of catalyzing a host of chemical reactions. For nearly every step in the intracellular metabolism of foods and the synthesis of the materials of which the body is built, there is a specific enzyme causing each specific reaction.

Various mammalian, plant, and bacterial enzymes are used for a variety of purposes.

MAMMALIAN ENZYMES

Hyaluronidase for Injection, N.F. (Alidase, Wydase)

Hyaluronidase for injection is a sterile, dry, soluble enzyme product obtained from mammalian testes. It hydrolyzes hyaluronic acid (cement substance of connective tissue) and increases the rate of absorption of fluids given subcutaneously. It is a *spreading factor* that increases the diffusion of fluid into the skin and connective tissue.

Therapeutic Uses. Hyaluronidase for injection is used (1) in hypodermoclysis, (2) with local anesthetics, (3) in urology with radiopaque dyes, (4) to aid reabsorption of hematomas, and (5) in some exacting surgical procedures (cosmetic facial, ophthalmological, etc.).

Dosage and Method of Administration. This enzyme is available in a dry, lyophilized form that is to be freshly dissolved in sterile physiological salt solution and injected into the tubing at the beginning of hypodermoclysis (subcutaneous infusion of fluids), or in other aqueous media. It is also available in a stable solution. The usual dose for hypodermoclysis is 150 U.S.P. units (15 to 1500 units).

Preparation

Hyaluronidase for Injection, U.S.P.   Vials or ampuls containing 150 and 1500 U.S.P. units

Trade names: Alidase; Diffusin; Enzodase; Hyalidase; Hyazyme; Hydase; Infiltrase; Kinetin; Laronase; Rondase; Wydase

Trypsin Crystallized, N.F. (Tryptar, Parenzyme)

Crystalline trypsin is a proteolytic, or protein-digesting enzyme preparation obtained from the mammalian pancreas. It is marketed in a dry form with an accompanying buffer solution. A *freshly prepared* solution is used for rapid and safe débridement of surfaces covered with necrotic tissue and abscess membranes, or for irrigation of such cavities as the pleural and nasal. The powder itself may be blown upon the involved surface (infected wounds, etc.), or capsules of it may be placed in poorly accessible sinus tracts, etc. Its greatest use lies in the liquefaction of coagulated blood and exudates and it is less frequently used in the digestion of fibrous tissue. It is irritating when inhaled as an aerosol for thinning viscous bronchial exudates. It is administered intramuscularly, orally, and (in milder cases) dissolved beneath the tongue for the treatment of thrombophlebitis (inflammatory clotting in veins), contusions with ecchymosis (extravasation of blood), varicose and other ulcers of the skin, and in severe bronchopulmonary disease. It digests only nonviable (nonliving) cells, their debris, bacteria, etc.

Side Effects. Trypsin may produce a local histamine-like effect with mild fever and increase in pulse rate. This may be combated by the use of an antihistamine. Used topically in wounds, it may cause a burning sensation. Administered intramuscularly, it may produce pain and induration. The enzyme should be removed from the pleural cavity and wounds after two hours, and the area cleansed.

Dosage and Administration. Trypsin is administered topically, sublingually, and intramuscularly. Wet dressings and irrigations should be repeated every three hours. Infiltration and instillation may be repeated twice daily. Trypsin in oil is stable; this and a solution in 5 per cent gelatin are injected deeply into the gluteal muscle, alternating the sites used. Patients with a history of hypersensitivity should receive a sensitivity test with a small dose. Allergic reactions may occur. Intramuscular doses of 2.5 to 5 mg., one to four times daily for up to eight days, with individualization and with caution against intravenous injection, are commonly employed. The 5-mg. buccal tablet for sublingual absorption can be used four times daily. The ointment is applied once or twice daily for two to four days. Antibacterial therapy with specific agents may be needed.

One brand of trypsin is labeled in units established by the maker, rather than in weight of pure enzyme. Package instructions for dosage should be followed.

Preparations

Trypsin Crystallized, N.F. (Lyophilized)	2500 N.F. units in 1 mg.; 25 mg. with 5-ml. vial of diluent; also 50,000 units in 10-ml. vials, 125,000 units in 20-ml. vials, and 250,000 units in 30-ml. vials
Trypsin in Oil	5 mg. in 1 ml., 5-ml. vials
Trypsin Buccal Tablets	5 mg.
Trypsin Ointments	Available with antibiotics or other bacteriocide

Trade names: Biotrase; Orenzyme; Parenzyme; Tryptar; Tryptest

Chymotrypsin (Chymar)

Chymotrypsin, a pancreatic enzyme similar to trypsin, is available in a solution in oil, with a dose of 0.5 ml. twice weekly if effective. An aqueous solution is also given intramuscularly at a dose of 0.5 to 1 ml. at the same intervals. A buccal tablet for sublingual absorption contains 10,000 units;

one tablet is given four times daily. An ointment is also available with hydrocortisone and neomycin added. It is reported to be useful in a number of types of skin conditions, ulcerations, and infections in the external ear canal.

Preparations

Chymotrypsin Solution in Oil (Injection)	5000 units in 1 ml., 5-ml. vials
Chymotrypsin Solution Aqueous (Injection)	5000 units in 1 ml., 5-ml. vials
Chymotrypsin Buccal Tablet	10,000 units
Chymotrypsin, Hydrocortisone, and Neomycin Ointment	10,000 units

Trade names: Chymar, Chymotest; Enzeon

Alpha Chymotrypsin (Alpha Chymar)

This pancreatic enzyme is similar to trypsin in origin and action but is used specifically for lysis (dissolving) of the zonular fibers of the suspensory ligament of the lens of the eye before the lens is surgically removed because of cataract. It is injected intraocularly prior to surgery. It is possible to remove the lens *within* its capsule and with greater ease after its use.

Preparation

Alpha Chymotrypsin (Lyophilized, Injection)	750 units, to be dissolved in 5 ml. of sterile saline

Pancreatic Dornase (Dornavac)

Deoxyribonuclease is an enzyme that splits into many smaller molecules the normal cellular constituent deoxyribonucleic acid, a complex organic material in cells, and also digests deoxyribonucleoprotein. Deoxyribonucleoprotein comprises between 30 and 70 per cent of the sediment of purulent material of bronchial and pulmonary discharge. The discharge is converted from a viscous exudate to a thinner, milky material, which is more readily expectorated when an aerosol of this enzyme is inhaled. Sensitivity may be rarely encountered.

Dosage and Administration. Pancreatic dornase is freshly dissolved in a sterile isotonic (physiological) solution of sodium chloride, 100,000 units in 2 ml., and administered by an aerosolizing apparatus. One or two milliliters may be inhaled once to three times daily for two to six weeks, if needed, and treatment repeated after a few days.

Preparation

Pancreatic Dornase (Lyophilized, Injection)	100,000 units

Fibrinolysin (Plasmin) (Actase, Thrombolysin)

Fibrinolysin dissolves fresh intravascular clots and is used with anticoagulants in the treatment of thrombophlebitis, phlebitis, and pulmonary embolism. It is given by intravenous infusion.

Fibrinuclease (Elase) is a combination of fibrinolysin and desoxyribonuclease used to lyse fibrin and liquefy pus. It aids in the removal of necrotic debris associated with vaginitis and cervicitis and of exudates from wounds, ulcers, and burns. It is applied topically and by irrigation. Solutions are prepared just before use to avoid loss of activity. Hyperemia may be noted.

Preparations

Fibrinuclease, dry material	Vials containing fibrinolysin, 25 units, and desoxyribonuclease, 15,000 units
Fibrinuclease Ointment	30 units fibrinolysin and 20,000 units desoxyribonuclease

Trade name: Elase

PLANT ENZYMES

Papain and Chymopapain

These potent proteolytic enzymes, or proteases, are present in the tropical fruit *Carica papaya*. They are available as aids to digestion, such as Caroid and Al-Caroid, in which they may substitute for pepsin in the gastric juice. They may also be used topically, as papain powder, which also contains chymopapain, for digesting mucinous, fibrinoid, and purulent crusts or discharges in wounds.

Preparations

Papain Powder	30 Gm., 2.2 kg.
Papain, Urea and Chlorophyll Ointment	30, 120 Gm.

Trade names: Caroid; Panafil

BACTERIAL ENZYMES

Streptokinase-Streptodornase (Varidase)

Streptokinase-streptodornase is a mixture of proteolytic enzymes derived from cultures of *Streptococcus hemolyticus*. Streptokinase causes a solution of fibrin; streptodornase is active against deoxyribonucleic acid, a component of pus, and produces liquefaction of the viscous, gel-like material. These enzymes are used together in solution.

Therapeutic Uses. Streptokinase-streptodornase is used to (1) liquefy clotted blood or fibrinous or purulent accumulations caused by injury or inflammation, (2) aid anti-infective drugs, and (3) stimulate healing. The preparation is used as a supplement in hemothorax, empyema, chronic suppuration in draining sinuses, infected wounds or ulcers, and osteomyelitis. It does not act on living cells and thus may be injected directly into body cavities or applied locally.

Preparation

Varidase Powder	24-ml. vials containing 100,000 units of streptokinase and 25,000 units of streptodornase; this is dissolved in 20 ml. of sterile saline before use

REVIEW QUESTIONS

1. *What are the principal features of, and phenomena occurring in, the allergic state?*
2. *Why is histamine thought to be involved in most allergic reactions?*
3. *Explain how the body supply of histamine does not cause any difficulty until it is released. What are its actions when released?*
4. *For what is histamine used? Name several antihistamine drugs and give their doses.*
5. *Describe the various effects of the antihistaminics.*
6. *By reviewing the sympathomimetic amines (Chap. 27) with the present chapter, choose the most desirable one or ones for dilating the bronchioles in asthma. Explain your choice or choices.*
7. *Describe the effects and methods of use of aminophylline.*
8. *Discuss the agents that decrease the thickness (tenacity) of mucoid secretions in the bronchial tree.*
9. *What enzymes are available for use in medicine? What are their particular applications? Must they always be freshly prepared?*

REFERENCES

HISTAMINE

Dragstedt, C. A.: "The Role of Histamine in Various Pathological Conditions and Methods for Controlling its Effects," *Quart. Bull. Northwestern Univ. M. School,* **19**:303, 1945.

————: "The Significance of Histamine in Anaphylaxis," *J. Allergy,* **16**:69, 1945.
Horton, B. T.: "The Use of Histamine in the Treatment of Specific Types of Headache," *J.A.M.A.,* **116**:377, 1941.
Selle, W. A.: "Histamine—Its Physiological, Pharmacological and Clinical Significance," *Texas Rep. Biol. & Med.,* **4**:138, 1946.

ANTIHISTAMINICS

Brown, F. R.: "The Use of Antihistamines in Allergic Disease," *New York J. Med.,* **56**:2711, 1956.
Council on Drugs: "Dexbrompheniramine Maleate (Disomer)," *J.A.M.A.,* **172**:242, 1960.
————: "Dexchlorpheniramine (Polaramine)," *J.A.M.A.,* **172**:242, 1960.

————: "Triprolidine Hydrochloride (Actidil)," *J.A.M.A.*, **172**:59, 1960.

Lipman, W. H.: "The Clinical Evaluation of Parabromdylamine Maleate (Dimetane)," *Ann. Allergy*, **17**:19, 1959.

MacLaren, W. R.: "Parabromdylamine Maleate, Chlorprophenpyridamine Maleate, and Tripelennamine Hydrochloride in Chronic Allergic Rhinitis," *J. Allergy*, **30**:235, 1959.

Michelson, A. L., and Lowell, F. C.: "Antihistaminic Drugs," *New England J. Med.*, **258**:994, 1958.

Olansky, S., and Olansky, M.: "Treatment of the Allergic Reaction with Dexbrompheniramine Maleate (Disomer)," *Current Therap. Res.*, **2**:81, 1960.

CYPROHEPTADINE

Bodi, T., *et al.*: "Clinical Use of a New Antihistamine and Antiserotonin Drug, Cyproheptadine," *Ann. Allergy*, **19**:386, 1961.

Stone, C. A., *et al.*: "Antiserotonin Antihistaminic Properties of Cyproheptadine," *J. Pharmacol. & Exper. Therap.*, **131**:73, 1961.

DIMETHPYRINDENE

Jacques, A. A.; and Fuchs, V. H.: "Dimethpyrindene, An Effective Antihistamine," *Louisiana Med. Soc.*, **113**:110, 1961.

METHDILAZINE

Arbesman, C. E.; and Ehrenreich, R.: "New Drugs in the Treatment of Allergies," *New York J. Med.*, **61**:219, 1961.

Spoto, A. P., Jr.; and Sieker, H. O.: "Treatment of Allergic Disorders with Methdilazine," *Ann. Allergy*, **18**:761, 1960.

BRONCHIAL ASTHMA

Levin, S. J.: "The Management of the Acute Attack of Asthma in Childhood; Special Reference to Short-Term Steroid Therapy," *A.M.A. J. Dis. Child.*, **97**:432, 1959.

Rowe, A. H., and Rowe, A. H., Jr.: "Bronchial Asthma—Its Treatment and Control," *J.A.M.A.*, **172**:1734, 1960.

Segal, M. S.: "Current Status of Therapy in Bronchial Asthma; Report to the Council," *J.A.M.A.*, **169**:1063, 1959.

AEROSOLS

Gibbs, G. E.: "Aerosol Therapy of Bronchopulmonary Disease of Childhood," *J. Omaha Mid-West Clin. Soc.*, **21**:5, 1960.

Seidel, J.: "Mucolytic Aerosol Therapy for Lipid Pneumonia," *J.A.M.A.*, **171**:1810, 1959.

ENZYMES

Burke, J. F., and Golden, T.: "A Clinical Evaluation of Enzymatic Debridement with Papain-Urea-Chlorophyllin Ointment," *Am. J. Surg.*, **95**:828, 1958.

Council on Drugs: "Buccal and Intramuscular Use of Streptokinase-Streptodornase (Varidase)," *J.A.M.A.*, **172**:701, 1960.

————: "Intramuscular Use of Crystalline Trypsin in Pulmonary Diseases," *J.A.M.A.*, **167**:1635, 1958.

Deaton, H. L., and Anlyan, W. G.: "Treatment of Thrombophlebitis with Streptokinase-Streptodornase," *J.A.M.A.*, **172**:1891, 1960.

Fletcher, A. P.; Alkjaersig, N.; Sawyer, W. D.; and Sherry, S.: "Evaluation of Human Fibrinolysin (Actase)," *J.A.M.A.*, **172**:912, 1960.

Liebowitz, D., and Riter, H., Jr.: "Anaphylactic Reaction to Chymotrypsin," *J.A.M.A.*, **172**:159, 1960.

Rob, C., and Singer, A.: "Debricin: A New Agent for Wound Debridement," *Brit. M. J.*, **2**:1069, 1959.

Simpson, D. G.: "Alpha-Chymotrypsin in Cataract Surgery," *Canad. M.A.J.*, **82**:767, 1960.

48

Toxicology

Toxicology is the scientific study of poisons—their source, chemical properties, actions, detection, and the treatment of conditions produced by them. A poison is a substance which, when introduced into the body in small quantities, may produce death or cause serious injury to one or more organs in the average healthy individual. It is often difficult to distinguish between drugs and poisons. All drugs are potential poisons, since overdosage may cause dangerous or fatal symptoms; and many poisons are useful drugs if they are administered in small doses. The margin of safety (the difference between the therapeutic and poisonous dose) may be extremely small in some cases. Some chemicals may be foods, drugs, or poisons, depending upon the amount ingested and the method of administration.

The nurse should be familiar with the symptoms and treatment of poisoning. She may be the first to see the patient and, by careful observation of the symptoms, may give much valuable information to the physician or, if death ensues, the toxicologist. The physician should be called immediately. In the meantime, the nurse should keep the patient warm and quiet, administer first-aid treatment, and remain as calm and collected as possible herself.

All evidence, such as (1) vomitus, (2) the first two gastric washings, (3) urine, (4) the stool passed, and (5) any foods or drugs that may have contributed to the symptoms, should be preserved in sealed, labeled containers. All may be used in identifying the poison. Diagnosis of poisoning is often very difficult because, although the toxic symptoms produced by overdosage with drugs are characteristic, they may be simulated by symptoms caused by disease. For example, poisoning with central nervous system stimulants may be mistaken for epilepsy, hypoglycemic convulsions for tetany, while symptoms caused by central nervous system depressants may simulate those that are caused by vascular accidents or brain tumors.

Occurrence of Poisoning.   Acute poisoning may be:

1. *Accidental.*   Accidental poisoning mostly occurs among young children who ingest substances found around the home, such as insecticides, cleaning fluids, and drugs. It may also occur among adults through attempts at self-medication, mistaking one drug for another, and clinical overdosage.

773

2. *Suicidal.* The substances most frequently used today for this purpose are carbon monoxide and the barbiturates.

3. *Criminal.* This form is not nearly so prevalent today as formerly.

Causes of Poisoning. Poisoning may occur by:

1. Inhalation of gases, volatile liquids, or dusts (e.g., carbon monoxide, carbon tetrachloride, lead dust).

2. Absorption through the skin (e.g., aniline dyes).

3. Overdosage with drugs by injection.

4. Ingestion of toxic materials.

Chronic Poisoning. This generally occurs as vocational or industrial poisoning among workers who inhale or absorb small amounts of a chemical over long periods of time. The harmful effects may be transient or permanent. This type of poisoning may also occur with prolonged treatment with drugs.

Acute Poisoning. *Accidental Poisoning in Children.* Each year over 1500 normal, healthy children in the United States die of acute accidental poisoning. There are also many who recover but remain crippled by lead encephalitis, liver or kidney damage, and esophageal stricture. One third of the accidental poisonings in children are due to the ingestion of drugs, and the commonest of these drugs are the salicylates (mostly aspirin, particularly the colored aspirin tablets containing sugar and a flavoring agent) and the barbiturates. Other dangerous substances are common household products such as insecticides, rat poison, bleaching agents, cleaning fluid, permanent-wave lotion, shampoo, nail-polish remover, antifreeze, detergents, furniture polish, and kerosene. The ingestion of kerosene is the cause of many deaths and sometimes occurs when this substance is kept in soft-drink bottles.

Most cases of accidental poisoning in children are preventable. However, when a child does swallow a poison, prompt and appropriate treatment may be lifesaving or prevent crippling.

Common Symptoms. The common symptoms of acute poisoning are as follows:

1. Nausea, vomiting, abdominal pain, diarrhea. SOURCE: many chemicals and drugs, food poisoning, black widow spider (abdominal pain, rigidity).

2. Corrosive burns on the lips, mouth, and throat. SOURCE: mineral acids, caustic alkali, oxalic acid, ammonia, bichloride of mercury, phenol, and fluorides.

3. Respiratory and circulatory symptoms such as cyanosis, shock, collapse, sudden loss of consciousness, and convulsions. SOURCE: lack of oxygen

(replacement by other gases, including odorless carbon monoxide, from decaying vegetables and fruit), many chemicals, and drugs.

4. Pupillary changes:

a. Mydriasis (dilated pupil). SOURCE: belladonna group, cocaine, nicotine, some anti-Parkinson's disease agents.

b. Miosis (constricted pupil). SOURCE: opium group, muscarine, physostigmine.

5. Respiratory paralysis. SOURCE: carbon monoxide, cyanides.

6. Skin discoloration:

a. Cyanosis (blue color around lips and fingernails). SOURCE: acetanilid, nitrobenzene, aniline, sulfa drugs, sodium nitrite, nitrate reduced in intestines to nitrite.

b. Jaundice (yellow color). SOURCE: arsenic, carbon tetrachloride, cinchophen.

c. Cherry red (color of blood). SOURCE: carbon monoxide.

7. Delirium. SOURCE: barbiturates, cocaine, opium, derivatives of atropine, lead, mercury.

8. Characteristic odor on the breath. SOURCE: chloroform, ether, phenol, and cyanides (differentiate acetone of diabetic acidosis).

Treatment. The specific treatment of acute poisoning is given in the discussion of the individual drugs. Most emergency treatment is symptomatic, and rapidity of action may result in the saving of a life or the prevention of disabling sequelae. The general principles for emergency treatment are as follows:

1. Identify the poison so that specific measures may be instituted with appropriate antidotes.

2. Remove most of the poison from the stomach by gastric lavage or emetics (1 tablespoon of mustard or 2 tablespoons of sodium chloride in a glass of warm water, or apomorphine). Children may be given a glass of milk, inverted, and gagged with the finger. Often emetics are of little or no value. Gastric lavage, however, is frequently lifesaving. When the stomach tube is used, antidotes and other substances (cathartics, when indicated) may be administered before removing the tube. Gastric lavage is contraindicated following ingestion of strong acids or caustic alkalies where passage of the stomach tube may cause perforation.

3. Administer a physiological antidote.

4. Institute supportive or restorative measures. These may be necessary even before the removal of the poison in order to keep the patient alive.

ANTIDOTES. Antidotes may be divided into two groups: chemical and physiological. The chemical antidotes administered orally, often by stomach tube, inactivate the poison in the stomach and prevent its absorption. The combination of the antidote and poison or the product formed may be a temporary one; hence it should be removed by gastric lavage. Common household substances used are milk and egg white, starch, strong tea, and coffee.

The chemical antidotes administered parenterally inactivate the poisons in the blood and tissues. Examples of these antidotes are dimercaprol (BAL), which is used in mercury, arsenic, gold, and cadmium poisoning; nitrites and thiosulfate, which are used in cyanide poisoning; and calcium versenate, which is used in lead poisoning.

Physiological antidotes combat or overcome the undesirable physiological effects produced by poisons. For example, respiratory stimulants will increase the amplitude and rate of respiration, which have been reduced by an overdose of a central nervous system depressant such as morphine. (See also Table 40, p. 783.)

SUPPORTIVE THERAPY.   Various measures should be instituted to maintain the vital processes of the body at a maximum functional level and to keep the patient alive while the poison is inactivated and excreted. This support includes the administration of oxygen for the treatment of shock, artificial respiration, circulatory and respiratory stimulants, and sedatives, when indicated.

In practically all forms of poisoning, death occurs due to cardiac paralysis or respiratory collapse.

POISONING WITH HEAVY METALS

MERCURY

Mercury poisoning may be either acute or chronic.

Acute Poisoning.   Acute mercury poisoning occurs most often from swallowing a solution of bichloride of mercury accidentally or with suicidal intent. Mercury may also be absorbed in toxic amounts through the skin and mucous membranes as well as through wounds.

Symptoms.   When a solution of a mercury salt is swallowed, there is a burning pain in the mouth, throat, and stomach. There are gum and tongue changes: a line across the gums denotes a deposit of mercury sulfide. There are a foul odor of the breath, excessive salivation, nausea, vomiting, bloody diarrhea, and tenesmus. Mercury salts are excreted by the kidneys, wherein they produce irritation of the tubules. Due to this action, albumin, blood cells, and casts appear in the urine. Extensive kidney damage may cause anuria and uremic poisoning. The pulse may be weak, thready, and irregular and the respiration shallow and irregular. Death due to collapse may occur rather quickly. Sometimes the patient may recover from the acute symptoms but die later from nephrosis and uremic poisoning.

Treatment. Skim milk or some protein is administered to precipitate the heavy metal. Fats should be avoided, since they would form mercury salts of fatty acids, which are soluble. The antidote is 1 pt. of skim milk, 50 Gm. of glucose, 20 Gm. of sodium bicarbonate, and three eggs. This causes precipitation of the poison and reduces further absorption. Mercury may also be adsorbed on activated charcoal. Dimercaprol (BAL) is administered intramuscularly to inactivate the mercury absorbed. Fluids are injected to maintain the volume and composition of the body fluids.

Chronic Poisoning. Exposure to small amounts of mercury over long periods of time will cause chronic poisoning. This may occur in workers in industries that use mercury salts. For example, mercury is used for smoothing rabbit fur in the manufacture of felt hats, and persons engaged in this occupation may become poisoned.

Symptoms. The symptoms are stomatitis (sore mouth), colitis, progressive renal damage, loss of appetite, gastrointestinal disturbances, anemia, and peripheral neuritis. The central nervous system may also be affected, as attested by the fact that behavior changes, mental depression, insomnia, and occasionally, hallucinations are observed. The treatment is symptomatic.

ARSENIC

Arsenic is present in many insecticides, rodenticides, paints, dyes, and cosmetics. The symptoms of acute arsenic poisoning are constriction of the throat, abdominal pain, vomiting, diarrhea, rice-water stools, bloody stools, convulsions or coma, or both.

Treatment. Arsenic poisoning is combated by gastric lavage with 1 per cent sodium thiosulfate, intramuscular administration of BAL, the administration of morphine for pain, stimulants, and treatment for shock.

LEAD

Chronic lead poisoning occurs in workers who handle lead or lead salts, such as white lead or type, over long periods of time. Painters, typesetters, and plumbers are often affected. The lead is absorbed from the skin, from the gastrointestinal tract when it is ingested with food contaminated by unclean hands, and by inhalation. Children are sometimes poisoned by chewing lead-painted objects.

Symptoms. The symptoms are nausea, metallic taste in the mouth, and bad breath. There is a line of lead sulfide on the gums. Lead colic (painter's colic), which consists of severe abdominal, cramplike pains, is a very characteristic symptom that may come on suddenly and last for several days.

Constipation and occasional vomiting occur. Anemia may be caused by the action of lead on the bone marrow. Muscular weakness of the extensor muscles of the hands and feet causes "hand drop" and "foot drop." Liver changes cause jaundice, and lead encephalitis causes sleeplessness, irritability, headache, and delirium.

In acute poisoning, severe appendicitis-like cramps, central nervous system disturbances, muscular twitchings, and convulsions may occur.

Treatment. *Acute Poisoning.* In acute poisoning, the stomach is washed out with warm water or 1 per cent sodium sulfate solution. Magnesium sulfate is administered as a cathartic. Morphine, atropine, and other antispasmodics are used to relieve pain. Shock therapy is instituted, and large amounts of calcium and phosphorus are administered. Calcium versenate is a safe and useful antidote in lead poisoning.

Chronic Poisoning. Lead colic is controlled by the intravenous administration of 10 ml. of a 10 per cent calcium gluconate solution. Atropine, nitrites, and papaverine are used as antispasmodics. Magnesium sulfate eliminates the unabsorbed lead. Excitement and convulsions are controlled by barbiturates. A diet high in calcium, phosphorus, vitamin D, and milk will cause the transfer of lead from the tissues to the bones. Large fluid intake ensures increased fluid output. Calcium versenate is used both in acute and chronic lead poisoning and as a prophylactic agent to prevent recurrence of symptoms in chronic poisoning.

CHELATING AGENTS

Chelating agents are organic compounds that unite with metal ions to form ring structures which are stable, soluble complexes. By their administration toxic metal ions may be removed from the body in a harmless form. Table 39 lists several of these agents and the heavy metals for which they are used with dosage and method of administration.

Dimercaprol, U.S.P., B.P., I.P. (BAL, British Anti-Lewisite)

Certain heavy metals combine with essential sulfhydryl (SH) groups in the receptor cells in the animal body and thus inactivate enzyme systems that depend on free SH groups for their action. BAL forms complexes with these metals, which are more stable than the complexes formed between the metal and the cell receptor. The metal-BAL complex is readily excreted.

Therapeutic Uses. BAL is useful in the treatment of poisoning or untoward reactions resulting from the administration of mercurials, arsenicals, and gold salts.

Dosage and Method of Administration. The intramuscular dose of 2.5 mg. per kilogram is repeated at four-hour intervals for a total of four

Table 39

Chelating Agents for Heavy Metal Poisoning

Chelating Agent	Antidote for Poisoning	Dosage and Method of Administration
Dimercaprol (BAL)	Arsenic Mercury Gold	I.m., 2.5 mg./kg. at 4- to 6-hr. intervals on each of first two days. Then reduced to two injections daily for a total of ten days.
Calcium Disodium Edetate (Calcium Disodium Versenate)	Lead	I.v., 1 Gm. in 250 to 500 ml. of 5 per cent dextrose solution by intravenous drip over 1 hr. twice daily for five days.
Penicillamine (Cuprimine) D-Acetyl-D,L Peni- cillamine	Copper Lead Iron Mercury	Orally, 250 mg. four times a day.
Deferoxamine (Desferal)	Iron	I.v., 400 to 600 mg. once or twice daily. In acute poisoning, 8 to 12 Gm. by gastric tube plus 2 Gm. i.m. or i.v.

to six injections on each of the first two days. The dosage then can be reduced to two injections daily for a total period of ten days or until complete recovery.

Preparation

Dimercaprol   Injection,   U.S.P.,   B.P.   300 mg. in 3 ml. in oil (I.P.)

Trade names: BAL; Dimersol; Sulphactin

Calcium Disodium Edetate, U.S.P.; Sodium Calcium Edetate, B.P.; Calcium Versenate (EDTA, Calcium Disodium Versenate)

This is a complex chemical compound that exchanges its calcium for lead ions in the blood to form a more stable, almost nonionic, water-soluble lead complex that is rapidly excreted intact in the urine. It can produce acute tubular necrosis principally of the convoluted tubules causing severe toxic and fatal effects.

Therapeutic Uses.   Calcium disodium edetate is used in the treatment of acute and chronic lead poisoning and in hypercalcemia.

Dosage and Method of Administration.   The contents of a 5-ml. (1-Gm.) ampul of calcium disodium edetate is diluted with 250 to 500 ml. of isotonic saline or sterile five per cent dextrose solution and administered by intravenous drip over a period of one hour. This dose is repeated twice daily for periods up to five days. Therapy is then interrupted for two days and followed by an additional five-day treatment, if necessary. The oral adult dose is 4 Gm. daily in divided doses.

Preparations

Calcium Disodium Edetate Injection,   5-ml. ampuls containing 1 Gm.
U.S.P.
Calcium Disodium Edetate Tablets   500 mg.
          Trade name: Calcium Disodium Versenate

Penicillamine (Cuprimine)

This derivative of penicillanic acid is a potent chelating agent useful in the treatment of Wilson's disease (hepatolenticular degeneration) which is caused by an inherited defect in copper metabolism. The symptoms of this disease are jaundice, pigmentation of the eye, ascites, and edema. Urinary secretion of copper is increased after the administration of this drug in Wilson's disease.

The oral dose is 250 mg. four times a day.

Preparation

Penicillamine Tablets   250 mg.
          Trade name: Cuprimine

Deferoxamine (Desferal) (see p. 505)

CARBON MONOXIDE POISONING

Carbon monoxide is formed by the incomplete combustion of carbon. Manufactured illuminating gas, automobile exhaust fumes, furnaces, and stoves are sources of this deadly gas. Carbon monoxide combines with hemoglobin to form carboxyhemoglobin, which does not readily take up oxygen and consequently blocks oxygen transport to the tissues. The mucous membranes, fingernails, and skin are cherry red in color. This gas is the cause of many cases of accidental and suicidal poisoning.

Symptoms. Small amounts of carbon monoxide may cause headache and vertigo. Transient weakness and dizziness may be the only symptoms before unconsciousness.

Treatment. Fresh air, artificial respiration, and oxygen are indicated. Circulatory and respiratory stimulants may be administered. The patient should be kept warm and quiet to minimize his need for oxygen.

CYANIDE POISONING

Cyanide, one of the most rapidly acting poisons, is used to fumigate ships and buildings and as an ingredient of silver and metal polishes. The poisoning is generally accidental. Firemen may be killed by cyanide liberated with the burning of celluloid.

Symptoms. There is a characteristic odor of bitter almonds on the breath. The cyanide ion inactivates the oxidative enzyme (cytochrome oxidase); thus, oxygen is not taken up by the tissue cells from oxyhemoglobin. The symptoms are giddiness, headache, cyanosis, and coma. Death results from respiratory paralysis.

Treatment. Inhalation of amyl nitrite is followed by the intravenous injection of 10 ml. of a 10 per cent solution of sodium nitrite. The nitrites produce methemoglobin, which in turn combines with cyanide to form non-toxic cyanmethemoglobin.

POISON CONTROL CENTERS

Accidental poisoning, particularly in children, is a very serious medical problem. In 1953, the first Poison Control Center was organized in Chicago. Since that time over 200 such centers have been established throughout the United States in over 40 states. About 90 per cent are located in hospitals. They supply up-to-date information concerning the identity of ingredients in trade-name products, current methods of treatment to physicians, and first-aid information to others. Some are mainly information centers and advice is often given by telephone. Other centers have facilities for the treatment of poisoning.

Analysis of the poisonings in 3926 cases show that about 55 per cent occurred as a result of the ingestion of medicines and that poisoning with aspirin was observed most frequently (more often in children than in older persons). Overdosage with barbiturates accounted for about one half of the deaths reported. Household preparations such as detergents, bleach, and disinfectants accounted for 14.3 per cent; pesticides, petroleum distillates, paints, and varnishes, 10.3 per cent. Cosmetics were the cause of about 3.5 per cent.

REVIEW QUESTIONS

1. *Discuss the things the nurse should do, with regard to aiding in the diagnosis of poisoning, when a very ill patient is brought to her clinical station.*
2. *What precautions could reduce poisoning in children?*
3. *List the household items that are poisonous if taken in sufficient quantities.*
4. *What poisons may discolor the skin? Constrict the pupils, dilate them? Cause a rigid abdomen with violent pain? Produce vomiting, abdominal pain without rigidity? Cause a healthy man to collapse soon after descending into a vat with potatoes therein? Cause death to several simultaneously in a home during the night?*

5. *When should a stomach tube not be employed following the ingestion of a poison?*
6. *Discuss the features of poisoning by bichloride of mercury. Discuss its specific, emergency, and supportive treatment.*
7. *Discuss lead poisoning, with regard to its acquisition, acute and chronic clinical symptoms and signs, laboratory findings, and methods of treating specifically as well as symptomatically.*
8. *Discuss poisoning by carbon monoxide and cyanide.*

REFERENCES

Arena, J. M.: "Accidental Poisoning in Children," *Ciba Clinical Symposia*, **3**:1, 1960.
———: "The Problem of Accidental Poisoning in Children as It Exists Today," *J.A.M.A.*, **159**:1537, 1955.
Bain, K.: "Deaths Due to Accidental Poisoning in Young Children," *J. Pediat.*, **44**:616, 1954.
Cann, H. M., and Verhulst, H. I.: "Control of Accidental Poisoning—A Progress Report," *J.A.M.A.*, **168**:717, 1958.
Line, F. G.: "Aspirin Poisoning in Children," *Tennessee M. A.*, **49**:307, 1956.
Mellins, R. B.; Christian, J. R.; and Bundensen, H. N.: "The Natural History of Poisoning in Children," *Pediatrics*, **17**:313, 1956.
Pearce, M. G.: "Emergency Service for the Poisoned," *Am. J. Nursing*, **63**:116, 1964.
Semsch, R. D.: "Acute Poisoning in Children," *Minnesota Med.*, **37**:362, 1954.
"Treatment of Acute Poisoning—2," *Brit. M. J.*, **2**:993, 1964.

HEAVY-METAL POISONING

"BAL in the treatment of Metallic Poisoning" (editorial), *J.A.M.A.*, **142**:488, 1950.
Cotter, L. H.: "Treatment of Lead Poisoning by Chelation," *J.A.M.A.*, **155**:906, 1954.
Foreman, H.; Hardy, H. L.; Shipman, T. L.; and Belknap, E. L.: "The Use of Calcium Ethylenediaminetetraacetate in Cases of Lead Intoxication," *A.M.A. Arch. Indust. Hyg.*, **7**:148, 1953.
Shiels, D. O.; Thomas, D. L. G.; and Kearley, E.: "Treatment of Lead Poisoning by Edathamil Calcium-Disodium," *A.M.A. Arch. Indust. Hyg.*, **13**:489, 1956.

— **Table 40** —

*Acute Poisoning in Children**

Poison	Common Source	Acute Symptoms	Treatment			Supportive
			Lavage	Antidote		
Strychnine	Cathartics, insecticides, rodenticides	Central nervous system stimulation, hyperreflexia, opisthotonos, convulsions	If no convulsion 1:10,000 potassium permanganate	No specific, use universal antidote		Sedation, oxygen
Arsenic	Insecticides, rodenticides, plant sprays, some paints	Constriction of throat, abdominal pain, projectile vomiting, diarrhea → rice-water stools → bloody stools, convulsions and/or coma	1% sodium thiosulfate	BAL		Morphine for pain, stimulants, treat for shock
Lye	Drano pipe cleaner, toilet bowl cleaner	Burning pain in mouth and stomach, mucous membranes soapy and ulcerated, bloody vomitus, collapse	No, and no emetic	Dilute vinegar solution or lemon juice, olive oil for pain		Fluids
Sodium hyposulfite or hypochlorite	Sani-Flush, Clorox, bleaching agents, washing powders	Vomiting, corrosive burns of lips, mouth, and tongue	Gastric lavage	No specific		Fluids
Salicylates	Aspirin, oil of wintergreen	Hyperpnea, listlessness, vomiting, dizziness, mental confusion, acidosis, hemorrhagic manifestations	Milk or 1:10,000 potassium permanganate	No specific, instill saline cathartic in stomach after lavage		Oral or parenteral fluids, watch electrolyte and acid-base balance

* Modified from Semsch, R.D.: "Acute Poisoning in Children," *Minnesota Med.,* **37**: 865, 1954.

Table 40 (*Continued*)

Acute Poisoning in Children

Poison	Common Source	Acute Symptoms	Lavage	Antidote	Supportive
				Treatment	
Barbiturates	Sedatives	Somnolence → stupor → coma, respiratory and circulatory collapse	If conscious	For use of analeptics see p. 319	Fluids, stimulants, oxygen, forced diuresis, artificial kidney
Hydrocarbons	Kerosene, gasoline, naphtha, benzene, cleaning fluids Fuel oil	Burning pain in mouth, nausea and vomiting, drowsiness, confusion, fever. Aspiration is common → bronchopneumonia	No	No specific	Oxygen, fluids, antibiotics
Fluoride	Insecticides	Excess salivation, abdominal pain, hematemesis, shallow respirations—respiratory collapse	Calcium chloride or milk	No specific	Fluids, calcium lactate i.v.
Carbon tetrachloride	Cleaning fluids, fire extinguishers, solvents for oils and fats	Nausea and vomiting, headache, inebriation, convulsions. Late effect is liver necrosis	1:10,000 potassium permanganate	No specific	Oxygen, fluids, high-protein and carbohydrate diet
Nicotine	Insecticides, plant sprays, tobacco, Black Flag	Nausea and vomiting, mental confusion, salivation, abdominal cramps, convulsions, coma, respiratory failure	Tannic acid or 1:10,000 potassium permanganate	No specific	Oxygen, stimulants
Mercury	Antiseptics, fireworks, insect spray, also tablets	Abdominal pain, vomiting, bloody diarrhea, circulatory collapse, kidney damage → oliguria → anuria	Copious amounts of milk, egg white	BAL	Fluids

Table 40 (*Continued*)

Acute Poisoning in Children

Poison	Common Source	Acute Symptoms	Treatment — Lavage	Treatment — Antidote	Treatment — Supportive
Aniline dye	Yellow and orange crayons, shoe polish	Apathy, dyspnea, cyanosis due to methemoglobinemia	Water	1% methylene blue i.v. (.2 ml./Kg.)	Oxygen, whole blood
Ammonia	Household ammonia	Burning in mouth and stomach, nausea and vomiting, abdominal pain, respiratory failure	No	Weak acids, olive oil	Fluids
Phosphorus	Rodenticides, roach poison, fireworks, imported matches*	Nausea and vomiting, abdominal pain, diarrhea, shock, garlic odor to breath, liver and kidney damage	2% copper sulfide, then 1:10,000 potassium permanganate	No specific	Fluids
Camphor	Camphorated oil, moth repellents†	Odor to breath, headache, excitement → delirium → convulsions	Water	No specific	Sedation, no opiates
DDT	Insecticides	Nausea and vomiting, weakness, vertigo, disorientation, coma	Water	No specific	Fluids, sedation, Ca gluconate
Cyanide	Rodenticides, metal polish, silver polish	Odor of bitter almonds on breath, giddiness, headache, cyanosis, coma acts rapidly	Early, 1:10,000 potassium permanganate	Immediate treatment may be of some value. Principle of treatment is to produce methemoglobin, which in turn combines with the cyanide to form nontoxic cyanmethemoglobin. Inhale amyl nitrate pearl. Follow with 10 ml. of 10% Na nitrite i.v. Sodium thiosulfate, 50%, 25 ml. i.v.	

*Matches made in the U.S.A. are now made with insoluble phosphorus trisulfide and are relatively harmless.

† Many moth repellents now contain paradichlorobenzene, which is relatively nontoxic.

XII
IMMUNITY AND IMMUNIZATION

In Section XII the processes by which individuals may develop or be given some degree of immunity or resistance to certain infectious diseases are described. The various types of immunity, both inherited and acquired, are briefly defined or discussed. This subject is taught as a separate course of nursing in some schools since it is not truly pharmacology. However, the nurse will under many circumstances administer "biologicals," the products to be described in this section, as frequently as other drugs described in this text. Therefore, the subject is sometimes included in courses of pharmacology and, for this reason, it is presented in this text.

In Chapter 49 certain principles and practical aspects of serums and vaccines, of toxins, antitoxins, and toxoids, and of antigens and antibodies will be discussed. Specific products available for use in providing in advance protection against several serious and often fatal infections, or in reducing their severity after they become established in the body will be considered.

49

Vaccines and Serums

TYPES OF IMMUNITY

Natural Immunity. Man is susceptible to infection only by certain microorganisms present in the world and has a *species immunity* to others that attack animals and other forms of life. Some races of men are less susceptible to certain specific infectious agents than others; for example, Caucasians, exposed to tuberculosis for many centuries, are appreciably more resistant to the disease than Afro-Americans and American Indians. This is an example of partial *racial immunity*. In addition, certain individuals exposed to an infectious agent, even in an epidemic or an endemic, may fail to contract the disease or to exhibit as severe a case as others. Thus, there is an *individual immunity* to many diseases affecting man. These various types of inherent, inborn resistance may be termed *natural immunity*. They are inherited by the individuals possessing them. When natural immunity is present, the tissues and circulating blood of the host or the intended host are not conducive to successful invasion by the infectious agent, or to the same degree as those of another host.

Acquired Immunity. In addition to any natural resistance to specific diseases which individuals may possess, they may acquire partial or complete protection against certain infectious disease. Such *acquired immunity* may come about through natural processes which may follow exposure to the infectious agent, whether overt disease accompanies the exposure or not. As a result of the subclinical or overt disease, substances may be produced within the body that can repel or moderate a subsequent attempted invasion by the same organism. Some of these substances may remain upon or within the wall of certain cells, and others may circulate in the tissue fluids and blood plasma. They can be demonstrated in the serum after clotting and separation of the serum from the contracted clot. They are known as *antibodies*, materials which are usually highly specific *against* invading organisms or their products. Antibodies are proteins made by certain cells of the host in response to the presence of foreign substances known as *antigens*. The latter may be the invading agents of infectious disease or chemicals derived from them. Antigens may also come from animals, plants, foods, and miscellaneous materials.

Passive Immunity. The antibodies against infectious agents produced

788

by some individuals or by animals may be concentrated and administered to patients for combating an infection. The use of antibodies constitutes *passive immunization* wherein the protective material, specific for a given infectious agent or group of closely related agents, is produced in another individual or animal and given thus "ready-made" to the patient.

Antiserum. The protective antibodies explained above in most cases are present in the serum of the animal or person who has produced them. Animals are repeatedly given small or increasing amounts of the particular antigen or infectious agent whereupon they may develop considerable quantities of antibodies, usually antitoxins. Administration of these antibodies in antisera provides immediate passive immunity to various diseases. They may abruptly improve the course of the disease process. They may also cause undesirable reactions such as allergic responses, anaphylaxis, anaphylactoid reactions, and serum sickness, to be described. In most cases the antibodies administered in antisera do not reside indefinitely in the recipient. The protection is temporary, often lasting for only a few months. The antibodies gradually lose their original potency by chemical change in the new host. The chief advantage of antisera, therefore, is the provision of immediate and, with sufficient dosage, quite high protection to a person exposed to or already having a serious infection. Antisera are not available for all diseases.

Active Immunity. A person may be caused to develop his own antibodies rather than receive them in antisera. For the development of such *active immunity* the antigens are injected into the subject. These antigens are either *vaccines* or *toxoids*.

Vaccines. Vaccines are suspensions of the infectious agents themselves that have been rendered incapable of multiplying in the host, or at least of causing the complete disease. They may be viruses, bacteria, or rickettsiae, treated in ways that render them safe and virtually harmless, yet allow them to serve as antigens and cause the active production of protective antibodies by the vaccinated individual. The latter thereby becomes resistant, partially or completely, to that disease in the event of subsequent exposure to its normally virulent, causative agent.

The disease agents used in vaccines have been made safe by exposing them to certain chemicals or by a process of *attenuation*. In this process, the infectious agents are allowed to grow on unnatural substances—in unnatural animal species, or in fertile incubated fowl eggs or embryos. Sometimes a small amount of the progeny of the agent is repeatedly removed from such environment and reinoculated into a new egg, animal, or other host. In some cases, such passage through dozens of abnormal hosts results in substantial decrease in virulence, to the point of producing no disease, or an extremely mild case, when the agent is finally harvested and administered to the person in whom immunization is to be produced.

Toxoids. Toxoids are altered toxins, the chemical materials poisonous to animals or man excreted by certain infectious agents or present in the microorganisms and released upon their death and disintegration. The excreted substances are known as *exotoxins* and the intracellular ones, *endotoxins*. Some toxins are extremely potent, minute amounts being capable of causing death. Active immunization against such powerful toxins would be laborious and could be dangerous if they were injected as antigens. Many such toxins can be altered chemically with reduction or abolition of their capability of causing toxic reactions, yet with preservation of their capacity to cause the body tissues to produce antitoxin against the original toxin. A widely used method of converting a deadly toxin into a virtually harmless toxoid is the treatment of the toxin with formaldehyde (Formalin). The protein of the toxin molecule is thereby *denatured*, or chemically altered in part so that it no longer can behave as it could originally. The toxoid can then be safely given, with rare exceptions, by injection on one or more occasions, with the gradual development of antitoxin in the tissues and blood of the person to be made resistant or immune to the specific disease or to its toxic effects.

Active immunization by the use of vaccines or toxoids requires a few weeks or months, depending upon the particular disease, because the host tissues must produce their own antibodies. These antibodies and antitoxins remain in the blood and tissues for longer periods of time when synthesized by the individual. Allergic reactions related to the injection of small amounts of blood protein from the donor animal are avoided in direct, active immunization.

When an individual is infected by or exposed to an agent against which he has been immunized, his antibodies and the specific antigens which caused their production meet in the blood, in the tissue fluids, or on tissue cell surfaces. One molecule of antigen combines with one molecule of antibody. An antibody usually will not react with an antigen of a different type. The affinity is so specific that it may be considered much as a lock and key for precision matching. The result of the *antigen-antibody reaction* is the neutralization of the antigen. It cannot then exert its toxic effect. Bacteria or viruses may thus be agglutinated, destroyed, or otherwise prevented from causing the usual damage. Toxins may be neutralized and made inert.

Summary.   Vaccines consisting of weakened (attenuated) or killed infectious agents, viruses or bacteria, may be injected or ingested for the production of *active immunity*. Several doses at weekly to monthly intervals are often required for the production of adequate protection. Antibodies are thus produced which can react with the original agent and render it ineffective for causing disease, or prevent the usual severity of infection. Toxoids, the safe, altered toxins of infectious agents, may be similarly used for the production of antitoxins in a subject who then develops active immunity against the specific toxin used.

Such antibodies or antitoxins can be derived from other individuals or from animals and administered to a subject for the establishment of immediate *passive immunity*. Materials of these types, including serum products and vaccines, are often called *biologicals*. Most of these medical products will be described in the ensuing pages, followed by descriptions of the general, untoward reactions which may occur with their use and the general methods of treating those reactions. The products must be kept under refrigeration at temperatures specified on their containers. This information and expiration dates are stamped upon cartons and labels as required by law.

VACCINES

Vaccines are employed for the prevention of specific diseases by the establishment of active immunity developed by the vaccinated individual.

Smallpox Vaccine, U.S.P., B.P.

Smallpox (variola major) is a serious and frequently fatal disease caused by the virus *variola*. Vaccines of virus (cowpox), which have been in use since the eighteenth century, are prepared by the attenuation process, calves being used as the experimental animals. The calf lymph is obtained on about the seventh day after the inoculation and is treated with glycerin as a preservative and antibacterial agent. After standing for four to six weeks, if free of bacteria, it is ready for use. Cowpox vaccine is called vaccinia, hence the name "vaccination." Calf lymph virus vaccine will probably be replaced by the vaccine made from virus grown in the allantoic sac of hen eggs. Successful vaccination against smallpox provides adequate protection within eight days, lasting for several years with gradual decrease of immunity.

Infants should be vaccinated before six months of age and before entering school. Vaccination should be repeated before or following known or possible exposure to smallpox. The deltoid muscle prominence of the upper arm is usually used for vaccination in boys and men, and the lateral portion of the thigh in girls and women.

Technique. One drop of smallpox vaccine is placed on the skin which has been cleansed with ether or acetone and allowed to dry. No germicidal solution should be used, for the virus may be inactivated thereby. A sterile solid needle is supplied for use in pressing the skin, held stretched with one hand, where the vaccine has been placed. The needle is held tangentially to the skin and pressed gently but firmly through the drop of vaccine into the epidermis of the skin. This is done 10 to 20 times but the area should not exceed 2 mm. in width. The excess vaccine should be removed but the area should not be covered. The parents should be instructed that the area around the vaccination may be washed but not the area itself. Parents should also be instructed that they should be sure that the child does not scratch the area.

Reactions. If an active vaccine is properly administered, one of three types of local reactions should occur: (1) *Primary* or *vaccinia* reaction, usually seen when there has been no previous vaccination, or when the immunity from a previous "take" has been largely lost. A papule appears on the third to the fifth day, which soon contains a fluid (vesicle formation) and is surrounded by a red zone called the areola. The lesion grows larger for one or two weeks, the top of the vesicle disintegrates, and an open ulcerated and weeping area exists until a crust forms. The latter becomes detached after the third week leaving a pink scar which becomes white and irregular over a period of two years. (2) *Accelerated* or *vaccinoid* reaction, a mild reaction occurring somewhat earlier, reaching a maximum within a week, and subsiding perhaps within two weeks. This modification of the vaccination results from partial immunity still existing from a previous vaccination. (3) *Immune* reaction or "early" response. This is a still milder reaction occurring within a few hours and becoming maximum within 10 to 72 hours. It may represent merely a sensitivity to previously administered virus and may *not* indicate immunity. It should be considered the latter only if the vaccine employed is known to be active and if the inoculation technique was proper. If the skin is not broken sufficiently for introducing the virus successfully, no reaction may occur, in which case the procedure should be repeated.

The vaccination site should be examined on three occasions: (1) on the second or third day for detecting an *early* reaction; (2) on the fifth to seventh day for noting *accelerated* or *vaccinoid* reaction; and (3) on the eighth or ninth day for observing a *primary* reaction or "take." Several mild to severe complications may infrequently follow smallpox vaccination, including eczematous lesions, secondary bacterial infections, gangrene at the site of inoculation, generalized vaccinia eruptions, spread of the lesion to adjacent skin, and, rarely, vaccinia encephalitis. These may be reduced in severity by the use of *vaccinal gamma globulin* available from Dr. C. Henry Kempe, Department of Pediatrics, University of Colorado Hospital, Denver, Colorado.

Smallpox vaccine is available in packages containing individual doses in sealed capillary tubes and a like number of sterile needles similarly sealed. A small rubber bulb is included for expressing the vaccine. Sterile precautions must be taken, following package instructions.

Preparation

Smallpox Vaccine, U.S.P.   Packages of 1, 5, and 10 capillary tubes

Poliomyelitis Vaccine, U.S.P., B.P.

An effective and safe vaccine for combating poliomyelitis has been sought for nearly a half century. Dr. J. F. Enders and his collaborators found in

1949 that the virus which causes this disease can be grown in tissues other than the brain and spinal cord, in which it produces its damage resulting in paralysis. This opened the way for the ultimate development of an effective vaccine by Dr. J. E. Salk and co-workers, using formaldehyde-killed viruses of three main types, grown in artificially cultured monkey kidney tissue. Extensive clinical use in 1954 indicated that a high degree of protection is provided by this vaccine against types 1, 2, and 3 viruses.

Vaccines made with living but attenuated virus of the three types have been made for oral use independently by the teams of Drs. A. B. Sabin, H. Koprowski, and H. Cox. These vaccines have been used extensively throughout the world with no present indication that the viruses may change to a virulent, form.

Dosage and Method of Administration.   For infants, children, and adults at least through the age of 40, three doses of 1 ml. each (killed-virus vaccine) are recommended for active immunization. The first two should be at least two but preferably four to six weeks apart, and the third, seven months later. Booster doses should be given every year until otherwise suggested after further study of the duration of protection. Either the subcutaneous or the intramuscular routes may be employed.

Preparation

Poliomyelitis Vaccine, U.S.P.   1-'and 9-ml. vials

Poliovirus Vaccine, Live, Oral, U.S.P., B.P. Types I, II, and III

Oral vaccines as originally developed by Dr. A. B. Sabin have been approved for immunization against three virus types of poliomyelitis. They provide a high degree of protection against types I, II, and III polioviruses, immunity occurring usually within seven to ten days after single doses of the separate vaccines. They usually produce both a local response in the epithelium of the gastrointestinal tract and a systemic one. Two frozen preparations are available as listed below and must be distinguished when administered.

Dosage and Administration.   The U.S. Public Health Service recommends that a dose consist of 200,000 to 500,000 Tissue Culture Infective Doses ($TCID_{50}$). This amount is contained in approximately three drops of the preconstituted diluted vaccine (not the concentrated form). It may be given on a small sugar cube, in water, in a syrup, or with food to infants over six weeks of age, to children, and to adults. The amount given to infants under six weeks of age is two drops of the preconstituted vaccine. Type I vaccine may be given first, followed by type II after four to six weeks. Type III is given after another six weeks. The vaccine should not be given during any acute illness other than minor respiratory infections nor within two weeks of tonsillectomy.

Preparations

Poliovirus Vaccine, Live, Oral, Types
I, II and III

Frozen Concentrate	5-ml. vials containing 100 doses (2 ml.), with calibrated dropper
Frozen Preconstituted Vaccine	5-ml. vials containing 10 doses (1.5 ml.), with calibrated dropper

Storage

Prolonged storage for both the concentrated and preconstituted form is safe for one year at a temperature of $-20°$ C., or below. After thawing and diluting, the vaccine is safe for seven days when refrigerated at temperatures of $2°$ to $5°$ C.

Influenza Virus Vaccine, U.S.P., B.P.

Influenza may be caused by one of several strains of influenza viruses. There are two or more A strains and two or more B strains. The known strains can be grown in the allantoic sac of the chick embryo, purified to a great extent, concentrated, and inactivated with formaldehyde or ultraviolet irradiation. The amount of virus of each strain is expressed in chicken cell agglutination (CCA) units, usually one or two hundred for each strain in each milliliter. Protection, established within one to two weeks, is not complete with present vaccines, but their use is recommended whenever outbreaks of the disease occur, or on an annual basis. Persons sensitive to egg, chicken, or chicken feathers should not be given vaccines of egg origin.

Dosage and Administration. Persons over 12 years of age not having been vaccinated within six months should receive subcutaneously or intramuscularly 1 ml. of a polyvalent (multiple-strain) vaccine, repeated after two or more weeks. Those vaccinated two to six months previously may be given one booster dose of 1 ml. Children under five years of age may receive intracutaneously or subcutaneously 0.1 ml., repeated in one week. Those between the ages of 5 and 12 may be given doses of 0.5 ml. similarly.

Preparation

Influenza Virus Vaccine, U.S.P.   1-, 5-, and 10-ml. vials

Rabies Vaccine, U.S.P., B.P.

Rabies, a serious, viral disease, may be produced by the bite, however trivial, of any animal harboring the infection. A number of wild and domesticated animals are known to have caused the disease in man. Any animal should be kept under close observation for ten days after it has bitten a person. If it has not died of its own infection in that time, it most probably does not have rabies and the bitten victim need not be given rabies vaccine, which was introduced by Dr. Louis Pasteur. If the animal dies, the brain must be examined by a pathologist; if the Negri bodies typical of rabies are found in brain cells, the victim must be vaccinated. Immunity can be established in a bitten man before the disease becomes manifest, since a few weeks or months may be required as the incubation period. If the neck or head is bitten, however, vaccination may be begun immediately.

The vaccine is a suspension of either finely ground brain virus harvested from infected duck embryos or of tissue of rabbits killed about six days after inoculation with rabies virus. The virus obtained from rabbits either is killed by phenol (Semple method) or is attenuated by freezing and rapid drying in a vacuum (Harris method). The virus from duck embryos is killed.

Complications.   Paralysis and death have occurred on rare occasions in persons who have received rabies vaccine. Postvaccinal encephalitis has occurred as often as once in 600 vaccinations, a higher ratio than the chances of contracting rabies after known dog bites in one area studied. The physician therefore uses considerable judgment before deciding upon the use of the vaccine unless rabies appear in the animal inflicting the wound. Antirabies horse serum is available and appears to be effective but causes serum sickness in up to one fifth of treated patients.

Dosage and Method of Administration.   The vaccine is prepared by several manufacturers in varying concentrations. The daily dose of a 5 per cent suspension is 2 ml. if the virus is killed and 1 ml. if "live." Package anl label instructions clearly state the daily dose of the. particular brand. Fourteen to twenty-one subcutaneous injections may be given in the loose tissue of the abdominal wall.

Preparation

Rabies Vaccine, U.S.P.   Vials of 7 and 14 doses (usually 0.5-, 1-, and 7-ml. vials)

Mumps Vaccine

Egg-grown mumps virus killed by ultraviolet irradiation or ether is moderately effective and may be given in two subcutaneous or intramuscular injections of 1 ml. each, at least a week apart, to children and adults. Sensitivity to egg or chicken products must be ruled out or great care taken in its presence. Immunity probably does not exceed two years.

Preparation

Mumps Vaccine   2- and 10-ml. vials

Yellow Fever Vaccine, U.S.P., B.P.

This vaccine is prepared from chick embryos inoculated with an attenuated strain which is safe and highly antigenic when administered as a living virus, frozen, dried, and resuspended. It is given subcutaneously as a single dose of 0.5 ml.

Preparation

Yellow Fever Vaccine, U.S.P.   5- and 10-dose ampuls

Measles Vaccine

Live Attenuated Measles Vaccine is prepared in chick-embryo tissue culture. The vaccine induces active immunity after a single dose and produces in the recipient a mild or noncommunicable measles infection. Although in the majority the symptoms are minimal, some persons experience fever of 103 F. beginning about the sixth day and lasting two to five days. However, they frequently experience relatively little disability. A modified measles rash is seen which, unlike true measles, begins with or after the subsidence of fever. A few persons develop mild cough, coryza, and Koplik's spots.

If standardized Immune Globulin is given in the recommended dose at the same time as the live attenuated vaccine, but at a different site and with a different syringe, clinical reactions to the vaccine are sharply reduced.

To date, there have been no reports of encephalitis or other serious reactions after administration of the live, attenuated vaccine to normal children. A few instances of convulsions, apparently of the febrile type and without known sequelae, have been recorded.

Inactivated Measles Vaccine is propagated on monkey or chick-embryo tissue culture, and subsequently inactivated, concentrated, and precipitated. Whether the protective effect of the vaccine persists beyond six months is not yet known.

It is thought that a combination of the two vaccines will improve their effectiveness.

Recommendations for Use.   The vaccines are indicated primarily for children without a history of measles. They should be administered at nine months of age or as soon thereafter as possible. Children under nine months of age frequently fail to respond to immunization because of the presence of residual maternal antibodies. The vaccines are rarely indicated in adults since all but a very few are immune.

Dosage and Method of Administration.   The live attenuated vaccine is administered subcutaneously in the upper arm in a dose of 0.5 ml. The dose of the inactivated vaccine is three intramuscular injections of 0.5 ml. each at approximately monthly intervals.

Preparations

Measles Virus Vaccine, Live, Attenuated   Vial containing 0.5 ml.
in lypholized form

Trade name: Rubeovax

Measles Vaccine Inactivated   Vial containing 0.5 ml.

Trade name: Vax Measles-K

Typhus Vaccine, U.S.P., B.P.

Epidemic, louse-born typhus is caused by a rickettsia (*R. prowazekii*) which may be grown in egg yolk sacs for vaccine production. The organisms are killed with formaldehyde. Two subcutaneous injections of the vaccine, 1 ml. each, should be given at seven- to ten-day intervals. The same total dose may be given to children in three or more separate amounts. A booster six months after the initial immunization is advocated.

Preparation

Typhus Vaccine, U.S.P.   1- and 20-ml. vials

Rocky Mountain Spotted Fever Vaccine

The rickettsia causing this disease, *R. rickettsiae,* is carried by ticks. Rickettsial vaccine is recommended for those who work in endemic areas at that time of the year when infected ticks reach maturity. Rickettsia vaccine is grown in chick embryos and is administered subcutaneously or intramuscularly. Adults are given three injections of 1 or 2 ml. each at weekly intervals. Children may receive half of these amounts.

Preparation

Rocky Mountain Spotted Fever Vaccine   3- and 20-ml. vials

Pertussis Vaccine, U.S.P., B.P.

Whooping cough, caused by the bacterium *Hemophilus pertussis,* is commonly combated by the subcutaneous injection of 0.5 ml. of pertussis vaccine (killed pertussis bacteria) weekly for three weeks in six-month-old infants. Immunization can be accomplished as early as one month after birth. Booster doses are advisable after two years, upon entry into a school, and under special situations thereafter. Package instructions may be followed for the dosage schedule. Pertussis Immune Human Serum, U.S.P., is described on page 802. Pertussis vaccine is combined with diphtheria and tetanus toxoids and with these and poliomyelitis vaccine. These preparations are described on page 800.

Preparations

Pertussis Vaccine, U.S.P.   7.5-ml. vials
Adsorbed Pertussis Vaccine, U.S.P.   7.5-ml. vials

Typhoid Vaccine, U.S.P., B.P.; Typhoid and Paratyphoid Vaccine, U.S.P., B.P.

"Triple typhoid" vaccine, containing killed bacteria of typhoid and paratyphoid A and B (TAB), provides a high but not complete degree of protection against all three infections. Typhoid Vaccine, U.S.P., is available for immunization against typhoid fever alone. The usual dose of either vaccine is three injections of 0.5 ml. 7 to 28 days apart. Children may receive smaller doses. Injections should be made subcutaneously above the deltoid muscle. Intracutaneous injections are made using smaller amounts on some occasions. Malaise, mild fever, chilliness, perspiration, and pain and swelling at the site of injection may occur. Booster doses every one or two years are advised for persons exposed to water and food likely to be contaminated with typhoid or paratyphoid organisms, or for patients with these diseases.

Preparations

Typhoid Vaccine, U.S.P.	0.5-, 1.5-, 5-, and 20-ml. vials
Typhoid and Paratyphoid Vaccine, U.S.P.	1.5-, 5-, 15-, and 20-ml. vials

Cholera Vaccine, U.S.P., B.P.

Killed cholera vibrios suspended in saline or another suitable solvent constitute this vaccine which is given subcutaneously, 0.5 ml., followed by 1 ml. in seven to ten days.

Preparation

Cholera Vaccine, U.S.P.	1.5- and 20-ml. vials

Plague Vaccine, U.S.P., B.P.

Containing killed plague bacilli, this vaccine is administered subcutaneously in two injections of 0.5 and 1 ml. seven to ten days apart.

Preparation

Plague Vaccine, U.S.P.	2- and 20-ml. vials

IMMUNIZING TOXINS AND TOXOIDS

Diphtheria Toxoid, U.S.P.; Diphtheria Vaccine, B.P.

The causative agent of diphtheria, *Corynebacterium diphtheriae*, secretes a potent exotoxin which is quite toxic to the victim of the disease and contributes materially to the morbidity and lethality of the infection. When the toxin itself, free of the bacteria, is injected into an animal or man, antibodies against it are produced, but the toxic effects of the antigen (the toxin) make it undesirable for use in man. The toxicity can be minimized and the antigen made quite tolerable to children by treating it with formaldehyde. It is then known as a toxoid (toxin-like), for it has been altered somewhat. It continues, however, to have good antigenic potency and causes the production in the body of adequate amounts of circulating antibodies against the natural toxin elaborated during infections. Diphtheria Toxoid, U.S.P., is the Formalin-treated toxin. Adsorbed Diphtheria Toxoid, U.S.P., is toxoid precipitated or adsorbed by the addition of alum or of aluminum hydroxide or phosphate. This process results in a more purified product with greater stability and fewer untoward reactions.

Infants should be immunized, preferably with alum-precipitated toxoid (APT), between the ages of 6 and 12 months or earlier if exposed. A booster should be given six months after the first inoculation and again upon entry into school. Immunity is not permanent, and if older children or adults are exposed, a Moloney skin test with plain toxoid, 0.1 ml. of a 1:20 dilution intracutaneously on the forearm, may be made for determining sensitivity to the toxoid. If no skin reaction occurs within 24 to 48 hours, toxoid or APT can be given as a booster or primary inoculation.

Dosage and Method of Administration.   Plain toxoid is given subcutaneously over the deltoid area in three injections of 0.5 or 1 ml. as specified on the particular label, three to four weeks apart. APT is given similarly in two such injections at an interval of four to six weeks.

In order to determine whether a person has immunity to diphtheria toxin and would thus probably not be suspectible to infection, a skin test known as the Schick test may be performed. Toxin which has been inactivated by heating between 70° and 85° C. for five minutes (Inactivated Diagnostic Diphtheria Toxin, U.S.P.) is injected intracutaneously in a dose of 0.1 ml. An absence of redness, swelling, etc., signifies adequate antibodies in the individual. A positive reaction denotes susceptibility.

Combinations of diphtheria toxoid with tetanus toxoid and pertussis vaccine are presented on page 800.

Preparations

Diphtheria Toxoid, U.S.P.	1.5-, 7.5-, and 15-ml. vials
Adsorbed Diphtheria Toxoid, U.S.P.	5-ml. vials
Inactivated Diagnostic Diphtheria Toxin, U.S.P.	1-, 5-, and 10-ml. vials

Tetanus Toxoid, U.S.P., B.P.

Tetanus, or "lockjaw," is an infection caused by the anaerobic bacillus, *Clostridium tetani,* which secretes an exotoxin that produces the major manifestations of the disease. Almost complete protection is afforded by active immunization with the formaldehyde-treated toxin, using three subcutaneous injections of 0.5 or 1 ml. as specified on particular labels three or four weeks apart. The more purified Adsorbed Tetanus Toxoid, U.S.P., which has been precipitated or adsorbed upon alum or aluminum hydroxide or phosphate, is given in two similar injections four to six weeks apart. Boosters are recommended within a year, at the time of injuries which may introduce tetanus bacilli, and at one- or two-year intervals, especially in those exposed to possible injuries. A skin test for sensitivity using 0.1 ml. of undiluted toxoid injected intradermally is often performed. If redness develops at the site of injection, daily administrations of fractions of the dose are carried out until the complete dose has been given. Tetanus antitoxin is discussed on page 801.

Preparations

Tetanus Toxoid, U.S.P.	1.5- and 7.5-ml. vials
Adsorbed Tetanus Toxoid, U.S.P.	1- and 5-ml. vials

COMBINATIONS OF ANTIGENS

We have had one example of the simultaneous vaccination with three antigens in the triple typhoid-paratyphoid A and B vaccine (p. 789). When desirable and permissible by reasons of safety and effectiveness, inoculation of several antigenic substances is performed with combined products. This avoids multiple injections for immunization against each disease. The following products are available with dosage regimens sufficiently close to the schedules specified for the individual items in the foregoing pages that they will not be separately listed here. In all cases, package directions should be followed unless altered by the physician.

Preparations

Adsorbed Diphtheria and Tetanus Toxoids, U.S.P., B.P.	1- and 5-ml. vials
Adsorbed Diphtheria and Tetanus Toxoids and Pertussis Vaccine, U.S.P., B.P.	1.5- and 7.5-ml. vials
Adsorbed Diphtheria and Tetanus Toxoids and Pertussis and Poliomyelitis Vaccine, Adsorbed	9-ml. vials

ANTITOXINS

The principles underlying the production of blood sera that contain antibodies that can be used in a patient for the protection against specific bacterial toxins (passive immunization) have been described on pages 788–89. Following a description of the more useful antitoxin preparations, a discussion of the dangers and untoward reactions which must be watched for will be given.

Diphtheria Antitoxin, U.S.P., B.P.

Diphtheria antitoxin is the refined and concentrated serum antibody globulin, usually obtained from the horse, and contains at least 500 antitoxin units per milliliter, based upon a standard. Antitoxin is used after an exposure to diphtheria if the subject is Schick-positive and cannot be observed daily, or upon early signs of the disease.

Dosage and Administration. For prophylaxis following exposure, 1000 units (500 to 2000) may be given intramuscularly or intravenously. For treatment of diphtheria, 20,000 units (10,000 to 80,000) may be administered with cautions to be described (pp. 802–3) and fully discussed in package literature.

Preparation

Diphtheria Antitoxin, U.S.P. 1,000, 5,000, 10,000, 20,000, and 40,000 units (vials)

Botulism Antitoxin, U.S.P.; Botulinum Antitoxin, B.P.

This combination of the two types (A and B) of antitoxins of equine origin is used in the treatment of toxemia known or suspected to be caused by *Clostridium botulinum*, the anaerobic species of bacteria that causes severe food poisoning.

Dosage. Intravenously, 10,000 units should be injected as early as possible and repeated at four-hour intervals as long as needed. The vials contain 10,000 units of each type, A and B.

Tetanus Antitoxin, U.S.P., B.P.

Tetanus antitoxin is usually of equine origin and is indicated immediately when wounds occur on the street or farm, around animals, or otherwise could be suspected of contamination by the bacillus of tetanus, unless tetanus toxoid (p. 799) has been given recently enough to be protective. The usual precautions for administering horse serum must be observed (p. 789). Antitoxin is also given when the disease is present.

Dosage and Administration. For prophylaxis, 1500 N.I.H. units (1500 to 5000) are given, and for therapy in established disease, 40,000 units (20,000 to 120,000) may be given. Smaller doses may be given subcutaneously or intramuscularly and higher ones intravenously.

Preparation

Tetanus Antitoxin, U.S.P. 1500, 3000, 5000, 10,000, and 20,000 N.I.H. units (vials)

Gas Gangrene Antitoxin, B.P.

The refined, concentrated equine, antibody globulins for protection against the toxins of two or more of the clostridia organisms are available. These organisms are anaerobes (they grow in the absence of oxygen) which produce gas and necrosis in the infected tissues. "Combined" antitoxin contains 10,000 units each of *Cl. perfringens* (*Cl. welchii*) and *Cl. septicum* (*vibrion septique*) antitoxins. Trivalent antitoxins include also 1500 units of *Cl. oedematiens* (*Cl. novyi*) antitoxin. Polyvalent antitoxins may also contain protection against *Cl. bifermentans* (*Cl. sordelli*), 1500 units, and *Cl. histolyticus*, 3000 units, in addition to the first three named above. These products are of greater importance in wartime, but are used in appropriate cases in civilian practice.

Dosage and Administration.   The several preparations described are available in vials containing in one therapeutic dose the amounts of antitoxins enumerated above. One to four vials may be given intramuscularly, although the intravenous route is usually preferred. Additional doses may be given in one to four hours. Sensitivity to horse serum must be ruled out or combated.

Tetanus–Gas Gangrene Antitoxin

Several preparations are available which combine tetanus antitoxin with two or more antitoxins in the gas gangrene group named above. Package literature specifies the dosage and the methods of administration.

Pertussis Immune Globulin, U.S.P.

This preparation is a sterile solution of globulins derived from the blood plasma obtained from persons who have recovered from pertussis and have been afebrile and free of signs of the disease for at least seven days. It is used prophylactically and therapeutically for whooping cough in infants and children.

Dosage and Administration.   Intramuscularly. Prophylactic, one or two injections of an amount recommended by the manufacturer at one-week intervals for two or more weeks. Therapeutic, two injections at one-day intervals.

REACTIONS TO VACCINES AND SERA

Reactions to Vaccines.   Persons in need of vaccines which are grown in chicken eggs should be asked about possible hypersensitivity to egg, chicken, or chicken feathers. The nurse may be the only one who makes such inquiry. In the presence of a history of hypersensitivity, such vaccines must not be given. This is true also of duck-egg vaccines. This precaution applies, therefore, to the vaccines of influenza, mumps, yellow fever, typhus, Rocky Mountain spotted fever, and rabies.

Local reactions to egg-grown vaccines are common. There may be transient stinging with redness, tenderness, and induration for up to 24 hours. Various vaccines may cause malaise, headache, backache, and fever. The minute amounts of penicillin or streptomycin present in some poliomyelitis vaccines have on rare occasions caused allergic reactions in persons hypersensitive to these agents. Dangerous specific reactions have already been described for some vaccines (e.g., rabies vaccine, p. 794). The various reactions to smallpox vaccine are discussed on page 792.

Reactions to Sera.   There are four main types of serum reactions. (1) *Serum Sickness.*   A subject receiving a first injection of horse serum may become febrile (up to 103° or 104° F.) within five to ten days or even as late as the fourth week. Urticaria (hives) usually follows; lymph glands may enlarge rather generally, especially above the site of injection. One or more joints may become enlarged and tender. A rash may appear. These manifestations may last for several hours and occasionally for a few days. They may recur one or more times but they are not fatal. Epinephrine is used in controlling serum sickness and other serum reactions (see pp. 450–54). (2) *Accelerated Reaction.*   The foregoing reactions may begin in two to five days and become more severe. This is more likely to occur in individuals who have previously received serum from the same species. (3) *Immediate Reaction.*   In a person who is highly sensitive to an animal serum, a severe and possibly lethal reaction can occur within a few minutes or hours after even a drop or two of diluted serum is received. This is called anaphylaxis or anaphylactic shock and is manifested by flushing, restlessness, dyspnea, cyanosis, edema of the lips and other facial tissues, urticaria, high fever (up to 108° F.), and sudden death. There may be local anaphylactic reaction called the *Arthus phenomenon* which may be associated with sloughing and gangrene. (4) *Thermal Reaction.*   Following serum administration by any parenteral route, but particularly the intramuscular, a febrile reaction may occur with chilliness followed by perspiration, all subsiding after one or more hours.

Prevention of Serum Reactions.   The present methods for refining serum have greatly reduced the former incidence and severity of reactions. Serum should not be used unless the indication is sufficiently great. *Ophthalmic tests,* in which 0.1 ml. of a 1:10 dilution of the serum is dropped into the conjunctival sac of one eye, may reveal with redness a sensitivity to the serum. A *skin test* using the same quantity of diluted serum injected intracutaneously (within the skin) may show redness around the wheal, indicating sensitivity. Negative ophthalmic and skin tests do not always mean an absence of sensitivity. The complete measures for preventing or treating serum reactions should be studied in courses in immunology and public health, for this is of utmost importance to avoid serious complications.

REVIEW QUESTIONS

1. *What factors contribute to natural immunity?*
2. *Describe two kinds of methods or events by which an individual may acquire immunity to a disease.*
3. *What is passive immunity and how does it differ from active immunization in rapidity of induction and in duration?*
4. *Discuss or define the following terms:*

Antigens	*Toxins*	*Accelerated serum reactions*
Antibodies	*Toxoids*	*Immediate serum reactions*
Antisera	*Attenuation*	*Sensitivity skin tests*
Vaccines	*Serum sickness*	*Ophthalmic testing*

5. *Describe the preferred technique for smallpox vaccination and the various possible reactions to it.*
6. *List the preparations available for active immunization against the following diseases and give the dosage schedules and any special precautions:*

Poliomyelitis	*Mumps*	*Diphtheria*
Influenza	*Typhus*	*Tetanus*
Yellow fever	*Pertussis*	*Rocky Mountain spotted fever*
Typhoid fever	*Cholera*	

7. *What is meant by a prophylactic and a therapeutic dose of an antiserum? Give those doses of the antisera used in protecting against the following diseases:*

Diphtheria	*Measles*
Tetanus	*Infectious hepatitis*
Poliomyelitis	*Pertussis*

REFERENCES

Adams, J. M.: *Newer Virus Diseases.* The Macmillan Company, New York, 1960.
The Control of Communicable Diseases in Man, 9th ed. The American Public Health Association, New York, 1960.
Top, F. H.: *Communicable and Infectious Diseases.* The C. V. Mosby Company, St. Louis, 1960.

SMALLPOX VACCINE

Cabasso, V. J., *et al.*: "Primary Response of Children to Glycerinated or Dried Smallpox Vaccine of Calf Lymph or Chick Embryo Origin," *Am. J. Pub. Health,* **44**:194, 1954.

POLIOMYELITIS VACCINE

Enders, J. F.; Weller, T. H.; and Robbins, F. C.: "Cultivation of the Lansing Strain of Poliomyelitis Virus in Cultures of Various Human Embryonic Tissues," *Science,* **108**:85, 1949.
Koprowski, H.; Jervis, G. A.; and Norton, T. W.: "Immune Responses in Human

Volunteers Upon Oral Administration of a Rodent-Adapted Strain of Polio-myelitis Virus," *Am. J. Hyg.*, **55**:108, 1952.

Krugman, S.; Warren, J.; Eiger, M. S.; Berman, P. H.; Michaels, R. H.; and Sabin, A. B.: "Immunization with Live Attenuated Poliovirus Vaccine," *Am. J. Dis. Child.*, **101**:38, 1961.

Paul, R. R.: "Status of Vaccination Against Poliomyelitis, with Particular Refer-ence to Oral Vaccination," *New England J. Med.*, **264**:651, 1961.

Sabin, A. B.: "Discussion of Attenuated Polio Viruses and Their Behavior in Human Beings," *New York Acad. Sc.*, **5**:113, 1957.

————: "Status of Field Trials with an Orally Administered, Live Attenuated Poliovirus Vaccine," *J.A.M.A.*, **171**:863, 1959.

Salk, J. E.; Bennett, B. L.; Lewis, L. J.; *et al.:* "Studies in Human Subjects on Active Immunization Against Poliomyelitis. I." *J.A.M.A.*, **151**:1081, 1953.

INFLUENZA VACCINE

Jensen, K. E.; Dunn, F. L.; and Robinson, R. Q.: "Influenza, 1957, a Variant and the Pandemic," *Progr. Med. Virol.*, **1**:165, 1958.

McLean, R. L.: *International Conference on Asian Influenza.* National Institutes of Health, U.S. Public Health Service, Bethesda, Md., Feb. 17, 1960.

RABIES VACCINE

Habel, K.: "Rabies Prophylaxis in Man," *Pub. Health Rep.*, **72**:667, 1957.

MUMPS VACCINE

Shaw, E. B.: Editorial. "Mumps Immunization," *J.A.M.A.*, **167**:1744, 1958.

MEASLES VACCINE

"Statement on the Status of Measles Vaccines," *J.A.M.A.*, **183**:120, 1963.

"The Status of Measles Vaccines," *Am. J. Nursing*, **63**:72, 1963.

ROCKY MOUNTAIN SPOTTED FEVER AND TYPHUS VACCINES

Cox, H. R.: "Cultivation of Rickettsiae of the Rocky Mountain Spotted Fever, Typhus and Q Fever Groups in the Embryonic Tissues of Developing Chicks," *Science*, **94**:399, 1941.

Fox, J. P.; Jordan, M. E.; and Gelfand, H. M.: "Immunization of Man Against Epidemic Typhus by Infection with Avirulent *Rickettsia prowazeki* Strain E. V." *J. Immunol.*, **79**:348, 1957.

PERTUSSIS AND DIPHTHERIA VACCINES

Bedson, S. P., *et al.:* "Prevention of Whooping Cough by Vaccination: Medical Research Council Investigation," *Brit. M. J.*, **1**:1463, 1951.

James, G.; Longshore, W. A., Jr.; and Hendry, J. L.: "Diphtheria Immunization Studies of Students in Urban High School," *Am. J. Hyg.*, **53**:178, 1951.

TETANUS TOXOID AND ANTITOXIN

Peterson, J. C.; Christie, A.; and Williams, W. C.: "Tetanus Immunization, Study of Duration of Primary Immunity and Response to Late Stimulating

Doses of Tetanus Toxoid," *Am. J. Dis. Child.*, **89**:295, 1955.
Spaeth, R.: "Serum Therapy of Tetanus," *Am. J. Dis. Child.*, **61**:1146, 1941.

SERUM REACTIONS

Kojis, F. G.: "Serum Sickness and Anaphylaxis," *Am. J. Dis. Child.*, **64**:93, 313, 1942.
Laurent, L. J. M., and Parish, H. J.: "Serum Reactions and Serum Sensitivity Tests," *Brit. M. J.*, **1**:1294, 1952.

APPENDIXES

APPENDIX

I *General References*

The following references may prove useful to students requiring greater description of the subject matter presented in this text.

Pharmacology

Beckman, H.: *Drugs, Their Nature, Action and Uses.* W. B. Saunders Company, Philadelphia and London, 1958.

———: *Pharmacology in Clinical Practice.* W. B. Saunders Company, Philadelphia, 1952.

Conn, H. F. (ed.) : *Current Therapy.* W. B. Saunders Company, Philadelphia, 1960.

Cutting, Windsor C.: *Handbook of Pharmacology,* 2nd ed. Appleton-Century-Crofts, New York, 1965.

Drill, V. A. (ed.) : *Pharmacology in Medicine,* 2nd ed. McGraw-Hill Book Company, Inc., New York, 1958.

Goodman, L. S., and Gilman, A.: *The Pharmacological Basis of Therapeutics,* 2nd ed. The Macmillan Company, New York, 1958.

Goth, Andres: *Medical Pharmacology,* 2nd ed. C. V. Mosby Co., St. Louis, 1964.

Grollman, A.: *Pharmacology and Therapeutics,* 4th ed. Lea & Febiger, Philadelphia, 1960.

Krantz, J. C., Jr., and Carr, C. J.: *Pharmacologic Principles of Medical Practice,* 6th ed. William & Wilkins Company, Baltimore, 1965.

Lewis, J. J.: *An Introduction to Pharmacology,* 2nd ed. Williams & Wilkins Company, Baltimore, 1963.

Marler, E. E. J.: *Pharmacological and Chemical Synonyms.* Excerpta Medica Foundation, Amsterdam, London, New York, 1961.

Wilson, A., and Schild, H. O.: *Clark's Applied Pharmacology,* 9th ed. Little, Brown and Company, Boston, 1959.

Physiology

Best, C. H., and Taylor, N. B.: *Physiological Basis of Medical Practice,* 6th ed. Williams & Wilkins Company, Baltimore, 1955.

Fulton, J. F. (ed.) : *A Textbook of Physiology,* 17th ed. W. B. Saunders Company, Philadelphia, 1955.

Kimber, D. C.; Gray, C. E.; Stackpole, C. E.; and Leavell, L. C.: *Anatomy and Physiology,* 14th ed. The Macmillan Company, New York, 1961.

Ruch, T. C., and Fulton, J. F.: *Medical Physiology and Biophysics.* W. B. Saunders Company, Philadelphia and London, 1960.

Youmans, W. B.: *Basic Medical Physiology.* Year Book Publishers, Inc., Chicago, 1952.

———: *Human Physiology.* The Macmillan Company, New York, 1954.

II *Glossary*

The following list of technical terms and their definitions is offered as a convenient source of information with the full realization that it cannot be made long enough to satisfy all needs. The text brings forward some terms used in the fields of anatomy, physiology, and biochemistry and introduces new ones used in pharmacology. The student nurse will find a medical dictionary very useful.

a

accommodation.   The adjustment of the lens of the eye, by changes in the tone (state of continuous contraction) of the ciliary muscle, in order to allow the focusing on the retina of light rays from near or far objects. Thus, blurred vision is avoided.

adhesions.   Abnormal union of tissues due to inflammation.

adrenergic.   Pertaining to (1) the fibers of the sympathetic nervous system that liberate epinephrine or norepinephrine at their endings (postganglionic) and produce effector responses; (2) a drug that accomplishes the same result. The term is synonymous with *sympathomimetic*.

adrenolytic.   A drug that obstructs the action of circulating epinephrine on effector cells of responsive tissues such as arterioles, etc.

adsorption.   The ability of a substance to attract and hold on its surface a thin layer of other substances (gases, liquids, or dissolved substances). Charcoal is an adsorbent.

amebicide.   An agent that causes the destruction of amebae.

anaerobic.   Pertaining to growth of microorganisms in the absence of oxygen.

analeptic.   A drug used to restore the respiration and arouse from unconsciousness.

analgesia.   The reduction of pain.

analog.   A part resembling another in function, but not in structure.

androgen.   A male sex hormone.

anesthesia.   Loss of sensation.

anodyne.   A substance that relieves pain upon local application.

anthelmintic.   An agent which paralyzes or kills intestinal worms.

antibiotic.   A substance produced by a mold or bacteria, which inhibits the growth of microorganisms.

antibiotic spectrum.   The range of activity of an antibiotic against different bacteria.

anticholinergic.   No practical distinction from *parasympatholytic*.

anticholinesterase.   An agent that destroys or temporarily inactivates the enzyme cholinesterase, which splits choline esters such as acetylcholine and

810

succinylcholine. It prolongs the action of acetylcholine, by protecting it from enzymatic hydrolysis into relatively inactive choline and acetate.

antidote. Drug for counteracting the effects of a poison.

antimetabolite. A substance having a chemical structure similar, but a pharmacological effect antagonistic, to an essential metabolite.

antipyretic. An agent that reduces elevated body temperature.

antiscorbutic. An agent used in the prevention or cure of scurvy.

antispasmodic. A substance that relieves spasmodic contraction of smooth muscle.

aromatic. Having a fragrant or spicy aroma and taste.

arrhythmia. An irregular rhythm of the heart beat; there are a number of different ones.

ascites. An abnormal accumulation of serous fluid in the peritoneal cavity.

asepsis. Absence of microorganisms that produce disease.

asthenia. Absence or loss of strength; muscular weakness; debility.

astringent. A substance that causes contraction of tissues of the body and stops bleeding and diarrhea.

ataraxics. A chemically unrelated group of drugs that promotes equanimity (calmness and composure) and is proving useful in treating certain mental and emotional disorders. Also, *ataractic.*

ataxia. Incoordination of muscular action.

atrophy. Decrease in size, and usually in function, of a structure (organ, gland, any tissue). Atrophy of the muscles occurs after their nerve supply is cut, as in apoplectic stroke.

b

bradycardia. Slow heart rate.

c

cardiospasm. Spasm of the musculature at the esophageal orifice (opening) of the stomach, preventing swallowed food from entering the stomach.

cardiotonic. An agent that exerts a favorable, so-called tonic, effect upon the heart.

carrier. A person who shows no symptoms of disease but who harbors and eliminates microorganisms that transmit disease to others.

cellulitis. A diffuse inflammation of connective tissue.

cholinergic. Pertains to (1) all postganglionic fibers of the parasympathetic nervous system and those in the sympathetic that liberate acetylcholine at their endings and thereby produce the responses associated with these nerves; (2) an agent that produces the above effects.

cholinolytic. No difference from *parasympatholytic.* Also synonymous with *anticholinergic.*

coma. Unconsciousness from which the patient cannot be roused.

comatose. In the condition of coma.

concentration. The relative amount of a substance dissolved in water or other solvent, as 10 per cent concentration of glucose (10 Gm. per 100 ml.).

congener. A drug or other chemical agent differing only moderately from a given compound. They come from (*-gen-*) the same parent substance or at least belong together (*con-*) because of certain similarities. The several sulfonamide drugs are, within limits, congeners of one another.

contraindication. A condition that prohibits the use of a drug or other measure. For example, digitalis is *contraindicated* in a certain heart disorder.

convulsions. Involuntary violent muscular contractions. They may be tonic (without relaxation) or clonic (with alternate contractions of opposite groups of muscles).

coordination. The harmonious activity and the proper sequence of events that work together to perform a certain function.

coryza. Inflammation of the mucous membranes of the nose; cold in the head.

cyanosis. A bluish tinge in the color of mucous membranes and skin.

cycloplegia. The paralysis (*-plegia*) of the circular (*cyclo-*) muscle, the ciliary muscle of the eye, allowing the lens to assume a relaxed, more flattened shape. Only distant objects can then be seen with some clarity.

cystitis. Inflammation of the urinary bladder.

cystography. The science of taking radiograms of the urinary bladder after the administration of a radiopaque substance.

d

decay. The spontaneous transformation of an isotope to one or more different isotopes, which is characterized by the emission of energy from the nucleus and has a measurable lifetime, a synonym for radioactive disintegration.

dehydration. The removal of water.

demulcent. An agent that soothes and relieves irritation, particularly of the mucous surfaces.

derivative. A substance derived or made from another substance, as homatropine is a derivative of atropine.

desquamate. To shed or scale off—as the skin in certain diseases.

detergent. A drug or chemical substance that lowers surface tension. Some are used for cleansing the skin, wounds, or ulcers.

disintegration. The spontaneous transformation of an isotope to one or more different isotopes which is characterized by the emission of energy from the nucleus and has a measurable lifetime. A synonym for radioactive disintegration.

diuretic. An agent that increases the volume of urine.

dyspnea. Labored or difficult breathing; may be faster than the normal 16 to 20 breaths per minute.

e

edema. The presence of a greater-than-normal amount of water and salts among the tissues and cells of the body; adj., *edematous*; old spelling, *oedema*.

embolus. A solid or oily substance that is moving or has moved through some part of the blood stream and lodges where it can go no farther because of narrowing of the stream. It is diagnosed by the difficulties it produces wherever it lodges, or at autopsy. It is usually a blood clot, having broken away from its original site. Oil droplets getting into the blood stream are *emboli* (plural). Great care is required to prevent the occasional injection, intended to be into a muscle, from being made into a vein.

emetic. An agent that produces vomiting. *Emesis* is the act of regurgitating food or fluid.

emollient. An agent used externally to soften the skin, or internally to soothe an irritated or inflamed surface.

empiric. That which is based on practical experience rather than scientific principles.

endemic. Peculiar to a particular locality, as a disease that occurs continually.

endometrium. The mucous membrane lining the uterus.

entity. An independently existing thing; a group of features that are so related as to make them the parts of a specific condition which can be given a name.

eosinophilia An increase in the number of eosinophil cells.

epidemic. The unusual prevalence of a contagious disease in a certain locality.

erythema. An abnormal redness of the skin owing to congestion and inflammation.

essential metabolite. A substance necessary for the growth, reproduction, and life of cells.

estrogen. A female sex hormone.

exophthalmos. An abnormal protrusion of the eyeball.

extravasation. The leakage of blood from any vessel into the surrounding spaces, or of medication in solution that is intended to be infused into a vein.

f

flaccid. Relaxed, soft, as a muscle. Also *flaccidity*, state of being relaxed, usually to greater-than-normal degree.

fluoroscope. An instrument used to view the form and motion of internal structures of the body by means of roentgen rays.

fungicide. An agent that kills or destroys fungi.

fungistatic. An agent inhibiting or preventing the growth of fungi.

fungus. A form of plant life, characterized by the absence of chlorophyll, that lives on dead or living substances.

g

ganglioplegic. An agent that blocks ganglia by prohibiting some or all nerve impulses from passing the synapse and on down the postganglionic neuron.

gavage. Administration of liquid through the stomach tube—washing out the stomach.

glabrous. Devoid of hairs, as the skin of the palms and soles.

glycogenesis. Formation of glucose in the liver.

glycogenolysis. The breaking down of glycogen into glucose.

gradient. Rising or descending by regular degrees.

griping. Abdominal pain due to spasmodic contractions of the bowel.

h

half-life. The amount of time required for 50 per cent of a given amount of a radioactive isotope to decay.

hemolysis. Rupture of red blood cell walls, liberating the hemoglobin. Also *hemolyze* and *hemolytic*.

hemostatic.   An agent that arrests hemorrhage.

hyperemia.   Greater-than-normal amount of blood in an area or part within capillaries which are all dilated and transporting blood. The part will thus be redder and warmer than usual.

hyperglycemia.   Greater-than-normal concentration of glucose in the blood.

hyperplasia.   An increase in the size of a tissue or an organ due to growth.

hypertrophy.   Greater-than-normal growth, as of the heart under loads greater than normal (hypertension, insufficient valves). Also overgrowth of any tissue (prostate, thyroid, uterus in pregnancy, etc.).

hypnotic.   An agent that induces sleep.

i

incidence.   The extent of occurrence.

indication.   In therapy this means the reason for giving a certain drug. Thus a certain agent is *indicated* in a particular disease.

indolent.   Slow to heal, causing little or no pain.

infarct.   In its most widely used meaning, an area in some part of the body that is damaged by the occlusion of its arterial blood supply, as occurs when a clot lodges therein or is formed in the vessel. *Infarction* is a broader term for this phenomenon.

infiltration.   The seepage or spread of a substance through intercellular (between cells) spaces, as a liquid administered through a needle. Local anesthetics are *infiltrated* around a nerve or group.

inflammation.   The reaction of tissues to irritation or injury by the production of redness, heat, swelling, and pain.

ingest.   To take food or drugs into the body.

innervation.   The supplying of a nerve or nerves to a given part. The part is *innervated* by a particular nerve or by several nerves.

insoluble.   Incapable of being dissolved in certain solvents.

interstitial.   Pertaining to the spaces between the cellular constituents of organs of the body.

intractable.   Unmanageable.

intradural.   Within the fibrous membrane forming the outer covering of the brain and spinal cord.

intraocular.   Within the eyeball.

intrathecally.   (1) Within any thecal membrane or a sheath; (2) usually refers to the theca vertebralis or the dura membrane of the spinal cord; hence the injection of a needle into the cerebrospinal fluid.

isotonic.   Pertains to a solution having the same osmotic pressure as blood, as 0.9 per cent sodium chloride (salt) solution or about 5 per cent glucose.

isotope.   Forms of an element which are alike in chemical reaction and atomic number but differ in atomic weight.

k

keratolytic.   An agent that causes a loosening or shedding of the epidermis.

l

labile.   Unstable; likely to change.

lacrimal.   Name of the tear gland above and to the outer side of the eyeball.

lesion. An injury or wound; localized structural change in the body due to injury or disease.

lethal. Pertaining to or causing death.

lethargy. A state of drowsiness or stupor.

leukopenia. A decrease below the normal number of leukocytes (white blood cells) in the blood.

lipids. Fats and fat-like substances.

lymphocytosis. An increase in the number of lymphocytes (a type of white blood cell).

m

malaise. A condition of bodily weakness frequently accompanied by loss of appetite, restlessness, and inactivity.

malfunctioning. Poor functioning, as in a diseased part.

mania. Excessive excitement with or without delusions.

meniscus. The concave upper surface of a column of liquid.

metabolism. The sum total of the chemical and physical processes that produce and maintain life in an organism or a single cell.

metabolite. A substance acted upon or produced in metabolism.

miosis. Constriction of the pupil, decrease in its diameter or size by the opposite events given for mydriasis.

miscible. Capable of being mixed.

moribund. In a dying condition.

motility. Capacity to move spontaneously.

mucosa. A mucous membrane lining a body cavity.

mydriasis. Dilatation of the pupil of the eye (relaxation of circular fibers of the iris or constriction of the radial fibers). The circular ones encircle the iris, and the radial ones are arranged like the spokes of a wheel. A *mydriatic* is a drug that produces the above effects.

myocardium. The muscular portion of the heart, which comprises nearly its entirety.

n

narcolepsy. Tendency to fall into a deep sleep of short duration.

necrosis. Death of cells of tissues.

neuritis. Inflammation of a nerve accompanied by hypersensitivity and pain.

neuromyal. Pertains to the synapse, at the muscle fiber, of the nerve to that muscle and the motor end-plate. Often also called *myoneural*.

o

objective. Pertaining to those findings that the physician can determine by his examinations. The reading of blood pressure, and the finding of a swelling are examples of the examiner's *objective* findings.

occlusion. The stopping up of a blood vessel or any hollow tube or passage, as by a clot, stone, tumor, inflammation, etc. Also "closing" in general, as the teeth when the two sets are apposed.

olfactory. Pertaining to the sense of smell.

opaque.   Not transparent; unable to transmit light.
ophthalmic.   Pertaining to the eye.
ophthalmoscope.   An instrument for viewing the interior of the eye.
orthostatic.   Standing upright.
oxytocic.   An agent that causes uterine contraction and thus promotes the rapidity of labor.

p

palpitation.   The patient's feeling of greater-than-normal heart rate and forcefulness; thus a subjective symptom as opposed to objective signs.
paralysis.   Loss of muscle function due to destruction or temporary inactivation, as by drugs, or nerves or nerve cells.
parasite.   An organism that lives on or in another organism (the host) from which it derives its nourishment.
parasympatholytic.   An agent that nullifies or reduces the responses to parasympathetic outflow (nerve volleys) by competing with acetylcholine for the receptor sites, which normally produce action by the structure (gland or smooth muscle).
parasympathomimetic.   An agent that produces the same type of responses as obtained by the parasympathetic nerves when they are stimulated.
parenteral.   Aside from the intestines or oral route; thus a method of administering a drug other than by swallowing or rectal suppository. Parenteral routes are subcutaneous, intravenous, intramuscular, and other special routes.
paresis.   Incomplete motor paralysis. Weakness of an arm or leg.
peripheral.   That part at or toward the outside. Opposed to central. The more distant, as *peripheral* resistance offered by the arterioles that act as "valves," or a dam through which the heart must pump blood under pressure. Also *peripheral* nervous system.
phagocytosis.   Ingestion of particles, principally bacteria, by certain cells.
plethora.   Overabundance.
prognosis.   The forecasting of the duration, course, and termination of the disease.
prophylactic.   Pertaining to the prevention of disease.
pruritus.   Itching.
psychoneurotic.   Emotional reactions characterized mainly by anxiety, which may be felt and expressed or controlled subconsciously.
psychosomatic.   A disorder that is caused by or influenced by the emotions.
psychotic disorder.   A severe mental disturbance characterized by disintegration of the personality and withdrawal from reality.
pyelography.   The science of taking roentgenograms of the kidneys and ureters after the administration of radiopaque media.
pylorospasm.   Spasm of the heavy ring of smooth muscle surrounding the pylorus, or lower right end of the stomach leading into the duodenum.

r

radioactive.   Any material which emits alpha particles, beta particles, and/or gamma rays.
radiopaque.   Not easily traversed by x-rays.

rationale. The reasons or justification for a particular measure, be it drug, physical, surgical, or other. Thus the *rationale* for using hexamethonium in a given patient.

renal. Relating to the kidneys.

rhinitis. Inflammation of mucous membrane of nose; acute rhinitis—coryza, cold in the head.

roentgen rays, or x-rays. The radiant energy of short wavelengths, discovered by Dr. Wilhelm Röntgen.

roentgenogram. A roentgen-ray record.

rubefacient. An agent that causes a reddening or mild irritation of the skin.

s

sedative. An agent that quiets activity.

sensory. Pertaining to sensation, as sensory nerves that convey various senses to the central nervous system.

sequelae (plural of *sequela*). Afterevents; conditions, usually complications, which are observed to follow therapeutic procedures, drugs, or diseases. Thus pneumonia may be a sequela of high abdominal surgery, and rashes and anemia are sequelae of exposure to certain poisons.

spasmogenic. Causing spastic contraction of smooth muscle.

steroid. A drug or compound having a particular structure: the sex hormones, vitamin D, and cholesterol.

subjective. Pertaining to a person's own feelings or awareness. Headache and pain are examples of *subjective* symptoms that are ordinarily beyond the physician's ability to diagnose. *See also* Objective.

sympatholytic. A drug that blocks or diminishes the usual effect of sympathetic nerve influence on tissues and smooth muscle of arterioles. Volleys of nerve impulses may arrive at the end organ or effector cells in various tissues but are unable to accomplish their usual activity.

sympathomimetic. A drug that simulates some of or all the activities of the functioning sympathetic nervous system.

synapse. The near touching of the terminal of one nerve and the receptor surface or end of another. The nerve impulse traverses the narrow space or substance between the two and may be relayed along the second neuron.

syncope. Fainting; sudden loss of consciousness.

syndrome. A group of features, such as the symptoms, signs, and laboratory data, which constitute the usual description of a disease. The term replaces the word "disease" when this designation is not appropriate.

systemic. Pertaining to (1) the entire body, as *systemic* medication *vs.* local action of a drug; (2) blood circulation in general other than the pulmonary circulation.

t

tachycardia. Rapid heart rate.

taeniacide. An agent that destroys tapeworms.

taeniafuge. An agent that expels tapeworms.

tension. (1) Mental or emotional strain. (2) Pressure, such as blood or intraocular pressure.

topical.   Pertaining to surface application or action.

trauma.   Injury, physical or biochemical; adj., *traumatic*.

u

urography.   Roentgenographic visualization of the urinary tract by the use of radiopaque media.

urticaria.   An allergic reaction of the skin characterized by the development of wheals which induce sensations of burning and itching.

v

vasoconstriction.   Narrowing of the lumen or bore of the arterioles. *Vasodilatation* is the opposite: relaxation of the encircling muscle fibers with increased lumen size.

vasomotor.   Regulating the constriction and dilatation of the blood vessels.

venereal.   Arising from or produced by sexual intercourse with an infected person.

vertigo.   A feeling that the earth is revolving about the patient or that he himself is moving in space.

vesicant.   An agent which causes blistering of the skin or mucous membranes.

viscid.   Adhesive; gluelike.

III Answers to Questions in Chapter 4

Write as small Roman numerals (p. 32):

		Answers			*Answers*
1.	8	viii	6.	49	il
2.	4	iv	7.	75	lxxv
3.	16	xvi	8.	52	lii
4.	60	lx	9.	90	xc
5.	35	xxxv	10.	87	lxxxvii

Write as Arabic numbers (p. 32):

		Answers			*Answers*
1.	iii	3	6.	xvi	16
2.	xx	20	7.	lxv	65
3.	xix	19	8.	xiv	14
4.	lx	60	9.	xxx	30
5.	iv	4	10.	lxxxi	81

Change improper fractions to mixed numbers (p. 33):

		Answers			*Answers*
1.	$18/5$	$3\frac{3}{5}$	6.	$7/3$	$2\frac{1}{3}$
2.	$89/7$	$12\frac{5}{7}$	7.	$43/5$	$8\frac{3}{5}$
3.	$13/6$	$2\frac{1}{6}$	8.	$60/8$	$7\frac{1}{2}$
4.	$21/4$	$5\frac{1}{4}$	9.	$77/5$	$15\frac{2}{5}$
5.	$39/4$	$9\frac{3}{4}$	10.	$11/3$	$3\frac{2}{3}$

Change mixed numbers to improper fractions (p. 34):

		Answers			*Answers*
1.	$6\frac{1}{6}$	$37/6$	6.	$5\frac{3}{4}$	$23/4$
2.	$7\frac{9}{10}$	$79/10$	7.	$66\frac{2}{3}$	$200/3$
3.	$8\frac{1}{2}$	$17/2$	8.	$7\frac{3}{8}$	$59/8$
4.	$9\frac{1}{8}$	$73/8$	9.	$33\frac{1}{3}$	$100/3$
5.	$40\frac{2}{5}$	$202/5$	10.	$2\frac{5}{6}$	$17/6$

Reduce the following fractions to their lowest terms (p. 34):

	Answers			*Answers*
1. $\frac{12}{60}$	$\frac{1}{5}$	6. $\frac{500}{2500}$		$\frac{1}{5}$
2. $\frac{6}{15}$	$\frac{2}{5}$	7. $\frac{6}{16}$		$\frac{3}{8}$
3. $\frac{27}{36}$	$\frac{3}{4}$	8. $\frac{12}{15}$		$\frac{4}{5}$
4. $\frac{5}{25}$	$\frac{1}{5}$	9. $\frac{8}{32}$		$\frac{1}{4}$
5. $\frac{4}{36}$	$\frac{1}{9}$	10. $\frac{5}{20}$		$\frac{1}{4}$

Change the following fractions to higher terms (p. 34):

	Answers			*Answers*
1. $\frac{5}{8}$	$\frac{30}{48}$	6. $\frac{5}{7}$		$\frac{25}{35}$
2. $\frac{3}{4}$	$\frac{18}{24}$	7. $\frac{1}{2}$		$\frac{10}{20}$
3. $\frac{1}{3}$	$\frac{3}{9}$	8. $\frac{1}{5}$		$\frac{6}{30}$
4. $\frac{4}{5}$	$\frac{12}{15}$	9. $\frac{3}{4}$		$\frac{6}{8}$
5. $\frac{2}{3}$	$\frac{8}{12}$	10. $\frac{5}{6}$		$\frac{30}{36}$

Simplify the following complex fractions (p. 35):

	Answers			*Answers*
1. $\dfrac{\frac{7}{9}}{\frac{3}{5}}$	$\frac{35}{27} = 1\frac{8}{27}$	6. $\dfrac{\frac{5}{11}}{\frac{1}{10}}$		$\frac{50}{11} = 4\frac{6}{11}$
2. $\dfrac{\frac{3}{8}}{\frac{4}{7}}$	$\frac{21}{32}$	7. $\dfrac{\frac{3}{16}}{\frac{5}{4}}$		$\frac{3}{20}$
3. $\dfrac{\frac{6}{7}}{\frac{2}{3}}$	$\frac{18}{14} = 1\frac{4}{14} = 1\frac{2}{7}$	8. $\dfrac{\frac{1}{3}}{\frac{4}{25}}$		$\frac{25}{12} = 2\frac{1}{12}$
4. $\dfrac{\frac{5}{3}}{\frac{1}{9}}$	$\frac{45}{3} = 15$	9. $\dfrac{\frac{1}{8}}{\frac{1}{2}}$		$\frac{2}{8} = \frac{1}{4}$
5. $\dfrac{\frac{3}{4}}{\frac{1}{2}}$	$\frac{6}{4} = 1\frac{1}{2}$	10. $\dfrac{\frac{9}{10}}{\frac{1}{4}}$		$\frac{36}{10} = 3\frac{6}{10} = 3\frac{3}{5}$

Change the following fractions to ones which have the same denominator (p. 35):

	Answers			*Answers*
1. $\frac{1}{2}$, $\frac{1}{4}$	$\frac{2}{4}$, $\frac{1}{4}$	6. $\frac{3}{5}$, $\frac{4}{10}$		$\frac{3}{5}$, $\frac{2}{5}$
2. $\frac{3}{4}$, $\frac{1}{8}$	$\frac{6}{8}$, $\frac{1}{8}$	7. $\frac{4}{5}$, $\frac{2}{20}$		$\frac{8}{10}$, $\frac{1}{10}$
3. $\frac{2}{3}$, $\frac{1}{15}$	$\frac{10}{15}$, $\frac{1}{15}$	8. $\frac{5}{6}$, $\frac{4}{12}$		$\frac{5}{6}$, $\frac{2}{6}$
4. $\frac{3}{8}$, $\frac{5}{16}$	$\frac{6}{16}$, $\frac{5}{16}$	9. $\frac{1}{2}$, $\frac{1}{3}$		$\frac{3}{6}$, $\frac{2}{6}$
5. $\frac{2}{7}$, $\frac{3}{14}$	$\frac{4}{14}$, $\frac{3}{14}$	10. $\frac{2}{3}$, $\frac{3}{5}$		$\frac{10}{15}$, $\frac{9}{15}$

Convert these fractions to one with LCD (p. 36):

	Answers
1. $\frac{1}{3}$, $\frac{3}{7}$, $\frac{4}{5}$	$\frac{35}{105}$, $\frac{45}{105}$, $\frac{84}{105}$
2. $\frac{5}{9}$, $\frac{3}{5}$, $\frac{2}{3}$	$\frac{25}{45}$, $\frac{27}{45}$, $\frac{30}{45}$
3. $\frac{1}{8}$, $\frac{3}{4}$, $\frac{3}{7}$	$\frac{7}{56}$, $\frac{42}{56}$, $\frac{24}{56}$

4. $\frac{1}{6}$, $\frac{4}{9}$, $\frac{3}{8}$ $\frac{12}{72}$, $\frac{32}{72}$, $\frac{27}{72}$
5. $\frac{2}{5}$, $\frac{3}{10}$, $\frac{2}{3}$ $\frac{12}{30}$, $\frac{9}{30}$, $\frac{20}{30}$
6. $\frac{2}{6}$, $\frac{3}{4}$, $\frac{4}{5}$ $\frac{20}{60}$, $\frac{45}{60}$, $\frac{48}{60}$
7. $\frac{1}{2}$, $\frac{4}{5}$, $\frac{2}{3}$ $\frac{15}{30}$, $\frac{24}{30}$, $\frac{20}{30}$
8. $\frac{4}{8}$, $\frac{3}{4}$, $\frac{5}{6}$ $\frac{6}{12}$, $\frac{9}{12}$, $\frac{10}{12}$
9. $\frac{4}{7}$, $\frac{5}{9}$, $\frac{2}{5}$ $\frac{180}{315}$, $\frac{175}{315}$, $\frac{126}{315}$
10. $\frac{3}{4}$, $\frac{2}{3}$, $\frac{3}{9}$ $\frac{9}{12}$, $\frac{8}{12}$, $\frac{4}{12}$

Add the following fractions and reduce the resulting fraction to the lowest terms (p. 37):

		Answers
1. $\frac{1}{4} + \frac{5}{8} + \frac{3}{4} + \frac{1}{6}$	$=$	$\frac{55}{24}$
2. $\frac{1}{6} + \frac{1}{3} + \frac{3}{4} + \frac{7}{12}$	$=$	$\frac{28}{12} = \frac{7}{3}$
3. $\frac{3}{8} + \frac{4}{32} + \frac{2}{3} + \frac{1}{4}$	$=$	$\frac{136}{96} = \frac{17}{12}$
4. $\frac{3}{5} + \frac{4}{10} + \frac{3}{4} + \frac{1}{2}$	$=$	$\frac{45}{20} = \frac{9}{4}$
5. $\frac{2}{3} + \frac{5}{12} + \frac{7}{16} + \frac{3}{4}$	$=$	$\frac{109}{48}$
6. $\frac{5}{6} + \frac{3}{5} + \frac{3}{4} + \frac{6}{15}$	$=$	$\frac{155}{60} = \frac{31}{12}$

Subtract the following fractions and reduce the resulting fractions to the lowest terms (p. 37):

		Answers
1. $\frac{7}{8} - \frac{2}{3}$	$=$	$\frac{5}{24}$
2. $\frac{4}{25} - \frac{2}{50}$	$=$	$\frac{3}{25}$
3. $\frac{3}{4} - \frac{1}{3}$	$=$	$\frac{5}{12}$
4. $\frac{5}{8} - \frac{1}{12}$	$=$	$\frac{13}{24}$
5. $\frac{5}{7} - \frac{1}{5}$	$=$	$\frac{18}{35}$
6. $\frac{13}{16} - \frac{4}{32}$	$=$	$\frac{11}{16}$

Multiply the following fractions and reduce the resulting fractions to the lowest terms (p. 38):

		Answers
1. $\frac{2}{3} \times \frac{7}{8}$	$=$	$\frac{7}{12}$
2. $\frac{3}{7} \times 4$	$=$	$\frac{12}{7}$
3. $\frac{3}{4} \times \frac{2}{3}$	$=$	$\frac{1}{2}$
4. $6 \times \frac{7}{8}$	$=$	$\frac{21}{4}$
5. $\frac{8}{9} \times \frac{4}{6}$	$=$	$\frac{16}{27}$
6. $\frac{1}{5} \times \frac{5}{6}$	$=$	$\frac{1}{6}$

Divide the following fractions and reduce the resulting fractions to the lowest terms (p. 38):

		Answers
1. $\frac{2}{3} \div 6$	$=$	$\frac{1}{9}$
2. $\frac{3}{4} \div \frac{2}{9}$	$=$	$\frac{27}{8}$
3. $\frac{1}{3} \div \frac{2}{5}$	$=$	$\frac{5}{6}$
4. $\frac{3}{8} \div \frac{1}{64}$	$=$	24
5. $\frac{1}{2} \div \frac{1}{3}$	$=$	$\frac{3}{2}$
6. $\frac{3}{4} \div 7$	$=$	$\frac{3}{28}$

Write in words the following decimal fractions (p. 39) :

Answers

1. 0.06   six hundredths
2. 0.004   four thousandths
3. 0.064   sixty-four thousandths
4. 12.598   twelve and five hundred ninety-eight thousandths
5. 318.07   three hundred eighteen and seven hundredths
6. 0.0162   one hundred sixty-two ten-thousandths

Add the following decimal fractions (p. 39) :

	Answers
1. 327.94, 8262.34, 287.05, 417.43	9294.76
2. 7.20, 9.736, 12.895, 0.25	30.081
3. 0.064, 0.001, 0.0002	0.0652
4. 17.756, 9.0623, 0.987, 0.0062	27.8115
5. 204.125, 14.321, 98.346, 452.06	768.852

Multiply the following decimal fractions (p. 40) :

		Answers
1. 234.43 × 0.256	=	60.01408
2. 12.42 × 213.89	=	2656.5138
3. 0.5 × 0.016	=	0.008
4. 0.7 × 0.008	=	0.0056
5. 0.5 × 0.4	=	0.2
6. 1.75 × 0.005	=	0.00875

Divide the following decimal fractions (p. 41) :

		Answers
1. 21 by 0.025	=	840
2. 639.028 by 98.312	=	6.5
3. 25.95 by 3.46	=	7.5
4. 16.15 by 4.25	=	3.8
5. 67 by 32.524	=	2.06
6. 3002 by 75.05	=	40

Divide the following numbers by each of the following—0.1, 0.01, 10, 100 (p. 41) :

Answers

7. 16.14	=	161.4	1614	1.614	0.1614
8. 50.65	=	506.5	5065	5.065	0.5065
9. 963.456	=	9634.56	96345.6	96.3456	9.63456
10. 0.568	=	5.68	56.8	0.0568	0.00568

Convert the following common fractions to decimal fractions (p. 41):

		Answers
1.	$3/4$	0.75
2.	$1/25$	0.04
3.	$5/9$	0.556
4.	$3/8$	0.375
5.	$6/17$	0.353
6.	$5/22$	0.227

Convert the following decimal fractions to common fractions (p. 41):

		Answers
1.	0.50	$\frac{50}{100} = \frac{1}{2}$
2.	0.45	$\frac{45}{100} = \frac{9}{20}$
3.	0.2045	$\frac{2045}{10,000} = \frac{409}{2000}$
4.	0.75	$\frac{75}{100} = \frac{3}{4}$
5.	0.04	$\frac{4}{100} = \frac{1}{25}$
6.	0.00654	$\frac{654}{100,000} = \frac{327}{50,000}$

Change the following ratios to per cent (p. 43):

		Answers
1.	1:1000	$\frac{1}{10}\%$
2.	3:5	60%
3.	1:500	$\frac{1}{5}\%$
4.	8:250	$3\frac{1}{5}\%$
5.	1:20	5%
6.	1:2	50%

Change the following percentages to ratio, decimal fractions, and common fractions (p. 43):

			Answers Decimal fractions	Common fractions
		Ratio		
1.	45%	45:100	.45	$\frac{45}{100}$ or $\frac{9}{20}$
2.	$\frac{1}{2}\%$	1:200	.005	$\frac{1}{200}$
3.	2%	2:100	.02	$\frac{2}{100}$ or $\frac{1}{50}$
4.	67%	67:100	.67	$\frac{67}{100}$
5.	$33\frac{1}{3}\%$	1:3	.333	$\frac{1}{3}$
6.	75%	3:4	.75	$\frac{75}{100}$ or $\frac{3}{4}$
7.	$\frac{3}{4}\%$	3:400	.0075	$\frac{3}{400}$
8.	89%	89:100	.89	$\frac{89}{100}$
9.	$\frac{1}{6}\%$	1:600	.00167	$\frac{1}{600}$
10.	68%	68:100	.68	$\frac{68}{100}$ or $\frac{17}{25}$

Change the following decimal fractions to per cent and ratio (p. 43):

	Answers	
	Per cent	*Ratio*
1. 0.3	30%	3:10
2. 0.75	75%	3:4
3. 0.532	53.2%	532:1000
4. 0.413	41.3%	413:1000
5. 0.8	80%	4:5
6. 0.5	50%	1:2

Change the following common fractions to per cent (p. 44):

	Answers
1. ⅞	87½%
2. ⅖	40%
3. ¾	75%
4. ⅔	66⅔%
5. 5⁄12	41⅔%
6. 7⁄15	46⅔%

Find a given per cent of the following numbers (p. 44):

	Answers
1. 5% of 650	32.5
2. ¼% of 25	0.0625
3. 10% of 3500	350
4. 0.1% of 2000	2
5. 1⅔% of 216	3.6
6. 12½% of 400	50

What per cent of (p. 44):

	Answers
1. 75 is 15	20%
2. 40 is 2	5%
3. 1.5 is 0.5	33⅓%
4. 9 is 3	33⅓%
5. 18 is 9	50%
6. 60 is 12	20%

Find the value of x (p. 44):

	Answers
1. $0.75:100::x:1000$	$x = 7.5$
2. $\dfrac{¼}{⅙} = \dfrac{x}{1}$	$x = \dfrac{3}{2}$
3. $8:4::x:9$	$x = 18$
4. $30:x::10:15$	$x = 45$
5. $0.1:10::x:3$	$x = 0.03$

Convert liters to milliliters (p. 47):

Answers

3.75 L.	3750 ml.
2.46 L.	2460 ml.
0.35 L.	350 ml.

Convert milliliters to liters (p. 47):

Answers

1753 ml.	1.753 L.
8736 ml.	8.736 L.
1500 ml.	1.5 L.

Convert grams to milligrams (p. 47):

Answers

0.350 Gm.	350 mg.
0.0015 Gm.	1.5 mg.
0.060 Gm.	60 mg.
0.001 Gm.	1 mg.
0.0003 Gm.	0.3 mg.

Convert milligrams to grams (p. 47):

Answers

30 mg.	0.03 Gm.
500 mg.	0.5 Gm.
0.4 mg.	0.0004 Gm.
0.05 mg.	0.00005 Gm.
2 mg.	0.002 Gm.

Convert to higher denominations (p. 49):

Answers

430 minims	7 drams and 10 minims
16 drams	2 ounces
18 ounces	1 pint and 2 ounces

Convert to lower denominations (p. 49):

Answers

6 fluid drams	360 minims
5½ fluid ounces	44 drams
2 pints	32 ounces
1½ quarts	3 pints

Convert the following metric quantities to their apothecaries' equivalents (p. 51):

Answers

1. 500 ml.	1 pint	6. 40 mg.	⅔ grain
2. 30 ml.	1 fluid ounce	7. 2 mg.	1⁄30 grain
3. 4 ml.	1 fluid dram	8. 15 Gm.	4 drams ½ ounce
4. 0.06 ml.	1 minim	9. 0.3 Gm.	5 grains
5. 0.1 ml.	1½ minims	10. 0.4 mg.	1⁄500 grain

Convert the following apothecaries' quantities to their metric equivalents (p. 52):

Answers

1. 1	quart	1000 ml.
2. 7	fluid ounces	210 ml.
3. 2½	fluid drams	10 ml.
4. 12	minims	0.75 ml.
5. ½	minim	0.03 ml.
6. 75	grains	5 Gm.

7. 10   grains   0.6 Gm. or 600 mg.
8. 2½ grains   0.15 Gm. or 150 mg.
9. ⅟₁₅₀ grain   0.4 mg.
10. ¼₀₀ grain   0.15 mg.

Conversion problems (p. 52):
1. 1 grain = 60 mg.; therefore 5 grains = 300 mg. per tablet. Since 600 mg. are required, you would need

$$\frac{600}{300} = 2 \ \text{(tablets)}$$

2. ⅙ grain to milligrams is ⅙ × 60 mg. per grain = 10 mg.

$$\frac{20}{10} = 2 \ \text{(tablets)}$$

3. ⅟₁₅₀ grain = 60 mg. per grain × ⅟₁₅₀ grain = 0.4 mg. Then one tablet is dispensed.
4. 1 pt. = 500 ml.

$$1{:}5000 = \frac{1 \ \text{Gm.}}{5000 \ \text{ml.}} :: \frac{x \ \text{Gm.}}{500 \ \text{ml.}}$$
$$x = 0.1 \ \text{Gm.}$$

Convert the following quantities to household equivalents (p. 53):

	Answers
6 fluid ounces	1 teacupful
30 ml.	2 tablespoonfuls
2 fluid drams	1 dessertspoonful
5 ml.	1 teaspoonful
240 ml.	1 glassful

Percentage problems (p. 57):

1. 20   Gm.
2. 8   tablets
3. 33   tablets
4. 3.75 tablets
5. 960 ml.

From full-strength drugs (pp. 58–59):

Drug	*Add water to:*
1. 0.5 Gm.	2500 ml.
2. 8.5 Gm.	1000 ml.
3. 60.0 Gm.	1500 ml.
4. 1400.0 ml.	2000 ml.

From tablets (p. 59):

Drug	Add water to:
1. 17 tablets	2000 ml.
2. 2 tablets	200 ml.
3. 1 tablet	1000 ml.

From stock solutions (p. 59):

Drug	Add water to:
1. 127 ml.	1500 ml.
2. 100 ml.	500 ml.
3. 714 ml.	1000 ml.
4. 200 ml.	1000 ml.

Tell how to measure the following doses (p. 62):

Measure	Dilute to	Administer
1. 10 minims	50 minims	45 minims
2. 5 minims	25 minims	15 minims
3. 5 minims	200 minims	5 minims
4. 5 minims	125 minims	5 minims
5. 20 minims		20 minims
5 minims	25 minims	15 minims
		15 minims of the dilution is added to 20 minims of the original solution

To prepare doses from tablets (p. 62):

Tablets	Dissolve in	Administer
1. 1 (gr. $\frac{1}{100}$)	2 ml.	1 ml.
2. 1 (gr. $\frac{1}{3}$)	2 ml.	1 ml.
3. 2 (gr. $\frac{1}{8}$)	15 minims	10 minims

To calculate doses using stock solutions (p. 62):

1. 0.5   ml.
2. 0.75 ml.
3. 0.3   ml.
4. 1.5   ml.

To prepare doses from full-strength drugs (p. 62):

Drug	Dissolve in	Administer
1. 500 mg.	2 ml.	1 ml.
2. 2,000,000 U.	5 ml.	1 ml.
20% solution remaining		

Problems (p. 63):

Units ordered	Strength of insulin used	Answers ml.	minims
U 15	U 40	0.4	6
U 10	U 40	0.25	4
U 35	U 80	0.4	7
U 45	U 80	0.6	9
U 25	U 40	0.6	10
U 16	U 40	0.4	6

Problems (pp. 64–65):

Doses for children
1.   200 mg.
2.   6 mg.
3.   100 mg.
4.   30 mg.
5.   250 mg.

Abbreviations used in orders and prescriptions (pp. 69–70):

1. Take two capsules twice a day.
2. One teaspoonful every four hours with water.
3. Three drops at once, one drop as needed.
4. One teaspoonful every four hours and at bedtime.
5. Apply ointment as directed.

Index

Trade-mark names are followed by the generic or approved name in parentheses.

Lucanthone in schistosomiasis, 225
Lugol's solution (strong iodine solution), 739
in hyperthyroidism, 676
Luminal (phenobarbital), 322
Lunar caustic (toughened silver nitrate), 738
Lunargen (mild silver protein), 738
Lupus erythematosis, adrenocorticosteroid in, 685
chloroquine in, 691
Luteal hormone, 614
Luteomersin (progesterone), 615
Lutestab (progesterone), 615
Lutesterone (progesterone), 615
Lutocylin (progesterone), 615
Lutocylol (ethisterone), 615
Lutoform (progesterone), 615
Lutogyl (progesterone), 615
oral (ethisterone), 615
Lutren (progesterone), 615
Lutrexin (lututrin), 607–8
Lututrin, 607–8
Lye, poisoning with, 783
Lymphoadenoma, 179, 188, 189
Lymphogranuloma inguinale, 108t., 148, 163
Lymphoma, malignant (Hodgkin's disease), 179
treatment of, 179
Lymphosarcoma (Hodgkin's disease), 179
Lynoral (ethinyl estradiol), 611
Lysergic acid diethylamide (hallucinogenic chemical), 353
Lysivane (ethopropazine), 373
Lysol (cresol emulsion), 741
Lysthenon (succinylcholine), 421
Lytic cocktail (hibernation, artificial), 301

M and B 800 (pentamidine), 226
Maalox (magnesium and aluminum hydroxide), 574
Maceration, 13
Macrocytic anemia of pregnancy, 509
Madribon (sulfadimethoxine), 165, 168, 173
Magmas, description of, 12
Magnacillin (fortified procaine penicillin G), 113
Magnesium and aluminum hydroxide suspension, 574
Magnesium, carbonate, 573, 590
citrate, 590
hydroxide mixture, 572, 590
oxide, 572, 590
sulfate, 590

trisilicate, 573
Malaria, 208–15
Male climacteric, 618
Male fern extract, 239
Malestrone (testosterone), 619
Malnutrition, chronic, 618
drugs used in, 621, 717
Mammalian enzymes, used as drugs, 766, 769
Mandelamine (methenamine mandelate), 648
Mannitol, 393
hexanitrate, 545
Mannomustine (nitrogen mustard), 189
MAO. See Monoamine oxidase inhibitors
Marc, definition of, 13
Marevan (warfarin), 518
Marezine (cyclizine), 378
Marihuana, 269–70
addiction to, 272
Tax Act of 1937, 29
Marplan (isocarboxazid), 350
Masenate (testosterone propionate), 619
Mastitis, cystic, 615
Mastodynia, 615
Mastoiditis, 155
Matromycin (oleandomycin), 122
Maxipen (phenethicillin), 114–15
McCollum, E. V., 714
Measles vaccine, 796–97
Measures, household, 52
Measuring medications, insulin, 62–63
oral, 59–62
Mebaral (mephobarbital), 316
in epilepsy, 363
Mebaroin, 363–64
Mebutamate, 558
Mecamylamine, 561
Mechlorethamine (nitrogen mustards), 188–89, 196t.
Mecholyl (methacholine), 471–72
Meclizine, 378
Meclozine (meclizine), 378
Mecostrin (dimethyltubocurarine), 418
Mecothane (bethanechol), 475
Medicated ointments, 725
Medications (oral), local for eye, 730
measurement of, 59–62
preparation of, 71–73
Medicine card, 72–73
Medicines. See Drug(s)
Medihalors, 83
Medinal (barbital), 321
Medomin (heptabarbital), 321
Medrol (methylprednisolone), 688
Medroxyprogesterone acetate, 616

Abbreviations of Latin Words Commonly Used in Orders and Prescriptions

Abbreviation	Latin Derivation	Meaning
āā	ana	of each
a.c.	ante cibum	before meals
ad	ad	to, up to
ad lib.	ad libitum	as desired
aq.	aqua	water
aq. dest.	aqua destillata	distilled water
amp.		ampul
b.i.d.	bis in die	twice a day
c.	cum	with
caps.	capsula	capsule
comp.	compositus	compound
cong.	Congium	a gallon
dil.	dilutus	dilute
E.C.		enteric coated ✔
elix.	elixir	elixir
et		and
ext.	extractum	extract
fl. or fld.	fluidus	fluid
Ft.	fiat	make
Gm.	gramme	gram
gr.	granum	grain
gtt.	gutta	a drop
h.	hora	hour
h.s.	hora somni	hour of sleep, or at bedtime
hypo		hypodermically
H.T.		hypodermic tablet
i.m.		intramuscularly
i.v.		intravenously
Lin.	linimentum	liniment
Lot.	lotio	lotion
M.	misce	mix
mist.	mistura	mixture